Handbook of
Cross-Cultural Neuropsychology

CRITICAL ISSUES IN NEUROPSYCHOLOGY

Series Editors

Antonio E. Puente
University of North Carolina at Wilmington

Cecil R. Reynolds
*Texas A&M University
and Bastrop Mental Health Associates*

Current Volumes in this Series

CONTEMPORARY APPROACHES TO NEUROPSYCHOLOGICAL ASSESSMENT
Edited by Gerald Goldstein and Theresa M. Incagnoli

DETECTION OF MALINGERING DURING HEAD INJURY LITIGATION
Edited by Cecil R. Reynolds

HANDBOOK OF CLINICAL CHILD NEUROPSYCHOLOGY, Second Edition
Edited by Cecil R. Reynolds and Elaine Fletcher-Janzen

HANDBOOK OF CROSS-CULTURAL NEUROPSYCHOLOGY
Edited by Elaine Fletcher-Janzen, Tony L. Strickland, and Cecil R. Reynolds

HANDBOOK OF NEUROPSYCHOLOGY AND AGING
Edited by Paul David Nussbaum

INTERNATIONAL HANDBOOK OF NEUROPSYCHOLOGICAL REHABILITATION
Edited by Anne-Lise Christensen and B. P. Uzzell

MEDICAL NEUROPSYCHOLOGY, Second Edition
Edited by Ralph E. Tarter, Meryl Butters, and Sue R. Beers

NEUROPSYCHOLOGICAL INTERPRETATION OF OBJECTIVE PSYCHOLOGICAL TESTS
Charles J. Golden, Patricia Espe-Pfeifer, and Jana Wachsler-Felder

NEUROPSYCHOTHERAPY AND COMMUNITY INTEGRATION
Brain Illness, Emotions, and Behavior
Tedd Judd

PRACTITIONER'S GUIDE TO EVALUATING CHANGE WITH INTELLECTUAL
ASSESSMENT INSTRUMENTS
Edited by Robert J. McCaffrey, Kevin Duff, and Holly J. Westervelt

PRACTITIONER'S GUIDE TO EVALUATING CHANGE WITH NEUROPSYCHOLOGICAL
ASSESSMENT INSTRUMENTS
Edited by Robert J. McCaffrey, Kevin Duff, and Holly J. Westervelt

RELIABILITY AND VALIDITY IN NEUROPSYCHOLOGICAL ASSESSMENT, Second Edition
Michael D. Franzen

A Continuation Order Plan is available for this series. A continuation order will bring delivery of each new volume immediately upon publication. Volumes are billed only upon actual shipment. For further information please contact the publisher.

Handbook of
Cross-Cultural Neuropsychology

Edited by

Elaine Fletcher-Janzen

University of Northern Colorado
Colorado Springs, Colorado

Tony L. Strickland

Drew University of Medicine and Science
Los Angeles, California and
UCLA School of Medicine
Los Angeles, California

and

Cecil R. Reynolds

Texas A&M University
College Station, Texas and
Bastrop Mental Health Associates
Bastrop, Texas

Kluwer Academic / Plenum Publishers
New York, Boston, Dordrecht, London, Moscow

Library of Congress Cataloging-in-Publication Data

Fletcher-Janzen, Elaine.
    Handbook of cross-cultural neuropsychology/Elaine Fletcher-Janzen, Tony L.
Strickland, and Cecil R. Reynolds
        p.   ; cm. — (Critical issues in neurpsychology)
    Includes bibliographical references and index.
    ISBN 0-306-46323-7
        1. Clinical neuropsychology—Cross-cultural studies.   I. Strickland, Tony L.   II.
Reynolds, Cecil R., 1952–   III. Title.   IV. Series.
        [DNLM: 1. Neuropsychology.   2. Cross-Cultural Comparison.   3. Ethnic
Groups—psychology.   4. Neuropsychological Tests. WL 103.5 F612h 2000]
    RC386.6.N48 F58 2000
    616.89—dc21
                                                                                    00-035713

ISBN 0-306-46323-7

©2000 Kluwer Academic / Plenum Publishers, New York
233 Spring Street, New York, N.Y. 10013

http://www.wkap.nl/

10 9 8 7 6 5 4 3 2 1

A C.I.P. record for this book is available from the Library of Congress.

Printed in the United States of America

Contributors

Cay Anderson-Hanley • Glens Falls Hospital, Glens Falls, New York 12801

Alfredo Ardila • Miami, Florida 33182

Kyle Brauer Boone • Harbor-UCLA Medical Center, Torrance, California 90509

Desiree A. Byrd • San Diego State University/University of California, San Diego, California 92616-2292

Jeffrey L. Cummings • UCLA School of Medicine, Los Angeles, California 90095; and Charles R. Drew University of Medicine and Science, Los Angeles, California 90059

Evan B. Drake • New York Presbyterian Hospital Cornell Medical Center, New York, New York 10021

Gwendolyn Evans • Walden House, Inc., San Francisco, California 94103

Jovier D. Evans • Department of Psychology, Indiana University-Purdue University, Indianapolis, Indiana 46202

Elaine Fletcher-Janzen • University of Northern Colorado, Colorado Springs, Colorado 80921

Charles J. Golden • Nova Southeastern University, Fort Lauderdale, Florida 33314

Gregory Gray • Charles R. Drew University of Medicine and Science, Los Angeles, California 90059; and UCLA School of Medicine, Los Angeles, California 90095

Christine R. Guzzard • University of Southern California, Los Angeles, California 90089

Robert K. Heaton • Department of Psychiatry, University of California, San Diego, California 92616-2292

Robyn S. Hess • University of Colorado at Denver, Denver, Colorado 80211

Hortencia Kayser • New Mexico State University, Las Cruces, New Mexico 88003-8001

Jeff King • Native American Counseling, Denver, Colorado 80222; and University of Denver, Denver, Colorado 80208

Antolin M. Llorente • Baylor College of Medicine, Houston, Texas 77030

Paul G. Longobardi • Charles R. Drew University of Medicine and Science, Los Angeles, California 90059; and UCLA School of Medicine, Los Angeles, California 90095

Chirstine M. LoPresti • UCLA School of Medicine, Los Angeles, California 90095

Po Lu • Harbor-UCLA Medical Center, Torrance, California 90509

Wendy B. Marlowe • Seattle, Washington 98104

S. Walden Miller • Department of Psychiatry, University of California, San Diego, California 92616-2292

Pamilla C. Morales • Texas A&M University, College Station, Texas 77843-4225

Hector F. Myers • UCLA School of Medicine, Los Angeles, California 90095

Nina A. Nabors • Eastern Michigan University, Ypsilanti, Michigan 48197

Lissette M. Perez • Texas A&M University, College Station, Texas 77843-4225

Antonio E. Puente • University of North Carolina-Wilmington, Wilmington, North Carolina 38406

Arnold D. Purisch • Irvine, California 92718

Cecil R. Reynolds • Texas A&M University, College Station, Texas 77843-4225; and Bastrop Mental Health Associates, Bastrop, Texas 78602

Robert L. Rhodes • New Mexico State University, Las Cruces, New Mexico 88003-8001

Paul Satz • UCLA School of Medicine, Los Angeles, California 90095; and Charles R. Drew University of Medicine and Science, Los Angeles, California 90059

Robert J. Sbordone • Irvine, California 92718

Tony L. Strickland • Charles R. Drew University of Medicine and Science, Los Angeles, California 90059; and UCLA School of Medicine, Los Angeles, California 90095

Ralph E. Tarter • University of Pittsburgh School of Pharmacy, Pittsburgh, Pennsylvania 15261

I. Maribel Taussig • University of Southern California, Los Angeles, California 90089

Rhiannon B. Thomas • Nova Southeastern University, Fort Lauderdale, Florida 33314

Jay M. Uomoto • Seattle Pacific University, Seattle, Washington 98119

Wilfred G. van Gorp • New York Presbyterian Hospital Cornell Medical Center, New York, New York 10021

Tony M. Wong • St. Mary's Hospital/University of Rochester, Rochester, New York 14611

Preface

"Human–egalitarian ideals, whose aims are group justice and reducing environmental inequality and privilege, must be tested against reality, as revealed by psychology and other social sciences."

James R. Flynn (1999, p. 5)

We have spent four years testing the concepts of neuropsychology and cultural competence against reality to produce this book. Quantum physicists tell us that "reality" is a very subjective entity. When physicists study particles they can either measure position or velocity but not both. The scientist makes a choice as to what he or she will observe (in this case, position or velocity) and, by doing so, incorporates subjective experience into the experiment. As we study brain–behavior relationships we also interject our subjective experiences into the experiment. We choose variables based on our worldview. If our worldview sustains the notion that all brain–behvaior interactions among humans are alike then we can conduct studies that ignore variables such as gender, age, socioeconomics, acculturation, and ethnicity.

In the past, the field of neuropsychology has settled comfortably into the notion that brains are alike. For example, inquiries into brain injury have shown that all brains go through grossly predictable stages of recovery and that brain injury survivors all tend to have problems with self-awareness postrecovery. On the other hand, there is another line of promising research studies that challenge the "universality" worldview and suggest ethnic (not racial) variances in relation to psychopharmacological agents. The other side of the brain–behavioral field of study has in the past been confined to a eurocentric worldview that supports a universal concept of behavior. In other words, all people will manifest the same behaviors to the same stimulus in the brain. Of course, this does not take into account that clinical psychology has been vigorously studying behavioral variances among different ethnic and socioeconomic groups for the past twenty years and has solid data to support the premise that culture influences health status. Brain–behavior relationships are interwoven and dependent on environmental influences. Groups of individuals who have a similar genetic makeup, socioeconomic status, ethnicity, acculturation, education, gender and so forth will manifest different responses to neuropsychological tests, treatment, and followup. The neuropsychologist of the new millennium will have to know what concepts are universal for his or her patients and what concepts are patient-specific.

This handbook is organized to give a broad neuropsychological overview of different patient populations present in the United States. Chapter 1 starts this volume with "Theoretical and Practical Issues in the Neuropsychological Assessment and Treatment of Culturally Dissimilar Patients." This chapter helps define "culture," explores American Psychological

Association ethical guidelines, and has practical suggestions for everyday clinical practice for the neuropsychologist. Chapter 2 studies the question of appropriate cross-cultural training in neuropsychology programs and residencies. This small introductory section sets the tone for evaluating data on neuropsychological assessment and treatment and the ethical mandates for cultural competence on the part of the practitioner. Part II of this volume is devoted to neuropsychological assessment and intervention with diverse groups of people. The reader will notice that some chapters have much more data-based information than others. This is probably due to the fact that most national health surveys and studies in the past two decades have focused on one or two ethnic groups. For those groups that have few historic data, the authors have had to go to other disciplines and try to extrapolate relational data. Part III is concerned with specific health populations such as brain injury, seizures, AIDS, and chronic illness in general. Part IV is a small section on research design and specific neuropsychological test instruments. Part V has been reserved for special topics such as the neuropsychological differential diagnosis of Spanish-speaking preschool children, forensic science, psychopathology, and ethnobiological responses to psychotropic medications.

For the most part, the chapters in this book are seminal. Many of the chapters focus on psychosocial aspects of neuropsychological assessment and treatment partly because of the abundance of data from cross-cultural psychology that cross over to neuropsychology and partly because research studies relative to brain–behavior relationships in a culturally competent way are scarce. Notwithstanding this lack of data, we decided to go forward with this volume because the field of neuropsychological inquiry into cultural aspects of assessment and treatment has to start somewhere.

It will probably be impossible for any reader to engage with this book and not find controversy. As in all cultural diversity training, trainers have long been aware of assisting trainees in identifying notions or concepts that trigger forceful emotion. It is difficult to read about syphilis experiments on African Americans, suicide rates for young Native Americans, lack of treatment for three-quarters of the world's seizure population and so forth, without having emotional responses. It may also be difficult to read criticisms of the neuropsychological assessment instruments that we have come to depend on, or criticisms of the status of general cultural competence of the profession of neuropsychology. There are many difficult questions asked in this volume and many difficult answers that may cause cognitive dissonance for the reader. In fact, this has been the case for ourselves as we edited and wrote this volume and we hope that it is the same for our readers because the field must move forward through meaningful discourse.

In terms of labels, we have tried to use ethnic labels that reflect the person's native origins. African American and black American are terms used interchangeably as are European/American/Anglo-American, and Latino/Hispanic American. We have avoided using the terms "minority" and "majority" where possible.

As with any volume that talks about cultural competence in detail, there is a chance that we will offend. This is not our intention. Many times in the past four years we have experienced differences of opinion among editors, editors and authors, and authors and authors. Most of the issues were resolved; some were not. We have intentionally tried to preserve the original intent of each author even when we, as editors, have found some of the concepts to be problematic or objectionable. It is very important that this volume of work represent the diversity of opinion and views of the neuropsychological community. In many ways, this volume is a diamond in the rough. Cross-cultural competency is new to neuropsychology and this volume reflects how we are wrestling with the ethical issues of cultural competency and its relationship to good treatment outcome. Therefore the first edition on this subject will probably stimulate more questions than it will answer. In fact, we invite the neuropsychological community to discuss and debate the issues presented in this volume.

There are many individuals to thank. First, we must thank Mariclaire Cloutier, our editor at Kluwer Academic / Plenum Publishers, who knowingly took on a project which can only be compared to "herding cats" with us as editors. Her patience is now legendary.

Elaine would like to thank David, Emma, and Leif for supporting the hours she was glued to the iMac and the much wringing of hands during this project. Elaine would also like to thank Tony Strickland and Cecil Reynolds for their courage, humor, and camaraderie.

Cecil notes the continued support from his companion on the journey through life and knows that he could not succeed without her continued support and her resilience. Thank you, Julia, for all you do that allows me to move ahead.

Tony would like to acknowledge the love and support of his family during this project, particularly his sons; also the Charles R. Drew University of Medicine and Science, which afforded him relief from duties as dean for research to complete the contributions to this book. The multifactorial approach to understanding brain–behavior relationships that this text unitizes is derived from the collective wisdom of many gifted teachers, colleagues, friends, and patients, and serves as an important step in the scholarly treatment of cross-cultural neuropsychology. As a result of these interactions, my life has been immeasurably enhanced.

We would also like to express our gratitude to the authors in this handbook. Their work, in many instances, is seminal and is representative of a commitment to ethical conduct and good treatment outcomes in the field of neuropsychology.

Elaine Fletcher-Janzen
Tony L. Strickland
Cecil R. Reynolds

Reference

Flynn, J. R. (1999). Searching for justice. *American Psychologist, 54,* 5–20.

Contents

III. Multicultural Aspects of Neuropsychological Assessment and Treatment of Special Populations

IV. Cross-Cultural Applications of Neuropsychological Assessment Instruments

V. Special Topics

I

Introduction

Theoretical and Practical Issues in the Neuropsychological Assessment and Treatment of Culturally Dissimilar Patients

TONY M. WONG, TONY L. STRICKLAND,
ELAINE FLETCHER-JANZEN, ALFREDO ARDILA,
AND CECIL R. REYNOLDS

Introduction

The American Psychological Association's (1993) "Guidelines for Providers of Psychological Services to Ethnic, Linguistic, and Culturally Diverse Populations" were developed in acknowledgment of the growing social presence of diverse cultural groups and of the need for psychological service providers to develop the awareness, knowledge, and skills necessary to work with those clients/patients whose cultural backgrounds may be different from that of the professional.

Within the specialty of neuropsychology, relatively few investigations have been sensitive to the analysis of cultural variables, and thus the limited understanding of the influence that cultural differences have on assessment and treatment is especially acute (Ardila, 1995). This has resulted in scant resources available to the clinical neuropsychologist who is interested in developing a better understanding of how to deal with cultural issues and variables. For example, in Lezak's (1995) *Neuropsychological Assessment* (3rd ed.), arguably one of the most familiar and authoritative books on neuropsychological assessment to American neuropsychologists, "race" is addressed in a rather brief and equivocal paragraph, and cultural

TONY M. WONG • St. Mary's Hospital/University of Rochester, Rochester, New York 14611.   TONY L. STRICKLAND • Charles R. Drew University of Medicine and Science, Los Angeles, California 90059; and UCLA School of Medicine, Los Angeles, California 90095.   ELAINE FLETCHER-JANZEN • University of Northern Colorado, Colorado Springs, Colorado 80921.   ALFREDO ARDILA • Miami, Florida 33182.   CECIL R. REYNOLDS • Texas A&M University, College Station, Texas 77843-4225, and Bastrop Mental Health Associates, Bastrop, Texas 78602.

Handbook of Cross-Cultural Neuropsychology, edited by Fletcher-Janzen, Strickland, and Reynolds. Kluwer Academic/Plenum Publishers, New York, 2000.

issues are discussed briefly in a two-paragraph section on "social and cultural variables," with somewhat dated references. Thus, an unfortunate and increasingly common situation has arisen recently, in which a clinical neuropsychologist is faced with evaluating or treating a patient whose cultural background or context is different from that of the professional, and the practitioner may not have the awareness, skills, knowledge, sensitivity, or resources available with which this cultural disparity can be bridged adequately in order that the necessary diagnosis, treatment, and recommendations can be offered.

The present volume was written to encourage and promote cross-cultural competency within the field of neuropsychology. Whereas most of the ensuing chapters will be dealing with specific cultural groups, neurobehavioral disorders, or instruments, the current chapter attempts to provide a more general framework by which to understand and to potentially ameliorate a situation where there is a cultural mismatch between the neuropsychologist and the patient. First, theoretical issues as they relate to cross-cultural neuropsychological assessment will be discussed. Given that one of the presumed overarching goals of high priority to both the clinical and research neuropsychologist is the reliable and valid assessment of neurocognitive function, the dearth of knowledge of cross-cultural variables in neuropsychology is a special concern. An exploration of this topic from a theoretical perspective should make it clear that the need to acquire cross-cultural competency in neuropsychology is rooted in the sound science that many neuropsychologists so proudly and ostensibly champion rather than in mere aesthetic or political appeal. Furthermore, other disciplines in psychology have not had problems in linking cultural competence with treatment outcome. Neuropsychologists are no less determined or mandated to produce good treatment outcome than any other clinicians in psychology. Secondly, practical considerations in cross-cultural neuropsychological assessment will be offered. During this transition period, while the entire field of neuropsychology hopefully acquires greater cross-cultural competency, there is a need for some general guidelines to help the practitioner provide adequate services to the patient who is of an unfamiliar cultural background.

Theoretical Issues

It is becoming increasingly clear that neuropsychological function, or at least the accurate measurement of it, is not independent of a number of culturally related variables. Although many neuropsychologists today would agree with this assertion, until significant advances are made in the study of the relationship between these variables and brain function, the net effect in the field is that these factors are treated with minimal attention. In this first section, various culturally related factors and their relevance to understanding brain function are identified and discussed. Also, neuropsychological measurement concepts (e.g., norms, instrumentation, etc.) that will need to be reexamined in light of cultural factors are addressed.

Culture

Culture is a broad and overarching concept that refers to a body of customary beliefs and social norms that are shared by a particular group of people. It includes behaviors, beliefs, values, and other shared elements. Some have defined it as "a way of the people," which includes beliefs and behaviors (Taussig & Ponton, 1996), as well as other social characteristics that are common to a group. Alternatively, it could be simply defined as the specific way of living of a human group. It is a complex entity, and can have ethnic, geographic, generational, linguistic, and social determinants. Unfortunately, culture is often used interchangeably with ethnicity or race and, to a lesser extent, with language. This is an all too common mistake and an oversimplification of culture as a variable that certainly has practical ramifications, but can also impede serious theoretical understanding and investigation in cross-cultural neuropsychology. As with all cases in empirical research, unless the relevant independent variable is defined and isolated, a moderating variable may lead to a confoundment and muddle the explanation of the results. For example, ethnic differences in neuropsychological performance that are attributed to group differences in neuropsychological function may actually be a function of cultural differences in expectations related to the assessment experience (e.g., Shepherd & Leathem, 1999), or of socioeconomic factors that determine access to health care (Centers for Disease Control and Prevention [CDC], 1993).

Having defined culture as an independent variable of interest in neuropsychology, it is also important to consider how this factor might affect the assessment of brain–behavior relationships. One legitimate avenue of inquiry has to do with the relationship between cross-cultural awareness/sensitivity and validity in neuropsychological assessment. Within the more general assessment literature, there has been active research and discussion of potential problems in diagnosis that can occur when cultural issues are ignored or minimized by the psychologist or when there is a cultural/ethnic mismatch between the professional and the patient (e.g., Hays, 1996; Russell, Fujino, Sue, Cheung, & Snowden, 1996; Westermeyer, 1987). These problems include poor rapport between the professional and client, overpathologizing of patient behavior or report, overestimation or underestimation of symptom significance, faulty attribution of symptom presentation, and misdiagnosis. The client's attitude toward the testing environment can also be a significant factor and an obstacle. While many individuals in Europe and North America commonly accept testing, this may not be the case for those from other countries and cultures (Ardila, 1995). Although the specific goals and emphases of assessment in neuropsychology (i.e., elucidation of brain–behavior relationships) are often different from those of more general clinical assessment (personality functioning, functional psychological diagnoses), the impact of subtle intercultural factors operating in the assessment situation, especially when there is a cultural/ethnic mismatch between the professional and the client, is no less important in the neuropsychological context. In fact, a cogent case can be made that, perhaps because of its relative youth as a clinical subspecialty and due to its ostensibly proud emphasis on its scientific foundations, neuropsychology has tended to underemphasize and underestimate the potential influence of cultural factors on valid assessment. This certainly has been the experience of the authors, who have participated in numerous neuropsychological case discussions over the years in various contexts and have rarely observed cultural factors systematically considered in a specific manner beyond the cursory caveat that, because of cultural factors, the normative data may not apply, following which they are, in fact, directly applied without further consideration.

Although the influence of cultural dynamics upon assessment remains a crucial area of research and education in neuropsychology, there are other means by which culture may affect neuropsychology. There has been a long history of research and debate, for example, on the relationship between handedness and culture (e.g., Ardila, Ardila, Bryden, Ostrosky, Rosselli, & Steenhuis, 1989; De Agostini, Khamis, Ahui, & Dellatolas, 1997; Hatta & Kawakami, 1994; Satz, Baymur, & Van der Vlugt, 1979; Teng, Lee, Yang, & Chang, 1976). Within experimental neuropsychology, there has been an intriguing line of research on culture-dependent variations of hemispheric specialization or lateral cerebral dominance (e.g., Cohen, Levy, & McShane, 1989; Gordon & Zatorre, 1981; Hatta, 1979; Hatta & Kawakami, 1997; Moss, Davidson, & Saron, 1985; Nishizawa, 1994; TenHouten, 1985). These investigations have particularly weighty and far-reaching implications, as they suggest that culture is not only a "soft" variable that has its effects upon the level of the process or practice of assessment but may have a direct impact upon the development and maturation of the brain and its behavioral manifestations. Of course, as is true with most factors, culture probably does not have a dichotomous influence upon brain and behavior, and it will be important for cross-cultural neuropsychological research to demonstrate at what levels cultural variables may have significant impact, and at which levels they may not. For example, in a study investigating the phenomenon of impaired self-awareness following brain injury in a sample of Japanese patients, Prigatano, Ogano, and Amakusa (1997) found that while cultural factors may influence self-reports of behavioral competency, patients across cultures with brain dysfunction appear to have reduced insight into their actual level of neuropsychological functioning. More studies of this type are needed in order to enhance cross-cultural understanding of many neuropsychological syndromes.

Current available neuropsychological tests and procedures also need to be reexamined for their cross-cultural appropriateness. As Ardila (1995) noted, a psychometric test represents a typical task or a paradigm that is assumed to be relevant to the examinee and some relevant clinical question by the examiner. From this perspective, most psychometric tests used currently by neuropsychologists are assumed to be relevant to those of European American background or culture, and may represent a different level of relevancy to those from other cultures. The California Verbal Learning Test (Delis, Kramer, Kaplan, & Ober, 1987) is a widely used verbal learning and memory test that offers a number of helpful indices to the neuropsychologist in differentiating various patterns of memory impairment that may be associated with different diagnoses. One of the supposedly appealing features of this test compared to other list learning tests is that the items are presented as a shopping list, an ostensibly more relevant paradigm to examinees, allowing for more direct inferences to be made in regards to the patient's approaches to everyday memory tasks (Delis et al., 1987). From a cross-cultural perspective, at least two questions are raised by the preceding supposition. First, does this assertion hold, even for majority culture patients, who would be European Americans native to the United States and for whom English is the first and primary language? That is, beyond its face validity, does this test truly possess an advantage over similar tests in terms of its relevancy and ultimate inferential power? Second, does the relevancy assumption hold true for patients from minority cultures? Note that this question is distinct from other legitimate questions or critiques that can be directed at this procedure from a cross-cultural perspective. For example, even if the shopping list paradigm is advantageous cross-culturally, what about the relative familiarity of the individual list items? The preceding is merely one example of the type of considerations that need to be directed toward most neuropsychological instruments in use today in order to determine their cross-cultural appropriateness, and extends beyond the more obvious differences that arise because of language. It is a common temptation for practitioners merely to provide a translation when faced with a cross-cultural/cross-linguistic situation. However, this method erroneously assumes that language is the only barrier to a valid assessment in such cases.

In summary, as the population of the United States becomes increasingly multicultural, neuropsychologists in both academic and clinical settings can ill-afford to continue minimizing the importance of cultural factors in theory as well as in practice. Just as with the larger discipline of psychology, where there has been a distinct gap between mainstream and cross-cultural psychologists (Clark, 1987), there is a similar, unfortunate indifference within a large portion of the subdiscipline of neuropsychology to the importance of cross-cultural factors in assessment and treatment. However, rapidly changing demographics in our society are forcing us to confront these issues more honestly and directly, lest both neuropsychological theory and practice quickly become irrelevant.

Ethnicity

Ethnicity is a concept that is somewhat distinct from culture. Whereas culture refers to common social beliefs and behaviors shared among a people, ethnicity is often considered to reflect group composition in which membership is based on common descent, physical characteristics, and heritage (Ardila, Rosselli, & Puente, 1994). In America, ethnicity is usually divided into five groups: Caucasian (or European American/Anglo American) and the four federally designated ethnic minority categories of African American, Hispanic/Latino Americans, American Indians/Alaskan Natives, and Asian/Pacific Islander Americans. This scheme is not without significant conceptual problems, as individuals may not fall clearly into one of the categories, and people of mixed racial/ethnic heritage are not easily denoted. Moreover, an immense heterogeneity within a category, especially in terms of culture and national origin, tends to be obscured by this rubric. For example, there are at least ten distinct groups under the category of Asian residing in the United States (U.S. Bureau of the Census, 1992), not including Pacific Islander Americans. One of these groups, Chinese, is comprised of individuals who may be from distinct cultures (e.g., China, Taiwan, Hong Kong) and whose primary language/dialect may be different (i.e., Mandarin, Cantonese). The challenge, then, from a neuropsychological perspective, is how to provide adequate services to the nonmajority patient whose ethnic background may be different from that of the professional, especially in light of the fact that virtually all of our familiar neuropsychological instruments were normed (albeit poorly in many circumstances) on subjects from the majority ethnic population. Also, as in the case of culture, little research to date has been conducted examining ethnicity as a variable in neuropsychology.

For the sake of simplicity and expediency, it would be tempting to argue that, apart from the roles of culture, language, socioeconomic status, and education as variables that are often confounded with ethnicity, ethnic background should not be a significant variable in neuropsychology. In other words, all other things being equal, brains should be alike across racial/ethnic categories. However, there is a growing scientific literature that raises serious questions regarding the validity of this assumption. This includes studies revealing interesting interethnic differences in responsivity to various medications, including psychotropics (e.g., Gray & Pi, in press; Lawson, 1996; Pi & Gray, 1998; Strickland, Ranganath, Lin, Poland, Mendoza, & Smith, 1991; Strickland, Stein, Lin, Risby, & Fong, 1997), illustrating and supporting the notion of varying pharmacogenetic, pharmokinetic, and pharmacodynamic differences that are modulated by ethnicity. Also, a recent study by Strickland et al. (1999) comparing learning and memory functioning among African American, European American, and Hispanic American chronic cocaine abusers, found preliminary results suggesting that the neurocognitive sequelae of cocaine abuse may be in part influenced by the ethnicity of the user. There are clear differences in patterns of performance on a variety of neuropsychological tests across ethnic groups, independent of overall level of performance (e.g., Reynolds, 1999; Reynolds, Willson, & Ramsay, 1999). All of these findings taken together support the intriguing notion that racial or ethnic background by itself may be a relevant factor neuropsychologically even when sociocultural differences are removed.

The complexity of ethnic or racial categorization potentially has serious ramifications for the development of a valid cross-cultural application of neuropsychology. The current status of the availability of viable normative data for neuropsychological instruments can be characterized as uneven, or spotty, at best, as could be gleaned from some of the following chapters in this volume (also see Mitrushina, Boone, & D'Elia, 1999). Although there has been more interest shown in the recent literature in collecting normative neuropsychological data for cultural/ethnic minority groups, the overall approach has been relatively unsystematic. Thus, while some studies involve multiple minority cultural groups but a limited set of neuropsychological tests/procedures (e.g., Kempler, Teng, Dick, Taussig, & Davis, 1998), others involve a more comprehensive test battery, but examine performance only within one ethnic minority group (e.g., Hauser, 1997; Jacobs, Sano, Albert, Schofield, Dooneief, & Stern, 1997). In terms of relative proportions, more neuropsychological data and research is currently available on African American and Hispanic/Latino American populations than on Asian American and Native American groups. It is suggested and recommended that the discipline of clinical neuropsychology determine whether the development of norms for a comprehensive set of neuropsychological tests/procedures assessing the major neurocognitive domains (e.g., attention/concentration, memory, visuospatial/visuomotor, and executive functions) for different ethnic groups and their major subgroups, stratified by age, education, gender, and acculturation is needed. Note that even if this admittedly ambitious goal were achieved, significant problems and questions would remain. This issue will only be resolved by studies of the cross-cultural validity of the interpretation of test scores based on homogeneous versus hetergeneous ethnic norms. In particular, the issue of the manner in which individuals who are not easily categorized from an ethnic perspective should be addressed neuropsychologically and resolved. However, until more applicable and comprehensive norms are developed, a viable cross-cultural neuropsychology cannot be realized.

Language

Despite the fact that most clinical neuropsychologists in North America are of European American descent and are fluent in English as their first and primary language, an increase in immigration to the United States of people who speak languages other than English has produced the increasingly more common situation where there is not only an ethnic/cultural difference inherent in the assessment setting, but also a significant linguistic barrier and mismatch. The neuropsychological evaluation of a non-English speaker by clinicians who have limited knowledge of the language of the examinee is not only risky, but could potentially be unethical (Artiola i Fortuny & Mullaney, 1998). The lack of linguistic competence on the part of the examiner not only places an obvious barrier to good communication and rapport with the examinee, it can seriously hamper effective neuropsychological assessment. As Artiola i Fortuny & Mullaney (1998) stated, "language is, in fact, a tool of assessment." Such an examiner would be less likely to detect abnormal prosody, unusual syntax, or other symptoms that might suggest a neurologically based language disorder. More generally, behavioral observations such as the patient's mood, affect, thought process, or functional attention might also be limited significantly or an examiner may greatly overinterpret normal language out of unfamiliarity.

Translation, even if done professionally and accurately, does not adequately remove problems created by the linguistic mismatch. Informal communication, important for rapport building and maximizing the patient's motivation and cooperation, may remain stilted, as many cultural idioms are difficult to translate. Cultural norms and values may influence interpreters themselves, and significant distortions in translation may occur (Marcos, 1979;

Sue & Sue, 1987). Similarly, standard instructions for formal tests and procedures may not be easily translated verbatim. Moreover, the very act of translating a standardized test violates the assumptions on which the test is normed, thus adding an additional potential source of variability besides that which culture, ethnicity, or other differences from the original normative group or procedure would contribute. Another problem in translating existing tests, which is often overlooked, is that the construct validity of most common interpretations may be lower or diminished for the cultural minority group. That is, most inventories, questionnaires, and diagnostic schemes do not take into account cross-cultural differences in the expression of symptoms. For example, a number of studies have shown the tendency for Asian Americans to report somatic complaints in depression, and that they are less likely to endorse dysphoric mood (Sue & Sue, 1987).

In summary, the neuropsychological assessment of nonnative English speakers raises many issues that are not easily resolved at this time. Ideally, in order to adequately serve the non–English-speaking population, more neuropsychologists who are fluent in foreign languages are needed, along with tests and procedures that are not only developed and normed in various native languages but are reliable and valid for those particular cultures. While this may appear to be an onerous and time-consuming task, from an empirically and scientifically honest perspective, there does not appear to be a viable alternative.

Age, Education, Gender, Socioeconomics, and Acculturation

There are other important variables of consideration in developing a viable cross-cultural neuropsychology. There has been a noticeable and valuable increase in attention directed toward aging in the last few decades within psychology as well as other disciplines. The publication of data from Mayo's Older American Normative Studies (Ivnik et al., 1992a,b) has been a significant contribution to the neuropsychological literature, and has helped practitioners to better assess the cognitive abilities of the elderly. While the elderly population may be in itself a distinct subculture, researchers and practitioners in neuropsychology should also consider the special needs or characteristics of older patients/clients from nondominant cultural backgrounds. Investigations of this type have begun to appear recently in the neuropsychological literature (e.g., Hauser, Morris, Heston, & Anderson, 1986; Jacobs et al., 1997; Lichtenberg, Ross, Youngblade, & Vangel, 1998), and will hopefully become part of a larger trend in this area. Hays (1996) proposed a creative model for the culturally responsive assessment of diverse older clients that might also be used in the neuropsychological context. Using cultural influences mentioned in the American Psychological Association's (1993) "Guidelines for Providers of Psychological Services to Ethnic, Linguistic, and Culturally Diverse Populations," she formed the slightly misspelled acronym ADRESSING (for *A*ge, *D*isability, *R*eligion, *E*thnicity, *S*ocial status, *S*exual orientation, *I*ndigenous heritage, *N*ational origin, and *G*ender) to provide a framework by which psychologists, especially of dominant cultural identities, can consider the impact of cultural factors on their clients. Readers may find this framework helpful for culturally responsive assessment of clients of all ages.

Education has been found to be significantly related to performance on most neuropsychological tests examined for this effect (Anderson, 1994; Spreen & Strauss, 1998). Cognitively intact patients with low levels of education can score lower than highly educated patients with mild impairments (Ardila, Rosselli, & Rosas, 1989). The neuropsychological evaluation of patients with very low levels of education can be particularly challenging. As to date there have been very few studies on how these patients perform on formal standardized test instruments (Ostrosky, Ardila, Rosselli, Lopez-Arango, & Uriel-Mendoza, 1998). Moreover, low levels of formal education (i.e., fewer than eight years) are much more common among immigrants from certain regions in the world, and thus the neuropsychologist who is not culturally competent and is asked to evaluate such a patient/client is faced with cultural dissimilarities at multiple levels. As with other factors mentioned in this chapter, more research needs to be conducted evaluating how those with low levels of education perform on established neuropsychological tests, and, more importantly, how assessment is best achieved with such cases.

There has been a long history of investigation into gender differences in both experimental and clinical neuropsychology. While the findings are often equivocal, enough differences have been revealed to consider gender a significant factor or category. Lateral asymmetry tends to be more subtle in women than in men (Levy & Heller, 1992). While tests of general intelligence do usually yield gender differences that are quite small (Heaton, Ryan, Grant, & Matthews, 1996), tests of specific abilities sometimes yield clinically significant gender advantages. For example, many reports suggest that males tend to perform better than females on visuospatial tests. Related to this, a substantial sex difference in mathematical reasoning ability in favor of boys has also been found (e.g., Benbow & Stanley, 1980, 1983). Considerations of possible gender differences will also be crucial in cross-cultural investigations of neuropsychology, as there are distinct social differences and biases related to gender among cultural groups. For example, many cultures have more clearly differentiated male and female roles and expectations compared to current American culture, such that a patient from a male-dominated culture may relate differently to a female neuropsychologist or "doctor," than to a male examiner. Gender can also be confounded by education level, as some of the more traditional, male-dominated societies tend to restrict educational opportunities for women.

Socioeconomic status is often a confounding variable in comparisons between ethnic groups (CDC, 1993; McKenzie & Crowcroft, 1994). When studies control for socioeconomic variables (in manifestation of disease and health problems), differences between ethnicities often disappear. In addition, within population subgroups, disease gradients according to socioeconomic status have been documented repeatedly (Flack et al., 1995). Indeed, the CDC (1993) has suggested that "additional measures of socioeconomic status and social groupings should be developed to avoid univariate analysis of race and ethnicity" (p. 14).

Another important moderator variable for consideration is the level of acculturation of the individuals being studied. Acculturation is not adequately measured by assessing ethnicity, race, or national origin (Mitchell, Scheier, & Baker, 1994). Acculturation can be assessed on a monolevel where the individual's level of retention of original culture is measured, or a bilevel where the individual's acquisition of dominant-society values and behaviors is also evaluated (Dana, 1993). There may be important differences between those newly arrived and United States-born individuals in terms of their attitudes and access toward health care, use of traditional medicines, sociocultural stress, treatment compliance, and obvious language issues.

Tests and Instrumentation

As suggested previously, in order for a valid cross-cultural neuropsychology to develop, validity and reliability of neuropsychological test performance will need to be demonstrated across cultures, genders, and other nominal groupings. Current practices, which include translating existing tests, using informal procedures, using less linguistically loaded tests, or just ignoring cultural variables, are not adequate and potentially deprive a significant portion of our patients of much needed and valuable services.

The Neuropsychologist and Cross-Cultural Competency

Neuropsychology is a relatively new clinical specialty within psychology. As such, much energy within the discipline has been directed toward defining the clinical neuropsychologist and what core education and training is needed to prepare the neuropsychologist for competent practice. Unfortunately, because of this, and due to the lack of adequate diversity within the specialty, a cogent rationale for the necessary development of cross-cultural competency within neuropsychology is rarely articulated. This has resulted in a relatively surface understanding and appreciation of multicultural and diversity issues, typically leading to vague and general aspirational statements, and leaving neuropsychologists considering such competency as an optimal preference to enlarge his or her professional repertoire. For example, in the policy statement emanating from the recent Houston Conference on Specialty Education and Training in Clinical Neuropsychology (Hannay et al., 1998), "cultural and individual differences and diversity" is recommended as an area of study under the Generic Psychology Core, and *"recognition* of multicultural issues" (italics ours) is listed under the Assessment and the Treatment and Interventions core skills sections. However, multicultural issues are not mentioned in the section on Internship Training in Clinical Neuropsychology nor in the section on Residency Education and Training in Clinical Neuropsychology. Note also that where multicultural issues are mentioned previously in the statement, they appear to be limited to a rather surface cognitive familiarity with the topic (i.e., recognition) as opposed to an integrated knowledge-skills package that needs to be trained and refined. Also illustrative is policy statement XIII on Diversity in Education and Training, which states, "The specialty of clinical neuropsychology should attempt to actively involve (sic) (enroll, recruit) individuals from diverse backgrounds at all levels of education and training in clinical neuropsychology." Without further clarification or expansion, this statement appears to promote only quantitative improvement in diversity. It may also serve to reinforce the all-too-familiar and flawed supposition that minority specialists are trained to serve minority patients. The more appropriate goal that needs to be articulated is that all neuropsychologists in this country should be trained for some minimal level of cross-cultural sensitivity and competency. The active recruitment and enrollment of individuals from diverse backgrounds at all levels of education and training serves that purpose by providing mentors and colleagues who would challenge the monocultural perspective inherent in the field. The current statement also lacks the broadness of inclusion that is necessary for real change to occur at a fundamental level. More specifically, diversity needs to be seriously and actively considered in venues beyond education and training, and in the administrative structures that have the resources and authority to carry out and enforce mandates in this area. Related to this, Chan (1989) argued that while in some cases Asian American faculty in American universities may have reputational power (recognition for scholarly work), they seldom have collegial (e.g., heading major committees) or administrative power (formal positions of authority within the university structure). Analogously, from a sociopolitical perspective, neuropsychology as a relatively new field may be barely ready to offer reputational power to ethnic-minority neuropsychologists, much less the collegial and administrative power that is necessary for true progress to occur.

As this chapter and volume suggest, cross-cultural competency is a necessary and fundamental skill for the neuropsychologist that cannot be ignored, especially given the rapidly changing demographics of our society. Thus, the authors' recommendation is that neuropsychology training programs and curricula include cross-cultural issues and sensitivity not only as required core knowledge, but also as an integrated part of clinical skills training. This would include assessment and intervention with patients of culturally dissimilar background relative to the examiner, accompanied by case discussion and supervision by those who are competent in this area. Likewise, internship and residency experiences should include a substantial amount of exposure and practice with patients of diverse backgrounds accompanied by cogent discussion of cross-cultural issues that may be inherent to a case. Board certification, which is supposed to assess advanced levels of competency in a specialty, should require that cross-cultural competency be demonstrated both on the written and oral portions of the examination (this of course assumes that the board examiners are competent and sensitive in this area themselves). For neuropsychologists who have already been trained or board-certified, provisions should be made for meaningful avenues of continuing education in cross-cultural issues. Perhaps one of the major professional organizations such as the Coalition of Clinical Practitioners in Neuropsychology (CCPN), Division of Clinical Neuropsychology of the APA, the International Neuropsychological Society, or the National Academy of Neuropsychology could develop, with recognized/established specialists in this area, regular intensive workshops on cross-cultural issues in neuropsychology.

It should also be noted that cultural competence is a process and not an end product. The assumption that formal courses and supervision in neuropsychology training programs will automatically satisfy adequate competency requirements for practitioners is invalid. The completion of specific courses in cultural diversity and ongoing supervision is the *minimum* prerequisite for competency. Cultural competence is a lifelong process that requires an ongoing self-analysis that questions one's own beliefs and value system and readily accepts differences in worldview from others. In turn, this flexible approach to the neuropsychologist–patient relationship is reflected in good treatment outcomes.

Practical Issues

The previous section established some of the major obstacles toward achieving a viable cross-cultural neuropsychology. Most of the goals mentioned earlier will take some time to achieve. Thus, a legitimate question that the neuropsychologist concerned with sound practice from a cross-cultural perspective might ask is, "So, what do I do now when I am asked to provide neuropsychological services to an individual with whose culture I am unfamiliar, or who speaks a language in which I am not fluent?" The remainder of this chapter offers some practical approaches to working with the culturally dissimilar patient during this transition period when a comprehensive cross-cultural neuropsychology does not exist, and adequate norms and procedures that are appropriate for a particular group may not yet be available. These should be viewed as more general guidelines, whereas some of the ensuing chapters on particular minority cultural groups might offer more specific help.

1. *Recognize, understand, and, if necessary, train for cross-cultural diversity and sensitivity.* This is fundamental and should be the starting point. Unfortunately, for whatever the reason, many professionals do not see the growing and undeniable need for this. As illustrated earlier, the need to develop an adequate cross-cultural neuropsychology is an empirical, scientific, and demographic reality, and should not be characterized as a political or aesthetic endeavor. Neuropsychologists should be familiar with the "Guidelines for Providers of Psychological Services to Ethnic, Linguistic, and Culturally Diverse Populations" (APA, 1993), which are not only aspirational guidelines strongly recommended for psychologists, but are based on empirical research regarding the need to consider cultural variables in providing

appropriate psychological services. The neuropsychologist who needs to enhance his or her cross-cultural knowledge and skills can take advantage of a number of avenues. Consultation and supervision with colleagues who are competent with the cultural issues in question is one legitimate method that is used whenever psychologists are dealing with areas in which they may not be competent. Continuing education courses or workshops on culture and diversity are offered from time to time and can be taken. Self-directed studies may be helpful to a certain extent, although if one is unfamiliar with the fundamental issues on this topic, a more structured or externally directed method is preferred.

2. *Be aware of cultural nuances, consider sociocultural influences on the patient's behavior, and try your best to naturally offer a culturally sensitive environment.* As is the case with most human social interaction, in cross-cultural interactions subtle differences in expected social behavior may lead to unintended offenses that interfere with fluid rapport. Hays (1996) notes, for example, that although the psychologist may intend to communicate friendliness by using first names, this may be perceived as presumptuous or disrespectful by older patients due to the generation-specific custom whereby people over 65 often prefer to be addressed by title. This may be even more of a perceived offense if ethnicity is also a factor (e.g., a young, European American therapist calling a 70-year-old, African American man "Charlie" instead of "Mr. Smith" upon initial contact). Neuropsychologists should also be aware of the phenomenon, well-established by social psychologists (e.g., Pettigrew, 1979), whereby people tend to attribute negative behaviors to internal, dispositional factors when evaluating others from a different sociocultural group, instead of considering external, situational factors. For example, before we conclude that the 29-year-old, unemployed, African American man who comes into the neuropsychology laboratory at the university's medical center for an evaluation at the behest of his primary physician was "sullen, defensive, and demonstrated performance suggestive of malingering," we should also seriously consider how situational and contextual factors may have contributed to this patient's behavior in the clinic. Perhaps the environment in which we, the professionals, are familiar and comfortable is especially unfamiliar and intimidating to patients from lower socioeconomic status backgrounds, which would make it difficult for them to be as open as we would want or expect. Perhaps he was told to "see this doctor," without much explanation or clarification, which would not generate eager anticipation or motivation on the part of the patient. In creating a culturally sensitive environment in your practice, it is also important to be authentic or natural. Using cultural jargon with which you are typically unfamiliar, though well intended, may come across as awkward, patronizing, humorous, and even insulting. Finally, it is especially helpful in cross-cultural situations to explain carefully the nature and purpose of a neuropsychological evaluation. This is an unfamiliar concept to many cultures, and to many languages, so the patient may not have any idea of what to expect, or just understands that he or she is seeing a "psychologist" and may erroneously assume that the professionals are not taking the physical problems seriously and attributing whatever the symptoms may be to psychiatric problems.

3. *A thorough clinical interview is helpful in identifying and understanding cultural nuances and differences.* While a good clinical interview is important in virtually all neuropsychological evaluations, this is especially true when the patient comes from a culturally dissimilar background, and extra time and effort may be required to acquire the information necessary to complete an accurate and valid evaluation. Discussing or exploring cultural issues and factors not only provides valuable information to the clinician, but also connotes respect and sensitivity to the patient. In ascertaining premorbid educational level, it is often helpful, if the patient was educated in a foreign country, to not only ask about the highest level of

education completed, but to also inquire about the nature and structure of the educational system, as well as societal norms and expectations regarding education for that culture.

4. *If the primary language of the patient is unfamiliar to the neuropsychologist, an earnest attempt should be made to refer the patient to another neuropsychologist in the region who can conduct the evaluation competently in that language.* This is an especially viable approach if one is practicing in a large urban area, where there is more multicultural diversity at the professional level. Even if you are not in an urban area, practicing in a rural area should not preclude an honest attempt at exhausting all possible and reasonable alternatives. This would include calling local colleagues for leads, consulting professional organizations (e.g., International Neuropsychological Society, National Academy of Neuropsychology, APA Committee on Ethnic Minority Affairs), and browsing directories for these organizations. Of course, there will be circumstances under which a fluent bilingual clinician will not be available.

5. *A referral should be considered if, even when language is not an issue, other cultural issues may be a hindrance to a competent evaluation.* Neuropsychologists, like the rest of the human population, are not immune to personal problems, impaired interpersonal/intrapersonal functioning, or both. This would include problems with racial prejudice or bias that would interfere with the adequate and competent provision of services to certain individuals. Neuropsychologists who have these difficulties have an ethical and professional responsibility to seek help for their problems and to refer patients that they would have difficulty serving to other neuropsychologists. This would also be consistent with section 1.13 of the Ethical Standards of the American Psychological Association's (1992) Ethical Principles of Psychologists and Code of Conduct, which addresses personal problems and conflicts.

6. *If at all possible, the use of translators or interpreters should be avoided.* It is often tempting to use a translator to help out in a situation where the patient does not speak English. However, there are several problems inherent in using a translator that would, in most cases, negate whatever benefit may be derived from using them. The addition of a third person to the interview and assessment situation by itself changes the dynamics of what is typically a dyadic interaction. Informal communication and conversation is more difficult and less natural. Using a translator brings in potential sources of distortion or bias of which the neuropsychologist may not be aware. For example, the translator may innocently help the patient with an answer or provide additional cues or instructions that are not part of standard procedure. For this reason, family members or other invested acquaintances of the patient should especially be avoided as translators. In cases where there are no reasonable alternatives, and a translator must be used, it is best to recruit individuals who are either professionally trained as translators or who have extensive experience with translating and interpreting. Moreover, it is very important to ascertain whether the translator is fluent in the particular dialect or variant of the target language, as well as familiar with the specific culture of the region the patient is from. For example, it may now be widely known to Westerners that an interpreter who is familiar with the Cantonese dialect of southern China may not be able to translate for an individual who is from northern China, where the predominant dialect is Mandarin. However, equally disparate, and less well known, is that this same interpreter may also be equally unable to translate for patients originally from the rural villages outside of Canton who speak the Toisan dialect, which was used by a majority of the immigrants from China who came to America during the first half of the 20th century. It is also very important that any interpreter, no matter how experienced or proficient, spend a preparation period or session with the neuropsychologist, so that he or she understand the special requirements and conditions of a neuropsychological evaluation session. In other words, it needs to be explained that test instructions should be

given verbatim if at all possible, and should there be any variations, they should be checked with the neuropsychologist before the actual translation occurs. Similarly, it should be made clear to the interpreter that no help or cues should be given to the patient unless they are directed by the neuropsychologist. To avoid misunderstanding, the translator should be aware ahead of time that the neuropsychologist will require a verbatim translation of virtually everything that is spoken during the session, as even informal banter and discussion may be potential sources of bias.

7. *Avoid the use of translated tests or instruments unless test score interpretations have been validated in the translated form.* As discussed previously, tests may not always be easily and smoothly translated. Also, even if accurate translation is assumed, construct validity of performance on the test for a specific population may not hold. If translated tests are used and they are not validated, they should only be used qualitatively and this should be addressed specifically in the report.

8. *A set of tests chosen judiciously with cross-cultural considerations in mind should be used.* There has been a small but noticeable increase in the publication of norms for certain cultural groups for some procedures in the neuropsychology literature. In addition, some norms have not yet been published, but have been presented at professional meetings, and can be obtained by contacting the authors. If applicable, these procedures should be used whenever possible, so that at least part of the evaluation can be based on empirical research pertaining to that particular group. Avoid tests/procedures that are obviously or are most likely biased against the culturally dissimilar patient. While it may be tempting to rely upon so-called "nonverbal" tests such as visuoperceptual or visuoconstructive procedures in the mistaken assumption that these are more culture-fair, in reality these tests are also often culture-biased. Bear in mind that neuropsychological testing can be perceived as unusual or even threatening in some cultural groups. Thus, some flexibility can be useful. Due to potential cultural bias, it is also appropriate to use multiple measures to assess the same cognitive function. In other words, use a more stringent criterion to determine probable impairment.

9. *Cross-cultural issues should be elucidated clearly in the evaluation report.* All relevant caveats related to cross-cultural issues should be stated clearly. It should be stated very clearly in the report that most, many, or all of the instruments or tests used in the neuropsychological evaluation were not normed or constructed for use with patients from this particular population. When using procedures in a nonnormative and qualitative fashion, the use of numerical cutoffs and normative statistics is inappropriate and misleading, and should be avoided. Unless clearly appropriate norms or standards are available, a conservative approach to interpretation should be used, one that errs with the benefit of the doubt to the patient. Circumstances and context will dictate whether a bias toward false positive or false negative error in diagnosis will be preferred.

Summary and Conclusions

The purpose of this chapter was to introduce the reader to some of the more general issues involved in the neuropsychological assessment of culturally dissimilar patients in preparation for some of the more specific chapters to follow. The need to develop a cross-culturally valid and sensitive approach in neuropsychology is undeniable, and is a growing empirical and demographic reality. For example, the U.S. Bureau of the Census (1996) reports that the Asian and Hispanic populations are the fastest growing groups in all regions, and their growth will be especially prominent in certain regions. For example, it is projected that by the year 2025,

Hispanics will comprise the largest ethnic group in California, with Asians being a substantial minority (21,232,000 Hispanics, 16,626,000 "Whites," and 8,564,000 Asians). It is clear that preparation for cross-cultural delivery of services for practitioners in such states will not be optional. While there is much to do toward this goal, and the task may not always be easy, there is not much of a choice if neuropsychology is to remain professionally and scientifically relevant as we enter the 21st century.

References

American Psychological Association (1992). Ethical principles of psychologists and code of conduct. *American Psychologist, 47,* 1597–1611.

American Psychological Association (1993). Guidelines for providers of psychological services to ethnic, linguistic, and culturally diverse populations. *American Psychologist, 48,* 45–48.

Anderson, R. M. (1994). *Practitioner's guide to clinical neuropsychology.* New York: Plenum.

Ardila, A. (1995). Directions of research in cross-cultural neuropsychology. *Journal of Clinical and Experimental Neuropsychology, 17,* 143–150.

Ardila, A., Rosselli, M., & Puente, A. (1994). *Neuropsychological evaluation of the Spanish speaker.* New York: Plenum.

Ardila, A., Rosselli, M., & Rosas, P. (1989). Neuropsychological assessment in illiterates: Visuospatial and memory abilities. *Brain and Cognition, 11,* 147–166.

Ardila, A., Ardila, O., Bryden, M.P., Ostrosky, F., Rosselli, M., & Steenhuis, R. (1989). *Neuropsychologia, 27,* 893–897.

Artiola i Fortuny, L., & Mullaney, H. (1998) Assessing patients whose language you do not know: Can the absurd be ethical? *The Clinical Neuropsychologist, 12,* 113–126.

Benbow, C. P., & Stanley, J. C. (1980). Sex differences in mathematical ability: Fact or artifact? *Science, 210,* 1262–1264.

Benbow, C. P., & Stanley, J. C. (1983). Sex differences in mathematical reasoning ability: More facts. *Science, 222,* 1029–1031.

Centers for Disease Control and Prevention (1993). Use of race and ethnicity in public health surveillance summary of the CDC/ATSDR workshop. *MMWR Weekly* (No. RR-10). Washington D.C.: Author.

Chan, S. (1989, November). Beyond affirmative action. *Change,* 48–51.

Clark, L. A. (1987). Mutual relevance of mainstream and cross-cultural psychology. *Journal of Consulting and Clinical Psychology, 55,* 461–470.

Cohen, H., & Levy, J. J., & McShane, D. (1989). Hemispheric specialization for speech and non-verbal stimuli in Chinese and French Canadian subjects. *Neuropsychologia, 27,* 241–245.

Dana, R. H. (1993). Multicultural assesment perspectives for professional psychology. Boston, MA: Allyn and Bacon.

De Agostini, M., Khamis, A. H., Ahui, A. M., & Dellatolas, G. (1997). Environmental influences in hand preference: An African point of view. *Brain and Cognition, 35*(2), 151–167.

Delis, D. C., Kramer, J. H., Kaplan, E., & Ober, B. A. (1987). *California Verbal Learning Test.* San Antonio, TX: The Psychological Corporation.

Flack, J. M., Amaro, H., Jenkins, W., Kunitz, S., Levy, J., Mixon, M., & Yu, E. (1995). Epidemiology of minority health. *Health Psychology, 14,* 592–600.

Gordon, D. P., & Zatorre, R. J. (1981). A right-ear advantage for dichotic listening in bilingual children. *Brain & Language, 13,* 389–396.

Gray, G. E., & Pi, E. H. (in press). Ethnicity and medication-induced movement disorders. *Journal of Practical Psychiatry and Behavioral Health.*

Hannay, H. J., Bieliauskas, L. A., Crosson, B. A., Hammeke, T. A., Hamsher, K. deS., & Koffler, S. P. (1998). Proceedings of the Houston Conference on Specialty Education and Training in Clinical Neuropsychology. *Archives of Clinical Neuropsychology, 13,* 157–250.

Hatta, T. (1979). Differences in laterality for recognition of nonverbal material by Japanese and English subjects. *Perceptual & Motor Skills, 48,* 917–918.

Hatta, T., & Kawakami, A. (1994). Cohort effects in the lateral preference of Japanese people. *Journal of General Psychology, 121,* 377–380.

Hatta, T., & Kawakami, A. (1997). Image generation and handedness: Is the hemi-imagery method valid for studying the hemisphere imagery generation process? *Neuropsychologia, 35,* 1499–1502.

Hauser, W. A. (1997). Incidence and prevalence. In J. Engel, and T. A. Pedley (Eds.), *Epilepsy: A comprehensive textbook* (pp. 47–57). Philadelphia: Lippincott-Raven.

Hauser, W. A., Morris, M. L., Heston, L. L., & Anderson, V. E. (1986). Seizures and myoclonus in patients with Alzheimer's disease. *Neurology, 36*, 1226–1230.

Hays, P. (1996). Culturally responsive assessment with diverse older clients. *Professional Psychology: Research and Practice, 27*, 188–193.

Heaton, R. K., Ryan, L., Grant, I., & Matthews, C. G. (1996). Demographic influences on neuropsychological test performance. In I. Grant, & K. M. Adams (Eds.), *Neuropsychological assessment of neuropsychiatric disorders* (2nd ed.). New York: Oxford University Press.

Ivnik, R. J., Malec, J. F., Smith, G. E., Tangalos, E. G., Peterson, R. C., Kokmen, E., & Kurland, L. T. (1992a). Mayo's Older American Normative Studies: WAIS-R norms for ages 56 to 97. *The Clinical Neuropsychologist, 6*, 1–30.

Ivnik, R. J., Malec, J. F., Smith, G. E., Tangalos, E. G., Peterson, R. C., Kokmen, E., & Kurland, L. T. (1992b). Mayo's Older American Normative Studies: WMS-R norms for ages 56 to 94. *The Clinical Neuropsychologist, 6*, 49–82.

Jacobs, D. M., Sano, M., Albert, S., Schofield, P., Dooneief, G, & Stern, Y. (1997). Cross-cultural neuropsychological assessment: A comparison of randomly selected, demographically matched cohorts of English- and Spanish-speaking older adults. *Journal of Clinical and Experimental Neuropsychology, 19*, 331–339.

Kempler, D., Teng, E. L., Dick, M., Taussig, I. M., & Davis, D. S. (1998). The effects of age, education, and ethnicity on verbal fluency. *Journal of the International Neuropsychological Society, 4*, 531–538.

Lawson, W. B. (1996). The art and science of the psychopharmacotherapy of African-Americans. *Mt. Sinai Journal of Medicine, 63*, 301–305.

Levy, J., & Heller, W. (1992). Gender differences in human neuropsychological function. In A. A. Gerall, H. Moltz, & I. L. Ward (Eds.), *Handbook of behavioral neurobiology: Vol. 11. Sexual differentiation*. New York: Plenum.

Lezak, M. D. (1995). *Neuropsychological assessment* (3rd ed). New York: Oxford University Press.

Lichtenberg, P. A., Ross, T.P., Youngblade, L., & Vangel, S. J. (1998). Normative studies research project test battery: Detection of dementia in African American and European American urban elderly patients. *The Clinical Neuropsychologist, 12*, 146–154.

Marcos, L. R. (1979). Effects of interpreters on the evaluation of psychopathology in non-English-speaking patients. *American Journal of Psychiatry, 136*, 171–174.

McKenzie, K. J., & Crowcroft, N. S. (1994). Race, ethnicity, culture, and science. *British Medical Journal, 39*, 286–287.

Mitchell, W. G., Scheier, L. M., & Baker, S. A. (1994). Psychosocial, behavioral and medical outcomes in children with epilepsy: A developmental risk factor model using longitudinal data. *Pediatrics, 94*, 471–477.

Mitrushina, M. N., Boone, K. B., & D'Elia, L. F. (1999). *Handbook of normative data for neuropsychological assessment*. Oxford: Oxford University Press.

Moss, E. M., Davidson, R. J., & Saron, C. (1985). Cross-cultural differences in hemisphericity: EEG asymmetry discriminates between Japanese and westerners. *Neuropsychologia, 23*, 131–135.

Nishizawa, S. (1994). Cross-cultural effects on hemispheric specialization reflected on a task requiring spatial discrimination of the thumb by Japanese and American students. *Perceptual & Motor Skills, 78*, 771–776.

Ostrosky, F., Ardila, A., Rosselli, M., Lopez-Arango, G., & Uriel-Mendoza, V. (1998). Neuropsychological test performance in illiterates. *Archives of Clinical Neuropsychology, 13*, 645–660.

Pettigrew, T. F. (1979). The ultimate attribution error: Extending Allport's cogitive analysis of prejudice. *Personality and Social Psychology Bulletin, 5*, 461–476.

Pi, E. H., & Gray, G. E. (1998). A cross-cultural perspective on psychopharmacology. *Essential Psychopharmacology, 2*, 233–260.

Prigatano, G. P., Ogano, M., & Amakusa, B. (1997). A cross-cultural study on impaired self-awareness in Japanese patients with brain dysfunction. *Neuropsychiatry, Neuropsychology, and Behavioral Neurology, 10*(2), 135–143.

Reynolds, C. R. (1999). Cultural bias in testing of intelligence and personality. In A. Bellack & M. Hersen (Series Eds.) & C. Belar (Vol. Ed.), *Comprehensive clinical psychology, Vol. 10: Sociocultural and individual differences* (pp. 33–56). New York: Pergamon.

Reynolds, C. R., Willson, V. L., & Ramsay, M. (1999). Intellectual differences among Mexican-Americans, Papagos, and whites, independent of "g". *Personality & Individual Differences, 27*, 1181–1187.

Russell, G. L., Fujino, D. C., Sue, S., Cheung, M., & Snowden, L. R. (1996). The effects of therapist-client ethnic match in the assessment of mental health functioning. *The Journal of Cross-Cultural Psychology, 27*, 598–615.

Satz, P., Baymur, L., & Van der Vlugt, H. (1979). Pathological left-handedness: Cross-cultural tests of a model. *Neuropsychologia, 17*, 77–81.

Shepherd, I. & Leathem, J. (1999). Factors affecting performance in cross-cultural neuropsychology: From a New Zealand bicultural perspective. *Journal of the International Neuropsychological Society, 5*, 83–84

Spreen, O. & Strauss, E. (1998). *Compendium of neuropsychological tests* (2nd ed.). New York: Oxford University Press.

Strickland, T. L., Ranganath, V., Lin, K., Poland, R., Mendoza, R., & Smith, M. (1991). Psychopharmacologic considerations in the treatment of black American populations. *Psychopharmacology Bulletin, 27,* 441–448.

Strickland, T. L., Stein, R., Lin, K.-M., Risby, E., & Fong, R. (1997). The pharmacologic treatment of anxiety and depression in African-Americans: Considerations for the general practitioner. *Archives of Family Medicine, 6,* 371–375.

Strickland, T. L., Wong, T. M., Andre, K., Gray, G. E., Miller, B., Alperson, B., Denison, E., Kinder, N., Mulligan, R., & Herrera, S. (1999). *Learning and memory functioning among substance abusers: differential ethnicity and sex effects.* Manuscript submitted for publication.

Sue, D., & Sue, S. (1987). Cultural factors in the clinical assessment of Asian Americans. *Journal of Consulting and Clinical Psychology, 55,* 479–487.

Taussig, I. M., & Ponton, M. (1996). Issues in neuropsychological assessment for Hispanic older adults: Cultural and linguistic factors. In G. Yeo & D. Gallagher-Thompson (Eds.), *Ethnicity & the dementias* (pp. 47–58). Washington D.C.: Taylor & Francis.

Teng, E. L., Lee, P. H., Yang, K., & Chang, P. V. (1976). Handedness in a Chinese population: Biological, social, and pathological factors. *Science, 193,* 1148–1150.

TenHouten, W. D. (1985). Right hemisphericity of Australian aboriginal children: Effects of culture, sex, and age on performances of closure and similarities tests. *International Journal of Neuroscience, 28*(1–2), 125–146.

U.S. Bureau of the Census. (1992). 1990 Census of population: General population characteristics. Washington, D.C.: Author.

U.S. Bureau of the Census. (1996). Demographic projections. Washington, D.C.: Author.

Westermeyer, J. (1987). Cultural factors in clinical assessment. *Journal of Consulting and Clinical Psychology, 55,* 471–478.

2

Neuropsychology Training

Ethnocultural Considerations in the Context of General Competency Training

WILFRED G. VAN GORP, HECTOR F. MYERS,
AND EVAN B. DRAKE

Introduction

Education and training in clinical neuropsychology have experienced a rapid development and crystallization over the past decade and a half, paralleling the explosive growth of the specialty. However, while there has been substantial growth in the specification of training requirements and competency guidelines in the specialty of clinical neuropsychology, meaningful integration of ethnocultural issues into the training curricula must be accomplished. In this chapter, we review the historical developments in generic training of neuropsychologists, then discuss the range of issues that the specialty of neuropsychology faces given the dramatic demographic changes that are occurring in our population that have implications for the education and training of neuropsychologists.

Historical Developments in Neuropsychology Training

It was not long after professionals (mostly psychologists, along with some neurologists and psychiatrists) began to formally meet and discuss issues of brain–behavior relationships, that attention was paid to training issues. In the late 1960s, a number of likeminded scientists coalesced to found the International Neuropsychological Society, with a membership of 175 in 1970 (Benton, 1987). During the 1970s, the International Neuropsychological Society took shape and grew substantially, and in 1980 the Division of Clinical Neuropsychology (Division 40) of the American Psychological Association (APA) was formally established. This division is now among the three largest divisions of the association.

As these events progressed in the 1970s and 1980s, it was not long before neuropsycholo-

WILFRED G. VAN GORP AND EVAN B. DRAKE • New York Presbyterian Hospital Cornell Medical Center, New York, New York 10021.　**HECTOR F. MYERS** • UCLA School of Medicine, Los Angeles, California 90095.

Handbook of Cross-Cultural Neuropsychology, edited by Fletcher-Janzen, Strickland, and Reynolds. Kluwer Academic / Plenum Publishers, New York, 2000.

gists began writing about the education and training of this new group of "formally educated" clinical neuropsychologists. In the mid-1980s, a joint task force of the International Neuropsychological Society and Division 40 of the APA met to discuss recommendations for training for clinical neuropsychologists. In 1987, the report of this task force was published. Soon thereafter, training programs began advertising their programs as following "INS/Division 40 guidelines" for training in neuropsychology. Despite the advance represented by the promulgation of these guidelines, they were brief, somewhat general, and lacked the detail that would later be needed.

During this same period, the number of formal education and training programs in neuropsychology grew exponentially. Various doctoral programs were established that specialized in training their students to become neuropsychologists (some research oriented, some scientist–practitioners). These included the University of Victoria, B.C., the City University of New York–Queens College, the University of Houston, and the joint University of California, San Diego–San Diego State University doctoral programs. These programs grew and matured, with the majority achieving APA-approved status.

During the same time, the number of predoctoral neuropsychology internships also increased considerably. This growth is documented in the publication, first in 1989, of a list of doctoral programs, internships, and postdoctoral fellowships, organized by Lloyd Cripe, Ph.D., and published in *The Clinical Neuropsychologist* (*TCN*). Between the first listing of the programs in existence in 1988 (Cripe, 1989) and the most recent listing 10 years later (Cripe, 1998), the number of doctoral programs listed grew from 24 to 38 (a 58% increase) and the number of internships grew from 36 to 52 (a 44% increase). However, as clearly stated in the Cripe listings, inclusion in this *TCN* roster was not a guarantee of the quality, breadth, or depth of training available at the individual programs.

Just as internships grew, the number of neuropsychology residency positions also increased during this period. (The term "residency" was formally initiated in 1998; before that, "post-doctoral fellowship" was generally used to specify postdoctoral specialty training). The lists published by Cripe (1989,1998) documented 41 postdoctoral fellowships (residencies) in 1988 and 80 in 1998, a remarkable increase of 95%. Residency programs in neuropsychology varied considerably in size, curriculum, clinical offerings, and research opportunities/requirements (more on this below).

After the publication of the INS/Division 40 guidelines for education and training in clinical neuropsychology, and the publication of Cripe listings of educational and training programs in neuropsychology, the next key event in the evolution of training was the publication of a series of articles on training in the inaugural issue of *TCN* in 1987. This volume included a collection of papers reviewing the development of the field (Benton, 1987); the Reports of the INS-Division 40 Task Force on Education, Accreditation, and Credentialing outlining guidelines for training in clinical neuropsychology at the graduate, internship, and postdoctoral level; a model of individual mentorship for individuals considering a respecialization in neuropsychology (Meier, 1987); and a review of the policies and procedures for becoming a diplomate in clinical neuropsychology from the American Board of Clinical Neuropsychology (Bieliauskas & Matthews, 1987). This collection of papers provided a generation of neuropsychologists with examples and documentation of traditional and nontraditional methods of education and training in the emerging specialty.

The next landmark event in this field came with the founding of the Association of Postdoctoral Programs in Clinical Neuropsychology (APPCN), a national organization that grew out of a Midwest consortium of educators in clinical neuropsychology. APPCN was founded as a collection of directors of neuropsychology postdoctoral programs, to ensure high uniform standards in the recruitment and training of clinical neuropsychologists. APPCN initially surveyed its members in order to insure conformity with INS/Division 40 guidelines, and soon began a path to eventual formal accreditation of residency programs. Under the direction of APPCN Presidents Tom Hammeke, Ph.D. and James Malec, Ph.D., the number of member programs has grown substantially. APPCN is still the primary force behind the establishment of uniform guidelines for what will ultimately be accreditation of clinical neuropsychology programs and serves as a coordinating body for the timing of postdoctoral residency offers from programs nationally each year.

As can be seen, these developments—many of which can be considered landmark events—occurred over a relatively brief period, fewer than 20 years. Another event, however, that was yet to occur propelled American clinical neuropsychology to the status of a formal specialty. In 1996, the American Psychological Association designated clinical neuropsychology as a formal specialty, the first such designation in 30 years and the first to be founded under the procedures established by the APA Commission for the Recognition of Specialties and Proficiencies in Professional Psychology (Meier, 1998). As a new specialty (just like clinical psychology, counseling, and school psychology in the past), it became clear that formal guidelines outlining the education and training of clinical neuropsychologists were now needed. This culminated in the Houston Conference. Held in Houston, Texas, over five days in September 1997, the Houston Conference consisted of 37 appointed delegates from all regions of the country, representing various viewpoints, employment settings, seniority, education and training models, cultures, and geographic locations of clinical neuropsychologists. Five representatives of the sponsoring neuropsychology organizations were also present. The selection process of delegates is detailed in the description of the Houston Conference, published in a single issue of the *Archives of Clinical Neuropsychology* (Hannay et al., 1998a).

The Houston Conference developed and published formal guidelines for the education and training of clinical neuropsychologists, from doctoral level graduate programs through internship and residency, with an eye toward future subspecialty postdoctoral fellowship training (Hannay et al., 1998b). The Houston Conference guidelines moved well beyond prior guidelines by establishing a competency-based model, with clearly delineated areas of study. In this model, all aspects of general neuropsychology and professional education should be integrated. This integration begins with doctoral level education and continues through internship and residency. Thus, one can attain competency in assessment by training and experience gained at the doctoral level (10%), as well as internship (40%), and residency (50%). Figure 1 outlines this model, which is given for purely illustrative purposes.

It can be seen that this model is both programmatic and competency-based. The programmatic level at which these various educational criteria are reached may vary, but the educational content may not. In this competency-based model, the prospective neuropsychologist may pursue a neuropsychology track in a doctoral program, or achieve a doctorate specifically in clinical neuropsychology. However, the model also allows an individual to enter a doctoral program in clinical psychology that provides training in "generic psychology and generic clinical cores." The guidelines recommend that the foundational understanding of brain-behavior relationships should be developed "to a considerable degree" at the graduate level. However, the document also allows for variability in this latter emphasis. The internship may or may not consist of or be housed within a primary neuropsychology program, but "should extend specialty preparation in science and professional practice in clinical neuropsychology" as well as allow for the completion of training "in the general practice of professional psychology." At entry to the internship, it is anticipated (though not required) that the applicant will have finished his or her doctoral dissertation before starting the internship program.

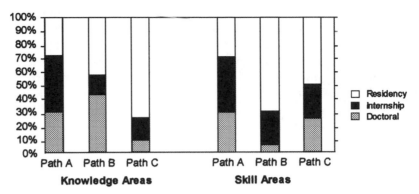

FIGURE 1. Possible education and training pathways under Houston Conference guidelines (adapted from Hannay et al., 1998b).

As managed care health plans move toward reimbursement for services provided by doctoral level providers, more and more internships will require candidates to have a doctorate prior to the start of the internship.

For the residency, a two-year period of fulltime education and training is expected, and this must occur on at least a halftime basis, in a "fixed site or on formally affiliated and geographically proximate training sites, with primarily on-site supervision." Thus, programs which espouse a model of training in which residents travel to one setting for a few weeks, then to another, and then another, would not meet the conditions of the Houston Conference. Similarly, training at weekend seminars as the primary means for specialization would not qualify under the Houston Conference. The residency program director is expected to be board certified in neuropsychology, a requirement echoed by APPCN. At the conclusion of the residency, the graduating resident is required to demonstrate competence as a clinical neuropsychologist through an examination or project (such as a published paper in a scientific journal, receipt of a grant, etc.).

It is anticipated that residency programs will soon be reviewed for accreditation by the APA or some other accrediting body. This has not yet occurred, because some issues unique to residency programs do not easily fit in with APA accreditation requirements, which have been traditionally oriented to the internship. For instance, the APA requires that multiple faculty train more than one resident. This is in contrast to the model residency program in APPCN, in which an apprenticeship model is used, with one or two faculty members training one resident. In addition, since most residency programs consist of a small number of residents, it is unclear whether their host institutions will agree to financially sponsor the relatively expensive accreditation process that APA currently requires. It is likely that these issues will be worked out, however, and readers of this chapter will be able to regard the preceding paragraphs as of historical interest, with accreditation of residency programs routine. We eagerly await that day.

Knowledge and Skill Base in Clinical Neuropsychology

The Houston Conference (1998) specified a minimum knowledge base that must be acquired in order to qualify as a clinical neuropsychologist. The knowledge base is divided into four areas. These include a generic psychology core (such as statistics, social psychology, and life span development), a generic clinical core (such as psychopathology, ethics, and intervention techniques), foundations for the study of brain-behavior relationships (such as functional neuroanatomy, neuroimaging, and neuropsychology of behavior), and foundations for the practice of clinical neuropsychology (such as neuropsychological assessment and professional issues in neuropsychology). The generic psychology core includes "cultural and individual differences and diversity" as a necessary area of knowledge.

The Houston Conference also outlines five skill areas that must be possessed by the clinical neuropsychologist, which may be acquired "through multiple pathways, not limited to courses, and may come through other documentable didactic methods." The skill areas are summarized as assessment, treatment and interventions, consultation, research, and teaching and supervision. It is notable that the skill areas of assessment and treatment/intervention include the requirement of "recognition of multicultural issues."

Education and Training: Practical Application

The student seeking a career as a neuropsychologist will pursue doctoral study in professional psychology, in either a program with a specialty in neuropsychology, or a general program with selected offerings. In addition to introductory neuropsychology courses (and those listed in the Houston Conference document), he or she will want to pursue courses in areas such as cognitive psychology, learning, and neuroscience. She or he will also undoubtedly pursue clinical practicum hours to develop basic clinical skills, learning the administration of neuropsychological tests, rationale for test selection, and elementary principles of test interpretation and report writing. Given the 10/40/50 division of education and training outlined by the Houston Conference, the graduate level is not considered the primary training ground for neuropsychologists.

As noted above, the Houston Conference allows for some programmatic flexibility in graduate training. Because it is a content and competency based model, the level at which knowledge is acquired (graduate program, internship, residency) may vary from individual to individual, as long as the educational criteria are eventually met. Thus, an individual who attended a graduate program that was more generally clinically oriented and that could only offer more basic training in neuropsychology might apply for internships that offer a dedicated neuropsychology track with didactic offerings in the specialized areas that were not available at the graduate level. In this example, 5% of training would occur at the graduate level and 45% occur at the internship level. Conversely, a student who has attended a doctoral program in neuropsychology that provided extensive neuropsychology practicum and coursework, might seek a more diversified internship that offered more general clinical training and didactics, as well as a rotation in neuropsychology (20% graduate training, 20% internship). Either of these possibilities is a viable pathway in the training of a clinical neuropsychologist.

The final phase of training as outlined in the Houston Conference is the residency program. In the 10/40/50 model of the Houston Conference, the residency program provides the balance of training in neuropsychology. Again, programs may be selected that fit the educational needs and career aspirations of the future neuropsychologist.

Ethnocultural Considerations in the Context of Generic Training

In the last two decades, we have seen a dramatic increase in the attention given to ethnocultural issues in psychology, especially in the developments in the field of minority mental health. These developments emerged in response to the need for more appropriate assessment tools, mental health services, research and training for psychologists given the dramatic changes in the U.S. population. Current census and future population projections into the 21st century clearly indicate that the U.S. is fast becoming a truly multicultural society with a significant percentage of nonwhites (U.S. Census Report, 1996). For example, population projections indicate that the U.S. population in July, 2001 will consist of 71.4% whites (non-Hispanics), 12.3% African Americans, 11.7% Latinos, 4.0% Asian/Pacific Islanders, and 0.8% Native Americans/Alaska Natives. The American Psychological Association has recognized the significance of these dramatic population changes and has played an active role in addressing these issues by cosponsoring a number of national conferences on research and training (Stricker et al., 1990; Myers, Wohlford, Guzman, & Echemendia, 1991; Wohlford, Myers, & Callan, 1993); modifying its guidelines for accreditation of training programs to include consideration of ethnocultural issues; modifying its ethical guidelines for the provision of psychological services; supporting programs to increase the recruitment, training and retention of more ethnic minority psychologists; and cohosting a National Multicultural Conference and Summit (Sue, Bingham, Porche-Burke, & Vasquez, 1999).

In addition, the National Institutes of Health, especially the National Institute of Mental Health, has increased its support for research on issues specific to racial/ethnic populations, including requiring the inclusion of racial/ethnic minorities and women in all NIH-funded studies.

These institutional changes have been driven by and occurred in conjunction with the growing body of psychological research on racial/ethnic populations that has begun to investigate the complex role that race/ethnicity, social class, and other sources of group differences can play in all aspects of psychological functioning. Unfortunately, these developments have occurred independent of and with little impact on the developments in the field of clinical neuropsychology. In fact, a careful perusal of the literature in neuropsychology and the more established training programs in neuropsychology indicate that more attention must be given to research and teaching to ethnocultural issues. Neuropsychology curricula evidence too little course content that would increase their trainees' appreciation of the potential impact these social status factors can have on the selection and interpretation of neuropsychological assessment measures, on the context of the assessments conducted, on the samples included in neuropsychological research, and on the conclusions drawn from research with limited or inadequately characterized study samples. These deficiencies in the literature reflect a lack of recognition that brain–behavior relationships always occur in social contexts, and that failure to adequately appreciate these contextual factors limits our ability to fully understand the behavioral phenomena we are studying. Social status defining factors such as race/ethnicity and social class exert powerful and complex effects on these brain–behavior relationships. Let's consider a few specific conceptual and methodological problems posed by these factors and which should be addressed in all neuropsychology training programs.

The Problem of Standardized Assessment Measures

The growing ethnocultural diversity in the population poses unique challenges to the field of clinical neuropsychology, especially with respect to the major tools of the trade. All neuropsychologists are required to develop considerable knowledge about the range of assessment measures that are the tools of the trade, and are required to have expertise in the selection, administration and interpretation of tests designed to answer specific questions about neuro-cognitive functioning and the possible bases for observed dysfunction. It is usually assumed that traditional "standardized" assessment tools provide an uncontaminated estimate of performance and ability (e.g., learning, problemsolving). As such, decisions based on the interpretation of these test results are taken as valid indicators of true performance and potential and are used in making critical decisions about people's lives and futures. Unfortunately, beyond superficial statements about "considerations of possible ethnic differences" in test performance, most neuropsychologists are ill equipped to understand or to give meaningful consideration of the real significance of this warning.

For example, and despite years of debate about "cultural biases" in testing, most of the measures included in standard neuropsychological batteries have never been standardized and demonstrated to be reliable and valid with diverse populations. Consequently, questions about their cross-cultural reliability and validity, and their specificity and sensitivity across diverse populations, remain open to debate. This is not to suggest that the measures used are invalid, but rather that many are of unknown validity, and there is considerable need for formal validation studies to be conducted using large samples with adequate representations of the diverse populations on whom the tests are to be used, so that valid performance norms can be established. Obviously, this is a challenge to the entire field and this ideal goal is not likely to be achieved anytime soon. Therefore, the challenge to training programs is to address these issues honestly and in depth so that trainees are cognizant of the potential limits in the utility of their measures when administered to racial/ethnic minority clients or research participants, and can take appropriate precautions in their conclusions and recommendations.

The Sociocultural Context of Testing

Race/ethnicity and social class can also exert powerful effects on test performance indirectly through their effects on the social context of testing. While considerable attention is given to standardizing test administration procedures to control method variance, we generally underestimate the potential differential effects that attributes of the setting and the tester can have on client performance. There is considerable research on interpersonal interactions between persons from different social classes and ethnic backgrounds. Although inconsistent in its findings (Graziano, Varca & Levy, 1982; Hanley & Barclay, 1979), this research indicates that examiner–client ethnicity, gender, and social class are not neutral factors and that test performance may be vulnerable to differences on these variables. These effects may also be greater when multiple sources of differences are present (e.g., a white male professional testing a low-income African American male teen), and may be more powerful with some race–gender pairings than with others (e.g., black male–white male dyads vs. white female–Asian or Latino male dyads) (Fuchs & Fuchs, 1989; Terrell, Terrell & Taylor, 1981).

There is also some provocative evidence from social psychology on the phenomenon of stereotype threat by Claude Steele and colleagues (Steele, 1998; Spencer, Steele, & Quinn, 1999; Steele & Aronson, 1998) that indicates that the test performance of African Americans and women is significantly lower when cueing of race or gender stereotypes occurs. These effects were observed even with such subtle cues as having respondents identify their ethnicity or gender.

Obviously, controlling for all of these variables is impractical and unrealistic, and perhaps even unjustified given the inconsistencies in some of the evidence to date. What is important, however, is to recognize the need for more studies that are designed to investigate these hypothesized effects and for neuropsychologists to be aware of their possible effects and to develop skills to minimize them, as well as to consider them in the interpretation of test results.

Another factor that is usually underappreciated is the differential effect that the test setting can have on performance. Skilled interviewers and examiners are well aware of the effects that even small changes in the room, in the testing set up, in the way the material is presented, in the style of interacting with the examinee can have on test performance. These subtle factors can be even more important the greater the social distance and power differentials between examiner and client. Therefore, attention needs to be given in assessment training to recognizing these issues and developing strategies for minimizing these potential sources of error.

Differential Exposures to Neurocognitive Compromising Agents and Events

There is general recognition in the field that there are significant ethnicity and social class differences in exposure to factors (e.g. toxic agents, poor education, inadequate nutrition) and events (e.g. accidents, violence) that can compromise neurocognitive functioning. For example, Amante, Van Houten, Grieve, Bader & Margules (1977) offer an ecological model to account for ethnic differences in IQ performance, noting that although ethnic differences in performance decreased when socioeconomic status (SES) is controlled, groups still differed on tests assessing different aspects of intelligence. This model postulates that neurological integrity differs along the SES continuum, and that the differential distribution of environmental risk factors across ethnic groups helps to account for the remaining black–white differences in performance despite comparable SES. However, it is important for trainees not to assume that these risk differentials are present simply on the basis of the race or social class of the client or to simply attribute lower test performance to ethnicity or to social class in an automatic, stereotypical fashion. Instead, trainees must be taught to specifically assess for exposure to these potential sources of variance and to systematically test for their effects in studies with participants from diverse ethnic and SES backgrounds.

Summary and Conclusions

Neuropsychology as a field and profession has grown dramatically in the last several decades, and parallel to this growth have been efforts to formalize and raise the standards of professional competency required. This has also led to the development of more predoctoral, postdoctoral and residency training programs. However, these developments have occurred independent of and with little integration of the other developments in psychology that address the growing challenges posed by the dramatic racial/ethnic diversification of the U.S. population. In this chapter we identify several of the challenges to the field that these population changes pose, and while no formal answers are offered, we underscore the need for more meaningful changes to be made in the curricula of neuropsychology training programs to address the issues raised here and to insure that graduates from these training programs actually meet the APA guidelines for responsible provision of psychological services. It is our impression that, at this juncture, the graduates from even the best training programs have not received the didactic and experiential training necessary to achieve even functional familiarity with ethnocultural issues, much less any meaningful level of expertise. We trust that focusing attention to these issues will stimulate more open and honest discussion of these challenges within the field and more efforts to incorporate these issues into the training curricula at all levels of graduate and professional training in neuropsychology.

ACKNOWLEDGMENTS.   This chapter was made possible in part by NIMH Grant 5T32-MH19998-02 to the first author.

References

Amante, D., Van Houten, V. M., Grieve, J. H., Bader, C. A., & Margules, P. H. (1977). Neuropsychological deficit, ethnicity, and socioeconomic status. *Journal of Consulting and Clinical Psychology*, *45*, 524–535.

Benton, A. (1987). Evolution of a clinical specialty. *The Clinical Neuropsychologist*, *1*, 5–8.

Bieliauskas, L. A., & Matthews, C. G. (1987). American Board of Clinical Neuropsychology: Policies and procedures. *The Clinical Neuropsychologist*, *1*, 21–28.

Cripe, L. (1989). Listing of training programs in clinical neuropsychology—1988. *The Clinical Neuropsychologist*, *3*, 116–128.

Cripe, L. I. (1998). Listing of training programs in clinical neuropsychology—1998. *The Clinical Neuropsychologist*, *12*, 365–448.

Fuchs, D., & Fuchs, L. S. (1989). Effects of examiner familiarity on Black, Caucasian, and Hispanic children: A meta-analysis. *Exceptional Children*, *55*, 303–308.

Graziano, W. G., Varca, P. E., & Levy, J. C. (1982). Race of examiner effects and the validity of intelligence tests. *Review of Educational Research*, *52*, 469–497.

Hanley, J. H. & Barclay, A. G. (1979). Sensitivity of the WISC and WISC-R to subject and examiner variables. *Journal of Black Psychology*, *5*, 79–84

Hannay, H. J., Bieliauskas, L. A., Crosson, B. A., Hammeke, T. A., Hamsher, K. deS., & Koffler, S. P. (1998a). Proceedings of the Houston Conference on Specialty Education and Training in Clinical Neuropsychology [Special issue]. *Archives of Clinical Neuropsychology*, *13*(2).

Hannay, H. J., Bieliauskas, L. A., Crosson, B. A., Hammeke, T. A., Hamsher, K. deS., & Koffler, S. P. (1998b). Proceedings of the Houston Conference on Specialty Education and Training in Clinical Neuropsychology: Policy statement. *Archives of Clinical Neuropsychology*, *13*, 160–166.

Meier, M. (1987). Continuing education: An alternative to respecialization in clinical neuropsychology. *The Clinical Neuropsychologist*, *1*, 9–20.

Meier, M. (1998). Developmental milestones in the specialty of clinical neuropsychology. *Archives of Clinical Neuropsychology*, *13*, 174–176.

Myers, H. F., Wohlford, P., Guzman, L. P., & Echemendia, R. (Eds.) (1991). *Ethnic minority perspectives on clinical training and services in psychology*. Washington, D.C.: American Psychological Association Press.

Spencer, S. J., Steele, C. M., & Quinn, D. M. (1999). Stereotype threat and women's math performance. *Journal of Experimental Social Psychology*, *35*, 4–28.

Steele, C. M. (1998). Stereotyping and its threat arc real. *American Psychologists*, *53*, 680–681.

Steele, C. M., & Aronson, J. (1998). Stereotype threat and the test performance of academically successful African Americans. In C. Jencks, M. Phillips, et. al., (Eds.), *The black–white test score gap* (pp. 401–427). Washington, D.C.: Brookings Institution.

Stricker, G., Davis-Russell, E., Bourg, E., Duran, E., Hammond, W. R., McHolland, J., Polite, K., & Vaughn, B. E. (1990). *Toward ethnic diversification in psychology education and training*. Washington, D.C.: American Psychological Association.

Sue, D. W., Bingham, R. P., Porche-Burke, L., & Vasquez, M. (1999). The diversification of psychology: A multicultural revolution. *American Psychologist*, *54*, 1061–1069.

Terrell, F, Terrell, S. L., Taylor, J. (1981). Effects of race examiner and cultural mistrust on the WAIS performance of Black students. *Journal of Consulting and Clinical Psychology*, *49*, 750–751.

U.S. Bureau of the Census (1996). *Resident population of the United States: Middle series projections, 1998–2005, by sex, race, and Hispanic origin, with median age*. Washington, D.C.: Author.

Wohlford, P., Myers, H. F., & Callan, J. (1993). *Services for the seriously mentally-ill: Public–academic linkages in services, research, and training*. Washington, D.C.: American Psychological Association.

II

Special Considerations in Neuropsychological Assessment and Intervention with Diverse Groups

3

Neuropsychological Assessment and Intervention with African Americans

NINA A. NABORS, JOVIER D. EVANS,
AND TONY L. STRICKLAND

Introduction

Attempts to address the impact of race and ethnicity on human behavior have increased in recent years. Race has been traditionally classified through genetically determined systems such as blood type or physical characteristics such as skin color (Kato, 1996). In its original definition developed to classify plants and animals, race was defined as an "inbreeding, geographically isolated population that differs in distinguishable physical traits from other members of the species" (Zuckerman, 1990). Social scientists attempted to take this definition and adapt it to the racial classification of human beings. The racial classification of human beings is generally fraught with problems, however, primarily due to a lack of empirically derived procedures to determine biologically distinct differences between different races. Ethnicity has been defined in several ways including national origin (i.e., Japanese American) and language (Hispanic American). Using this classification says little about the possible similarities between individuals within an ethnic classification. As with race, ethnicity has also been used to refer to distinguishing physical characteristics between groups of people. This has led to the tendency to use race and ethnicity interchangeably, further increasing the confusion. These differences in definition tend to decrease the ability to compare research findings across studies and have led to either a tendency to avoid using racial or ethnic categories altogether or to superficial use of the classification. As opposed to a more narrow biological classification, ethnicity has been more recently viewed as a "sociocultural" construction determined by the rules of the culture (Kato, 1996). A sociocultural definition of

NINA A. NABORS • Department of Psychology, Eastern Michigan University, Ypsilanti, Michigan 48197. JOVIER D. EVANS • Department of Psychology, Indiana University-Purdue University, Indianapolis, Indiana 46202. TONY L. STRICKLAND • Charles R. Drew University of Medicine and Science, Los Angeles, California 90059; and UCLA School of Medicine, Los Angeles, California 90095.

Handbook of Cross-Cultural Neuropsychology, edited by Fletcher-Janzen, Strickland, and Reynolds. Kluwer Academic/Plenum Publishers, New York, 2000.

ethnicity focuses more on the values, customs, and rules that the members of an ethnic group share. Sociocultural definitions of ethnicity also recognize that a group of pepople may share the experience of being a minority (i.e., similar treatment at the hands of the majority society due to physical characteristics). This chapter will utilize black and African American inter-changeably to refer to Americans who share common ancestral descent from people indige-nous to sub-Saharan Africa (Jackson & Sellers, 1996). This definition relates to the socio-cultural aspects of being black or African American.

African Americans are a growing proportion of American society. Estimated to be 12% of the population in 1993, the current predictions of African American growth by the year 2050 are to between 14% and 17% of the population (Kottak & Kozaitis, 1999). African Americans are at increased risk of dementia and other neurological conditions. Incidence rates of traumatic brain injury (Rosenthal et al., 1996; Whitman, Coonley-Hoganson, & Desai, 1984), stroke (Giles, Kittner, Hebel, Losonczy, & Sherwin, 1995), and spinal cord injury (Devivo, Rutt, Black, Go, & Stover, 1992) have increased more rapidly in the African American populations than in the general population. Thus African Americans are increasingly in need of neuropsychological assessment and intervention.

Unfortunately, current neuropsychological practices are less than optimal to effectively assess and treat African Americans. There is a limited understanding of the impact of culture, race, and social class on test development and test performance (Heaton, Ryan, Grant & Matthews, 1996; Helms, 1997). Furthermore, the effects of learning styles, test-taking atti-tudes, and information processing strategies on test performance and test interpretation are also absent. The lack of test norms specific to African Americans often lead to a tendency to overpathologize African Americans (Heaton et al., 1996; Manly et al., 1998; Palmer, Olivarez, Wilson & Fordyce, 1989). These issues have significant implications for diagnosis and treat-ment. This chapter will address important issues for more culturally sensitive assessment and intervention, and provide specific guidelines for working with African American populations.

Intellectual Assessment

Many studies over the years have compared African American performance to European American performance on cognitive ability measures. African Americans have consistently scored approximately one standard deviation lower than European Americans on a number of verbally laden standard intellectual measures (Kaufman, McLean, & Reynolds, 1988; Rey-nolds, Kaufman, & McLean, 1987; Vincent, 1991). African Americans' scores were lowest on measures of verbal and visuospatial abilities (i.e., Vocabulary and Block Design of the Wechsler scales). Vocabulary and Block Design subtests are most often used to estimate IQ due to the high correlation with Verbal and Performance IQ. Utilizing this estimated IQ with African Americans, however, can lead to an underestimate of their Full Scale IQ. Research on the appropriate use of short forms of the Wechsler scales with African Americans (i.e., which subtests most accurately reflect Full Scale IQ) is needed. Several theories have been proposed as to why African Americans tend to score lower on standard intellectual measures than European Americans (Heaton et al., 1996; Helms, 1997; Herrnstein & Murray, 1994; Jensen, 1969). Environmental factors such as level of education, socioeconomic status (SES), and culture appear to be critical factors in these IQ differences.

Researchers have addressed the impact of the environment on intellectual performance. Krohn and Lamp (1989) compared the performance of African American and European

American preschool children on intellectual and achievement measures (Stanford Binet 4th edition and Kaufman Assessment Battery for Children [K-ABC]). The usual one-standard-deviation difference between the two groups of children disappeared after controlling for SES. The African American children, however, continued to score significantly lower on the achievement scale of the K-ABC, which suggests that SES and level of education may be distinct factors. Similarly, Vincent (1991) addressed intellectual performance (Wechsler scales, Stanford Binet, Raven's Progressive Matrices, and Kaufman Assessment Battery for Children) between black and white children pre- and post-1980. While he documented the usual differences of one standard deviation between black and white adults and children on intellectual measures prior to 1980, the differences in intellectual performance after 1980 shrank to one-half a standard deviation between black and white children. This suggests that improvements in education and SES have positively affected intellectual performance for black children.

Some researchers make the distinction between knowledge-based and processing-dependent measures and have found knowledge-based tests to be more influenced by exposure. Development of vocabulary, for instance, is significantly influenced by communication patterns in the home environment. Moreover, a significant relationship has been found between frequency and diversity of words used in the home and SES (Hart & Risley, 1995; Huttenlocher, Haight, Bryk, Seltzer & Lyons, 1991). African American and European American children were given language-based tests (oral scales from the Woodcock Johnson Psychoeducational Battery) and process dependent tasks (nonword repetition task, competing language processing task, revised token test) (Campbell, Dollaghan, Needleman, & Janosky, 1997). The African American childrens' performance was significantly lower on the oral language scales, but there were no differences between the two groups on the process-dependent tasks.

Grubb and Dozier (1989) compared black and white college students' performance on measures of intelligence (WAIS-R), memory (drum learning tasks), and abstract reasoning (Category test). They found the usual differences on the intelligence measure, but found that these differences became nonsignificant after controlling for number of siblings in the home, occupation level of father, combined level of parents' education, and income. These studies indicate that education and SES may have a significant impact on performance on intellectual measures. The differences found in intellectual performance on standardized measures between African Americans and European Americans, however, may be due to more than education and SES since African Americans continue to perform significantly lower than European Americans across education levels (Kaufman et al., 1988; Reynolds et al., 1987). The answer may be the influence of culture.

In summary, the gap in intellectual performance between African American and European American children appears to be decreasing. Intellectual performance of African Americans appears to be moderated by several variables including education and SES. In addition, African Americans tend to perform better on process-dependent tasks rather than knowledge-based tasks.

Education

Education is an important factor in neuropsychological test performance. Reynolds and colleagues (1987) reported a two-standard-deviation discrepancy between college-educated participants and participants with an eighth-grade education on measures of intellectual functioning (Wechsler scales). Specifically, education appears to be related not only to verbal subtests such as Vocabulary, Information, Comprehension, Similarities, Arithmetic, and Digit Span, but also to performance measures such as Digit Symbol. Level of education was least correlated with Object Assembly, Picture Completion, and Picture Arrangement. Education also influenced performance on the neuropsychological measures for older African Americans (Callahan et al., 1996; Unverzagt et al., 1996). The higher the education levels, the better the performance on neuropsychological measures. Unverzagt and colleagues (1996) found that education most influenced performance on the Mini-Mental State Examination, Boston Naming, Animal Fluency, Constructional Praxis, and, to a lesser extent, delayed recall and recognition. Norms for neuropsychological measures corrected for education levels have been developed (Heaton, Grant, & Matthews, 1991). Current methods for determining education, however, are inadequate at best. For example, years of education indicate little about the quality of the educational experience (Helms, 1997). There are significant discrepancies between educational environments in terms of resources dedicated to such factors as quality of equipment (i.e., textbooks, computers, and microscopes), environmental hazards (lead, asbestos), and safety concerns (violence, drugs). African Americans are more likely to receive an inferior education (Helms, 1997), which may also affect their performance on neuropsychological measures.

In short, education has a significant impact on cognitive ability performance. Therefore, strategies to assess quality of education and its impact on cognitive test performance need to be a priority for those assessing cognitive abilities.

Socioeconomic Status (SES)

SES has also been addressed mostly at a superficial level (Helms, 1997). SES refers to the amount and quality of economic resources available to an individual. These are usually measured through income, education, and occupational attainment. Generally, years of education have been used as a proxy measure of SES (i.e., the higher the education level, the higher the presumed SES). As mentioned earlier, assessing education is problematic in itself. African Americans tend to have a different socioeconomic structure than that of the majority society (Wyche, 1996). SES has improved for African Americans in dual-income, college-educated households. Unfortunately, African Americans do not reap the same benefits from education as European Americans. African Americans tend to have lower incomes regardless of education, occupation, and geographic region. More importantly, African Americans tend to have significantly fewer assets compared to European Americans. Other than their homes and other material possessions, African Americans tend to have comparatively little equity such as stocks, bonds, and real estate, making comparisons across income level problematic. In addition, researchers have looked at the quality of neighborhoods as a measure of class when assessing the SES of African Americans. African Americans from several income levels, however, may live in the same neighborhood (Wyche, 1996). Using superficial measures of SES with little understanding of the complex factors related to SES for African Americans leads to inaccurate measurements at best. Consequently, African Americans are assumed to have access to more economic resources than they do.

The meaning and impact of SES may differ in the African American community from the majority society. Future research needs to address the complexity of SES within ethnic groups and how this interaction affects access to resources. This research could then lead to more accurate ways of measuring the impact of SES on cognitive ability performance.

African American Culture

For the purposes of this chapter we adapt Kottak and Kozaitis's definition of culture. Culture is defined as a way of life (traditions, customs) transmitted through learning that plays a vital role in molding the beliefs and behavior of the people exposed to them (Kottak & Kozaitis, 1999). Culture has two general components: objective and subjective (Cushner, 1999). Objective culture includes tangible components such as foods, clothing, names for things, and artifacts, which are easily identified. Subjective culture, which is the larger component, refers to intangibles such as attitudes, values, beliefs, and practices that are much more difficult to identify. Culture is taught both directly (rules, values) and indirectly (observation, modeling). Thus, culture affects every aspect of human behavior including attitudes and perceptions of normalcy. Culture affects definitions of ability and performance as well as tests to determine ability. Many neuropsychologists currently acknowledge the possible impact of education and SES on standardized measures of intelligence and achievement, but the significance of culture is less well known. It is often believed that most assessment measures utilized by neuropsychologists are culture-free, particularly the "nonverbal" measures (Heaton et al., 1996). African Americans, however, have been found to exhibit lower scores on measures of visual naming, abstract reasoning, computerized simple and choice reaction times, speed of information processing, tactile visual discrimination, attention/working memory, and verbal and nonverbal learning and memory compared to European Americans (Heverly, Isaac, & Hynd, 1986; Johnson-Selfridge, Zalewski, & Abourdarham, 1998; Manly et al., 1998; Nabors, Vangel & Lichtenberg, 1997; Roberts & Hamsher, 1984; Welsh et al., 1995). This suggests that even purportedly culture-free tests may exhibit culture bias. Attempts to develop culture-free tests are problematic in that they continue to include content that may not be familiar across different cultures (Helms, 1997). Techniques such as using a panel of experts, for example, may inadvertently bias the measure. Presumably, the panel of experts has significant exposure to the majority culture themselves and thus may be less able to determine what information people with less exposure have or have not learned.

While researchers have begun to address the impact of culture on test performance, specifically as it applies to language differences (Chan, 1991; Gomez, Piedmont, & Fleming, 1992), a paucity of research exists on the impact of African American culture on test performance. This is due, in part, to the myth that African Americans do not have a separate culture from the majority American society (Landrine & Klonoff, 1994). Apparently, African Americans have the same exposure to the majority culture as European Americans and therefore should be expected to achieve at the same level when opportunities such as education and SES are equal. This logic is faulty on two levels. First, it is highly unlikely in this largely segregated society that all, or even most, African Americans have a significant exposure to the majority culture (Helms, 1997). Culture is transmitted in several ways including in the home, school, place of worship, work, and leisure pursuits. African Americans, whose lives are more segregated in these areas, will experience less exposure to the cultural values of the majority society. To some extent, this may explain the idea that African Americans across educational, socioeconomic levels, or both may continue to perform lower on particular cognitive ability measures than their counterparts from the majority society. Secondly, theorists have addressed factors that may be unique to the African American culture. Common values associated with African American culture include communal focus (i.e., extended family, flexible family roles), expressive creativity (oral expression), and focus on knowledge for practical, utilitarian, and relevant purposes (Grubb & Dozier, 1989; Helms, 1997; Willis, 1989). These values may have an impact on the learning styles of African Americans which are not assessed through the currently available standardized cognitive measures. African Americans may perform better on measures of contextual interpretation, improvisation and creativity, and memory for essence rather than facts (Willis, 1989). The smallest differences between blacks and whites on the Wechsler scales commonly occur on Picture Arrangement, Digit Symbol, and Digit Span, subtests which may tap creativity, improvisation, and contextual interpretation (Helms, 1997).

In summary, all cognitive measures are affected by culture, but the current understanding of the impact of culture on test development and test performance is limited. African American culture may emphasize values that affect cognitive performance, but these values are not currently assessed in typical measures of cognitive ability. In order to determine how well African Americans will perform on traditional measures of cognitive ability, level of exposure, acculturation to European American culture, or both must be assessed.

Acculturation

"Acculturation measures the level at which an individual participates in the values, language and practice of his/her own ethnic community versus those of the majority culture" (Manly et al., 1998). Landrine and Klonoff (1994) developed the African American Acculturation Scale (AAAS) to assess the level of acculturation among African Americans. The scale addresses several practices including religious beliefs, traditional black family structure, socialization, and traditional health beliefs. This 74-item scale reliably discriminated among blacks, whites, Hispanics, and Asians. In addition, the acculturation score was independent of gender, social class, and education. As with other acculturation measures, the AAAS could be useful for assessing the impact of acculturation on cognitive performance.

Recently, Manly and colleagues (1998) assessed the impact of acculturation on neuropsychological test performance of African Americans. One hundred seventy neurologically normal African Americans were administered an expanded version of the Halstead–Reitan Neuropsychological Battery (HRB) (Heaton et al., 1991; Reitan & Wolfson, 1993). Comparing the scores to the published HRB norms (predominantly European American sample), the African Americans were significantly impaired on the majority of the tests, with 10 of the 16 tests showing at least a 30% impairment rate for the group. Acculturation, as measured by the AAAS-short form (Landrine & Klonoff, 1995), accounted for a significant proportion of the variance in the majority of the measures. After controlling for acculturation and demographics (age, education, and sex), less acculturated individuals continued to exhibit lower scores on WAIS-R Information and the Boston Naming Test. In a second study, Manly and colleagues (1998) compared the neuropsychological performance on demographically matched HIV-positive African American and white participants. African Americans scored significantly lower on measures of attention–working memory (PASAT), verbal and nonverbal learning (Story and Figure Learning Tests), abstraction (Category Test and Trails B), visuospatial ability (WAIS-R Block Design), and speed of information processing. After controlling for acculturation, differences between the two groups became nonsignificant on a number of tasks including the Category Test, Trails B time, Vocabulary, Block Design, and the Figure Learning Test. The group difference remained for verbal learning. Acculturation was not related to performance on Trails A, WAIS-R Digit Symbol and Digit Span, PASAT, Story and Figure Retention, Sensory Perceptual Exam, and Grooved Pegboard. These results indicate that acculturation accounts for some of the variance in neuropsychological test performance. The fact that the participants continued to exhibit lower performance on knowledge-based measures (WAIS-R Information and Boston Naming) after controlling for acculturation and other demographics suggests either that current measures of education or acculturation do not adequately account for these variables or that there are others factors involved in cognitive performance that have not been addressed.

A major criticism of current attempts to assess acculturation is that acculturation is usually measured only on a nominal level such as generation in country, language preference, SES, and level of education. Thus, most acculturation measures assess the amount of adaptation an individual has to the majority culture rather than measuring how acculturated they are to their culture of origin. In addition, there has been less of an attempt to measure how these demographic variables influence the learning of the majority culture (Helms, 1997). The AAAS distinguished between African Americans and members of other ethnic groups, but research to determine exactly how these variables relate to learning the majority culture are needed. For example, does a high level of acculturation within one's own ethnic group imply less acculturation into the majority society? What about those individuals who are truly bicultural (equally immersed in both the culture of origin and the culture of the majority society)? Are bicultural individuals as acculturated to the information necessary to perform well on cognitive ability measures as individuals raised in the majority society? It is important to address these and many other questions when assessing the impact of culture on cognitive test performance.

While limited in scope, current acculturation measures may be useful in assessing the impact of culture on cognitive ability tests. This suggests that when working with an African American population, using the AAAS or other measures of acculturation as a moderating variable is necessary to decrease the possibility of overpathologizing due to lower test scores.

Impact of Racism

In addition to culture, education, and SES, other variables may affect performance on tests of cognitive ability for African Americans. The impact of racism on test performance has rarely been addressed. Cultural mistrust is an often-discussed factor in the relationship between African Americans and majority institutions (i.e., health care and educational systems). Lingering suspicions of majority institutions abound among African Americans, particularly since the Tuskegee syphilis experiment. The Tuskegee syphilis project is a well-known example of the types of abuses that have taken place in the name of science. The long-term effects of syphilis were studied in African American men for approximately 40 years without the benefit of the most effective and available cure. This and other examples of "experimentation" on African Americans have led to a cultural mistrust of majority institutions.

How does cultural mistrust affect cognitive test performance? Terrell, Terrell, and Taylor (1981) assessed the cultural mistrust of 100 black college students using the Cultural Mistrust Inventory, a 48-item measure which addresses the extent to which blacks trust whites in various situations. Examples of items which are scored on a likert scale of strongly agree to strongly disagree include "Blacks should be wary of a White person who tries to be friendly" and "Black parents should teach their children not to trust White teachers." The students were separated into two groups based on their scores: a tendency to mistrust whites and a tendency to trust whites. Half of each group (high and low mistrust) were randomly assigned to either a white or a black examiner who administered the WAIS. There was no main effect for either level of cultural mistrust or race of examiner. Interestingly, the researchers reported that black students in the high mistrust group who were examined by white examiners scored significantly lower on the WAIS than the high mistrust group examined by black examiners. In addition, black students in the low mistrust group examined by white examiners scored significantly higher than the high mistrust group examined by white examiners. Predictably, all four groups scored lower than expected based on level of education. The results of this study point to the possible effects of cultural mistrust on cognitive test performance. Individuals with higher levels of cultural mistrust may not perform as well with white examiners for several possible reasons. The individual may believe that the examiner has a racial bias regarding cognitive test performance or that the examiner may use the information from the cognitive evaluation in a negative fashion. In addition, internalized oppression (i.e., the internal belief that African Americans are less intelligent) may lead to higher anxiety in testing situations leading to lower test performance.

The impact of racism (specifically, internalized oppression) on cognitive test performance has been indirectly studied by Steele (1997). Steele theorizes that negative stereotypes regarding cognitive test performance lower cognitive performance for those invested in the domain to be tested. This was tested with black and white college students from an Ivy League university. It was assumed that the students were invested in a college education as they were attending such a prestigious and competitive institution. The students were given a test composed of difficult items from the Graduate Record Examination verbal exam. Half of the students in each group were told that the test measured intellectual ability and half were told it measured problem solving with no mention of its relationship to ability. The black students who were told the test measured intellectual ability exhibited significantly lower performance compared to the white students, while the black students in the nonability group performed equally to the white students. This result was replicated when, under the same conditions, all students were told this was a problem-solving task, but with half of the students asked to record their race on a demographic form just before taking the test. Steele's conclusion is that the salience of a racial stereotype (that blacks are intellectually inferior) is enough to depress African American performance on cognitive ability measures. The effect of racial stereotypes on cognitive test performance for African Americans (particularly in light of the recent success of *The Bell Curve* [Herrnstein & Murray, 1994]) warrants further study.

In conclusion, various demographic factors impact neuropsychological performance. Educational level and SES exhibit significant effects on cognitive ability performance. The patterns related to the impact of education and SES in African American samples, however, may diverge from similar studies done with European American samples. In addition, cultural immersion (i.e., level of acculturation) and cultural mistrust have also been found to affect cognitive performance of African Americans. Level of motivation, test anxiety, ability to work quickly, and the tendency to guess when in doubt about answers which may be related to both cultural immersion and cultural mistrust may differentially affect cognitive test performance as well (Aiken, 1997; Helms, 1997).

Intervention

Intervention is not often addressed in neuropsychology, yet it is an important component of the profession. African Americans with neurologic conditions are treated in rehabilitation settings, inpatient psychiatry, day treatment programs, VA hospitals, and other treatment settings. Many of the same issues discussed in assessing African Americans are pertinent to treatment (Brown et al., 1991). Cultural mistrust and attitudes about psychological treatment may affect the participation of African Americans. Studies have addressed the barriers to successful treatment outcomes for African Americans including language, lack of resources, and perception of racism leading to noncompliance (Jackson, Stephens, & Smith, 1997; Millet, Sullivan, Schwebel, & Myers, 1996; Robinson, 1989). Rosenthal and colleagues (1996) addressed the impact of ethnicity on functional outcome and community integration following traumatic brain injury. They found that ethnic minorities tended to have less community integration one year postinjury. While they discussed the possibility of less access to resources (transportation, funding sources) as possible mechanisms for the lower functional outcomes, other possibilities involve cultural mistrust and the impact of racism which may have led to lower follow-up rates for ethnic minorities in the study.

Similarly, Russell and colleagues (Russell, Fujino, Sue, Cheung & Snowden, 1996) addressed the impact of therapist–client matching in assessment of mental health functioning. They found that ethnically matched therapists tended to judge their clients as exhibiting higher mental health functioning than nonethnically matched therapists. These effects remained for African American and Asian American clients even after controlling for age, gender, referral source, and other demographic variables. This study suggests that the impact of culture needs to be addressed in more detail in treatment outcome studies. Measures such as the Outcome Questionnaire (which has been found to reliably assess treatment outcomes for African Americans; Nebeker, Lambert & Huefner, 1995) and the Schedule of Racist Events (a measure of the impact of racism on psychological functioning) (Landrine & Klonoff, 1996) may be useful. In addressing the needs of African Americans specifically, attention has also been recently focused on offering more culturally relevant intervention approaches such as the Afrocentric approaches utilized in substance abuse and other mental health treatment (Jackson et al., 1997; Plummer, 1996).

Traditionally, cultural mistrust and the stigma of mental disturbance may have led to lower psychological outcomes and less participation in health research. Culturally relevant approaches to intervention with African Americans could ameliorate these cultural barriers to treatment.

Current Applications and Future Directions

The following guidelines are important in neuropsychological assessment and intervention with African Americans.

1. Use African American norms for specific neuropsychological measures when they are available.
2. Add an acculturation measure such as the AAAS to the neuropsychological battery. If the client/patient appears to be less acculturated to the majority society, then the neuropsychological test scores must be viewed with caution.
3. Know the research, specifically which neuropsychological measures are less culturally biased.
4. Obtain detailed information about education and SES during the interview. In cases where it is clear that the client/patient was raised with less access to resources, then the test results must be viewed with caution.
5. Increase your knowledge of the African American culture. Specifically, learn which cultural values affect cognitive ability measures. Work to become a culturally competent provider.

For the future, the most pressing need is to develop norms for common neuropsychological measures across cognitive domains. Appropriate norms would lead to less overpathologizing of African Americans and more appropriate diagnosis and treatment. Secondly, level of acculturation needs to be routinely measured and controlled in cognitive assessment of African Americans. Of course these only superficially address the issue of assessment and intervention of African Americans. Research must focus on the impact of culture on test performance and how acculturation interacts with education and SES. SES and level of education need to be more robustly defined and their effects on test development and test measurement addressed. Finally and perhaps most importantly, there is a desperate need for education and training of neuropsychologists of color. This would not only address the impact of culture and cultural mistrust, but could also lead to further education and research related to the impact of ethnicity and culture on test performance. Training regarding the impact of ethnicity and culture needs to begin at the graduate level for all students and continue throughout neuropsychological preparation. It needs to become a part of the standard requirement for specialty licensing as well, to ensure that these cultural myths of objective neuropsychological measures are addressed at all levels.

References

Aiken, L. R. (1997). *Psychological testing and assessment*. Boston: Allyn and Bacon.

Brown, A., Campbell, A., Wood, D., Hastings, A., Lewis-Jack, O., Dennis, G., Ford-Booker, P., Hicks, L., Adeshoye, A., Weir, R., & Davis, T. (1991). Neuropsychological studies of blacks with cerebrovascular disorders: A preliminary investigation. *Journal of the National Medical Association, 83*, 217–224.

Callahan, C. M., Hall, K. S., Hui. S. L., Musick, B. S., Unverzagt, F. W., & Hendric, H. C. (1996). Relationship of age, education, and occupation with dementia among a community-based sample of African Americans. *Archives of Neurology, 53*, 134–146.

Campbell, T., Dollaghan, C., Needleman, H., & Janosky, J. (1997). Reducing bias in language assessment: Processing-dependent measures. *Journal of Speech and Hearing Research, 40*, 519–525.

Chan, J. (1991). Are the western-type mental tests measuring Chinese mental faculties? *Bulletin of the Hong Kong Psychological Society*, Jan–Jul (n26–27), 59–70. (Abstract from Melvyl File: PsychINFO).

Cushner, K. (1999). *Human diversity in action: Developing multicultural competencies for the classroom*. Boston: McGraw-Hill.

Devivo, M. J., Rutt, R. D., Black, K. J., Go, B. K., & Stover, S. L. (1992). Trends in spinal cord injury demographics and treatment outcomes between 1973 and 1986. *Archives of Physical Medicine and Rehabilitation, 73*, 424–430.

Giles, W. H., Kittner, S. J., Hebel, J. R., Losonczy, K. G., & Sherwin, R. W. (1995). Determinants of black–white differences in the risk of cerebral infarction. *Archives of Internal Medicine, 155*, 1319–1324.

Gomez, F. C., Jr., Piedmont, R. L., & Fleming, M. Z. (1992). Factor analysis of the Spanish version of the WAIS: The Escala de Inteligencia Wechsler para Adultos (EIWA). *Psychological Assessment, 4*, 317–321.

Grubb, H. J., & Dozier, A. (1989). Too busy to learn: A "competing behaviors" explanation of cross-cultural differences in academic ascendancy based on the cultural distance hypothesis. *Journal of Black Psychology, 16*, 23–45.

Hart, B., & Risley, T. R. (1995). *Meaningful differences in the everyday experiences of young American children*. Baltimore: Paul H. Brookes.

Heaton, R. K., Grant, I., & Matthews, C. G. (1991). *Comprehensive norms for an expanded Halstead–Reitan Battery: Demographic corrections, research findings and clinical applications*. Odessa, FL: Psychological Assessment Resources.

Heaton, R. K., Ryan, L., Grant, I., & Matthews, C. G. (1996). Demographic influences on neuropsychological test performance. In I. Grant. & K. M. Adams (Eds.), *Neuropsychological assessment of neuropsychiatric disorder*, 2nd ed. (pp. 141–163). New York: Oxford University Press.

Helms, J. E. (1997). The triple quandary of race, culture, and social class in standardized cognitive ability testing. In D. P. Flanagan, J. L. Genshaft, & P. L. Harrison (Eds.), *Contemporary intellectual assessment* (pp. 517–532). New York: Guilford.

Herrnstein, R. A., & Murray, C. (1994). *The bell curve: Intelligence and class structure in American life*. New York: Free Press.

Heverly, L. L., Isaac, W., & Hynd, G. W. (1986). Neurodevelopmental and racial differences in tactile visual (cross modal) discrimination in normal black and white children. *Archives of Clinical Neuropsychology, 1*, 139–145.

Huttenlocher, J., Haight, W., Bryk, A., Seltzer, M., & Lyons, T. (1991). Early vocabulary growth: Relation to language input and gender. *Developmental Psychology, 27*, 236–248.

Jackson, J. S., & Sellers, S. L. (1996). African-American health over the life course: A multidimensional framework. In P. M. Kato, & T. Mann (Eds.), *Handbook of diversity issues in health psychology* (pp. 301–317). New York: Plenum.

Jackson, M. S., Stephens, R. C., & Smith, R. L. (1997). Afrocentric treatment in residential substance abuse care. *Journal of Substance Abuse Treatment, 14*, 87–92.

Jensen, A. R. (1969). *Bias in mental testing*. New York: Free Press.

Johnson-Selfridge, M. T., Zalewski, C., & Abourdarham, J. F. (1998). The relationship between ethnicity and word fluency. *Archives of Clinical Neuropsychology, 13*, 319–325.

Kato, P. (1996). On nothing and everything: The relationship between ethnicity and health. In P. M. Kato, & T. Mann (Eds.), *Handbook of diversity issues in health psychology* (pp. 287–300). New York: Plenum.

Kaufman, A. S., McLean, J. E., & Reynolds, C. R. (1988). Sex, race, residence, region and education differences on the 11 WAIS-R subtests. *Journal of Clinical Psychology, 44*, 231–248.

Kottak, C. P., & Kozaitis, K. A. (1999). *On being different: Diversity and multiculturalism in the North American mainstream*. New York: McGraw-Hill.

Krohn, E. J., & Lamp, R. E. (1989). Concurrent validity of the Stanford-Binet 4th edition and the K-ABC for head start children. *Journal of School Psychology, 27*, 59–67.

Landrine, H., & Klonoff, E. A. (1994). The African American Acculturation Scale: Development, reliability and validity. *Journal of Black Psychology, 20*, 104–127.

Landrine, H., & Klonoff, E. A. (1995). The African American Acculturation Scale II: Cross validation and short form. *Journal of Black Psychology, 21*, 124–152.

Landrine, H., & Klonoff, E. A. (1996). The Schedule of Racist Events. *Journal of Black Psychology, 22*, 144–168.

Manly, J. J., Miller, W., Heaton, R. K., Byrd, D., Reilly, J., Velasquez, R. J., Sacuezo, D. P., & Grant, I. (1998). The effect of African American acculturation on neuropsychological test performance in normal and HIV positive individuals. *Journal of International Neuropsychological Society, 4*, 291–302.

Millet, P. E., Sullivan, B. F., Schwebel, A. I., & Myers, L. J. (1996). Black Americans and white Americans views of the etiology and treatment of mental health problems. *Community Mental Health Journal, 32*, 235–242.

Nabors, N. A., Vangel, S. J., Lichtenberg, P. A, & Walsh, P. (1997). Normative and clinical utility of the Hooper Visual Organization Test with medical inpatients. *Journal of Clinical Geropsychology, 3*, 191–198.

Nebeker, R. S., Lambert, M. J., & Huefner, J. C. (1995). Ethnic differences on the Outcome Questionnaire. *Psychological Reports, 77*, 875–879.

Palmer, D. J., Olivarez, A., Wilson, V., & Fordyce, T. (1989). Ethnicity and language dominance: Influence on the prediction of achievement based on intelligence scores in nonreferred and referred samples. *Learning Disability Quarterly, 12*, 261–274.

Plummer, D. L. (1996). Developing culturally responsive psychosocial rehabilitative programs for African Americans. *Psychiatric Rehabilitation Journal, 19*, 38–43.

Reitan, R. M., & Wolfson, D. (1993). *The Halstead–Reitan Neuropsychological Test Battery* (2nd ed.). Tuscon, AZ: Neuropsychology Press.

Reynolds, C. R., Kaufman, A. S., & McLean, J. E. (1987). Demographic characteristics and IQ among adults: Analysis of the WAIS-R standardization sample as a function of the stratification variables. *Journal of School Psychology, 25*, 323–342.

Roberts, R. J., & Hamsher, K. D. (1984). Effects of minority status on facial recognition and naming performance. *Journal of Clinical Psychology, 40*, 539–540.

Robinson, J. B. (1989). Clinical treatment of black families. *Social Work, 34*, 323–329.

Rosenthal, M., Dijkers, M., Harrison-Felix, C., Nabors, N., Witol, A., Young, M., & Englander, J. (1996). Impact of minority status on functional outcome and community integration following traumatic brain injury. *Journal of Head Trauma Rehabilitation, 11*, 40–57.

Russell, G. L., Fujino, D. C., Sue, S., Cheung, M. K., & Snowden, L. R. (1996). Effects of therapist–client match in assessment of mental health functioning. *Journal of Cross-Cultural Psychology, 27*, 598–615.

Steele, C. M. (1997). A threat in the air: How stereotypes shape intellectual identity and performance. *American Psychologist, 52*, 613–629.

Terrell, F., Terrell, S. L., & Taylor, J. (1981). Effects of race of examiner and cultural mistrust on the WAIS performance of black students. *Journal of Consulting and Clinical Psychology, 49*, 750–751.

Unverzagt, F. W., Hall, K. S., Torke, A. M., Rediger, J. D., Mercado, N., Gureje, O., Osuntokun, B. O., & Hendrie, H. C. (1996). Effects of age, education and gender on CERAD neuropsychological test performance in an African American sample. *The Clinical Neuropsychologist, 10*, 180–190.

Vincent, K. R. (1991). Black–white IQ differences: Does age make the difference? *Journal of Clinical Psychology, 47*, 266–270.

Welsh, K. A., Fillenbaum, G., Wilkson, W., & Heyman, A., Mohs, R. C., Stern, Y., Harrell, L., Edland, S. D., & Beekly, D. (1995). Neuropsychological test performance in African American and white patients with Alzheimers disease. *Neurology, 45*, 2207–2211.

Whitman, S., Coonley-Hoganson, R., & Desai, B. T. (1984). Comparative head trauma in two socioeconomically different Chicago-area communities: A population study. *American Journal of Epidemiology, 4*, 570–580.

Willis, M. G. (1989). Learning styles of African American children: A review of the literature and interventions. *Journal of Black Psychology, 16*, 47–65.

Wyche, K. F. (1996). Conceptualizations of social class in African American women: Congruence of client and therapist definitions. In M. Hill & E. D. Rothblum (Eds.), *Classism and feminist therapy: Counting costs* (pp. 35–43). New York: Haworth.

Zuckerman, M. (1990). Some dubious premises in research and theory on racial differences. *American Psychologist, 45*, 1297–1303.

4

Neuropsychological Assessment and Intervention with Asian Americans

TONY M. WONG

Introduction

The relative lack of serious consideration of cultural variables as a relevant factor in neuropsychology has led to a shortage of adequate knowledge and skills necessary for a viable cross-cultural neuropsychology (Ardila, 1995; Ardila, Rosselli, & Puente, 1994; Wong, Strickland, Fletcher-Janzen, Ardila, & Reynolds, Chapter 1, this volume). This has become even more apparent in recent years, as practitioners are being asked more frequently to evaluate patients who are of different ethnic, cultural, or language backgrounds than themselves, and are finding few resources to aid them. Clinical neuropsychologists, in particular, rely heavily on tests and procedures that are standardized and validated in order to reliably assess neurocognitive and neurobehavioral function, yet they find few such instruments available to evaluate the culturally dissimilar patient. However, assessment at some level must proceed. Though it is clear that, ultimately, more systematic research in cross-cultural neuropsychology is necessary (Ardila, 1995) as our society becomes more culturally and ethnically diverse, the immediacy of the clinical neuropsychologist's need for increased understanding and direction in this domain becomes more acute.

In this chapter, the neuropsychological assessment and intervention of one of the most rapidly growing ethnic-minority groups in the United States, Asian Americans, will be considered. Demographic trends and issues will be addressed first, as this is a very heterogenous group that defies simple generalizations. Second, some of the major cultural and cross-cultural issues relevant to the neuropsychological assessment and intervention of Asian Americans will be discussed. Finally, suggestions and strategies that will help clinical neuropsychologists who are asked to evaluate an Asian American patient will be offered. Due to the heterogeneity of the Asian American group and culture (32 distinct cultural groups according to the 1990 census), a pan-Asian approach will be adopted for this chapter. That is, the focus

TONY M. WONG • St. Mary's Hospital/University of Rochester, Rochester, New York 14611.

Handbook of Cross-Cultural Neuropsychology, edited by Fletcher-Janzen, Strickland, and Reynolds. Kluwer Academic/Plenum Publishers, New York, 2000.

will be on generally what is common across the Asian subgroups. However, neither the similarities nor implied differences should be taken too literally or rigidly, as the unique histories of each of the 32 groups as well as those of the individuals need to be considered when evaluating or working with an individual from a particular subgroup. Readers are encouraged to consult references and resources for specific cultural subgroups when working with an individual from that group.

Demographics and Characteristics

In the United States, ethnicity is officially divided into five groups. In addition to the majority white/Caucasian (or European American), there are four federally designated ethnic minority groups: black (or African American), Hispanic/Latino American, Native American Indian/Alaska Native, and Asian/Pacific Islander American. People who are of mixed racial/ ethnic heritage do not fit easily into this scheme, and thus this typology has been subject to some criticism. According to the U.S. Bureau of the Census (1996), the Asian/Pacific Islander group is the fastest growing group in all regions of this country, and is projected to have the greatest gains in the West during the period 1995 to 2025, amounting to an increase of 7 million people in that region or 56% of the total added to the U.S. Asian American populaton. Asian Americans will remain particularly concentrated in California, where it is projected that by 2025, 41 percent of the nation's 21 million Asian Americans will reside. Other states that will have high proportions of Asian Americans, in descending order, are New York, Hawaii, Texas, and New Jersey. Regardless of region, though, most Asian and Pacific Islanders live in or around metropolitan areas. In 1991, 49% of this group lived in suburbs, and 45% lived in central cities (U.S. Bureau of the Census, 1993).

Because clinical neuropsychology, like clinical psychology, is concerned with individual differences, the term "Asian American" can be misleading, as it can obscure the fact that this is a quite varied, heterogeneous group. Asian America is comprised of those whose cultural and ethnic heritage is from Asia or the Pacific Islands, which encompasses a broad range of geography and peoples. Although there are similarities in racial features and culture among the Asian groups, there are also distinctive differences. In America, Asian Indians, Chinese, Filipinos, Japanese, Koreans, and Vietnamese make up nearly 90% of the census classification of Asian and Pacific Islander (Hing, 1993), but Cambodians, Hmong, Indonesians, Laotians, Pakistanis, Samoans, and Tongans have also begun to establish sizeable communities here and cannot be ignored. As an example of the fundamental heterogeneity of the group, it is noteworthy that not all necessarily agree with the grouping of Asian Indians and Filipinos along with the rest of the Asian subgroups, due to their unique racial features, distinctive cultures, or geographic distance from the rest of Asia (Hing, 1993).

As with Hispanic or Latino Americans, the sociological makeup of Asian Americans has been influenced significantly by immigration policies and patterns, and related factors. For example, most of the Chinese who immigrated to California in the 19th century came from a particular region in Guangdong (Kwangtung) province, mainly rural villages outside of Guangzhou (Canton), and spoke a similar rural Chinese dialect. Primarily farmers and manual laborers who were relatively uneducated, they left their wives and children in China and came to America looking for economic opportunity, working on the railroads and joining the "gold rush" communities in California in the late 1800s. Isolated and segregated due to various exclusionary laws that made it particularly difficult for Chinese women to immigrate to America, and subjected to constant racial discrimination and violence, these immigrants formed rather insular bachelor societies that were fairly resistant to acculturation. The significance of this brief (and admittedly oversimplified) history is that most of the elderly Chinese today who have lived in America since the early 20th century need to be understood in that context from an educational, linguistic, and psychological perspective. In contrast, Chinese who have immigrated during the latter part of the 20th century, when the immigration laws were more relaxed and the host society was more accepting, are a more heterogeneous group, socioeconomically and educationally, and speak a variety of dialects. Each of the other Asian groups in America has its unique history accounting for its particular present sociological character.

Despite the popular stereotype of Asians as a hardworking, successful "model minority" in America who suffer few social ills compared to other groups (Chan, 1991; Hing, 1993; Suzuki, 1989), this perception obscures the reality of the true variability underlying this group. For instance, although statistics from the 1990 census show that the household income for Asian and Pacific Islanders was higher on average than that of whites, this actually reflected the fact that the Asian families tended to have more wage earners in their families than the whites. When per capita income was evaluated, it was found that whites had the higher income. Consistent with this, in 1990, 11% of Asian and Pacific Islander fami013 lived in poverty, compared to 8% for whites (U.S. Bureau of the Census, 1992). Census data also show that Asians and Pacific Islanders obtain higher educational attainment as a group than whites. However, others have shown that there is a high degree of variability behind this.

In summary, Asian Americans form a remarkably diverse group in America, with multiple intergroup and intragroup differences. In working with patients or clients of Asian heritage, it will be important to be sensitive to these differences in order to establish a good rapport or working relationship. As with any group or individual from that group, stereotyping or rigidly adhering to a group trend to describe/understand the individual is counterproductive and should be avoided.

Cultural Factors in the Neuropsychological Assessment and Intervention with Asian Americans

In this section, cultural factors that need to be appreciated and considered when evaluating or treating an Asian American patient will be discussed. Although most of these issues can be found in working with culturally dissimilar patients of any background, the focus will be on the aspects of those factors that might be especially applicable to Asian patients.

Intercultural Issues

In the typical, modal neuropsychological evaluation, the professional and the patient are from the same general cultural milieu and culture is not a very prominent issue. However, when there is a cultural mismatch between the neuropsychologist and the patient, it is crucial to consider how cultural differences or issues may influence the interaction between them, and, ultimately, the assessment. The ignorance of these factors can lead to poor rapport between professional and client, and to misdiagnosis. Overestimation or underestimation of psychopathology can occur. The necessity of competent, intercultural assessment has been a growing need and subject of strong debate in the psychological literature (e.g., Clark, 1987; Hays, 1996; Jones & Thorne, 1987; Westermeyer, 1987). Likewise, potential subtle intercultural factors may indeed influence the neuropsychological assessment process in ways that might invalidate or obscure the correct diagnosis or conclusions. Neuropsychologists depend not only on tests that are valid and reliable in assessing/measuring brain function indirectly through what is essentially a behavior sample, but also on reasonable motivation and effort on the part of the patient in order to avoid misattributing poor performance to impaired neurologic function. Thus, good rapport, communication, and understanding generally helps the neuropsychologist to obtain a valid evaluation. What are some of the culturally based attitudes, norms, or social expectations common to the Asian American that might influence this process? The purpose of this section is to examine some of these factors and consider how they might impact the delivery of neuropsychological services.

Acculturation and Immigration

Determining the Asian American's level of acculturation, or familiarity and identification with the host majority culture, can be valuable in guiding the direction and viability of the neuropsychological evaluation as well as the broader clinical assessment. Generally, the younger one has emigrated from the country of origin, and the longer one has stayed and acclimated to the United States and its prevailing culture, the more one is acculturated. As mentioned earlier, the more highly acculturated the patient, the more comfortable the neuropsychologist might be with using tests and procedures that were normed on majority culture populations. From a broader perspective, the more highly acculturated or "Americanized" patient would be more similar to the average European American patient in terms of the general expectations, and the prevailing sociocultural norms governing social interaction that one brings to the neuropsychological evaluation. The Japanese have distinguished themselves from other immigrant groups, including Asian ones, by naming each successive generation in the United States (Tempo & Saito, 1996). The *issei* refers to the first generation Japanese immigrant, the *nisei* are the American-born second generation, and the *sansei*, *yonsei*, and *gosei* are the third, fourth, and fifth generations, respectively. In general, and in theory, each generation represents a different blend of attachment or identification to traditional Japanese values and culture, versus the newer, American culture. While the other Asian cultures have not labeled their successive American generations as formally, it is not the label itself that assigns primary cultural identification. That is, one can assume that, aside from individual differences and preferences, the third generation Chinese American, like the Japanese American *sansei* probably has interests and values that are more Western or American in nature than they are Eastern, or Chinese.

Conceptualization of Mental Health and Helping Issues

As mentioned earlier, the view of Asians as a "model minority" in American society suggests that Asians are somewhat immune to social ills, including problems of psychological adjustment. However, while some of the earlier studies on the subject showed that Asians tended to underutilize mental health services relative to other groups, subsequent research has found evidence that the prevalence of psychopathology among Asian Americans is not extraordinarily low (e.g., Sue, Sue, & Takeuchi, 1995), and that other factors need to be considered to explain low utilization. There is also evidence that, while Asian Americans may be low utilizers of mental health services, they may be more disturbed than others by the time they seek services (Durvasula & Sue, 1996). Related to this, as Sue and Sue (1987) note, while negative reactions to emotional problems exist in the general public, the amount of shame and stigmatization associated with these difficulties is greater among Asian American groups. This may also help explain why, as Sue and Sue reviewed the literature, they found that Asians were more likely to complain of somatic symptoms in depression than of dysphoric mood, and that Asian Americans tend to conceptualize mental health problems as being caused by organic factors. Similarly, and ironically, Elliot, Di Minno, Lam, and Tu (1996) discuss the tendency for Chinese to view dementia as mental illness, and, because of strong feelings of shame and stigmatization, tend to avoid seeking help from medical professionals for their loved ones.

A related cultural factor is the Asians' help-seeking pattern. Because of the more traditional Asian's emphasis on the family system, help from unrelated strangers is typically a last resort, especially for the more stigmatizing and personal problems. Thus, help is sought, and is expected to be sought, from the immediate family first, then the extended family, followed by the immediate community (geographically in the country of origin, and ethnoculturally in the United States), and then beyond. In America, what this also means is that in some Asian groups, such as the Chinese, traditional treatments and medicines may be sought either before or in conjunction with Western medical treatment. Understanding this cultural preference might help the professional to assess and understand the Asian patient's possible ambivalence toward neuropsychological services.

The Family System

In contrast to modern Western culture, in which the individual is the most fundamental and important organism, and independence, individuation, and self-advancement are desired and admired, the traditional Asian's most important and fundamental unit is the family or extended family. In this system, the interests of the individual are subjugated to the greater goals and interests of the family unit. Along with individuality, emotions are also to be moderated and controlled, and conformity and mutual dependence valued. The system is also hierarchical, and thus filial piety, respect for the elderly, and respect for authority are all high values in this structure. Knowing this characteristic aspect of many Asian cultures will help the professional to understand the basis for some of the decisions and conflicts that may occur in a neuropsychological context. For instance, despite the recommendations of the neuropsychologist and the referring primary physician that an elderly Asian woman be placed in a nursing home due to her pronounced behavioral and cognitive impairments secondary to a rather aggressive lobar dementia, her eldest son decides to take her home with him, even though he has a family with three children. What may seem incredibly inconvenient and unwise from the cultural context of the professionals may have been a natural choice from that of the Asian son.

Interactions with Health Professionals

While Asian Americans may appear to be submissive and deferential, this is in large part due to unwritten cultural rules and expectations in regards to role relationships. Thus, an Asian American patient, conforming to a somewhat traditional and rigid perspective on roles, will be quite respectful, cooperative, and acquiescent to the "expert" health professional. Little eye contact will be made, as this is perceived as a challenging gesture that is rude and disrespectful. The clinical neuropsychologist working with an Asian American patient will have to remember that, despite this somewhat disarming initial or general presentation, there may be an underlying culturally based misunderstanding or mistrust of how this "psychologist" can help. Sue and Zane (1987) provided a framework by which to understand the role of culture in psychotherapy that may be helpful here. Under that framework, health professionals have to consider two major issues that will determine whether the Asian American patient will feel that continued assistance from the health service provider is worth pursuing. The first issue is the credibility of the service provider, which is related both to the ascribed status of the provider as well as his or her achieved status. Status is ascribed according to age, gender, and expertise (credentials, experience, educational background). Thus high ascribed status would be given to someone who is male, older, and is the director of the clinic or is a well-known expert in his field. Of course, the individual neuropsychologist has little immediate control over his or her ascribed status. However, achieved status is dependent on skills that are perceived as competent by the patient, and instills hope and confidence in the professional. This is precisely where cultural competence on the part of the neuropsychologist is helpful in engaging the Asian American patient. The second issue has to do with the patient experiencing some direct and immediate benefit, or a "gift" from the health professional. As Sue and Zane (1987) explain, gift-giving is a common ritual in interpersonal relationships among Asians. Examples of gifts in the mental health context that may also apply in the neuropsychological context are: immediate reduction in the experience of anxiety or depression; normalization of feelings or experiences; or cognitive clarity in the midst of a state of confusion. While the issues of credibility and gift-giving may also be important with other cultural groups (as well as the majority culture), the critical difference is that, because of the cultural unfamiliarity of psychologically related services to Asians, credibility needs to be established quickly, and a gift given immediately in order to engage the patient and prevent attrition, noncompliance, or both.

The above represent only a few examples of some of the more common culturally based Asian American attitudes and preferences that may help neuropsychologists understand the cultural context of their patients' reactions and interactions with neuropsychology. For example, it might be very important to explain carefully to an Asian patient being evaluated secondary to attention and memory difficulties, and who is not very acculturated, what are the nature and purpose of neuropsychology, as he or she might only understand the "psychologist" part of neuropsychologist, stirring up culturally based anxieties. The result might be that the patient might actually welcome the evaluation, as it now appears more "medical" to him and is more consistent with his cultural conceptualization of the basis of mental-type problems. Conversely, the patient might be quite resistant to the finding or suggestion that the pattern and nature of his memory problems appear more consistent with a behavioral or psychiatrically based etiology than a neurologic one.

Testing and Measurement Issues

That most tests and procedures used by neuropsychologists are best normed for use with English-speaking European Americans can be a vexing problem when any patient who deviates from this category is to be evaluated. However, the marked heterogeneity of the Asian American group, especially in terms of language and specific culture/ethnicity, presents an even greater challenge to both the researcher and the clinician in defining a reasonable normative base with appropriate stratification. It is likely for this reason that there are even fewer normed cross-cultural instruments for use with Asian Americans than there have been recently for other ethnic/cultural groups, such as African Americans and Hispanic/Latino Americans, that are not quite as varied. Thus, the clinician today who needs to perform a comprehensive neuropsychological examination on an Asian American patient/client would be hard-pressed to assemble a set of procedures with appropriate norms to assess all the major cognitive domains.

The difficulty of assessing an Asian American patient, from an instrumentation perspective, may also vary according to the neuropsychologist's approach or philosophy to testing. For example, many North American neuropsychologists employ a fixed battery approach, using a standardized and invariant battery of procedures across most patients and situations. One of the major advantages of this approach, according to these practitioners, is that repetitive use of a fixed battery facilitates comparability across patients and situations as well as the development of internal norms. The Halstead–Reitan Neuropsychological Battery (HRNB) (Reitan & Wolfson, 1985) and the Luria–Nebraska Neuropsychological Battery (LNNB) (Golden, Purisch, & Hammeke, 1985) are examples of such batteries that are popularly used with this approach. Neuropsychologists using this approach may be especially stymied when given the task of evaluating an Asian American patient, particularly one who is not acculturated or assimilated into the American culture. Although Chinese versions of the HRNB (Doerr & Storrie, 1981; Yao-Xian, 1986) and the LNNB (Yun, Yao-Xian, & Matthews, 1987) have been developed, these are not widely available and cannot be used easily by non-Chinese speaking neuropsychologists or psychometrists. Also, extensive validation, which is the hallmark of fixed batteries, has not been ensured in these cases. Finally, these versions only apply to one out of the many Asian subgroups. Clinical neuropsychologists who take a flexible battery approach, where a specific collection of tests and procedures are chosen case by case, may appear to have a slight advantage over the fixed battery practitioners when assessing patients of Asian descent. Theoretically, under this approach, a brief battery can be assembled by finding the few tests or procedures that might be normed for a particular Asian subgroup, and then selecting some familiar instruments that, although normed on non-Asian samples, are less dependent on language for performance. However, this rarely is feasible in practice. First, there are very few tests available, published or otherwise, that are normed for use with Asian groups. The ones that do exist are normed for a specific subgroup, and by definition are not appropriate for other Asian groups. Second, while the use of "nonverbal" tests, or tests that are ostensibly less language-dependent (e.g., block design type tests, Rey–Osterrieth figure, etc.), may certainly be the only reasonable alternative at this time when not much else is available, these procedures are by no means known to be "culture-free" nor "culture-fair," as they also have not been normed on minority groups.

One can reasonably argue that, provided that the Asian American to be examined is highly acculturated, meaning that he or she is native to America and is highly assimilated into American culture, European American norms can be used. While this is an appealing rationale, and is based on the theory that cross-cultural differences in neuropsychological performance are related primarily to cultural differences, and not ethnic factors, it is an assumption that ultimately may not hold true (Strickland et al., 1999; Wong et al., Chapter 1, this volume). Although on a practical level there may be no other choice in the interim but to take this approach with our more acculturated English-speaking patients, there needs to be a systematic effort at collecting comprehensive norms for this group with familiar instruments.

The more difficult challenge has to deal with evaluating Asian patients who are less acculturated and do not speak English fluently. Although there might be a temptation to use a translator or interpreter in this situation, there are a number of liabilities with this approach that result in the high probability that the clinician would obtain inaccurate, distorted information and data (Artiola i Fortuny & Mullaney, 1998; Sue & Sue, 1987; Wong et al., Chapter 1, this volume). Even if the translation was impeccable, and the presence of another party was absolutely nonintrusive, or even if a neuropsychologist who was matched in ethnicity, language, and culture was to examine the patient, a fundamental issue/problem still remains. That is what standardized instruments are available for the client or patient. In most cases, the answer would be "none." The next best thing might be for the linguistically and culturally matched bilingual neuropsychologist (and this might be impossible to find at this point for some of the Asian subgroups) to administer some familiar neuropsychological tests with translation. However, this too is not completely adequate, as even accurately translated tests that were originally normed with one cultural group may not have construct validity when used with another cultural group (Sue & Sue, 1987; Wong et al., Chapter 1, this volume).

As suggested, there is a tremendous void in terms of available neuropsychological tests and procedures with appropriate norms for the various Asian American groups. While it may not be practically possible to achieve this goal for all of the subgroups, there needs to be a systematic and concentrated effort at collecting appropriate norms with a wide variety of tests/procedures that can assess neurocognitive abilities comprehensively for at least some of larger Asian subgroups. There do seem to be promising efforts under way. For example, Hsieh and Riley (1997) collected normative data on four attentional tests in the People's Republic of China. The normative group was recruited across a broad range of occupational and educational categories, and the data were stratified by age groups. Kim and Kang (1999) developed the Korean-California Verbal Learning Test based on the California Verbal Learning Test (Delis, Kramer, Kaplan, & Ober, 1987) and presented age and sex stratified normative data based on the performance of 357 Korean subjects. Also, Kempler, Teng, Dick, Taussig, and Davis (1998) examined performance on a verbal fluency task by Chinese, Hispanic, and Vietnamese immigrants, along with white and African American English speakers. More reearch like this, especially when evaluated and published in refereed journals, would be especially helpful. Concomitantly, more neuropsychologists who are also culturally and linguistically competent to work with some of the Asian groups are needed.

Suggestions on Working with Asian Americans

The following are intended as some general guidelines or principles that neuropsychologists might find helpful in working with Asian Americans. They should not be used rigidly or inflexibly. As discussed earlier, Asian Americans are a very variable and heterogeneous group, and it is important that one takes the time and effort to understand and to learn more about the specific group as well as the individual from that group. Irresponsible stereotyping would only create more of a barrier between the professional and the patient, and would further complicate and invalidate the assessment or treatment.

Fundamentals and Preparation

1. *Make a commitment to increasing cross-cultural competency.* Given the increasing cultural diversity of patients that we will encounter, and given that the extant research shows that a cultural mismatch may lead to errors and distortion in diagnosis, there should be a high priority placed on cross-cultural competency. As Sue (1988) aptly put, in reviewing the research on therapist–client match and outcome, "ethnic or racial match in treatment is more of a moral/ethical concern, whereas cultural match is more of an empirical one."

2. *Take concrete steps toward increasing cross-cultural competency.* There are many alternatives one can follow. Continuing education courses on cultural issues/diversity might be available from time to time. Consult with or even arrange for supervision

from colleagues who might be more knowledgeable in this area. Nowadays, books abound on Asian studies and Asian American issues.

3. *Determine the patient's primary cultural identity.* That is, find out what the country of origin is, the primary language or dialect, and the level of acculturation. This will help in determining what approach you might take in the neuropsychological assessment (or whether you might be able to do it at all). For more suggestions and detail on what to do if an interpreter is needed and how best to proceed with an evaluation, see Chapter 1 in this volume by Wong et al.).

4. *Avoid stereotyping.* As with all groups, there are behaviors, customs, or beliefs that might be of greater frequency or probability as a whole for the particular group, but there will inevitably be variability and individual differences. Use knowledge of cultural characteristics or tendencies to help you understand what you might encounter when working with that group. Stereotyping is not only offensive and distancing, but in a situation where neuropsychological tests are not used in a standard fashion and cannot be interpreted in a straightforward manner, such bias can further skew the results or their interpretation.

Facilitative Behaviors with Asian American Clients

1. *Be aware of and show respect for cultural nuances.* What the Westerner may intend as openness and friendliness through a casual approach may be perceived as rude and disrespectful by an Asian who is not very acculturated. Interestingly, what Hays (1996) described as a generation-specific custom of addressing people by their titles applies not only to the elderly, but also to younger people in more formal settings for Asians. So, unless the patient is highly acculturated, or unless you are invited to addresss the person by first name, it is safer and more sensitive from a cross-cultural perspective to use a title. Direct eye contact, another behavior valued by Americans, which for them connotes positive attention or focus, may also be perceived as challenging and disrespectful by some Asians.

2. *Be aware of and sensitive regarding cultural taboos.* For example, talking about things that might be considered "bad luck," such as death, dying, or accidents too freely might hinder rapport. Talking about very personal or private issues, such as sex, too quickly can also be a problem. If it is impossible to avoid because you need to as part of your interview, be very discreet and acknowledge the cultural awkwardness of discussing the topic, and also be ready to explain why it is necessary to discuss the particular topic at that time.

3. *Establish rapport with the patient.* While this is certainly important with all patients, this is especially important with Asian patients who are not highly acculturated. They may be somewhat uncomfortable with or wary of a "psychologist," and they may be doubtful of your ability to help. Related to this, until rapport and trust are established, it is probably better for the professional to be more active and direct in approach, rather than passive. Respect can be communicated and rapport established by showing active curiosity in that patient's cultural perspective.

4. *Respect and facilitate cultural preferences that are not harmful.* For instance, Chinese patients or their family members will commonly seek out traditional Chinese remedies or medicines if they feel that Western style medicine has not worked rapidly enough. Instead of a blanket denial, which will be perceived as one culture's values pitted

against another's, one can attempt to work out a compromise by offering to find out whether the physician is willing to allow the patient to take the Chinese medicine as long as it has been evaluated by the lab to ensure that it does not have any harmful effects or is contraindicated by the medicine that has been prescribed.

5. *Reassure confidentiality.* While confidentiality is of paramount importance for all psychologists in their work with patients, it is important for the Asian patient to be reassured of this due to the Asian cultural value of the hierarchical family unit. For example, especially for the Asian patient who is lower in the family hierarchy (e.g., a younger sister), she may not be accustomed to having her thoughts and feelings validated and protected.

Other Considerations and Suggestions

1. *Be aware of your own stimulus value to the Asian patient.* Recall that authority, which includes professional "experts," is to be respected in the traditional Asian worldview. Therefore, what may appear to you to be only your recommendations or preferences will be taken very seriously by the patient.
2. *Remember the importance of the family unit in Asian culture.* This means that there may be high expectations of family involvement and information exchange, which may challenge the customary boundaries of confidentiality.

Summary and Conclusion

Despite being the most rapidly growing ethnic minority in the United States, by virtue of its marked heterogeneity in language, acculturation, and country of origin, Asian Americans are also one of the most challenging groups to assess neuropsychologically. While there are some general cultural similarities among Asians that were discussed in this chapter, there are also enough differences that a simple, unifying description is impossible. As with some of the other ethnic minority groups in America, the empirical reality is that the need for more suitable neuropsychological instruments and approaches that can be used with Asian Americans is rapidly becoming more acute. Along with the need for more validated neuropsychological instruments for use with Asians, there is also an equally acute need for the training of more neuropsychologists who are culturally and linguistically compatible with at least the major or larger Asian groups in America.

References

Ardila, A. (1995). Directions of research in cross-cultural neuropsychology. *Journal of Clinical and Experimental Neuropsychology, 17,* 143–150.

Ardila, A., Rosselli, M., & Puente, A. (1994). *Neuropsychological evaluation of the Spanish speaker.* New York: Plenum.

Artiola i Fortuny, L., & Mullaney, H. (1998) Assessing patients whose language you do not know: Can the absurd be ethical? *The Clinical Neuropsychologist, 12,* 113–126.

Chan, S. (1991). *Asian Americans: An interpretive history.* Boston: Twayne.

Clark, L. A. (1987). Mutual relevance of mainstream and cross-cultural psychology. *Journal of Consulting and Clinical Psychology, 55,* 461–470.

Delis, D. C., Kramer, J. H., Kaplan, E., & Ober, B.A. (1987). *California Verbal Learning Test.* San Antonio, TX: The Psychological Corporation.

Doerr, H. O., & Storrie, M. C. (1981). Neuropsychological testing in the People's Republic of China: The Halstead–Reitan Seattle/Changsha project. *Clinical Neuropsychology, 4*, 49–52.

Durvasula, R. & Sue, S. (1996). Severity of disturbance among Asian American outpatients. *Cultural Diversity & Mental Health, 2*(1), 43–51.

Elliot, K. S., Di Minno, M., Lam, D., Tu, A. M. (1996). Working with Chinese families in the context of dementia. In G. Yeo & D. Gallagher-Thompson (Eds.), *Ethnicity & the dementias* (pp. 89–108). Washington D.C.: Taylor & Francis.

Golden, C.J., Purisch, A. D., & Hammeke, T. A. (1985). *Luria–Nebraska Neuropsychological Battery: Forms I & II: Manual.* Los Angeles: Western Psychological Services.

Hays, P. (1996). Culturally responsive assessment with diverse older clients. *Professional Psychology: Research and Practice, 27*, 188–193.

Hing, B. O. (1993). *Making and remaking Asian America through immigration policy, 1850–1990.* Stanford, CA: Stanford University Press.

Hsieh, S., & Riley, N. (1997, November). *Neuropsychological performance in the People's Republic of China: Age and educational norms for four attention tasks.* Presented at the National Academy of Neuropsychology, Las Vegas, NV.

Jones, E. E., & Thorne, A. (1987). Rediscovery of the subject: Intercultural approaches to clinical assessment. *Journal of Consulting and Clinical Psychology, 55*, 488–495.

Kempler, D., Teng, E. L., Dick, M., Taussig, I. M., & Davis, D. S. (1998). The effects of age, education, and ethnicity on verbal fluency. *Journal of the International Neuropsychological Society, 4*, 531–538.

Kim, J. K., & Kang, Y. (1999, February). *The Korean-California Verbal Learning Test (K-CVLT): A standardization.* Presented at the International Neuropsychological Society, Boston, MA.

Reitan, R., & Wolfson, D. (1985). *The Halstead–Reitan neuropsychological test battery.* Tempe, AZ: Neuropsychology Press.

Strickland, T. L., Wong, T. M., Andre, K., Gray, G. E., Miller, B., Alperson, B., Denison, E., Kinder, N., Mulligan, R., & Herrera, S. (1999). *Learning and memory functioning among substance abusers: differential ethnicity and sex effects.* Manuscript submitted for publication.

Sue, D., & Sue, S. (1987). Cultural factors in the clinical assessment of Asian Americans. *Journal of Consulting and Clinical Psychology, 55*, 479–487.

Sue, S. (1988). Psychotherapeutic services for ethnic minorities: Two decades of research findings. *American Psychologist, 43*, 301–308.

Sue., S., Sue, D. W., & Takeuchi, D. T. (1995). Psychopathology among Asian Americans: A model minority? *Cultural Diversity & Mental Health, 1*(1), 39–51.

Sue, S., & Zane, N. (1987). The role of culture and cultural techniques in psychotherapy. A critique and reformulation. *American Psychologist, 42*, 37–45.

Suzuki, B. H. (1989, November). Asian Americans as the "model minority." *Change,* 13–19.

Tempo, P. M., & Saito, A. (1996). Techniques of working with Japanese American families. In G. Yeo & D. Gallagher-Thompson (Eds.), *Ethnicity & the dementias* (pp. 109–122). Washington D.C.: Taylor & Francis.

U.S. Bureau of the Census. (1992). *1990 Census of population: General population characteristics.* Washington, D.C.: Author.

U.S. Bureau of the Census (1993). *Asian and Pacific Islander Americans: A profile* (SB/93-12). Washington, D.C.: Author

U.S. Bureau of the Census. (1996). *Demographic projections.* Washington, D.C.: Author.

Westermeyer, J. (1987). Cultural factors in clinical assessment. *Journal of Consulting and Clinical Psychology, 55*, 471–478.

Wong, T. M., Strickland, T. L., Fletcher-Janzen, E., Ardila, A., & Reynolds, C. R. (2000). Theoretical and practical issues in the neuropsychological treatment of culturally dissimilar patients. This volume.

Yao-Xian, G. (1986). The Chinese revision of the Halstead–Reitan Neuropsychological Test Battery for adults. *Acta Psychologica Sinica, 18*, 433–442.

Yun, X., Yao-Xian, G., & Matthews, J. R. (1987). The Luria–Nebraska Neuropsychological Battery revised in China. *Journal of Clinical Psychology, 9*, 97–101.

5

Neuropsychological Assessment of Gays and Lesbians

PAMILLA C. MORALES

Neuropsychological Aspects of Gays and Lesbians

The study of the neuropsychological aspects of gays and lesbians is in its infancy. Currently there is no research on this group in terms of differences in brain structure or neurochemistry. They are a group of people embedded in all cultures, races, and ethnic groups. The sexual orientation of the individual makes no difference in the neuropsychological results; however, when the assessment is completed and the results are provided to the individual and his or her support system(s), the sexual orientation of the client may have a profound effect on the outcome of treatment. The specific external stressors that affect homosexuals will influence how this information will be assimilated into their lives. This chapter will explore and address the complex issues of neuropsychological assessment of gays and lesbians and how psychosocial issues affect the neuropsychological assessment. It is suggested that the clinician go beyond the traditional assessment procedures and explore with the client and their support system(s) how their sexual orientation will affect the assessment and rehabilitation.

Gays and Lesbians

According to *Webster's Dictionary* (1984), homosexuality is defined as "the manifestation of sexual desire toward a member of one's own sex." Heterosexuality is defined as "the manifestation of sexual desire toward a member of the opposite sex." A bisexual is a person who " is sexually oriented toward both sexes."

Male homosexuals are often called "gay," female homosexuals lesbians, and heterosexual men and women "straight." Although often referred to as an "alternate lifestyle" there is no gay or lesbian lifestyle and gay and lesbian behavioral patterns are as varied as those of heterosexual people. However, many gay men and lesbian women report being aware at an early age that they were different from their peers (Coleman, 1982).

Throughout history the homosexual's place in society has ranged from public toleration to total abhorrence and violent persecution (Fassinger, 1991). The level of toleration often

PAMILLA C. MORALES • Texas A&M University, College Station, Texas 77843-4225.

Handbook of Cross-Cultural Neuropsychology, edited by Fletcher-Janzen, Strickland, and Reynolds. Kluwer Academic/Plenum Publishers, New York, 2000.

varied considerably between different class levels within the same societies. In some societies, bisexuality was common and for many people homosexuality was a behavior and perhaps a proclivity, but not a defining trait (LaMar & Kite, 1998). To this day, many people maintain that homosexual behavior exists but that homosexuals, as such, do not (Anonymous, 1996). In the United States this behavioral view is now mainly espoused by two diverse groups: right-wing antigay activists, who believe that everyone is naturally heterosexual, and left-wing progay activists, who believe that sexual categories themselves are cramping and repressive (Anonymous, 1996).

Prior to the late 19th century and the beginnings of modern psychiatry, homosexuality, whether condemned or accepted, was defined in moral terminology. With the work of Freud and his successors and the scientization of sexuality, homosexuality, in scientific/medical circles, became a pathological diagnosis and was considered a sign of a disturbed personality (Atkinson & Hackett, 1988). Homosexuality then came to be seen as a vice and a disease simultaneously and was considered the fault of the people afflicted with it.

In the United States over the past 30 years change has come in three overlapping phases. First, in many places homosexuality was struck from lists of crimes and illnesses. Homosexuality, second, ceased to be shameful, and third, it became an identity of a self-aware minority (Anonymous, 1996).

Research conducted on lesbians and gay men promoted the belief that homosexuality was an illness (Buhrke, Ben-Ezra, Hurely, & Ruprecht, 1992; Morin, 1977; Watters, 1986). In 1973 the American Psychiatric Association removed homosexuality from its list of mental disorders, resulting from a gradual change in the attitudes of researchers regarding gay men and lesbians (Flores, O'Brien, & McDermott, 1995). However, stereotypes and stigma continue to persist (Buhrke et al., 1992).

The fact that the term "sexual orientation" has become a descriptor is indicative of changes in professional approaches to homosexuality. To refer to homosexuality as an orientation implies that it is a neutral trait or disposition, like left-handedness: not changeable, or at least not changeable without deforming the individual's personality; not innately harmful, though perhaps inconvenient; and not itself chosen. This latest view is a radical redefinition wholly divorced from its predecessors in that it treats homosexuality as both fundamentally distinct from the heterosexual majority and at the same time quite normal (Anonymous, 1996).

Homosexual Theories

Many genetic, neuroendrocrinological, and sociobiological theories have attempted to explain the development of sexual orientation.

A large-scale study of several hundred male and female homosexuals (Bell, Weinberg, & Hammersmith, 1981) attempted to assess the effects of childhood experiences, specifically interactions between the child and parents. This research indicated that there were no correlations for types of parent–child interactions and homosexuality. Neither domineering mothers or submissive fathers created homosexuality; rather, the best predictor of adult homosexuality was a self-report of homosexual feelings, which usually preceded homosexual activity by approximately three years.

Other research has focused on differences in levels of gonadal hormones and the possibility that male homosexuality might be caused as a result of varying levels of hormones, although research to date has shown that well-adjusted male homosexuals have normal levels of gonadal hormones (Tourney, 1975).

Another path of neuroendocrinological research has been the study of androgens. Androgens are hormones that increase the growth of male physical qualities. Adrenogenital syndrome is characterized by a deficit in the release of the hormone cortisol from the adrenal cortices, which results in adrenal hyperactivity and the excessive release of adrenal androgens. This has little effect on the development of males, other than accelerating the onset of their puberty, but it has major effects on the development of genetic females (Pinel, 1993). Cortisone-treated adrenogenital teenage girls typically display a high degree of tomboyishness and little interest in maternity. They prefer boys clothes, play mainly with boys, show little interest in handling babies and tend to daydream about future careers rather than motherhood. It is important not to lose sight of the fact that many teenage girls not treated with cortisone also display similar characteristics and that this behavior is considered normal (Pinel, 1993).

Females who have adrenogenital syndrome appear to lag behind normal females in dating and marriage, possibly because of the delayed onset of their menstrual cycle, but in all other respects their sexual interests appear normal, with most of these females reporting to be heterosexual, although one study has reported a slight tendency toward bisexuality (Ehrhardt & Meyer-Bahlburg, 1981).

Gladue, Green, and Hellman (1984) examined the response of the anterior pituitary gland to estradiol. Researchers injected adult male homosexuals, male heterosexuals, and female heterosexuals with estrogen. The blood levels of luteinizing hormone (LH) in the women showed a dramatic rise, those of the heterosexual men did not, and the change in blood levels of LH in the homosexual men was intermediate, showing a statistically significant increase, but one smaller than that of the women. Results suggest that the homosexual men's pituitary glands may have received less exposure to androgens during some critical stage of prenatal development and that this decreased exposure may have increased the likelihood of developing a preference for male sex partners later in life. However, there are many other confounding variables that may play a role in homosexual development and this research was far from conclusive.

It has been hypothesized that prenatal hormone levels influence the sexual orientation of adult humans. However, the effects of hormones on the development of sexual orientation has been very difficult to investigate. The strongest support for this view comes from the quasi-experimental study of Ehrhardt et al. (1985). They interviewed adult women whose mothers had been exposed to diethylstilbestrol during pregnancy. The subjects' responses indicated that they were significantly more attracted sexually to women than was a group of matched control subjects. Ehrhardt and her colleagues concluded that prenatal estrogen exposure does encourage homosexuality and bisexuality in women, but that it is relatively weak.

Other results that support the theory of prenatal hormone levels come from studies of twins. Bailey and Pillard (1991) identified a group of male homosexuals who had twin brothers. Fifty-two percent of the monozygotic twin brothers and 22% of the dizygotic twin brothers were homosexual. Again, the evidence is weak, but there does appear to be a link in genetic factors.

LeVay (1991) compared the postmortem neuroanatomy of three groups of subjects: heterosexual men, homosexual men, and women who were assumed to be heterosexual. LeVay confirmed a previous report (Allen, Hines, Shryne, & Gorski, 1989) that the third interstitial nucleus of the anterior hypothalamus is more than twice as large in heterosexual men than in women. In addition, he found that it is more than twice as large in heterosexual men than in homosexual men. However, third factors may have been responsible for these differences as many of the homosexual brains in LeVay's study came from men who had died of AIDS and its complications.

There is no conclusive evidence that exposure to prenatal androgens affects a person's sexual behavior during adulthood (Carlson, 1986; Pinel, 1993). However, it is possible that androgens do have an effect on the human brain that could subsequently influence sexual behavior. Research has not been conclusive in proving this as a theory of homosexuality. If homosexuality does have a physiological cause, it is more likely to be a more subtle difference in brain structure caused by the presence or absence of prenatal androgenization. This subtle difference may or may not be significant. It could influence future ways of conducting neuropsychological assessments with gays and lesbians, however, to date this difference, if it exists, has not been identified.

To date there is no definitive evidence that the neurological development of homosexuals is any different than the neurological development of heterosexuals. Therefore the practitioner should approach the neuropsychological assessment in the same manner that he or she approaches heterosexuals. The assessment approach should be dependent upon the neuropsychological question. However, there are external factors that the practitioner should bear in mind when assessing gay and lesbian clients. These factors include psychosocial issues and family interaction.

Family Interaction

Family interaction refers to the network of relationships that exists within a family and how an individual is influenced by those relationships. The family is a unit of many simultaneous interactions and it can have profound effects upon the individual with a traumatic brain injury. Within a systems perspective, the different relationships that exist within families are referred to as subsystems (Turnbull & Turnbull, 1991).

Extended Family Subsystem

The extended family subsystem is composed of family and individual interactions with parents, relatives, friends and professionals. Family cohesion represents both the close emotional bonds that members have with each other, as well as the level of independence or autonomy that individuals experience within the family system. Families vary tremendously in the size and richness of their support system network and this is especially true among homosexuals who may or may not have extended family support (Turnbull & Turnbull, 1991).

Homosexuals who are single will interact with their parents as adult children. For the single person the familial support provided often depends upon the past relationship, the receptivity to the individual's homosexuality, and how open the parents are to caring for an adult child with a traumatic brain injury. If the parents were unaware of the individual's homosexuality, this could be a major issue for the individual and the family along with the information of the individual's brain injury.

The Marital Subsystem

The marital subsystem consists of interactions between husbands and wives and for the homosexual couple, their identified partners (Turnbull & Turnbull, 1991). Within the homosexual marital subsystem these unions are not legally recognized and therefore are not protected under the same guidelines as heterosexual unions. This can cause significant difficulty when medical authorization by a legally recognized guardian is required. Often the partner does not have the legal authorization to determine medical procedures or to make any medical decisions. In some cases this may revert back to the nuclear family, which may or may not have a working relationship with the homosexual partner. Neuropsychologists need to be aware that conflicts may arise between the nuclear family and the homosexual partner in terms of medical procedures and care. It will be important for the neuropsychologist to know the dynamics that exist between the homosexual couple and the extended family and what limitations exist for the partner. This will indicate how much authority the partner will have, to what degree he or she will be involved with the care of the person with traumatic brain injury, and to what degree the neuropsychologist will involve the partner.

Parental Subsystem

Another subsystem is the parental subsystem that is composed of interactions between parents and their child or children (Turnbull & Turnbull, 1991). This subsystem would consist of homosexual couples and their children. The presence of a parent with a disability such as a brain injury will affect parental roles in multiple ways and the parent–child relationship will be shaped accordingly. A major issue for both parents and children is the learning of new roles and expectations and developing support systems to deal with the losses that occur in the relationships. Some of these losses are compensated for by the other spouse/partner, who must assume double responsibility. This subsystem may be compounded for the homosexual. For the homosexual couple with children, the child or children within the relationship may be the legal responsibility of the partner with traumatic head injury, while the other partner may have no legal custodial rights. The partner with a traumatic brain injury may not be able to function independently and as a result may require supervision and assistance in caring for their child or children, placing additional pressure on the noninjured partner. Another issue may be that the partner with traumatic brain injury may not be the custodial parent and may have been in a previous heterosexual relationship. Care must be taken by the clinician to assess the relationship between the children, previous spouse, and the noninjured partner when assessing the roles, duties, and functions that each individual will be able to perform. Many of the adjustment issues and much of the emotional distress is attributable not to individual pathology but to a sudden and dramatic disruption of family roles and role relationships.

Head Injuries and the Family System

Traumatic brain injury often has a tremendous impact upon family members. Among heterosexual couples there are reports of disproportionately high rates of divorce and marital disharmony (Gath, 1977; Murphy, 1982). Rosenbaum and Najenson (1976) found that wives of men with head injuries were more depressed than wives of men with spinal cord injuries and men without injuries. No research currently documents the impact that traumatic brain injury has on homosexual couples, however, it can be assumed that as a result of initial societal pressure upon the relationship, with the additional stress of an injured partner, that these couples would experience more marital discord and more breakups than heterosexual couples. The financial burdens and medical expenses of brain injuries are staggering and because of the legalities of homosexual marriages this can add exceptional stress to the couple, who are often unable to list their partners on their health insurance policies.

The neuropsychologist need make no special alterations in consultation with the client and their families when working with gay men and lesbians. Naturally the clinician will be well served by taking into account the individuals involved and their emotional capacities to understand the nature and severity of the head injury. The fact of a client's sexual orientation is simply a component of the complete assessment. The physical involvement usually can be seen and dealt with first; the cognitive communication impairments and the social and behavioral changes that often accompany the physical problems are experienced over a longer period and are not as well understood (DePompei & Zarski, 1989). An assessment of family resources, perceptions of the injury, and coping patterns should be completed. Family resources encompass two aspects: 1) strengths of individual family members that can be utilized to help the injured person, and 2) the family's ability to use existing support systems such as support groups, friends, extended family members, and religious organizations, as well as being able to take advantage of new systems (Zarski, DePompei, West, & Hall, 1988). Assessment of the family's/partner's perception of the injury may be accomplished by asking all family members to explain verbally and in writing how they understand the impact of the injury (DePompei & Zarski, 1991). Positive coping patterns include: 1) maintaining an optimistic definition of the situation, 2) developing social support, and 3) understanding the medical situation (DePompei & Zarski, 1991). The family/partner that is unable to cope with the situation creates resistance to medical recommendations and often increases family conflict (DePompei & Zarski, 1991). Family coping patterns can be observed in behaviors of denial, blame, overcompensation, and too much tolerance (DePompei, Zarski, & Hall, 1988). These behaviors are readily observable within the family's interactions. The following is a list designed by DePompei and Zarski (1991) that can help to identify poor coping patterns.

1. What is the family's explanation of how this injury occurred? Look for issues of blame, religious affiliation, and family mythology which can include punishment especially if the family was uncomfortable with the individual's sexual orientation.
2. Who is the best person in the family to direct the care of the member with a head injury? If the family has a strong internal locus of control, the family may want a specific member to be a spokesperson and contact person. If the family has a strong external locus of control, members may feel the medical team should always be in charge and may feel anger and resentment if they must assume responsibility for the brain injured person. Again, consideration of the homosexual partner must be taken into account as the family may want something different from what the partner wants or may attempt to exclude the partner altogether.
3. What is the family's ethnic and or religious background, as it may influence beliefs about the rehabilitation process? McGoldrick, Pearce, and Giordona (1982) indicate that families tend to have different cultural identities that may dictate who will be responsible for care of the person, what the role of extended family will be, and how the medical team will be involved in the planning process. This process can be further complicated with the aspect of homosexuality.

Assessment Procedures for Working with Gay and Lesbian Individuals with Traumatic Brain Injury

1. Determine the physical problems that may interfere with completing a formal assessment and accommodate wherever possible, this includes modifying test administration if necessary.
2. Assess the cognitive–communicative competencies of the person and how well the person believes they are communicating with family/support systems.
3. Be aware that gays and lesbians may have difficulty responding to questions about significant others phrased in terms of the opposite gender.
4. Occasionally items may not be accurately interpretable for gays and lesbians as a result of lack of an appropriate norm group.

5. Obtain a personal perception from the injured person of family structure, roles, and rules and how this may change as a result of the injury.
6. Observe interactions among family/support systems when the brain-injured person is present.
7. Ask the person to share his or her ideas about who should be in charge of decisions regarding treatment and rehabilitation.
8. Assess how the injury may affect the person's sexuality and how these changes may affect his or her lifestyle.

Basic Neuropsychological Assessment with Gay and Lesbian Clients

Mental Status and Memory Assessment

A determination of the patient's level of alertness, attention, and concentration is a prerequisite to any type of neuropsychological assessment. Mental status and memory assessment serve several purposes. The first is that this type of testing will determine the presence, extent, or type of memory disorder, and, second, it provides an assessment of alertness, attention, and concentration.

Language Assessment

A complete neuropsychological evaluation includes an assessment of the patient's ability to comprehend, process, and express language. Neuropsychologists should utilize a brief screening device for detecting language disorders. The common characteristic of all measures of language function is the presentation of stimuli to the patient in order to assess his or her ability to comprehend, retain, or express information via speech, gestures, or writing. The assessment of language is very important in the evaluation procedure and contributes to the overall picture formulated concerning the abilities and level of functioning of the patient. Aphasia is one of the few symptoms that can be considered definitely indicative of cerebral pathology. In right-handed persons, the pathology will almost invariably be situated in the left cerebral hemisphere.

The type of language disorder can also assist in localizing the lesion responsible. Halting, telegraphic speech with relatively normal comprehension and right-sided weakness is a pattern seen with lesions in the left cerebral hemisphere in the region of the third frontal convolution. A lesion in the posterior temporal–inferior parietal area may be present if the speech is fluent, but dysphasic, with poor comprehension, and there is no presence of motor weakness on the right side. If both syndromes are present, either a widespread lesion which affects both anterior and posterior speech areas or, perhaps, a disconnection of the anterior and posterior centers exists.

Handedness and Motor Functions Assessment

The determination of handedness is the first step in evaluating the patient's motor functions. The traditional manner of determining handedness involves observation of the patient's performance of such activities as writing, using tools, throwing a ball, or opening a door. The evaluation of motor functions proceeds from gross to more refined motor skills. There are three specific areas that should be evaluated: strength of grip, and finger and foot tapping speed.

Strength of grip can be determined by the use of a hand dynamometer which will accurately measure manual grip strength in kilograms. The clinician should be careful to not over-interpret strength of grip as any weakness may not be directly related to brain dysfunction.

Finger and foot tapping speed are measured by comparing the relative efficiency of the two sides of the body, and by comparing the patient's relative proficiency on the two tasks. Patients with fairly deep or extensive lesions which interrupt efferent pathways from the motor cortex will evidence deficits with both finger and foot. Finger tapping reflects the speed and consistency with which an individual can carry out a simple, repetitive finger movement that is utilized in basic activities such as eating and dressing. Foot tapping speed may indicate the patient's proficiency in walking, climbing stairs, or driving.

Sensory and Perceptual Assessment

Cortical sensory functions include finger recognition, tactile perception of symbols, and tactile recognition of three dimensional objects. In addition, two-point texture and weight discriminations require cortical analysis. The ability to detect and identify bilateral simultaneous sensory stimuli also requires higher level integration. Basic sensory functions such as unilateral detection of pain, temperature, vibration, sound, or light are not ordinarily considered "cortical" in nature.

Brain lesions which impinge upon the visual system result in characteristic alterations in the visual field. Depending on the location of the lesion, the patient may lose all vision in one eye or portions of the visual fields in both eyes.

Auditory perception is the ability to detect and discriminate among auditory signals. This ability is a prerequisite for normal verbal communication. Therefore, the clinician must assess the patient's ability to perform auditory discriminations prior to evaluating verbal–intellectual skills.

Many types of sensory perceptual functions can be evaluated on the Halstead–Reitan Battery. Tactile perception is the evaluation of the basic ability to detect light touch to the back of either hand or to hand and face simultaneously, along with the ability to recognize other double simultaneous stimulation. Failure to detect stimuli on one side of the body or the other is suggestive of postcentral dysfunction in the contralateral cerebral hemisphere.

Finger recognition refers to the ability to correctly identify each of one's fingers by touch alone. This ability is tested by first blindfolding the patient and then by lightly touching each finger on each hand. Failure to correctly identify which finger is being touched may indicate dysfunction in the parietal cortex contralateral to the side which evidenced deficit.

Tactile symbol recognition measures the ability to perceive linguistic or numbered symbols which are traced on the skin, which is termed graphesthesia. Testing is carried out by tracing numbers or letters on the palm of the hand or fingertips.

Tactile form recognition measures the ability to recognize both objects and shapes by touch alone and is termed sterognosis. Testing typically consists of presenting the blindfolded patient with various objects or shapes which he or she is required to name.

Intellectual and Academic Achievement Assessment

The evaluation of cognitive functions is an integral part of the neuropsychological evaluation. The ability to recall specific information on command, as well as to comprehend the significance of social situations, to reason abstractly, or to express ideas clearly are among the abilities evaluated by psychometric intelligence tests.

Special Issues in Neuropsychological Assessment of Gays and Lesbians

Sexuality after Traumatic Brain Injury

Significant sexual dysfunction is not uncommon after traumatic brain injury. Lishman (1973) found that decreases in libido seemed to correlate with the severity of brain injury. The research indicates that traumatic brain injury typically results in alterations in sexual behavior, as well as function, and most typically these changes are more pronounced with more severe injuries (Lezak, 1986; Sbordone, 1984; Zasler & Kreutzer, 1991).

Sexuality is an example of integrative function, requiring the integration of physical, cognitive, and psychobehavioral components in order to be adequately expressed (Zasler & Kreutzer, 1991). Sensitivity is important in regards to sexuality and disability on the part of the gay or lesbian person with traumatic brain injury and the family. Professionals and family members must overcome any and all emotional roadblocks that prevent them from accepting that a person with a brain injury can be, and generally is, a sexual being. This is especially important when working with gays and lesbians for whom their sexuality is a part of their identity. All must learn to accept this fact in terms of sexual rights along with day-to-day functioning.

Dating can be and generally is a very anxiety-provoking experience for people with brain injury, particularly when they have more significant neurophysical or cognitive–behavioral deficits (Zasler & Kreutzer, 1991). This issue becomes more complicated for homosexuals who must also confront the stigmatizing effects of their sexual orientation. Single people should be encouraged, as appropriate, to pursue normal interactions with their peers of either gender. Typically, many of these people feel that as a result of their injuries they will be unable to find a compatible companion (Zasler & Kreutzer, 1991).

Sexual problems following traumatic brain injury can occur in the context of two types of family situations: individuals in established preinjury relationships, and individuals residing with their nuclear family. In either case, psychological as well as physical difficulties may contribute to sexual problems. In some cases, the person with a traumatic brain injury may experience psychological difficulties that manifest themselves in organic dysfunction (Zasler & Kreutzer, 1991). This individual may no longer be able to rely on previously established patterns of sexual functioning and must adapt and compensate for physical/psychological problems. Often people with traumatic brain injury have difficulty maintaining emotional stability. This difficulty can negatively affect the way they process information, creating problems in their ability to adapt to and compensate for the differences in their sexual functioning (Zasler & Kreutzer, 1991). Additionally, their sexual partners may have difficulty adjusting to the emotional and physical changes that their partners have experienced and grieve their previous stable preinjury relationships. Noninjured partners are also faced with the challenges of changing roles and are forced to provide care. These changes in roles often have pronounced effects on relationships. The stresses of caregiving and changing roles often permeate relationships with ambivalence, adversity, or both, further exacerbating emotional and psychological problems, increasing sexual dysfunction.

Individuals in Established Relationships

Research among heterosexual couples has found that after a brain injury many of these relationships experience extreme distress and often dissolve (Jacobs, 1988). Individuals in previously established relationships may find difficulty experiencing sexual satisfaction as a result of diminished frequency of intercourse, physical dysfunction, or both which may stem from emotional as well as physical problems encountered by either or both partners in the relationship (Zasler & Kreutzer, 1991). Those couples who are able to sustain relationships following injury are presented with long-term challenges to the maintenance of their relationships. The financial, physical, and emotional consequences of head trauma serve as major stressors to committed relationships and family activities. Priorities in relationships shift, with activities oriented toward stress reduction being assigned high priority relative to achievement of sexual satisfaction (Zasler & Kreutzer, 1991). Role changes in the family arising from the injury can affect the willingness of partners to engage in sexual activity. Preinjury, committed relationships were likely to have involved relatively equitable sharing of responsibilities among two people in normal adult roles. Following the injury, the partner who has been traumatized is likely to have far fewer responsibilities and to become more dependent on the partner without injury. Financially, the family may become entirely dependent on the non-injured partner's income.

Often with brain injuries there are many characterological changes that can affect the committed relationship. Lezak (1986) indicated that common characterological alterations subsequent to brain injury include self-centeredness and immaturity. Mauss-Clum and Ryan (1981) in their survey of family members, found that nearly 50% or more of persons with brain injury displayed childish behaviors including dependency, impatience, decreased self-control, self-centeredness, and inappropriate public behavior. Partners are often forced into taking a parental role and must restrict activities, give regular feedback about appropriate and inappropriate behavior, provide assistance with activities of daily living, and ensure that their partner follows the recommendations of professionals (Zasler & Kreutzer, 1991). The adverse personality changes of the brain-injured partner, combined with the increased stresses on the caregiver, detract from the familiarity and intimacy that underlie a satisfying sexual relationship (Zasler & Kreutzer, 1991).

Single Individuals Living with Parents

Epidemiological research on traumatic brain injury indicates that a majority of people with severe injuries are single (Jacobs, 1988; Kozloff, 1987). Currently no statistics are available indicating the number of homosexuals with traumatic brain injuries and whether these people are single or in relationships. For the single person, the effects of injury often cause previously successful relationships to dissolve (Zasler & Kreutzer, 1991). Individuals who did not have relationships prior to their injury often have difficulty establishing relationships postinjury. Adverse characterological, intellectual, and physical changes, as well as negative societal attitudes toward persons with disabilities, contribute to difficulties establishing satisfying relationships.

People with head injury become more dependent on their families following injury (Jacobs, 1988). Single, previously independent people living with their parents as a result of their injury must reestablish themselves and adapt to the loss of autonomy and privacy. For homosexuals family attitudes toward their sexual orientation make this particularly problematic. They may find it very difficult to maintain sexual relationships or establish new relationships. Some of these problems may stem from nonacceptance of their homosexuality by their parents or the individuals' embarrassment about continuing their previous sexual freedom with same-gender partners. Homosexuals may not have the privacy to bring partners home and may be forced to rely on other types of arrangements such as the partner's home or motel/hotel accommodations. These situations and attitudes may exacerbate sexual problems that stem from individuals' searching for suitable partners as well as coping with the aftereffects of their injuries and the possibility of diminished physical capabilities.

Research has indicated that social network density increases over time postinjury, with a corresponding decrease in the size of the network (Zasler & Kreutzer, 1991). People with head injury become more socially isolated, have fewer friends, and rely more heavily on remaining support systems for emotional and physical needs. Family members are often ill-prepared to assist the single person with brain injury in coping with sexual and social problems arising from injury. This is especially true for homosexuals who often must cope with the lack of support of their sexual identities. Parents have little experience addressing sexual concerns with their gay/lesbian children. Hesitancy to discuss sexual concerns with parents may reflect the person's belief that such a role is inappropriate for parents; concerns that parents may be critical; or deterioration in the parent–child relationship, which may arise from perceived insensitivity, misunderstanding, and overprotectiveness (Zasler & Kreutzer, 1991). Parents may convey discomfort because of their own issues surrounding their children's sexual identities and negative feelings toward homosexuality.

Other difficulties may be lack of opportunities for meeting people, physical problems (fatigability, seizures), parental overprotectiveness, or the lack of transportation. Family members may be unwilling to provide transportation for the homosexual individual and may already feel overwhelmed by the caretaking responsibilities, along with feeling uncomfortable with their child's sexual orientation (Zasler & Kreutzer, 1991).

The clinician should be aware and sensitive to the issues of sexual orientation and help the family acknowledge the importance of the person's sexual and emotional needs relative to other areas of rehabilitation.

AIDS Dementia Complex among Homosexual Men

Acquired immune deficiency syndrome (AIDS) and its related conditions are caused by the human immunodeficiency virus (HIV). HIV affects both the central nervous system and the peripheral nervous system. HIV is responsible for the destruction of the body's immune system. The virus enters the brain and other organs throughout the body, resulting in compromised movement, memory, and body functions.

AIDS has emerged as a health problem of enormous magnitude and complexity. Of the estimated 1.5 to 2 million Americans infected with human immunodeficiency virus, approximately 30% will progress to AIDS in 5 to 6 years. In 1997 49% of the reported AIDS cases were among homosexual men (Centers for Disease Control and Prevention [CDC], 1997). HIV and the AIDS dementia complex (ADC) are emerging as significant health issues among homosexual men.

Researchers have found that one of the many complications of AIDS is neurological disease (Gansler & Klein, 1992; Kaemingk & Kaszniak, 1988). Navia, Jordan, and Price (1986) reported that over 50% of AIDS patients showed some cognitive, motor, and/or psychological changes in the course of their illness. About 70–90% of adult AIDS patients have some neurological impairment (Koppel, Worinser, Tuchman, Maayan, Hwelett, & Daras, 1985; Levy, Bredesen, & Rosenblum, 1985; Levy & Bredesen, 1988; Snider et al., 1983). Upon autopsy 70–80% of AIDS patients have HIV-related neuropathy (Moskowitz, Hensley, Chan,

Gregorios & Conley, 1984). Navia, Cho, Petito, and Price (1986) reported that out of 70 autopsied adult AIDS patients, fewer than 10% of the brains were histologically normal. Abnormalities were divided into three discontinuous but sometimes overlapping groups: diffuse pallor of white matter, multinucleated cell encephalitis, and vascular myelopathy. Diffuse pallor of white matter was the most common histopathological finding.

Neurological disease in the HIV-positive individual can be caused by an opportunistic infection, such as toxoplasmosis or cryptococcal meningitis, or from direct HIV infection of the central nervous system. The fungus *Cryptococcus neoformans* is found in soil. The fungus is aerosolized and inhaled and is contained in the lungs. In immunosuppressed individuals the fungus can cause disseminated infection and accounts for 5–8% of all opportunistic infections in AIDS. The most common presentation of *Cryptococcus* is meningitis. Beginning symptoms are fever, nonspecific fatigue, nausea, and vomiting. Headache may be diffuse, frontal, or temporal. Encephalitis may occur with altered mental status, subtle behavioral changes, memory loss, and confusion. *Cryptococcus* affects the white matter and subcortical structures of the brain. Brain computed tomography (CT) or magnetic resonance imaging (MRI) may show the occasional focal granulomas associated with *Cryptococcus*.

Toxoplasma gondii is a protozoan which causes only a mild or asymptomatic infection when it infects normal hosts. Cats and other animals serve as a reservoir for the organism that is spread to humans via ingestion of contaminated soil, water, food, and raw or undercooked meat. In the United States, it is believed that approximately 50% of the population has been infected with *Toxoplasma* or is *Toxoplasma* seropositive. Onset of symptoms for immunosuppressed individuals is generally localized to intracranial disease with headaches, confusion, fevers, lethargy, seizures, and poor coordination or gait. The onset of symptoms varies and can be slow and insidious or rapid and dramatic. Toxoplasmic encephalitis will develop in 30% of AIDS patients who are seropositive for *Toxoplasma*. Focal neurologic changes such as hemiparesis, ataxia, cranial nerve palsies, sensory deficits, aphasia, and hemianopia are the most common signs. MRI scans are more sensitive than CT. When CT is performed, lesions are most evident after double-dose delayed contrast study. Multiple ring-enhancing lesions may be noted, especially in the white matter or basal ganglia.

Direct infection of the brain and central nervous system (CNS) takes place through specific brain cells that have surface molecules similar to the CD4 antigen on T4 lymphocytes and are receptive to HIV infection. In other brain cells, an alternative receptor for HIV has been identified which is a glycolipid that can mediate HIV infection. In addition to these brain cells, HIV-infected monocytes can migrate to the brain, become tissue macrophages, and release HIV to infect adjacent cells.

CD4 counts have become important in terms of classification of HIV progression. As HIV infects CD4 cells (T-helper cells), the absolute count of CD4 cells drops and is an indicator of the status of the HIV-infected person's immune system. The CDC has classified individuals into three basic groups: CD4 > 500, which indicates that the immune system is relatively intact and individuals are at low risk for opportunistic infections; CD4 < 500 but > 200, which indicates that the immune system is being compromised and individuals are at low- to moderate-risk for opportunistic infections; and finally, CD4 < 200, which indicates that individuals have AIDS and are at high risk for opportunistic infection.

The exact mechanisms by which HIV gains access to the central nervous system is as yet unknown, however, infection of the brain is the ultimate conclusion. The exact evolution of HIV–CNS symptomatology is variable. Some people experience intermittent cerebral spinal fluid abnormalities without symptoms, others experience chronic meningitis with headaches, while others experience acute or chronic inflammatory demyelination. At autopsy individuals with AIDS show atrophy, white matter pallor, and modest loss of neurons. Cellular changes within the brain include an invasion of macrophages, clusters of microglial and giant cell formation. ADC is the most frequent disease resulting from direct HIV infection of the CNS. ADC is a significant cause of disability among those in the advanced stages of the disease. Research has shown that HIV causes brain damage by a cytotoxic factor secreted by some HIV-infected macrophages that is responsible for some of the neurologic damage. The major neuropathological effects of HIV infection occur in the white matter of the brain, the thalamus, and the basal ganglia. Once an individual experiences severe dementia, his or her mean survival time ranges from one to six months. ADC is a clinical diagnosis with a variable course which includes symptoms in three different areas: cognitive, behavioral, and motor symptoms (Boccellari et al., 1993).

Petito, Cho, Lehman, Navia, and Price (1986) characterized AIDS dementia as having insidious onset and gradual progression in most cases and affecting intellectual and motor functions, although it is notable that virtually none of the early reports concerning AIDS dementia or ADC contained any objective measurements or data on these functions. Though the frequency and severity of brain histopathology correlate with the degree and duration of clinical dementia, autopsy examinations may find little CNS damage in proportion to the neurological impairment during life (Navia et al., 1986). Recently, there have been increasing attempts to determine the incidence and nature of the cognitive, motor, and behavioral changes in HIV-positive people.

Early manifestations of dementia may be mistaken for depression or may be seen as secondary to systemic illness. Memory loss, difficulties concentrating, and mental slowing were frequently reported early cognitive impairments in 46 patients with progressive dementia studied by Navia et al. (1986). Patients also reported motor impairments including unsteady gait, leg weakness, loss of coordination, impaired handwriting, and tremor. Finally, some patients described changes in behavior such as depression, apathy, agitation, and confusion.

Signs related to these early symptoms were detected on both mental status and neurologic examinations. The mental status examinations revealed psychomotor slowing and difficulty with the serial sevens task or tasks designed to test recent memory in some patients. The neurologic examinations showed cases of rapid movement impairment, gait ataxia and/or leg weakness, hyperflexia, dysarthria, and impairment of smooth pursuit eye movement.

Early cognitive symptoms of ADC include difficulties with concentration and memory, forgetfulness, recent memory loss, loss of concentration and slowness of thought, and a general slowing of mental function. Common behavioral symptoms include social withdrawal and a generalized apathy. Early motor problems can include difficulty with balance, clumsiness slurring of speech, loss of balance, deterioration of handwriting, and impaired motor function and leg weakness.

Late symptoms of ADC are characterized by loss of speech, extreme fatigue, muscle weakness, bladder and bowel incontinence, headache, seizures, coma, and finally death. Approximately 95% of patients with ADC have HIV antibodies in their cerebral spinal fluid. The late manifestations in Navia et al. (1986) patients included moderate to severe dementia, and confusion. Psychomotor slowing with verbal response delays and near or absolute mutism accompanied by a vacant stare were common.

An early diagnosis of ADC is difficult because the early signs of neurologic disease are very similar to the symptoms of clinical depression. Information presented by the National Institute of Allergy and Infectious Diseases indicated that asymptomatic HIV-infected individuals generally do not demonstrate mental impairment. The onset of mental impairment begins sometime after the HIV-infected person becomes symptomatic.

Neurological impairment will emerge as a major health care problem for HIV-positive individuals and their families as the burden of care for these people will often rest with the family, as is the case for people with other types of dementia, specifically Alzheimer's. HIV dementia, unlike Alzheimer's, is a rapid progressive disease which leaves individuals quickly incapacitated, with death in approximately three to six months. As a result of the rapid progression, adequate care and guidelines for these individuals has been largely ignored. The issue quickly resolves itself with the death of the individual.

Neuropsychological Assessment in ADC

The first assessment that should be conducted is a brief mental screening. Many mental-screening exams exist, but the Mini-Mental State Examination (MMSE) is the most widely utilized. The MMSE is used in epidemiological studies and community surveys, and forms part of the Diagnostic Interview Schedule (Tombaugh & McIntyre, 1992). In addition, it serves as one of the tests recommended by the National Institute of Neurological and Communicative Disorders and Stroke and the Alzheimer's Disease and Related Disorders Association (Folstein, Folstein & McHugh, 1975).

The MMSE consists of a variety of questions such as: What is the year? Where are we? Serial sevens, and so forth. The MMSE has a maximum score of 30 points, and can be administered in 5–10 minutes. The questions typically have been grouped into seven categories, each rationally representing a different cognitive domain or function: orientation to time (5 points), orientation to place (5 points), registration of three words (3 points), attention and calculation (5 points), recall of three words (3 points), language (8 points), and visual construction (1 point).

A score of 23 or less has generally been accepted as indicating the presence of cognitive impairment. This cutoff score evolved from research findings. Many researchers have further grouped the cognitive impairment into three levels: 24–30, no cognitive impairment; 18–23, mild cognitive impairment; and 0–17, severe cognitive impairment. MMSE scores are also frequently used to classify dementia patients as mild, moderate, or severe.

The reliability of the MMSE is approximately .96 for internal consistency, test–retest is .95. The validity of the MMSE has been measured in sensitivity and specificity. The sensitivity of the MMSE refers to its ability to correctly identify individuals who have been classified as cognitively impaired, whereas specificity refers to the its ability to correctly identify individuals who previously have been classified as cognitively intact (i.e., true negatives/total number of cognitively intact cases). Both of these measures have indicated that the MMSE is able to correctly identify cognitively impaired individuals 85% of the time with 87% specificity.

The following assessment battery is recommended if the mental screening suggests that neurological impairment may exist, which would be an MMSE score between 18–23. These assessment instruments have been utilized with great success by this writer in detailing the deficits in people with possible ADC.

Attentional capacities
Digit cancellation
Trails A
WAIS-III Digit Span

Spatial processing
WAIS-III Block Design
WAIS-III Object Assembly
Figure and Key copies from Reitan–
    Indiana AST
Trails A&B

General intelligence
WAIS-III Vocabulary
WAIS-III Similarities
WAIS-III Block Design
WAIS-III Object Assembly
Raven's Standard Progressive Matrices
Language
Reitan–Indiana Aphasia Screening Test
Controlled Oral Word Association Test–FAS and
    Animal Naming

Memory
Rey Auditory Verbal Learning Test
Wechsler Memory Scale—Revised
    Visual Reproduction I & II
Symbol-Digit Modalities Test
Complex cognition
Wisconsin Card Sorting Test
Trails B
Motor speed and coordination
Finger Tapping
Symbol-Digit Modalities Test
Depression
Beck Depression Inventory

Conclusion

Homosexuality has been loaded with every kind of significance, from pathological disease to moral vice. A gradual change in awareness and attitudes has come in the past thirty years, but stereotypes and stigma have continued and research in every arena within this group lags behind. Currently there is no known physiological difference between heterosexuals and homosexuals. The essential neuropsychological assessment is basically the same. However, when creating a treatment plan the neuropsychologist should take into consideration the effect of sexual orientation upon the individual's support system and social needs. Two specific areas that are different are family interactions and sexuality. As a result of society's view of homosexuality, family interaction may be complicated depending upon the degree of acceptance of the individual's sexual orientation previous to neurological injury or impairment. Sexuality is a part of the homosexual's identity and should be incorporated into the results provided to the individual and their support system(s). The homosexual individual may have to make significant changes in his or her life to adapt and compensate for physical/psychological/ characterological changes as a result of neurological impairment. A specific area that has affected gay men has been HIV and ADC. Many individuals infected with HIV will experience severe neurological impairments and ADC is becoming a major health care problem for the families and support systems. In conclusion, neuropsychologists need to be sensitive and aware of the large variety of special psychosocial issues when working with gay and lesbian clients. Care must be taken when conducting a neuropsychological assessment and information should be provided to the families and partners in detail surrounding the issues and extent of their neurological impairments. If sexual orientation is ignored, the assessment will be incomplete and the information provided will not be as informative in terms of daily functioning.

References

Allen, L. S., Hines, M., Shryne, J. E., & Gorski, R. A. (1989). Two sexually dimorphic cell groups in the human brain. *Journal of Neuroscience, 9,* 497–506.

Atkinson, D. R., & Hackett, C. (1988). *Counseling non-ethnic American minorities.* Springfield, IL: Charles C Thomas.

Anonymous (1996). It's normal to be queer. *The Economist,* January 6–12, 68–70.

Bailey, M. J., & Pillard, R. C. (1991). A genetic study of male sexual orientation. *Archives of General Psychiatry, 48*, 1089–1096.

Bell, A. P., Weinberg, M. S., & Hammersmith, S. K. (1981). *Sexual preference: Its development in men and women.* Bloomington: Indiana University Press.

Boccellari, A. A., Dilley, J. W., Chambers, D. B., Yingling, C.D., Tauber, M. A., Moss, A. R., & Osmond, D. H. (1993). Immune function and neuropsychological performance in HIV-1 infected homosexual men. *Journal of Acquired Immune Deficiency Syndromes, 6*, 592–601.

Buhrke, R. A., Ben-Ezra, L. A., Hurley, M. E., & Ruprecht, L. J. (1992). Content analysis and methodological critique of articles concerning lesbian and gay male issues in counseling journals. *Journal of Counseling Psychology, 39*, 91–99.

Carlson, N. R. (1986). *Physiology of behavior* (3rd ed.). London: Allyn & Bacon.

Centers for Disease Control and Prevention (1997). *HIV/AIDS surveillance report, 9*(2), 1–44.

Coleman, E. (1982). Developmental stages of the coming out process. *Journal of Homosexuality, 7*, 31–43.

DePompei, R. & Zarski, J. J. (1989). Families, head injury, and cognitive–communicative impairments: Issues for family counseling. *Topics in Language Disorders, 9*(2), 78–89.

DePompei, R. & Zarski, J. J. (1991). Assessment of the family. In J. M. Williams & T. Kay (Eds.), *Head injury: A family matter* (pp. 37–63). London: Brookes.

DePompei, R., Zarski, J. J., & Hall, D. E. (1988). A systems approach to understanding CHI family functioning. *Cognitive Rehabilitation*, March/April, 6–10.

Ehrhardt, A. A., & Meyer-Bahlburg, H. F. L. (1981). Effects of prenatal sex hormones on gender-related behavior. *Science, 211*, 1312–1318.

Ehrhardt, A. A., Meyer-Bahlburg, H. F. L., Rosen, L. R., Feldman, J. F., Verdiano, N. P. Zimmerman, I., & McEwen, B. S. (1985). Sexual orientation after prenatal exposure to exogenous estrogen. *Archives of Sexual Behavior, 14*, 57–77.

Flores, L. Y., O'Brien, K. M. & McDermott, D. (1995, August). *Counseling psychology trainees' perceived efficacy in counseling lesbian and gay clients.* Poster session presented at the annual meeting of the American Psychological Association, New York.

Fassinger, R. E. (1991). The hidden minority. *The Counseling Psychologist, 19*(2), 157–177.

Folstein, M. F., Folstein, S. E., & McHugh, P. R. (1975). Mini-Mental State: A practical method for grading the cognitive state of outpatients for the clinician. *The Journal of Psychiatric Research, 12*, 189–198.

Gansler, D. A. & Klein, W. L. (1992). Human immunodeficiency virus encephalopathy and other neuropsychological consequences of HIV infection. In R. F. White (Ed.), *Clinical syndromes in adult neuropsychology: The practitioner's handbook.* New York: Elsevier.

Gath, A. (1977). The impact of an abnormal child upon the parents. *British Journal of Psychiatry, 130*, 405–410.

Gladue, B. A., Green, R., & Hellman, R. E. (1984). Neuroendocrine response to estrogen and sexual orientation. *Science, 225*, 1496–1499.

Jacobs, H. E. (1988). The Los Angeles head injury survey: Procedures and initial findings. *Archives of Physical Medicine and Rehabilitation, 69*, 425–431.

Kaemingk, K. L. & Kaszniak, A. W. (1988). Neuropsychological aspects of human immunodeficiency virus infection. *The Clinical Neuropsycholgist, 3*, 309–320.

Koppel, B. S., Worinser, G. P., Tuchman, A. J., Maayan, S., Hwelett, D., & Daras, M. (1985) Central nervous system involvement in patients with acquired immune deficiency syndrome (AIDS). *Acta Neurologica Scandinavica, 71*, 337–353.

Kozloff, R. (1987). Networks of social support and the outcome from severe head injury. *Journal of Head Trauma Rehabilitation, 2*(3), 14–23.

LaMar, L. & Kite, M. (1998). Sex differences in attitudes toward gay men and lesbians: A multidimensional perspective. *Journal of Sex Research, 35*(2), 189–196.

LeVay, S. (1991). A difference in hypothalamic structure between heterosexual and homosexual men. *Science, 253*, 1034–1037.

Levy, R. M., Bredesen, D. E., & Rosenblum, M. L. (1985). Neurological manifestations of the acquired immunodeficiency syndrome (AIDS): Experience at UCSF and review of the literature. *Journal of Neurosurgery, 62*, 475–495.

Levy, R. M. & Bredesen, D. E. (1988). Central nervous system dysfunction in acquired immunodeficiency syndrome. In M. L. Rosenblum, R. M. Levy, & D. E. Bredesen (Eds.), *AIDS and the nervous system.* New York: Raven.

Lezak, M. D. (1986). Psychological implications of traumatic brain damage for the patient's family. *Rehabilitation Psychology, 31*, 241–250.

Lishman, W. A. (1973). The psychiatric sequelae of head injury: A review. *Psychological Medicine, 3*, 304–318.

Navia, B. A., Cho, E. S., Petito, C. K., & Price, R. W. (1986). The AIDS dementia complex II neuropathology. *Annals of Neurology, 19*, 525–535.

Navia, B. A. & Price, R. (1986). Dementia complicating AIDS. *Psychiatric Annals, 16*(3), 158–166.

Navia, B. A., Jordan, B. O., & Price, R. W. (1986). The AIDS dementia complex: I. Clinical features. *Annals of Neurology, 19*, 517–524.

Mauss-Clum, N., & Ryan, M. (1981). Brain injury and the family. *Journal of Neurosurgical Nursing, 13*(4), 165–169.

McGoldrick, M., Pearce, J. K., & Giordano, J. (1982). *Ethnicity and family therapy*. New York: Guilford.

Morin, S. F. (1977). Heterosexual bias in psychological research on lesbianism and male homosexuality. *American Psychologist, 32*, 629–637.

Moskowitz, L. B., Hensley, G. T., Chan, J. C., Gregorios, J., & Conley, F. K. (1984). The neuropathology of acquired immune deficiency syndrome. *Archives of Pathology and Laboratory Medicine, 108*, 867–872.

Murphy, A. T. (1982). The family with a handicapped child: A review of the literature. *Developmental and Behavioral Pediatrics, 3*(2), 73–82.

Petito, C. K., Cho, E. S., Lehman, W., Navia, B. A. & Price, R. W. (1986). Neuropathology of acquired immunodeficiency syndrome (AIDS): An autopsy review. *Journal of Neuropathology and Experimental Neurology, 45*, 635–646.

Pinel, J. P. J. (1993). *Biopsychology* (2nd ed.). London: Allyn & Bacon.

Rosenbaum, M., & Najenson, T. (1976). Changes in life patterns and symptoms of low mood as reported by wives of severely brain-injured soldiers. *Journal of Consulting and Clinical Psychology, 44*, 831–888.

Sbordone, R. J. (1984). Rehabilitative neuropsychological approach for severe traumatic brain-injured patients. *Professional Psychology Research & Practice, 15*, 165–175.

Snider, W. D., Simpson, D. M., Nielsen, S., Gold, J. W. M., Netroka, C. E. & Posner, J. B. (1983). Neurological complications of acquired immune deficiency syndrome: Analysis of 50 patients. *Annals of Neurology, 14*, 403–418.

Tombaugh, T. N. & McIntyre, N. J. (1992). The mini-mental state examination: A comprehensive review. *Journal of the American Geriatrics Society, 40*, 922–935.

Tourney, G. (1975). Hormonal relationships in homosexual men. *American Journal of Psychiatry, 132*, 288–290.

Turnbull, A. P., & Turnbull, H. R., III (1991). Understanding families from a systems perspective. In J. M. Williams & T. Kay (Eds.), *Head injury: A family matter* (pp. 37–63). London: Brookes.

Watters, A. T. (1986). Heterosexual bias in psychological research on lesbianism and male homosexuality (1979–1983), utilizing the bibliographic and system of Morin (1977). *Journal of Homosexuality, 13*, 35–49.

Webster's Dictionary (1984). (Library ed.). New York: Chatham River.

Zarski, J. J., DePompei, R., West, J., & Hall, D. G. (1988). Chronic illness: Stressors, the adjustment process and family focused interventions. *Journal of Mental Health Counseling, 10*(2), 145–158.

Zasler, N. D. & Kreutzer, J. S. (1991). Family and sexuality after traumatic brain injury. In J. M. Williams & T. Kay (Eds.), *Head injury: A family matter* (pp. 253–270). London: Brookes.

6

Gender Effects in Neuropsychological Assessment

KYLE BRAUER BOONE AND PO LU

Several publications have reviewed the effects of gender on individual neuropsychological measures, however, to date there has been no review of the impact of gender on a wide range of neuropsychological tests. This type of information is critical in that to the extent that there are gender differences on cognitive measures, test normative data must be stratified by sex, otherwise the available norms will render inaccurate results; that is, they will overpathologize the scores of the underperforming gender and at the same time fail to detect true declines in the gender with the higher baseline.

This chapter will review structural and physiological differences between male and female brains, and then summarize the available literature on gender differences on commonly used neuropsychological instruments.

Gender Differences in Brain Structure and Physiology

Brain Weight and Size

Studies in brain size and weight have consistently revealed that men possess larger brains than women (Ankney, 1992; Breedlove, 1994; Gur et al., 1991; Reiss et al., 1996; Todd et al., 1995; Willerman, Schultz, Rutledge, & Bigler, 1992). Gender differences in brain weight emerge early in childhood, beginning in the second year of life. The weight of the developing male brain increases faster than that of the female brain, reaching its full adult value by about age 5 (Giedd et al., 1996; Reiss et al., 1996; Todd et al., 1995). Because men also have larger bodies, some researchers have proposed that gender differences disappear after statistically correcting for body size (measured as height, body mass, or estimated surface area) (Breedlove, 1994; Lewontin et al., 1984). Others report contradictory findings and demonstrate that the gender differences remain even after adjusting for body size (Ankney, 1992; Gur et al., 1991; Willerman et al., 1992). Measures of brain volume using magnetic resonance imaging

KYLE BRAUER BOONE AND **PO LU** • Harbor-UCLA Medical Center, Torrance, California 90509.

Handbook of Cross-Cultural Neuropsychology, edited by Fletcher-Janzen, Strickland, and Reynolds. Kluwer Academic / Plenum Publishers, New York, 2000.

(MRI) have also corroborated the finding of a gender difference in adult brain size favoring men (Andreasen et al., 1993; Gur et al., 1991; Schlaepfer et al., 1995). The prevailing consensus appears to be that sex differences in brain size may be reduced by covarying for variables representative of body size, but no single measure will normalize brain weight sufficiently to eliminate the male advantage (Breedlove, 1994).

The functional significance of brain size in terms of cognitive abilities is less clearly understood. It is generally recognized that brain size in weight or volume is positively associated with measures of intelligence (Andreasen et al., 1993; Reiss et al., 1996; Rushton & Ankney, 1996; Willerman et al., 1992). However, the finding that women have proportionately smaller brains than men but demonstrate no comparable differences in intelligence presents a paradox.

Reiss et al. (1996) emphasized that only a relatively small amount of variance in intelligence can be accounted for by the size of the brain; therefore, brain size may be just one of many factors related to human intelligence. In addition, Reiss and colleagues (1996) also reported that only gray matter showed a significant positive relationship with intelligence. Research has shown that no gender differences exist in the cortical surface area and that women appear to have greater cortical neuron-packing density, both of which imply that the number of information processing modules are comparable between men and women, enabling sex-equivalent capacities in general ability (Willerman et al., 1992). Of interest, even though overall percentage of gray matter in the brain did not differ between genders, MRI has revealed that women have significantly greater gray matter in the dorsolateral prefrontal cortex (DLPFC) and superior temporal gyrus (STG), two cortical areas closely linked to higher order verbal function (Schlaepfer et al., 1995). In contrast, the male advantage in brain size may allow enhanced function on visual-perceptual tasks, analogous to computers requiring substantially more memory to run visual/graphic programs (Ankney, 1992).

Corpus Callosum

The corpus callosum, the main fiber tract connecting the cortical regions of the two cerebral hemispheres, consists of neuronal axons and is an important structure involved in interhemispheric communication and coordination of left and right cerebral functions. In addition to its functional importance, this structure is often studied due to its relatively clear anatomical boundaries and ease of obtaining direct measurements through postmortem brain specimens and MRI (Witelson, 1990). The corpus callosum more than triples its size over the lifespan with the majority of the growth occurring during infancy and childhood (Witelson & Kigar, 1988). It is hypothesized that the course of callosal development parallels the myelination of callosal fibers. An initial growth spurt occurs from birth to age 2, followed by a marked decline in growth rate until about age 10 when full adult size is reached, coinciding with the completion of callosal myelination (Witelson & Kigar, 1988). No reliable sex differences have been found up through this stage of callosal development (Witelson & Kigar, 1988).

Studies examining sex differences in the midsagittal area of the adult corpus callosum have reported contradictory findings. Some investigators failed to find a gender difference in the absolute size of the callosum (Allen, Richey, Chai, & Gorski, 1991; deLacoste-Utamsing & Holloway, 1982). However, Witelson (1989) reported the results from a number of studies demonstrating that the callosal area tends to be larger in men than women, but most of them failed to show a statistically significant difference. One study found that callosal size is proportionate to brain size, and when brain size was statistically controlled, the gender difference disappeared (Witelson, 1989).

Instead of examining the corpus callosum in its entirety, several studies divided the structure into seven distinct subregions with each region analyzed separately. The splenium, defined as the posterior one-fifth of the overall length of the callosum, contains fibers connecting the occipital lobes and the inferior regions of the temporal lobe, allowing for interhemispheric transfer of visual information (deLacoste-Utamsing & Holloway, 1982; Witelson, 1990). deLacoste-Utamsing and Holloway (1982) found this subregion qualitatively to be more bulbous and wider and quantitatively larger in area in females relative to males, a finding that was supported by Allen et al. (1991). However, other studies have failed to replicate these gender differences (Witelson, 1989).

Another region that yielded intriguing results is the isthmus, defined as the posterior one-third minus the posterior one-fifth of the length of the callosum (Witelson, 1989). The isthmus has been found to be clearly larger in women and the difference is even more striking when considered relative to the generally larger callosal area in men. This region houses fibers from posterior superior temporal as well as posterior parietal regions and is part of an anatomical network with cortical regions relevant to language and visuospatial skills (Witelson, 1989, 1990). In addition to differences in size, the isthmus is also associated with sex differences in hand preference, often considered a reflection of asymmetric control of behavior (Kimura & Harshman, 1984). In males, the isthmus was 60% larger in individuals who are characterized as nonconsistent right-handers compared to those who are consistent right-handers, but no associations in hand preference and isthmus area exist among females (Witelson, 1990). The gender differences in callosum morphology, specifically the area of the isthmus, and their relationship to handedness suggest that the isthmus serves as the neuroanatomical basis for hemisphere specialization and the differences in lateralization of functions between males and females (Witelson, 1990). The finding that representation of speech and language functions in the left frontal regions and bihemispheric representation of some language skills in posterior cortical regions is greater in women is compatible with sex differences in callosal anatomy.

Cerebral Blood Flow and Glucose Metabolism

Activity of the human brain can be examined in vivo through various functional neuroimaging techniques such as the ^{133}Xe inhalation method, positron emission tomography, and single proton emission tomography, which assess regional cerebral blood flow (CBF) and metabolic rate of glucose utilization. The level and rate of these two indices of neural activity provide information regarding function of the cerebral cortex and can potentially establish a connection between brain activity and cognitive abilities.

Most studies investigating the relationship between gender differences and regional CBF consistently report that, at rest, women exhibit a higher level and rate of global CBF than men (Gur & Gur, 1990; Gur et al., 1982; Mathew, Wilson, & Tart, 1986; Rodriguez, Warkentin, Risberg, & Rosadini, 1988). No overall hemispheric differences in blood flow was found in either sex, but when specific regions were examined, men possessed higher blood flow in the right frontal lobe. No such asymmetrical difference in this area was identified in the females. When neuroimaging has been conducted during performance of cognitive tasks, increased rate in blood flow was observed to be greater in the left hemisphere during the performance of a verbal task and greater in the right during the performance of a spatial task, but no gender differences were found (Gur et al., 1982; Wendt & Risberg, 1994).

Cerebral glucose metabolism, another measure of neural activity, is thought to be highly coupled with CBF (Baxter et al., 1987; Gur et al., 1995), leading to the expectation that gender differences comparable to those observed in CBF would be found (Baxter et al., 1987).

However, the majority of studies failed to document gender differences in global or regional glucose metabolism (Azari, Rapoport, Grady, & DeCarli, 1992; Gur et al., 1995; Haier & Benbow, 1995; Mansour, Haier, & Buchsbaum, 1996). Some did demonstrate a trend toward greater brain metabolic activity in females but the differences were not statistically significant (Andreasen et al., 1993). Analysis of sex differences in the regional distribution of metabolic activity revealed that men and women are fundamentally similar, though three specific regions were identified to have greater glucose metabolic rate in women: the left posterior cingulate gyrus (Gur et al.,1995), posterior corpus collosum (Gur et al., 1995), and the orbital–frontal region including somatosensory cortices (Andreason, Zametkin, Guo, Baldwin, & Cohen, 1994; Azari et al., 1992; Gur et al., 1995). Of interest, gender differences in glucose metabolism in various neuroanatomical regions may be elicited/activated during the performance of a cognitive task (Mansour et al., 1996). For example, glucose metabolism of the temporal lobe was found to be statistically related to the performance of a mathematical reasoning task in males while no such association was found in females (Haier & Benbow, 1995).

Gender Differences in Cognition

Given the structural and physiological differences in male and female brains, the question arises as to whether there are functional differences in cognitive ability between the sexes. The experimental psychological literature on cognition in men and women have suggested rather consistently that men show an advantage in spatial skills (especially involving mental rotation) and math, while women exhibit a superiority in verbal skills (for reviews see Halpern & Crothers, 1997; Levy & Heller, 1992; Maccoby & Jacklin, 1974). However, it is unclear whether these laboratory findings translate to the "real world" of clinical assessment. The subsequent section will review the available literature on gender differences on commonly used neuropsychological instruments with the tests grouped according to cognitive domain.

Intelligence

Few gender differences have been observed on tests of intelligence, an expected finding given that tests such as the Stanford-Binet and Wechsler scales were specifically constructed to minimize sex differences (Matarazzo, 1972). Snow and Weinstock (1990) have reviewed the literature on gender differences on the Wechsler-Bellevue, WAIS, and WAIS-R, and conclude that in terms of overall IQ scores and IQ discrepancy scores, there is a tendency for males to obtain slightly higher Verbal IQs, but there are no differences on PIQ or FSIQ or VIQ–PIQ discrepancy. Regarding individual subtest scores, a male advantage has been reported for the Information (Saykin et al., 1995; Snow & Weinstock, 1990), Arithmetic, Picture Completion, and Block Design subtests (Snow & Weinstock, 1990), although the differences amounted to only one-third of a standard deviation. In contrast, some studies have found a female advantage for Digit Symbol (Ponton et al., 1996; Snow & Weinstock, 1990), although other studies have failed to replicate this finding in low education samples (Mazaux et al., 1995).

Language

1. *Boston Naming Test*: Most studies have failed to show a gender effect on Boston Naming Test performance (Fastenau, Denburg, & Mauer, 1998; Ivnik, Malec, Smith, & Tangalos, 1996; LaBarge, Edwards, & Knesevich, 1986, Saykin et al., 1995). However, a slight

male advantage was observed in an investigation of Spanish-speaking subjects using a translated and modified version of the test (Ponton et al., 1996), and both male (Welch, Doineau, Johnson, & King, 1996) and female (Ganguli et al., 1991) advantages have been observed in older samples.

2. *Speech Sounds Perception Test*: The available literature has failed to reveal any gender differences in test performance (Seidenberg et al., 1984; Yeudall, Reddon, Gill, & Stefanyk, 1987).

Visual Perceptual/Spatial Skills

1. *Rey–Osterrieth Complex Figure*: The research data either suggest no gender differences (Berry, Allen, & Schmitt, 1991; Bennett-Levy, 1984; Boone, Lesser, Hill-Gutierrez, & Berman, 1993; Browers et al., 1984) or a slight male advantage (Ardila & Rosselli, 1989; Ardila, Rosselli, & Rosas, 1989; King, 1981; Rosselli & Ardila, 1991). Ardila et al. (1989) initially reported that the superiority of males was only confined to subjects with no formal education, however, this relationship was not corroborated in a larger sample of older subjects (Rosselli & Ardila, 1991). Of interest, most of the studies which reported sex effects collected data on Spanish-speaking subjects from Colombia, and it is possible that cultural and educational factors contributed to the sex effects observed.

2. *Tactual Performance Test*: Most publications suggest that there is no difference between males and females on TPT performance (Dodrill, 1979; Filskov & Catanese, 1986; Fromm-Auch & Yeudall, 1983; King et al., 1978; Pauker, 1980; Thompson et al. 1987; Yeudall et al., 1987). On the other hand, Heaton et al. (1986) reported that males outperformed females on total time, although the amount of variance in test scores accounted for by sex was minimal (1%; Heaton et al. 1991). Ernst (1987) documented better male performance in his sample of elderly subjects averaging less than 12 years of education on memory, localization, and all time scores except dominant hand. Conversely, other reports have suggested that women score better than men on memory (Fabian, Jenkins, & Parsons, 1981), localization (Chavez, Schwartz, & Brandon, 1982), or both scores (Gordon & O'Dell, 1983), although Gordon and O'Dell (1983) comment that the sex differences they observed were not of "practical significance."

3. *Hooper Visual Organization Test*: The sparse literature on the Hooper VOT suggests no effect of gender on test performance (Hilgert & Treloar, 1985).

4. *Judgment of Line Orientation*: Again the limited literature fails to reveal any impact of gender on test performance (Saykin et al., 1995).

Verbal Memory

1. *Rey Auditory Verbal Learning Test*: The available data tend to reveal an advantage for women on this measure (Bleecker, Bolla-Wilson, Agnew, & Meyers, 1988; Bolla-Wilson & Bleecker, 1986; Geffen, Moar, O'Hanlon, & Clark, 1990; Vakil & Blachstein, 1997), although a few studies have failed to document this relationship (Savage & Gouvier, 1992; Wiens, McMinn, & Crossen, 1988). Of interest, most of the studies which documented a female superiority examined an older sample, and Bleecker and colleagues (1988) in fact observed that the gender differences on the RAVLT increased with age; specifically, women in the age group 40–49 averaged one more word than men on Trial V while women aged 80–89 averaged two more words than their male counterparts. The studies that failed to document gender differences either contained a small subset of women subjects (e.g., 13%; Wiens et al.,

1988) or had very unusual variability in performance across cells (Savage & Gouvier, 1992), and thus may have had limited power to detect gender differences. Taken as a whole, the data suggest that there is a small female advantage in RAVLT performance which doubles in size in the elderly.

2. *California Verbal Learning Test*: Most studies have suggested that women might display an advantage on most CVLT scores (Delis, Kramer, Kaplan, & Ober, 1987; Kramer, Delis, & Daniel, 1988; Wiens, Tindall, & Crossen, 1994), with gender accounting for up to 10% of test score variance. However, others have failed to document a female superiority (Saykin et al., 1995).

3. *Wechsler Memory Scales-Logical Memory subtest*: The literature fails to reveal any effect of gender on test performance (Saykin et al., 1995).

Nonverbal/Visual Memory

1. *Wechsler Memory Scales-Visual Reproduction subtest*: While some authors have found a slight superiority of men on this task (Ivison, 1977), others have found no gender differences (Saykin et al., 1995; Trahan, Quintana, Willingham, & Goethe, 1988).

2. *Rey–Osterrieth Complex Figure*: No effect of gender has been observed in 3-minute delayed recall of the Rey–Osterrieth (Boone, Lesser, Hill-Gutierrez, & Berman, 1993).

3. *Continuous Visual Memory Test*: No significant gender effects have been documented for either the acquisition or delayed recognition portions of the CVMT (Trahan & Quintana, 1990).

4. *Benton Visual Retention Test*: Similarly, gender has not been found to be related to performance on the Benton Visual Retention Test (Coman et al., 1999).

Motor Strength, Speed, and Dexterity

1. *Dynamometer*: Available literature suggests that the dynamometer (or grip strength) is the one neuropsychological motor test most affected by gender (Heaton et al., 1991). Men have been found to consistently outperform women (Bornstein, 1985; Ernst, 1988; Fromm-Auch & Yeudall, 1983; Koffler & Zehler, 1985; Rounsaville, Jones, Novelly, & Kleber, 1982; Yeudall et al., 1987) with scores achieved by men on average 50% greater than those displayed by women.

2. *Grooved Pegboard*: Some minor gender differences have been reported for Grooved Pegboard with women outperforming men by approximately 4 to 7 seconds with both hands (Bornstein, 1985; Heaton et al., 1991; Polubinski & Melamed, 1986; Ruff & Parker, 1993); gender accounts for approximately 3 to 4 % of test score variance (Heaton et al., 1991).

3. *Finger Tapping*: The existing literature is consistent in documenting a male advantage on finger tapping speed of approximately 3 to 6 taps (Bornstein, 1985; Brandon, Chavez, & Bennett, 1986; Buckelew & Hannay, 1986; Chavez, Trautt, Brandon, & Steyaert, 1983; Dodrill, 1979; Echternacht, 1981; Filskov & Catanese, 1986; Fromm-Auch & Yeudall, 1983; Gordon & O'Dell, 1983; Harris, Cross, & VanNieuwkerk, 1981; Heaton et al., 1991; Hoffman, 1969; King et al., 1978; McKeever & Abramson, 1991; Morrison, Gregory, & Paul, 1979; Ruff & Parker, 1993; Saykin et al., 1995; Trautt, Chavez, Brandon, & Steyaert, 1983; Yeudall et al., 1987).

4. *Purdue Pegboard*: Similar to findings observed for Grooved Pegboard, females have been found to outperform males on the Purdue Pegboard (Yeudall, Fromm, Reddon, & Stefanyk, 1986).

Attention and Information Processing Speed

1. *Symbol Digit Modalities*: The literature suggests that females demonstrate a slight advantage (Yeudall et al., 1986).

2. *Seashore Rhythm Test*: The majority of investigators have not found sex to be related to test performance (Bornstein, 1985; Dodrill, 1979; Fromm-Auch & Yeudall, 1983; Heaton et al., 1991; Reitan & Wolfson, 1989; Yeudall et al., 1987). Only Young and Delay (1993) report a small but significant gender difference in favor of males which they indicate may be a function of education, IQ differences, or altered scoring procedures utilizing signal detection theory.

Executive/Problem-Solving Skills

1. *Auditory Consonant Trigrams*: No differences in performance between men and women have been found in the two studies to address this issue (Boone, 1999; Stuss, Stethem, & Poirier, 1987).

2. *Stroop Test*: Most studies have failed to observe an effect of gender on Stroop performance (Boone et al., 1999; Connor, Fanzen, & Sharp, 1988; Houx, Jolles, & Vreeling, 1993; Saykin et al., 1995; Swerdlow, Fillon, Geyer, & Bratt, 1995; Trenerry, Crosson, DeBoe, & Leber, 1989) although some have reported a female advantage confined to color naming (Golden, 1978; Jensen & Rohwer, 1966; Strickland, D'Elia, James, & Stein, 1997; Stroop, 1935) or word reading (Strickland et al., 1997); no studies have documented a gender effect on the color-interference section.

3. *Trailmaking*: The literature on sex differences in TMT scores has generally indicated that there are no gender effects (Dodrill, 1979; Ernst, 1987; Fromm-Auch & Yeudall, 1983; Heaton et al., 1986, 1991; Ivnik et al., 1996; Saykin et al., 1995; Stuss et al., 1987; Yeudall et al., 1987). The five studies which found sex effects differed as to which sex performed better, and the differences in performance between the sexes were small: Portin, Saarijarvi, Joukamaa, and Salokangas (1995) and Giovagnoli et al. (1996) reported superiority of men on part A and Davies (1968) found that men scored higher than women on part B; in contrast, Ganguli and colleagues (1991) observed a female advantage for part A, and Bornstein (1985) reported that women outperformed men on both test sections.

4. *Verbal Fluency/Word Generation*: The literature on the impact of gender on word generation is split fairly evenly with half of the studies observing a slight female advantage but the other investigations failing to detect any gender differences. Specifically, Bolla, Lindgren, Bonaccorsy, and Bleeker (1990), Gaddes and Crockett (1975), Ruff, Light, Parker, and Levin (1996), Veroff (1980), and Ganguli and colleagues (1991) documented superior word generation ability in women, while Cauthen (1978), Ripich, Petrill, Whitehouse, and Ziol (1995), Yeudall et al. (1986, 1987), Saykin et al. (1995), Boone (1999), and Thombaugh, Kozak, and Rees (1999) did not observe any gender differences. When gender differences were found, they were small; for example, on the FAS task, Bolla et al. (1990) reported that women averaged 2 to 4 words more than men.

Level of education may moderate the effect of gender on word generation; Ruff and colleagues (1996) reported that scores of men and women were comparable for educational levels up to and including 15 years of formal schooling, but that women with 16 or more years of education significantly outperformed men, averaging 5 more words.

5. *Wisconsin Card Sorting Test*: Boone and colleagues (1993) reported that middle-aged and older women outperformed men in terms of number of categories, errors, perseverative responses, percent perseverative errors, percent conceptual level responses, and trials to first

category. Specifically, women averaged one more category and had a 20% increase in percent conceptual level responding along with one-third fewer errors, perseverative responses, and percent perseverative errors, and one quarter fewer trials to first category. In a subsequent publication examining the relative contribution of age, education, gender, IQ, and health status to WCST performance, gender was found to be a predictor of number of categories, percent conceptual level responses, and number of errors, accounting for between 4% and 5% of test score variance (Boone, 1999).

However, other investigators examining primarily younger populations have failed to document sex differences (Heaton et al., 1993; Saykin et al., 1995; Yeudall et al., 1986).

6. *Design Fluency*: No gender differences have been reported in performance on figural fluency tasks (Lee et al., 1997).

7. *Category Test*: In general, no significant sex differences have been noted in Category Test performance (Dodrill, 1979; Fromm-Auch & Yeudall, 1983; Heaton et al., 1986, 1991; Kupke, 1983; Pauker, 1980; Saykin et al., 1995; Seidenberg et al., 1984; Yeudall et al., 1987), although Ernst (1987) reported that in his elderly sample averaging fewer than 12 years of education, men performed slightly better than women on the booklet version of the test.

8. *Paced Auditory Serial Addition Test*: The available literature has failed to document any gender differences on this measure (Wiens, Fuller, & Crossen, 1997).

Summary and Conclusions

Despite the evidence of structural and physiological differences between male and female brains, there are few detectable differences between the sexes on standard cognitive measures. Males appear to have a slight advantage on math skills (WAIS/WAIS-R Arithmetic subtest), fund of general information (WAIS/WAIS-R Information subtest), and select visual perceptual/spatial tasks (WAIS/WAIS-R Picture Completion and Block Design subtests), while females may show a minor advantage on rote verbal memory tasks (Rey Auditory Verbal Learning Test, California Verbal Learning Test), select executive skills (verbal fluency–FAS, Wisconsin Card Sorting Test), and rapid eye–hand coordination (Digit Symbol/Symbol Digit, Grooved Pegboard, Purdue Pegboard). This suggests that from an evolutionary standpoint, the cognitive demands made by the environment were for the most part highly comparable for both genders, causing male and female humans to develop very similar cognitive skills despite differences in brain structure and physiology (Levy & Heller, 1992). In contrast, there are prominent differences between the sexes in motor strength (Grip Strength/Dynamometer) in favor of men, with men also showing a more minor advantage in repetitive motor speed (Finger Tapping), suggesting that environmental demands have historically dictated that male survival depended on strength and, to a lesser extent, speed.

An interesting finding which emerged from this review was that the superiority of women in rote verbal memory and select executive skills was either confined to or more pronounced in elderly women versus elderly men. There are several possible factors which may contribute to a preservation of select cognitive skills in older women as compared to older men.

First, there is evidence that estrogen enhances and protects verbal skills. To the extent that older women receive estrogen replacement therapy, their verbal skills (fluency and memory) are higher than those of older women without estrogen replacement as well as those of older men (Lindman et al., 1998).

Second, a precipitous increase in ventricular volume, an indicator of brain atrophy, begins in the fifth decade in men but not until the sixth decade in women (although once the atrophy process begins, velocity increases with age more rapidly in women than in men; Murphy, DeCarli, McIntosh, & Daly, 1996). Thus, the earlier onset of brain atrophy in men may lead to a divergence in cognitive abilities between the sexes in older age.

Finally, comparison of studies conducted in the 1970s and later as compared to data collected on prior decades has suggested that gender differences in cognition have declined over the last 30 years, perhaps due to changes in parental socialization practices or more equitable school environments. As a result, measurement of cognitive skills in older cohorts could be expected to reveal greater differences between the sexes than that observed in younger generations.

In conclusion, the available literature would suggest that use and selection of normative data for clinical interpretation of neuropsychological tests requires consideration of gender for motor strength and dexterity measures, and perhaps for math, fund of general information, verbal memory, eye–hand speed/coordination, and select executive tasks, especially in older populations.

References

Allen, L. S., Richey, M. F., Chai, Y. M., & Gorski, R. A. (1991). Sex differences in the corpus callosum of the living human being. *Journal of Neuroscience, 11*, 933–942.

Andreasen, N. C., Flaum, M., Swayze, V. W., O'Leary, D. S., Alliger, R., Cohen, G., Ehrhardt, J., & Yuh, W. T. (1993). Intelligence and brain structure in normal individuals. *Journal of Psychiatry, 150*, 130–134.

Andreason, P. J., Zametkin, A. J., Guo, A. C., Baldwin, P., & Cohen, R. M. (1994). Gender-related differences in regional cerebral glucose metabolism in normal volunteers. *Psychiatry Research, 51*, 175–183.

Ankney, C. D. (1992). Sex differences in relative brain size: The mismeasure of woman, too? *Intelligence, 16*, 329–336.

Ardila, A., & Rosselli, M. (1989). Neuropsychological characteristics of normal aging. *Developmental Neuropsychology, 5*, 307–320.

Ardila, A., Rosselli, M., & Rosas, P. (1989). Neuropsychological assessment in illiterates: Visuospatial and memory abilities. *Brain and Cognition, 11*, 147–166.

Azari, N. P., Rapoport, S. I., Grady, C. L., & DeCarli, C. (1992). Gender differences in correlations of cerebral glucose metabolic rates in young normal adults. *Brain Research, 574*, 198–208.

Baxter, L. R., Mazziotta, J. C., Phelps, M. E., Selin, C. E., Guze, B. H., & Fairbanks, L. (1987). Cerebral glucose metabolic rates in normal human females versus normal males. *Psychiatry Research, 21*, 237–245.

Bennett-Levy, J. (1984). Determinants of performance on the Rey–Osterrieth Complex Figure Test: An analysis, and a new technique for single-case assessment. *British Journal of Clinical Psychology, 23*, 109–119.

Berenbaum, S. A., Baxter, L., Seidenberg, M., & Hermann, B. (1997). Role of the hippocampus in sex differences in verbal memory: Memory outcome following left anterior temporal lobectomy. *Neuropsychology, 11*, 585–591.

Berry, D. T. R., Allen, R. S., & Schmitt, F. A. (1991). Rey–Osterrieth Complex Figure: Psychometric characteristics in a geriatric sample. *The Clinical Neuropsychologist, 5*, 143–153.

Bleecker, M. L., Bolla-Wilson, K., Agnew, J., & Meyers, D. A. (1988). Age-related sex differences in verbal memory. *Journal of Clinical Psychology, 44*, 403–411.

Bolla, K. I., Lindgren, K. N., Bonaccorsy, C., & Bleecker, M. L. (1990). Predictors of verbal fluency (FAS) in the healthy elderly. *Journal of Clinical Psychology, 46*, 623–628.

Bolla-Wilson, K., & Bleecker, M. L. (1986). Influence of verbal intelligence, sex, age, and education on the Rey Auditory Verbal Learning Test. *Developmental Neuropsychology, 2*, 203–211.

Boone, K. B., Ghaffarian, S., Lesser, I. M., Hill-Gutierrez, E., & Berman, N. (1993). Wisconsin Card Sorting Test performance in healthy, older adults: Relationship to age, sex, education and IQ. *Journal of Clinical Psychology, 49*, 54–60.

Boone, K. B., Lesser, I. M., Hill-Gutierrez, E., Berman, N. (1993). Rey–Osterrieth complex figure performance in healthy, older adults: Relationship to age, education, sex, and IQ. *The Clinical Neuropsychologist, 7*, 22–28.

Boone, K. B. (1999). Clinical neuropsychological assessment of executive functions: Impact of age, education, gender, intellectual level, and vascular status on executive test scores. In B. L. Miller and J. L. Cummings (Eds.), *The frontal lobes.* New York: Guilford.

Bornstein, R. A. (1985). Normative data on selected neuropsychological measures from a nonclinical sample. *Journal of Clinical Psychology, 41*, 651–659.

Brandon, A. D., Chavez, E. L., & Bennett, T. L. (1986). A comparative evaluation of two neuropsychological finger tapping instruments: Halstead–Reitan and Western Psychological Services. *International Journal of Clinical Neuropsychology, 8*, 64–65.

Breedlove, S. M. (1994). Sexual differentiation of the human nervous system. *Annual Review of Psychology, 45*, 389–418.

Brouwers, P., Cox, C., Martin, A., Chase T., & Fedio, P. (1984). Differential perceptual-spatial impairment in Huntington's and Alzheimer's dementia. *Archives of Neurology, 41*, 1073–1076.

Buckelew, S. P., & Hannay, H. G. (1986). Relationships among anxiety, defensiveness, sex, task difficulty, and performance on various neuropsychological tasks. *Perceptual and Motor Skills, 63*, 711–718.

Cauthen, N. R. (1978). Verbal fluency: Normative data. *Journal of Clinical Psychology, 34*, 126–129.

Chavez, E. L., Schwartz, M. M., & Brandon, A. (1982). Effects of sex of subject and method of block presentaton the Tactual Performance Test. *Journal of Consulting and Clinical Psychology, 50*, 600–601.

Chavez, E. L., Trautt, G. M., Brandon, A., & Steyaert, J. (1983). Effects of test anxiety and sex of subject on neuropsychological test performance: Finger Tapping, Trail Making, Digit Span and Digit Symbol tests. *Perceptual and Motor Skills, 56*, 923–929.

Cohen, Andres, & Smolen, as cited in Mitrushina, M. N., Boone, K. B., & D'Elia, L. F. (1999). *Handbook of normative data for neuropsychological assessment.* New York: Oxford University Press.

Coman, E., Moses, J. A. Jr., Kraemer, H. C., Friedman, L., Benton, A. L., & Yesavage, J. (1999). Geriatric performance on Benton Visual Retention Test: Demographic and diagnostic considerations. *The Clinical Neuropsychologist, 13*, 66–77.

Connor, A., Fanzen, M. D., & Sharp, B. (1988). Effects of practice and differential instructions on Stroop performance. *International Journal of Clinical Neuropsychology, 10*, 1–4.

Davies, A. D. (1968). The influence of age on Trail Making Test performance. *Journal of Clinical Psychology, 24*, 96–98.

deLacoste-Utamsing, C., & Holloway, R. L. (1982). Sexual dimorphism in the human corpus callosum. *Science, 216*, 1431–1432.

Delis, D. C., Kramer, J. H., Kaplan, E., & Ober, B. A. (1987). *The California Verbal Learning Test.* New York: Psychological Corporation.

Dodrill, C. B. (1979). Sex differences on the Halstead–Reitan Neuropsychological Battery and on the neuropsychological measures. *Journal of Clinical Psychology, 35*, 236–241.

Echternacht, R. (1981). Neuropsychological assessment of motor functioning: The Finger Tapping Test: Data on adult, female, inpatient psychiatric population. *Clinical Neuropsychology, 3*, 8–9.

Ernst, J. (1987). Neuropsychological problem-solving skills in the elderly. *Psychology & Aging, 2*, 363–365.

Ernst, J. (1988). Languate, grip strength, sensory-perceptual, and receptive skills in a normal elderly sample. *The Clinical Neuropsychologist, 2*, 30–40.

Fabian, M. S., Jenkins, R. L., & Parsons, O. A. (1981). Gender, alcoholism, and neuropsychological functioning. *Journal of Consulting and Clinical Psychology, 49*, 138–140.

Fastenau, P. S., Denburg, N. L., & Mauer, B. A. (1997). Parallel short forms for the Boston Naming Test: Psychometric properties and norms for older adults. *Journal of Clinical and Experimental Neuropsychology, 20*, 828–834.

Fastenau, P. S., Denburg, N. L., & Hufford, B. J. (1999). Adult norms for the Rey–Osterrieth Complex Figure Test and for supplemental recognition and matching trials from the Extended Complex Figure Test. *The Clinical Neuropsychologist, 13*, 30–47.

Filskov, S. B., & Catanese, R. A. (1986). Effects of sex and handedness on neuropsychological testing. In S. B. Filskov & T. J. Boll (Eds.). *Handbook of clinical neuropsychology* (vol. 2. New York: Wiley.

Fromm-Auch, D., & Yeudall, L. T. (1983). Normative data for the Halstead-Reitan Neuropsychological Tests. *Journal of Clinical Neuropsychology, 5*, 221–238.

Gaddes, W. H., & Crockett, D. J. (1975). The Spreen-Benton Aphasia Tests, normative data as a measure of normal language development. *Brain and Language, 2*, 257–280.

Ganguli, M., Ratcliff, G., Huff, F. J., Belle, S., Kancel, M. J., Fischer, L., Seaberg, E. C., & Kuller, L. H. (1991). Effects of age, gender, and education on cognitive tests in a rural elderly community sample. Norms from the Monongahela Valley Independent Elders Survey. *Neuroepidemiology, 10*, 45–52.

Geffen, G., Moar, K. J., O'Hanlon, A. P., & Clark, C. R. (1990). Performance measures of 16- to 86-year-old males and females on the Auditory Verbal Learning Test. *The Clinical Neuropsychologist, 4*, 45–63.

Giedd, F. N., Snell, J. W., Lange, N., Rajapakse, J. C., Casey, B. J., Kozuch, P. L., Vaituzis, A. C., Vauss, Y. C., Hamburger, S. D., Kaysen, D., & Rapoport, J.L. (1996). Quantitative magnetic resonance imaging of human brain development: Ages 4–18. *Cerebral Cortex, 6*, 551–560.

Giovagnoli, A. R., Pesce, D., Mascheroni, S., Simoncelli, M., Laiacona, M., & Capitani, E. (1996). Trail making test: Normative values from 287 normal adults controls. *Italian Journal of Neurological Sciences, 17*, 305–309.

Golden, C. (1978). *Stroop Color and Word Test: Manual for clinical and experimental uses.* Chicago: Stoelting.

Gordon, N. G., & O'Dell, J. W. (1983). Sex differences in neurospychological performance. *Perceptual and Motor Skills, 56,* 126.

Gur, R. E., & Gur, R. C. (1990). Gender differences in regional blood flow. *Schizophrenia Bulletin, 16,* 247–254.

Gur, R. C., Gur, R. E., Obrist, W. D., Hungerbuhler, J. P., Younkin, D., Rosen, A. D., Skolnick, B. E., & Reivich, M. (1982). Sex and handedness differences in cerebral blood flow during rest and cognitive activity. *Science, 217,* 659–661.

Gur, R. C., Mozley, L. H., Mozley, P. D., Resnick, S. M., Karp, J. S., Alavi, A., Arnold, S. E., & Gur, R. E. (1995). Sex differences in regional cerebral glucose metabolism during a resting state. *Science, 267,* 528–531.

Gur, R. C., Mozley, P. D., Resnick, S. M., Gottlieb, G. L., Kohn, M., Zimmerman, R., Herman, G., Atlas, S., Grossman, R., & Berretta, D. (1991). Gender differences in age effect on brain atrophy measured by magnetic resonance imaging. *Proceedings of the National Academy of Science, USA, 88,* 2845–2849.

Haier, R. J., & Benbow, C. P. (1995). Sex differences and lateralization in temporal lobe glucose metabolism during mathematical reasoning. *Developmental Neuropsychology, 11,* 405–414.

Halpern, D. F., & Crothers, M. (1997). Sex, sexual orientation, and cognition. In L. Ellis, & L. Ebertz (Eds.). *Sexual orientation: Toward biological understanding* (pp. 181–197). Westport, CT: Praeger.

Harris, M., Cross, H, & VanNieuwkerk, R. (1981). The effects of state depression, induced depression and sex on the Finger Tapping and Tactual Performance Tests. *Clinical Neuropsychology, 3,* 28–34.

Heaton, R. K., Grant, I., & Matthews, C. G. (1986). Differences in neuropsychological test performance associated with age, education, and sex. In I. Grant & K. Adams (Eds.), *Neuropsychological assessment of neuropsychiatric disorders* (pp. 100–120). New York: Oxford University Press.

Heaton, R. K., Grant, I., & Matthews, C. G. (1991). *Comprehensive norms for an expanded Halstead–Reitan Neuropsychological Battery: Demographic corrections, research findings, and clinical applications.* Odessa, FL: Psychological Assessment Resources.

Heaton, R. K., Chelune, G. J., Talley, J. L., Kay, G. G., & Curtiss, G. (1993). *Wisconsin Card Sorting Test manual.* Odessa, FL: Psychological Assessment Resources.

Hilgert, L. D., & Treloar, J. H. (1985). The relationship of the Hooper Visual Organization Test to sex, age, and intelligence of elementary school children. *Measurement and Evaluation in Counseling and Development, 17,* 203–206.

Hoffman, D. T. (1969). Sex difference in preferred finger tapping rates. *Perceptual and Motor Skills, 29,* 676.

Houx, P. J., Jolles, J., & Vreeling, F. W. (1993). Stroop interference: Aging effects assessed with the Stroop Color-Word Test. *Experimental Aging Research, 19,* 209–224.

Ivison, D. (1977). The Wechsler Memory Scale: Preliminary findings toward an Australian standardization. *Australian Psychologist, 12,* 303–312.

Ivnik, R. J., Malec, J. F., Smith, G. E., & Tangalos, E. G. (1996). Neuropsychological tests' norms above age 55: COWAT, BNT, MAE, Token, WRAT-R Reading, AMNART, STROOP, TMT, and JLO. *Clinical Neuropsycyhologist, 10,* 262–278.

Jensen, A. R., & Rohwer, W. D. (1966). The Stroop Color-Word Test: A review. *Acta Psychologica, Amsterdam, 25,* 36–93.

Kimura, D., & Harshman, R. A. (1984). Sex differences in brain organization for verbal and non-verbal functions. *Progress in Brain Research, 61,* 423–441.

King, G. D., Hannay, H. J., Masek, B. J., & Burns, J. W. (1978). Effects of anxiety and sex on neuropsychological tests. *Journal of Consulting and Clinical Psychology, 46,* 375–376.

King, M. C. (1981). Effects of non-focal brain dysfunction on visual memory. *Journal of Clinical Psychology, 37,* 638–643.

Koffler, S. P., & Zehler, D. (1985). Normative data for the hand dynamometer. *Perceptual and Motor Skills, 61,* 589–590.

Kramer, J. H., Delis, D. C., & Daniel, M. (1988). Sex differences in verbal learning. *Journal of Clinical Psychology, 44,* 907–915.

Kupke, T. (1983). Effects of subject sex, examiner sex, and test apparatus on Halstead Category and Tactual Performance Tests. *Journal of Consulting and Clinical Psychology, 51,* 624–626.

LaBarge, E., Edwards, D., & Knesevich, J. W. (1986). Performance of normal elderly on the Boston Naming Test. *Brain and Language, 27,* 380–384.

Lee, G. P., Strauss, E., Loring, D. W., McCloskey, L., Haworth, J. M., & Lehman, R. A. W. (1997). Sensitivity of figural fluency on the Five-Point Test to focal neurological dysfunction. *The Clinical Neuropsychologist, 11,* 59–68.

Levy, J., & Heller, W. (1992). Gender differences in human neuropsychological function. In A. A. Gerall, H. Moltz, & L. W. Ingeborg (Eds.), *Sexual differentation. Handbook of behavioral neurobiology* (vol. 11, pp. 245–274). New York: Plenum.

Lewontin, R. C., Rose, D., & Kamin, L. J. (1984). *Not in our genes*, New York: Pantheon.

Lindman, K., Boone, K., Lesser, I., & Miller, B. (1998). Does estrogen replacement therapy protect cognitive ability in postmenopausal women? Poster presented at the 1998 International Neuropsychological Society Meeting in Honolulu, Hawaii.

Maccoby, E. E., & Jacklin, C. N. (1974). *The psychology of sex differences*. Stanford, CA: Stanford University Press.

Mansour, C. S., Haier, R. J., & Buchsbaum, M. S. (1996). Gender comparisons of cerebral glucose metabolic rate in healthy adults during a cognitive task. *Personality and Individual Differences, 20,* 183–191.

Matarazzo, J. D. (1972). *Wechsler measurement and appraisal of adult intelligence* (5th ed.). New York: Oxford University Press.

Mathew, R. J., Wilson, W. H., & Tant, S. R. (1986). Determinants of resting regional cerebral blood flow in normal subjects. *Biological Psychiatry, 21,* 907–914.

Mazaux, J. M., Dartigues, J. F., Letenneur, L., Darriet, D., Wiart, L., Gagnon, M., Commenges, D., & Boller, F. (1995). Visuo-spatial attention and psychomotor performance in elderly community residents: Effects of age, gender, and education. *Journal of Clinical and Experimental Neuropsychology, 17,* 71–81.

McKeever, W. F., & Abramson, M. (1991). Halstead and Halstead–Reitan norms for Finger Tapping Test are severely biased against females and left-handers. *Journal of Clinical and Experimental Neuropsychology, 13,* 91.

Morrison, M. W., Gregory, R. J., & Paul, J. J. (1979). Reliability of the Finger Tapping Test and a note on sex differences. *Perceptual and Motor Skills, 48,* 139–142.

Murphy, D. G. M., DeCarli, C., McIntosh, A. R., & Daly, E. (1996). Sex differences in human brain morphometry and metabolism: An in vivo quantitative magnetic resonance imaging and positron emission tomography study on the effect of aging. *Archives of General Psychiatry, 53,* 585–594.

Pauker, J. D. (1980). *Norms for the Halstead–Reitan Neuropsychological Test Battery based on a nonclinical adult sample*. Address presented at the meeting of the Canadian Psychological Association, Calgary, Alberta, Canada.

Polubinski, J. P., & Melamed, L. E. (1986). Examination of the sex difference on a symbol digit substitution test. *Perceptual and Motor Skills, 62,* 975–982.

Ponton, M. O., Satz, P., Herrera, L., Ortiz, F., Urrutia, C., Young, R., D'Elia, L., Furst, C., & Namerow, N. (1996). Normative data stratified by age and education for the Neuropsychological Screening Battery for Hispanics (NeSBHIS): Initial report. *Journal of the International Neuropsychological Society, 2,* 96–104.

Portin, R., Saarijarvi, S., Joukamaa, M., & Salokangas, R. K. R. (1995). Education, gender, and cognitive performance in a 62-year-old normal population: Results from the Turva Project. *Psychological Medicine, 25,* 1295–1298.

Reiss, A. L., Abrams, M. T., Singer, H. S., Ross, J. L., & Denckla, M. B. (1996). Brain development, gender and IQ in children. A volumetric imaging study. *Brain, 119,* 1763–1774.

Reitan, R. M., & Wolfson, D. (1989). The seashore rhythm test and brain functions. *The Clinical Neuropsychologist, 3,* 70–78.

Ripich, D. N., Petrill, S. A., Whitehouse, P. J., & Ziol, E. W., et al. (1995). Gender differences in language of AD patients: A longitudinal study. *Neurology, 45,* 299–302.

Rodriguez, G., Warkentin, S., Risberg, J., & Rosadini, G. (1988). Sex differences in regional cerebral blood flow. *Journal of Cerebral Blood Flow and Metabolism, 8,* 783–789.

Rosselli, M., & Ardila, A. (1991). Effects of age, education, and gender on the Rey–Osterrieth Complex Figure. *The Clinical Neuropsychologist, 5,* 370–376.

Rounsaville, B. J., Jones, C., Novelly, R. A., & Kleber, H. (1982). Neuropsychological functioning in opiate addicts. *The Journal of Nervous and Mental Disease, 170,* 209–216.

Ruff, R. M., Light, R. H., Parker, S. B., & Levin, H. S. (1996). Benton Controlled Oral Word Association Test: Reliability and updated norms. *Archives of Clinical Neuropsychology, 11,* 329–338.

Ruff, R. M., & Parker, S. B. (1993). Gender- and age-specific changes in motor speed and eye-hand coordination in adults: Normative values for the Finger Tapping and Grooved Pegboard tests. *Perceptual and Motor Skills, 76,* 1219–1230.

Rushton, J. P., & Ankney, C. D. (1996). Brain size and cognitive ability: Correlations with age, sex, social class, and race. *Psychonomic Bulletin and Review, 3,* 21–36.

Savage, R. M., & Gouvier, W. D. (1992). Rey Auditory Verbal Learning Test: The effects of age and gender, and norms for delayed recall and story recognition trials. *Archives of Clinical Neuropsychology, 7,* 407–414.

Saykin, A. J., Gur, R. C., Gur, R. E., Shtasel, D. L., Flanner, K. A., Mozley, L. H., Malamut, B., Watson, B., & Mozley, P. D. (1995). Normative neuropsychological test performance: Effects of age, education, gender and ethnicity. *Applied Neuropsychology, 2,* 79–88.

Schlaepfer, T. E., Harris, G. J., Tien, A. Y., Peng, L., Lee, S., & Pearlson, G. D. (1995). Structural differences in the cerebral cortex of healthy female and male subjects: A magnetic resonance imaging study. *Psychiatry Research, 61,* 129–135.

Seidenberg, M., Gamache, M. P., Smith, M., Sackellares, J. C., Beck, N. C., Giordani, B., Berent, S., & Boll, T. (1984).

Subject variables and performance on the Halstead Neuropsychological Test Battery: A multivariate analysis. *Journal of Consulting and Clinical Psychology, 52,* 658–662.

Snow, W. G., & Weinstock, J. (1990). Sex differences among non-brain-damaged adults on the Wechsler Adult Intelligence Scales: A review of the literature. *Journal of Clinical and Experimental Neuropsychology, 12,* 873–886.

Strickland, T. L., D'Elia, L. F., James, R., & Stein, R. (1997). Stroop color-word performance of African Americans. *The Clinical Neuropsychologist, 11,* 87–90.

Stroop, J. R. (1935). Studies of interference in serial verbal reactions. *Journal of Experimental Psychology, 18,* 643–662.

Stuss, D. T., Stethem, L. L., & Poirier, C. A. (1987). Comparison of three tests of attention and rapid information processing across six age groups. *The Clinical Neuropsychologist, 1,* 139–152.

Swerdlow, N. R., Filion, D., Geyer, M. A., & Braff, D. L. (1995). "Normal" personality correlates of sensorimotor, cognitive, and visuospatial gating. *Biological Psychiatry, 37,* 286–299.

Thompson, L. L., Heaton, K. R., Matthews, C. G., & Grant, I. (1987). Comparisons of preferred and nonpreferred hand performance on four neuropsychological motor tasks. *The Clinical Neuropsychologist, 1,* 324–334.

Todd, R. D., Swarzenski, B., Rossi, P. G., & Visconti, P. (1995). Structural and functional development of the human brain. In D. Cicchetti, & D. J. Cohen (Eds.). *Developmental psychopathology, Vol. 1: Theory and methods* (pp. 161–194). New York: Wiley.

Tombaugh, T., Kozak, J., & Rees, L. (1999). Normative data stratified by age and education for two measures of verbal fluency: FAS and Animal Naming. *Archives of Clinical Neuropsychology, 14,* 167–177.

Trahan, D. E., & Quintana, J. W. (1990). Analysis of gender effects upon verbal and visual memory performance in adults. *Archives of Clinical Neuropsychology, 5,* 325–334.

Trahan, D. E., Quintana, J. W., Willingham, A. C., & Goethe, K. E. (1988). The Visual Reproduction subtest: Standardization and clinical validation of a delayed recall procedure. *Neuropsychology, 2,* 29–39.

Trautt, G. M., Chavez, E. L., Brandon, A. D., & Steyaert, J. (1983). Effects of test anxiety and sex of subject on neuropsychological test performance: Finger Tapping, Trail Making, Digit Span, and Digit Symbol Tests. *Perceptual and Motor Skills, 56,* 923–929.

Trenerry, M., Crosson, B., DeBoe, J., & Leber, W. (1989). *Stroop Neuropsychological Screening Test, Manual.* Odessa, FL: Psychological Assessment Resources.

Vakil, E., & Blachstein, H. (1997). Rey AVLT: Developmental norms for adults and the sensitivity of difference memory measures to age. *The Clinical Neuropsychologist, 11,* 356–369.

Veroff, A. E. (1980). The neuropsychology of aging: Qualitative analysis of visual reproductions. *Psychological Research, 41,* 259–268.

Welch, L. W., Doineau, D., Johnson, S., & King, D. (1996). Educational and gender normative data for the Boston Naming Test in a group of older adults. *Brain and Language, 53,* 260–266.

Wendt, P. E., & Risberg, J. (1994). Cortical activation during visual spatial processing: Relation between hemispheric asymmetry of blood flow and performance. *Brain and Cognition, 24,* 87–103.

Wiens, A. N., Fuller, K. H., & Crossen, J. R. (1997). Paced Auditory Serial Addition Test: Adult norms and moderator variables. *Journal of Clinical and Experimental Neuropsychology, 19,* 473–483.

Wiens, A. N., McMinn, M. R., & Crossen, J. R. (1988). Rey Auditory-Verbal Learning Test: Development of norms for healthy young adults. *The Clinical Neuropsychologist, 2,* 67–87.

Wiens, A. D., Tindall, A. G., & Crossen, J. R. (1994). California Verbal Learning Test: A normative data study. *Neuropsychologist, 8,* 75–90.

Willerman, L., Schultz, R., Rutledge, J. N., & Bigler, E. D. (1992). Hemisphere size asymmetry predicts relative verbal and nonverbal intelligence differently in the sexes: An MRI study of structure-function relations. *Intelligence, 16,* 315–328.

Witelson, S. F. (1989). Hand and sex differences in the isthmus and genu of the human corpus callosum. A postmortem morphological study. *Brain, 112,* 799–835.

Witelson, S. F. (1990). Structural correlates of cognition in the human brain. In A. B. Scheibel & A. F. Wechsler (Eds.). *Neurobiology of higher cognitive function. UCLA forum in medical sciences* (No. 29). (pp. 167–183). New York: Guilford.

Witelson, S. F., & Kigar, D. L. (1988). Anatomical development of the corpus callosum in humans: A review with reference to sex and cognition. In D. L. Molfese & S. J. Segalowitz (Eds.), *Brain lateralization in children: Developmental implications* (pp. 35–57). New York: Guilford.

Yeudall, L. T., Fromm, D., Reddon, J. R., & Stefanyk, W. O. (1986). Normative data stratified by age and sex for 12 neuropsychological tests. *Journal of Clinical Psychology, 42,* 918–946.

Yeudall, L. T., Reddon, J. R., Gill, D. M., & Stefanyk, W. O. (1987). Normative data for the Halstead-Reitan neuropsychological tests stratified by age and sex. *Journal of Clinical Psychology, 43,* 346–367.

Young, K. L., & Delay, E. R. (1993). Seashore Rhythm Test: Comparison of signal detection theory and standard scoring procedures. *Archives of Clinical Neuropsychology, 8,* 111–121.

7

Neuropsychological Assessment of Hispanics

ANTONIO E. PUENTE AND ALFREDO ARDILA

In a volume on cultural aspects of clinical neuropsychology, a reader living in the United States, or for that matter the Americas, would certainly expect to find a chapter on Hispanics. Hispanics represent not only the fastest growing ethnic minority in the United States but represent a unique challenge to those who have a traditional view of ethnic minorities (i.e., ethnic minorities are essentially all African American). Hispanics represent an important challenge to those working in the field of clinical neuropsychology and it is the purpose of this chapter to explain not only those challenges but also their potential solutions.

The chapter begins by defining Hispanic emphasizing what is traditionally considered to be "Hispanic," such as language differences. In addition, less obvious issues are explored as well including educational, economic, religious, and psychological variables. This approach provides a foundation for addressing potential cultural differences between Hispanics and other groups, including other ethnic minorities, in neuropsychological abilities and performance. The second section focuses on neuropsychological research on Hispanics and clinical knowledge. A review of the literature, including the problems and limitations of existing knowledge, is considered. The third section comprises the major portion of the chapter. This section addresses such issues as heterogeneity of Hispanics, translation of tests, data and norms, cultural and cognitive equivalence, and the use of time. The fourth section focuses on potential solutions to these problems. This section includes the need for more research, personnel, understanding, public policy, and support from test publishers. The rationale for the preceding concerns is based not just on sociopolitical foundations but on the consideration of clinical experience and the scientific literature. The chapter ends with a summary and direction, both for short and long term possibilities.

The authors' intention is to synthesize existing concepts and research. It is important to note that the existing literature is not extensive. Further, some of the previously published work that will be considered is anecdotal, clinical, or theoretical. The critical question underlying the neuropsychological assessment of Hispanics is whether English and Spanish tests are actually measuring the same variables.

ANTONIO E. PUENTE • University of North Carolina-Wilmington, Wilmington, North Carolina 38406. **ALFREDO ARDILA** • Miami, Florida 33182.

Handbook of Cross-Cultural Neuropsychology, edited by Fletcher-Janzen, Strickland, and Reynolds. Kluwer Academic/Plenum Publishers, New York, 2000.

Defining Hispanic

Merriam-Webster's Collegiate Dictionary defines the term Hispanic as relating to the people, speech, or culture of Spain and Portugal, or Latin America. The *Diccionario de la Lengua Española* (The Dictionary of the Spanish Language, [Real Academia Española, 1984]), edited by the Royal Spanish Academy, defines the word Hispanic as pertaining to (or relative to) Spain or the nations of Latin America. Seemingly, there is a basic agreement in terminology, even though according to *Merriam-Webster's Collegiate Dictionary*, Portugal and Brazil would be included as Hispanic nations. Hispanic is usually defined in the United States as a person whose primary (or, in some cases, secondary) language is Spanish. Further, there is an assumption that their heritage is of Spanish origin with their eventual roots being traceable back to Spain. Few, if any other, variables are factored into the definition of this ethnic group. These assumptions are misleading, maybe even incorrect. As a consequence, several important issues that help define Hispanic will be considered prior to addressing the primary focus of this chapter, the neuropsychology of the Spanish speaker.

According to the U.S. Bureau of the Census (1999) the total Hispanic population of the U.S. currently accounts for over 29 million people (11% of the total U.S. population). Of these Hispanics, 63% are of Mexican origin, 14.4% are of Central and South American origin, 10.6% are mainland Puerto Ricans (residents of Puerto Rico are not included in these statistics), 4.2% are of Cuban ancestry, and 7.4% are classified as being of "Other origin." The distribution of the Hispanic population in the United States, however, is quite uneven. Mexicans are concentrated in the southwestern states, especially California and Texas. Puerto Ricans mostly live in New York. In south Florida it is estimated that over half of the Hispanic population is Cuban. Taking into account not only the significant number of Spanish speakers, but also the fact that there is one Spanish-speaking associate state (Puerto Rico), the United States can be regarded, to a certain extent, as a partially Spanish-speaking country.

Heterogeneity

Hispanics are not a unified ethnic group. One could easily divide this group into individuals living or from the Iberian peninsula (i.e., Spain) and those living in or from the Americas. Those from Spain tend in many respects to be more similar to other Europeans than to Latin Americans. It is anticipated that the commonality will be further enhanced with the development of the European Union. In contrast, Hispanics in the United States have a form of the Spanish language, customs, and behaviors more akin with Latin American countries.

Hispanics living in or from the Americas could be further subdivided into two groups; North America (excepting Mexico) versus Mexico, Central and South America. Individuals living in or from the United States and Canada are more likely to have some knowledge of English and the American way of living. This could include an understanding of standardized testing, the importance of time and time-based productivity, and competition in academic situations. Thus, although data is lacking in this area, Hispanics from the United States are more likely than their Mexican, Central, and South American counterparts to appear similar to North American cohorts on standardized testing.

Individuals living in Latin America (i.e., Mexico, Central and South America) should also be further subdivided into subcultural groups. For the initial work on the translation of the Wechsler scales, a panel of experts from a variety of Latin-American countries subdivided Latin Americans into the following categories: Caribbean (e.g., Cuba), Mexican, Central American (e.g., Panama), and South American (e.g., Argentina). It was the belief of the working group that some minor language differences existed between these groups. Further, there are small yet important differences in food, dress, and customs that prevent an easy and justifiable generalization across all subgroups.

Regionalisms or vernacular idiosyncrasies with respect to vocabulary exist in the use of Spanish. This is valid with any large language including English, Chinese, Russian, and so forth. Spanish is the primary language spoken in at least nineteen countries within the Western Hemisphere. Given the expansive geographic distribution and the huge number of speakers (some 400 million), regionalisms in vocabulary usage are common. Each country will also have its own slang terms that are commonly used in conversational speech. Minor phonological variations are also noted. In many Spanish-speaking areas S and Z as well as LL and Y correspond to a single phoneme. The affricate /ch/ sometimes becomes the fricative /sh/. Regional variations in the production of other phonemes are also found. Nonetheless, in general Spanish is a well unified language, and there is a standard Spanish (as there is also a standard English) that is easily understood by any Spanish speaker.

Confounding Variables

Hispanics are an ethnic group, like African Americans, Asian Americans, and Native Americans. Unlike those groups, however, Hispanics are not a race. In fact, Hispanics, although mainly Caucasians, also include people of color, including Native Americans, Asians, and blacks. Thus, Hispanics are multiracial and, depending on the area of interest, one race might be more represented than another (Shorris, 1992).

For a number of reasons, ranging from economic to sociopolitical, Hispanics have not achieved the level of educational attainment typically seen in the United States even when compared to other ethnic groups (Shorris, 1992). This decreased educational attainment holds true for both Hispanics living in and outside of the United States, regardless of their country of origin. There is growing evidence both in the neuropsychological literature (e.g., Lezak, 1995; Spreen & Strauss, 1998) in general, and with Hispanics in particular (e.g., Ardila, Rosselli, & Puente, 1994), that education plays an important role in the expression of brain function. Non–brain-damaged Hispanic illiterates appeared neuropsychologically highly similar to a portion of educated, brain-damaged persons (Ardila et al., 1994). Recent data in the United States (U.S. Bureau of the Census, 1999) suggest that Hispanics drop out of school almost three times as much as both their white counterparts (i.e., Anglo- or European Americans) as well as African Americans. In addition, Hispanics in the United States tend to start school later than average relative to other groups, and exit much earlier (Shorris, 1992). In the context of neuropsychological assessment of Hispanics education has to be carefully understood.

When testing people of low educational levels a significant error is frequently found, so in psychology as in neuropsychology: When normalizing psychological and neuropsychological instruments, people with 10 years of education and below are most frequently considered a homogenous educational group. Research has demonstrated that the educational effect on neuropsychological test performance is not a linear effect. Differences between zero and three years of education are usually highly significant; differences between three and six years of education can be lower; between six and nine are even lower, and so on. Virtually no differences are found between, for example, 12 and 15 years of education. This means the educational effect represents a kind of negatively accelerated curve, tending toward a plateau (Ardila, 1998a; Ostrosky, Ardila, Rosselli, Lopez-Arango, & Uriel-Mendoza, 1998). As a consequence, it is frankly erroneous to consider people with fewer than 10 years of education a homogenous group.

Religion and the understanding of the physical causes of diseases are similarly important variables. As a consequence, understanding and acceptance of neuropsychological assessment can be affected. However, the impact of religion on everyday life is extremely variable among Hispanics. For many Hispanics religion is simply a non-existing issue in life or it is just formally maintained as part of the culture. Many other Hispanics, on the other hand, view disease as something God has given them and could, with prayer and support, take back. Thus, appreciation of even the basic reasons for a neuropsychological assessment may be missing in this population of individuals.

Psychologists often misunderstand customs and traditions, especially as they pertain to psychological assessment. There are several important factors that are rarely appreciated (e.g., Perez-Arce & Puente, 1996; Puente & Salazar, 1998). These include time, relationship to examiner, and competitiveness. Time in Hispanic cultures is often something to be cherished, appreciated, and not necessarily conquered. Speed may not be so important: Good products are usually the result of a careful process, and quality and rush may be contradictory. Productivity and speed are often seen as less crucial by Hispanics, as enjoying life is more useful. Time is something, for example, that one spends together with friends and family. In contrast, other Americans have very intensive exposure and training in testing. For them, testing is a challenge and one is expected to perform his or her best and quickly. For Hispanics, it may be more important to be courteous with the examiner and establish a good rapport rather than perform well. It may be significant to have the opportunity to talk and interchange ideas. That is, the personal relationship with the examiner may be more important than the results of the evaluation. Competitiveness is also viewed with suspicion. Cooperation and social ability are by far more important. For example, in Hispanic cultures being "educated" implies having social skills, not necessarily educational attainment. In fact, it is not uncommon for an individual with a college degree to be thought of as uneducated because of arrogance and unpoliteness. Further, education in Latin American countries is not synonymous with the United States. For example, a college degree in Latin America equals a master's degree in the United States, both in the scope of education and the number of years of college required.

Acculturation

Another very critical, if not the most critical, factor in the neuropsychological assessment of Hispanics is acculturation. This concept is broadly defined as an individual's ability to understand and maneuver outside the culture that he or she was raised in and are most familiar with (Berry, 1997). The underlying question is, What is the criterion? In other words, What is being measured? It could be argued that the ultimate criterion in neuropsychological measurement is whether the patient has the ability to understand and answer the question correctly enough so that the examiner finds the answer to be generally "normal." This criterion is quite different from whether a brain injury actually exists. In other words, the issue ends up being whether the patient can perform the task, and nothing more. Hence, what could be measured in a neuropsychological evaluation may actually be acculturation of the patient. If the patient understands the value of time, and time is used to assess brain function (as is often the case), then the uninjured individual will respond in the allocated time. If the first premise is not true, the patient comes across as being brain-damaged (Ardila et al., 1994). Hispanics might not have understood that they had to respond as quickly as possible (something very "foreign" to them). To ignore this important concern will surely result in exaggeration of false positives.

Degree of acculturation is quite variable among Hispanics in the United States. Patterns of behavior, beliefs, and values among Hispanics living in the United States, however, tend to become progressively more similar to the middle-class American standards over time (Shorris, 1992). Thus, Hispanics living in the United States present mixed patterns of behaviors and eventually integrate their Latin values with the middle-class American values. Sometimes integration is not easy and conflict results.

Bilingualism

Bilingualism in general represents a rather complex phenomenon, but Spanish–English bilingualism in the United States is an extremely complex issue. Bilingualism in general depends upon the specific cultural context. The type of relationship between both culture groups represents one of the most the crucial points. For Hispanics in the United States, Spanish and English are not in conflict and the "rules of the game" are clear enough: English is the official language, Spanish is the informal one. But, combinations of Spanish, English and "Spanglish" (mixture of Spanish and English due to borrowings and code-switchings) are found. These combinations occur with regard to age of acquisition, proficiency (oral and written), preference (likely correlated with the degree of cultural identification), and patterns of use (English, Spanish, and any type of combination and mixture can be imagined) (Ardila, 1998b). The language spoken at home and at work can be English, Spanish, or any type of mixture of both.

Several distinctions have been proposed for grouping bilinguals. The distinction between early and late bilingualism seems to be the simplest one and the most extensively used (Manuel-Dupont, Ardila, Rosselli, & Puente, 1992). Early bilingual means the individual learned the second language before the age of about 12. Later acquisition of a second language will be mediated through the first language, and second language learning will be incomplete. The distinction among coordinate, compound, and subordinate bilingualism also has been extensively used. The coordinate bilingual is an early bilingual who can function as a native speaker of each language. These distinctions, though useful, are insufficient, as a particular bilingual can be classified in more than one group. There are many factors capable of affecting the ability to speak and understand a second language, but also there is the factor that bilingualism appears under quite different contexts and diverse circumstances.

Some variables are considered crucial to pinpoint the degree of bilingualism: age and sequence of acquisition, method of acquisition, schooling language, contexts of the two languages, patterns of use of the two languages, personal and social attitudes toward each language, and even individual differences in verbal abilities (Ardila, 1998b). However, these are only general variables and many variations can be found.

1. The age, sequence, and method of acquisition are not necessarily correlated with the degree of mastery of each language. As an example, many Hispanics in the United States initially learned Spanish in their native countries and used only Spanish until the age of five or six. Later, these people moved to the United States, and years later, they have serious difficulty speaking Spanish whereas they speak English fluently.

2. Schooling language can be indeed a highly significant and decisive variable. In fact, it may be the most crucial variable. Nonetheless, many children attend classes in English but communicate among each other in Spanish. And in general, the degree of exposure to either language can be extremely variable (e.g., home language, TV, neighbors, friends).

3. Personal and social attitudes toward the two languages can present significant variations. Some Hispanics in the United States consider that what is really important is to

learn proper English; Spanish matters considerably less, if at all. Others consider it important to maintain proficiency in Spanish. Thus, they expect their children not only to learn to speak Spanish, but also to read, to write, and even to appreciate Spanish language literature. A significant percentage of Hispanics falls between these two anchors. Their location in this spectrum is probably related to the degree of cultural identification, the type of links maintained with the native countries, their age, the community in which they live, and so forth. Again, significant heterogeneity exists in bilingual abilities.

4. Individual differences in the ability to learn a second language has not been a frequent topic in bilingualism literature (Kilborn, 1994). But evidently, very significant differences have been observed in the ability to learn and use not only a first, but also a second language.

Linguistic idiosyncrasies may influence the results in psychological and neuropsychological testing. For an example, spelling is not used in testing in Spanish—or in any language relying on a phonological writing, such as Italian or Russian. The overtrained ability to spell observed in English speakers has some general linguistic consequences. The use of spelled abbreviations is common in English, but not in Spanish. No native Spanish speaker would read UCLA as U, C, L, A, but /ukla/. Understanding abbreviated words such as MS or ADHD is extremely hard for Spanish speakers, and an intermediate decoding process ("multiple sclerosis," "attention deficit hyperactivity disorder") is usually required. This strong tendency to "spell" in English is observed even when saying numbers (345 is three, four, five). Spanish speakers prefer to cluster (345 is three hundred forty-five). English speakers do better in single digit span (about 7 digits) than Spanish speakers (about 5.2 digits), and it could be conjectured that Spanish speakers would do better in multiple-digit span (e.g., 34, 76, etc.). Interestingly, using bilingual subjects, digit span was found larger (closer to the English norm) when performing in English, and shorter (closer to the Spanish norm) when performing this test in Spanish (Ardila et al., in press).

Most Hispanics in the United States are bilinguals to different degrees, and quite often bilinguals may be at a significant disadvantage when tested in either language (Ardila et al., in press). A bilingual can be considered not just as the speaker of two different languages, but as the speaker of an extended language (Grosjean, 1989). Both languages can be active languages. As a matter of fact, their functional language can be either Spanish or English, or a mixture of both. Interference between the languages is expected to be high. *To use either Spanish or English testing materials and norms can penalize United States Spanish–English bilinguals.* Unfortunately, a clear solution to this difficult situation is not yet available.

Three procedures, however, could at least reduce the *bilingualism effect* in psychological and neuropsychological testing.

1. Have special norms for Spanish–English bilinguals. This solution does not seem easy, taking into consideration the tremendous heterogeneity of United States bilingualism.
2. The examiner could be a bilingual mastering a similar type of biligualism. Testing could be performed in Spanish, English, and any combination of both languages. Instructions and answers in either language or any mixture of both languages could be acceptable; both English and Spanish norms could be used, preferring the one favoring the subject.
3. Scores could be adjusted to neutralize the penalizing effect of bilingualism. The problem here is that we do not know how much the test scores should be adjusted in order to achieve reasonable validity. Of course, it depends on the test, the idio-

syncrasies of the client's bilingualism, and the testing situation, including the examiner's language.

None of these three solutions alone or combined seems easy to effect. Regardless, when testing United States Hispanic bilinguals, it should be emphasized that *current results are not necessarily reflecting the real individual's abilities, and his/her real performance may be higher than observed.* Obviously, in any neuropsychological report on a bilingual, the degree of bilingualism should be reported. An estimate could be arrived at by considering the age of acquisition of the second language, schooling language, use of both languages in everyday life, language used in testing, and norms used. Caution regarding bilingual issues needs to be inserted within the context of the report as well.

Neuropsychological Assessment of Hispanics

The focus of this section of the chapter will be on a review of the literature. Unfortunately, some of the existing literature is based on anecdotal or case studies, theoretical orientation, or both rather than comprehensive data gathering and analysis. Many studies are conducted and published outside the United States so their applicability to the United States is in question. For example, in Spain, several programs of research exist including those in Barcelona (Junque), Granada (Perez), Madrid (Cespedes, Iruarrizaga, Tobal, & Cano). In Latin America, research is often carried out by non-psychologists (including neurologists) and issues of culture and ethnicity are not as central to their concerns. Further, Hispanics are not an ethnic group in Mexico and Central and South America, as they represent the majority.

As the Catalan group in Barcelona remains relatively isolated from the rest of Spain, the other regions (e.g., Andalucia) of Spain remain relatively isolated from each other. In Latin America, the traditional neuropsychological group has been the Latin American Society of Neuropsychology (SLAN). They have attempted to publish a journal but for numerous reasons it does not appear to be widely distributed or indexed by the major abstracting services. Another group (Asociacion Latinoamericana de Neuropsicologia, ALAN) was formed in April 1999 with the inaugural meeting held in Cartagena, Colombia. An important reason for the development of an alternative organization for Latin America appears to be the issue of the journal. *Neuropsicologia, Neuropsiquiatria y Neurociencias* started publishing in 1999. However, neuropsychology is viewed more from a multidisciplinary perspective in Latin America than it is in the United States. For example, in Barcelona, Spain, neurologists have primarily developed the neuropsychological research and clinical programs. One of the first published Spanish neuropsychological tests, which came from Barcelona and resembled the Luria–Nebraska Neuropsychological Battery, was developed by a team led by a neurologist.

This multidisciplinary pattern is in sharp contrast to the United States where neuropsychology is closely aligned with psychology. For example, the Hispanic Neuropsychological Society is a loosely formed group that meets at either one of the two main neuropsychological meetings held each year: the National Academy of Neuropsychology (NAN) and the International Neuropsychological Society (INS). With bylaws, elected officers, and dues the group has served mostly as a network of professionals, mostly Hispanic, interested in the neuropsychological assessment of the Spanish-speaking patient. Numerous individuals including Alfredo Ardila, Rusen Echemendia, Josette Harris, Tedd Judd, Patricia Linn-Fuentes, Gloria Morote, Patricia Perez-Arce, Marcel Ponton, Antonio Puente, and Monica Rosselli helped organize this society.

Unfortunately, however, out of the estimated 4,000 neuropsychologists in the United States, it is our estimate (based on our experience and the membership of the Hispanic Neuropsychological Society) that fewer than 50 neuropsychologists could be considered either bilingual or bicultural. Further, almost all of these neuropsychologists (as evidenced by the membership of the Hispanic Neuropsychological Society) are practitioners rather than researchers. This paucity of academicians may help explain the paucity in the research literature.

Methodological Problems

It is not uncommon to assume that testing Hispanics involves simply the translation of a test into Spanish. The assumption is that the major problem in adapting the test is simply the language. Indeed, this approach is typically used to assess Hispanics. For example, the Minnesota Multiphasic Personality Inventory (MMPI), which is the most common test used by neuropsychologists (Camara, Nathan & Puente, in press), has been translated into Spanish. However, the Spanish is intended to be applicable to all Hispanic subgroups and there are no norms associated with the test. In this section, the numerous methodological problems facing a simple translation of tests will be discussed. The issues to be considered include translation, translators, sampling and norms, cultural meaningfulness, and cognitive equivalence.

Translation

The most common assumption involving the application of psychological tests to Spanish speakers is that all that is needed for the test to be used with a Spanish speaker is a translation of the text (Echmendia, Harris, Congett, Diaz, & Puente, 1997). Anecdotal evidence obtained from members of the Hispanic Neuropsychological Society reveals that most members have idiosyncratic translations that they have adapted for their own personal use or, in many cases, special tests are "translated" as the test is being administered, much like what would be done in an interview. Based on what our colleagues tell us at the annual meetings, standardized procedures are rarely used (in part because, for example, norms are not available). Numerous authors have described these procedures but in this case the suggestions by Brislin (1983) are used. While we consider the approach of Brislin to be traditional, there are several reasons for pursuing this approach. First, some of the early research started on the neuropsychology of Hispanics used this conceptual framework. Secondly, the use of back-translation insures a safeguard of potential mistakes in the initial translation. However, it is important to emphasize that back-translations should provide a general, rather than a specific check on the initial translation. Avoiding a back-translation places undue emphasizes on the original translation.

According to Brislin, there are several basic steps that should be used:

1. Initial translation
2. Back translation
3. Resolution of differences between the original English version and the resulting Spanish version

More recently, Muniz and Hambleton (1996) published a summary of the International Test Commission's guidelines for the translation and adaptation of tests. The ethical guidelines are as follows:

- General guidelines for professional behavior
- Competence
- Responsibility
- Safety of the test materials
- Confidentiality

The general guidelines for appropriate use of tests include:

1. Understanding the testing situation
2. Selection of the appropriate tests
3. Consideration of potential biases
4. Adequate preparation for the testing situation
5. Adequate use of the tests
6. Appropriate scoring methods
7. Appropriate interpretation
8. Appropriate communication of findings
9. Revision of the test

Appropriate translation and adaptation requires much time and expertise. For example, in the translation of the Luria-Nebraska Neuropsychological Battery (Puente, Cespedes, Iruarrizaga, Cano, & Tobal, 2000) care had to be taken to use personnel versed in both languages; what Harris, Cullum, and Puente (1995) have called balanced-bilinguals. In addition, those individuals had to have expertise not just in Spanish but also in psychology. While it is not difficult to find balanced-bilinguals, it is difficult to find individuals who are truly bilingual and have the psychological knowledge necessary to understand the subtleties of testing. Also, the resolution of discrepancies of the original and initial translation require special understanding of issues that will later be addressed under the rubric of cognitive equivalence.

Another problem of a serious nature in working with Hispanics is that, as discussed previously, this ethnic group actually includes different subgroups (Shorris, 1992). As in the case with the Luria–Nebraska, the initial translation would have worked well with Cubans and Puerto Ricans because a Cuban completed it. The second translation, completed by Spaniards, would have been adequate for Castillian speakers. The final translation attempted to blend not only the those two translations but also use words and phrases that were generic to Spanish speakers. This required avoiding specific terminology that would be applicable to one culture. Standard Spanish was used, and this is indeed the best solution in developing and translating testing instruments. The problem of translating became even more evident in the initial efforts of translating the Wechsler intelligence scales into Spanish (Puente & Salazar, 1998).

A final issue is that a translation is not just a translation. Sometimes the intention is, for example, to have the similar number in Spanish represent a number in English. Translating digits is a very difficult task. *Eight* in English is one syllable whereas in Spanish *ocho* is two syllables. Furthermore, sometimes a literal translation simply does not make sense. The Luria–Nebraska has numerous proverbs and phrases, such as "the golden egg," which literally make no sense when translated. Hence, care must be taken to address the criterion in question.

Translators

If a test is published in English, then one could easily and incorrectly assume that all that is necessary is to use a translator. This simple approach is riddled with unforeseen difficulties.

Translators are not necessarily well versed in psychology or medical principles. As a consequence, very literal but nonsensical translations are produced. Thus, the patient views the question as literally not making any sense. Further, the translator might speak Spanish but be unfamiliar with Spanish culture. Next, there is the issue of time. If an item is to be timed, timing may get convoluted with figuring out the translation. Rapport is decreased when a third party acts as an intervening variable. Hence, the patient may view the evaluation and evaluator in a less trusting manner. Finally, subtleties will be missed if a translator is used. This could range from immediate nonverbal cues to more complex language responses, which are bound to be "translated out" when the final response is provided.

Norms and Sampling

Neuropsychological tests require a reference value. This reference value is typically in the form of a normative table. This is one reason why flexible batteries are often considered to be problematic. In other words, how does a unique set of tests compare between patients. Whereas neuropsychological tests have traditionally been weak in this regard, Golden, Purisch, and Hammeke (1979) provided norms for the Luria–Nebraska whereas both Reitan (Reitan & Wolfson, 1994) and more recently Heaton and colleagues (Heaton, Grant, & Matthews, 1991) have provided useful norms for the Halstead–Reitan Battery. Almost all tests published by the major publishing houses now include normative data.

Perusal of all of these normative sources, including two recent compendium books (Mitrushina, Boone, & D'Elia, 1999; Spreen & Strauss, 1998), suggests that while age and education (though not always) are taken into account, ethnic status almost always is not considered. As discussed earlier, this omission may reflect the overall belief that ethnic status or culture is not important in understanding brain function and dysfunction. However, as argued in this chapter, in the rest of this volume, and in other scholarly publication outlets, this omission introduces unnecessary error into the evaluation procedure.

If this premise is held to be true, then most neuropsychological tests provide faulty reference values. Samples that are used for normative tables rarely include ethnic status. This is indeed the case with the two historically used batteries in neuropsychology, the Halstead–Reitan and the Luria–Nebraska, as well as all the tests that are most frequently used by neuropsychologists (from a large-scaled survey completed by Camara, Nathan, & Puente, in press). One could argue that because ethnicity is not reported in the sampling procedure, the norms could be considered invalid.

Another related issue is that most neuropsychological tests do not have norms in Spanish. Few commercially available tests in Spanish contain Spanish-speaking norms. The Wechsler scales have been translated and have norms. However, the norms are from Puerto Rico only. Ardila, Rosselli, and Puente (1994) include in their book norms for over a dozen different tests. However, with most of the tests, the sample is limited to individuals living in Colombia. Further, most of the individuals representing the normative sample are over the age of 50. However, one particularly positive aspect of this set of norms is the inclusion of both literates and illiterates. Ponton and colleagues (Ponton, Satz, Herrera, & Ortiz, 1998) have recently published norms for a screening test. The norms, obtained from residents in Los Angeles, may prove to be more promising in that a variety of ethnic groups are included. However, as with other normative samples, no norms are found for the different Hispanic subgroups proposed in this chapter. This pattern is found also with other studies, such as Harris, Cullum, and Puente (1995) which reported preliminary results of a Spanish translation of the California Verbal

Learning Test. Loewenstein and colleagues (Loewenstein, Rubert, Arguelles, & Duara, 1995b) have also worked to develop norms for Spanish speakers, especially for older populations.

Maybe it is unreasonable to expect norms for different Hispanic subgroups when (1) most neuropsychological tests are not adequately translated into Spanish, and (2) norms are not typically available. However, the goal of ethnic-group sampling and normative reference values should be considered as new studies are being formulated.

Cultural Meaningfulness

When administering and/or translating tests developed in a specific culture to a different cultural context, the issue of equivalence in cultural meaningfulness and relevance should be addressed. Items developed in a cultural context do not have the same relevance when translated to another culture. The Boston Naming Test is a good example. Several of the figures are simply unfamiliar and meaningless for Hispanics (e.g., the beaver is a North American animal), whereas others have a quite different degree of familiarity (e.g., igloo, frequently interpreted as an oven by Hispanics). Igloo is a very easy and familiar word for English speakers because it is used at the elementary school for learning the sound /i/). Several stories in the Picture Arrangement subtest of the WAIS are perceived by Hispanics as strange and rare. Cultural familiarity and meaningfulness can result in differences in performance.

Cognitive Equivalence

Assuming that all the preceding variables are held constant, then the real question becomes whether English and Spanish tests are measuring the same thing. In the section "Translation," the question of translation equivalence was addressed and the example of *eight* and *ocho*—one versus two syllables—was presented. When a test is translated the value of the test depends not on whether a translation is viable from a language perspective but, instead, from a cognitive one. Before a translation is completed or before a test is administered a clear understanding must be had of what is to be measured. This requires that the underlying factor for each item, scale, and test be understood. As Anderson (1996) has indicated, most tests measure a variety of things—ranging from immediate attention to verbal articulation to recognition and recall. Rarely does a test measure just one cognitive domain. The obvious step is to determine what is the most important or salient variable that needs to be measured and then proceed accordingly. In addition, one must then be careful that the item is of equal difficulty. For example, one of the most common tests for fluency in English is the F, A, S, whereas in Ardila, Rosselli, and Puente (1994) norms are provided for this test, because the frequency of occurrence for these letters is not the same in English as in Spanish. In the tests requiring digits in the WAIS and WISC, the question is whether the task is to remember a single-digit number or a single-digit number with a specified number of syllables. Interestingly, when a letter fluency test is administered to Hispanics, they mainly report nouns, and occasionally adjectives and verbs, but do not say grammatical words. English speakers report grammatical words in the letter fluency test (M. Rosselli & A. Ardila, unpublished manuscript). The reason for this difference is unclear, but it may suggest a subtle difference in the internal representation of words, i.e., what is understood as a word and how semantic nets are constructed. It may be conjectured that this difference relates to the clearer distinction between grammatical elements existing in Spanish relative to English. Outcome studies will determine the answer to these questions. For now, clinical experience and theoretical speculation provide the necessary framework from which to consider these important questions.

Interviewing

Unfortunately, a comprehensive review of the psychological literature revealed that no empirical articles were published on interviewing Hispanics in neuropsychological evaluations. The few articles that exist are based on clinical, anecdotal, or theoretical perspectives. For example, Puente and Perez (2000) have provided some background for structuring interviewing. Considering the complexities associated with cultural issues and the possibility of missing key elements in the interview, a structured approach will increase the likelihood of addressing the important issues in question. However, it is important to appreciate the importance of establishing rapport and explaining the purpose of the evaluation to Hispanics. This need is based on prior limited encounters with mental or medical professionals. Further, mental concerns may be private matters which are family and religious focused. Thus, opening up to a stranger is abnormal. And when opening up involves talking about personal issues (such as memory), the interview will hold special challenges and difficulties for the professional. Frequently, intellectual or cognitive testing may be perceived by the patient as aversive. In Latin America, highly educated people usually dislike, and try to avoid, testing. Intellectual testing may be even be perceived as humiliating and disrespectful of privacy. "Are you taking me for stupid?" is frequently the implicit message of some Hispanics when rejecting testing. People with little education, on the other hand, may be afraid and embarrassed when tested. In consequence, testing can be much more effective if performed in a flexible and informal way rather than using a rigid and highly standardized situation.

Testing

As previously mentioned, there are few research programs associated with neuropsychological assessment. A review of the neuropsychological testing literature reveals four cities; Denver, Los Angeles, Miami, and Wilmington, North Carolina. In Denver, Harris has focused on the development of a Spanish version of the California Verbal Learning Test. In Los Angeles, Ponton and Taussig, in separate and collaborative efforts, have published important information on Spanish speakers. In Miami, the work of Ardila and Rosselli as well as Loewenstein and colleagues (primarily with the elderly) has been ongoing for over a decade. In Wilmington, Puente and colleagues (primarily from universities in Madrid and Granada, Spain) have worked on a variety of issues including the translation and adaptation of the Wechsler scales (especially with Ardila and Harris, from Colorado). This section reviews the existing literature and ongoing research efforts on the neuropsychological testing of the Spanish speaker.

One of the first publications in the literature (Dergan, 1987) reflected the ongoing status of Hispanic neuropsychological assessment. In an article in *Avances en Psicologica Clinica Latinamericana*, Dergan describes an initial translation of the Luria–Nebraska Neuropsychological Battery. Although the translation violates many of the principles previously outlined in this chapter and no empirical data are reported, this article could be considered the first in the field. During the 1980s, a series of articles by Ardila and colleagues began to appear in the literature (e.g., Ardila & Rosselli, 1989; Ostrosky, Canseco, Quintana, Narvarro, & Ardila, 1985). Ardila's primary collaborators have been Monica Rosselli in Colombia and Miami, and Ostrosky in Mexico City. However, it was not until 1989 that L. Bernard first reported that "blacks" and Hispanics of average intellectual functioning but from poor academic backgrounds (and no reported brain impairment) exhibited scores that were in the impaired range.

A series of studies was conducted by Ardila and colleagues examining the relationship of education and sociocultural status on brain functioning. As early as 1989, Ardila and colleagues (Ardila, Bryden, & Ostrosky, 1989) reported on the incidence of handedness in adolescent and adult Amazonian jungle residents. Also, Rosselli, Ardila, Florez, and Castro (1990) reported normative data on a Spanish translation of the Boston Diagnostic Aphasia Examination. This type of work resulted in the publication of *Neuropsychological Evaluation of the Spanish Speaker* by Ardila, Rosselli, and Puente (1994). The book was the first comprehensive publication to present a variety of neuropsychological tests across several cognitive domains that were translated into Spanish, ranging from tests of attention to visuopraxic abilities. The test results were stratified according to age and education. As previously discussed, both of these variables were associated with neuropsychological performance. It is interesting to note that some of the tests and test materials (e.g., Wechsler Memory Scale) could not be reproduced in the book due to copyright restrictions. The group has continued to publish extensively with their primary base of operation being Miami.

Another successful research program, also in Miami, has been that of Loewenstein. In a series of studies during the 1990s (Loewenstein, Arguelles, Arguelles, & Linn-Fuentes, 1994; Loewenstein, Duara, Arguelles, & Arguelles, 1995a; Loewenstein et al., 1995b) Loewenstein and colleagues have focused on developing neuropsychological instruments applicable to elderly Spanish speakers. They have reported the WAIS Block Design and Digit Symbol subtests along with the Mini-Mental State Examination were strong predictors of functional capacity. They have also been supporters of the use of culturally reduced or limited tests for assessing neuropsychological functioning. For example, Loewenstein et al. (1995a) reported that the Fuld Object Memory Evaluation was a useful tool for detecting dementia in Spanish speakers.

Taussig and Ponton have also published another series of studies. Using a customized translation of the WAIS-R, Taussig and colleagues (Taussig, Mack, & Henderson, 1996) reported good differentiation of controls to mildly-to-moderately demented Spanish speakers. Ponton, Satz, Herrera, Ortiz, et al. (1996) have provided normative data on 300 Hispanic subjects ranging from the age of 16 to 75 for the newly developed Neuropsychological Screening Battery for Hispanics. Gender, age, and education associations were seen for a variety of neuropsychological tests.

A series of unrelated articles have been published during the second half of the 1990s involving verbal fluency and learning. Harris, Cullum, and Puente (1995) investigated the effect of bilingualism on verbal learning and memory, using a scientifically constructed Spanish translation (most existing Spanish forms are not scientifically constructed) of the California Verbal Learning Test. A total of 44 Hispanics bilingual and 22 monolingual English speakers participated in this study. When groups were assessed in their dominant language, no significant differences were found.

Perri, Naplin, and Carpenter (1995) reported on the development of the Perri Test of Verbal Learning and Memory (in Spanish). The test consists of a 16-word list composed of 4 categories of 4 words each together with a 40-word recognition list. Normative data for 100 Spanish-speaking adults ranging from 15 to 70 years of age were presented. Hence, it appears that verbal learning and memory can be measured with appropriately translated and standardized instruments. However, it is important to note that verbal memory is more complicated than might initially appear and that normative data are inconclusive at this point. For example, Olazaran, Jacobs, and Stern (1996) reported that the differences in the number of syllables per digit string might have been responsible for an observed decrement in Spanish speakers on the WAIS-R digit span. More recently, Kempler, Teng, Dick, Taussig, and Davis (1998) have reported cross-ethnic differences (between Vietnamese and Spanish speakers) for fluency measures.

Other studies are apparently in progress. For example, Munges (1996) reported a work in progress at the University of California at Davis. The study focused on the development of a battery with strong psychometric characteristics in both English and Spanish across 12 different cognitive domains. The ongoing work of Stricks, Pittman, Jacobs, Sano, and Stern (1998) probably best reflects the current status of the field. In their attempt to obtain norms for English and Spanish-speaking elderly, a battery of neuropsychological tests was administered to almost 1,000 participants. Their findings indicate, as do many of the studies reviewed in this chapter, that age, education, and language are associated with neuropsychological test performance. What is important to note, however, is that there is increasing evidence to suggest that nonverbal tests are not culturally reduced. Indeed, it has long been held true that tests that are translated are high in cultural confound. However, increasing evidence has been recently reported that identifies similar problems, possibly even at a lower level, in tests that are nonverbal.

Interpretation

Most of the research reviewed, whether theoretical, clinical, or empirical, focused on the appropriate development of neuropsychological instruments. However, interpretation is the important element of the standardized neuropsychological assessment.

Taking information out of context invariably will result in increased error variance. Taking psychometric data without regard to the issues previously addressed is incorrect and unethical. For example, care must be taken to understand the limits of the test, the patient, and the evaluator in determining what the psychometric findings really mean. Hence, the clinician has to work doubly hard to appreciate the unusual nuances that are being faced with the Hispanic neuropsychological patient. However, the psychometric results must be framed in a complex biopsychosocial context (see Puente & McCaffrey, 1992). This would include not only an appreciation of the limits of the test but an understanding of the purpose of the examination (e.g., learning disability placement) and the context of the patient at the time of the evaluation (e.g., how many years in the United States). Arnold, Montgomery, Castaneda, and Longoria (1994) reported on the association of acculturation to performance on the Halstead–Reitan Neuropsychological Battery. The authors reported that acculturation levels correlated with the results of the following: Tactual Performance Test, the Seashore Rhythm Test, and the Halstead Category Test.

As argued previously (Puente & Perez, 2000), the issue in question may not necessarily be the neuropsychological status of the patient. The question may be whether the patient cognitively acculturated into the culture from which the principles are being derived for the foundation of the evaluation. As discussed earlier, many neuropsychological tests are timed. For Hispanics, time is not the same thing as for North Americans (Shorris, 1992). Hence, one would expect to see a greater percentage of false positives in situations when the psychometric results are not interpreted in a broad biopsychosocial context.

Suggestions and Potential Solutions

Neuropsychologists are beginning to address the problems that arise from the ever-expanding population of Hispanics in both the United States and Latin America. However, Hispanics as an ethnic group pose challenges that could serve as a foundation for conceptualizing the understanding of other ethnic minorities both in and outside the United States.

Development of a Hispanic neuropsychology would serve but a small amount of what is needed to understand the neuropsychological function of minority individuals living in a majority culture (on any continent). In this section, several issues are presented that might assist not only in increasing the knowledge necessary to address the neuropsychological evaluation of the Spanish speaker but to lay the framework for larger issues involving cultural neuropsychology. It is anticipated that this foundation would, in turn, later serve as a starting point for expanding neuropsychological knowledge beyond the clinical to the more theoretical. Specifically, a more comprehensive understanding of culture and neuropsychology should serve as an initial step for questioning the possibility of the role of neuropsychological function in evolutionary focus. The work of Sperry (1994), Wilson (1995), and others provide glimpses into the kinds of questions that heretofore neuropsychology has not considered. For example, Does a commonality across cultures in neuropsychological functioning, or neuropsychological "g," exist? What role does culture play in shaping brain functioning across the life-span? Is neuropsychological function nothing more than the cognitive expression of cultural traits? And, if so, could neuropsychological analysis be nothing more than measuring cognitive acculturation? Could neuropsychological knowledge serve to understand more than an individual's cognitive and emotional status after brain injury? Could neuropsychological knowledge be the starting point for a more comprehensive understanding of the human condition? After all, with over a century of research, psychology has yet to produce much more than a strong methodology. "Why" questions have lagged way behind "how" questions. Conceivably, neuropsychology, especially from a cultural context, could serve to address these heretofore unanswered questions.

There is little question that neuropsychology is a very traditional psychological specialty. Most members of APA's Division 40, Clinical Neuropsychology, are white men, and in proportions not typical of other APA divisions (Puente & Marcotte, in press). Considering the mix of ethnic minorities in the population at large, it would seem that increasing the number of ethnic minorities in the field would be an obvious process for the field to encourage. Echemendia, Harris, Congett, and Puente (1997) reported that neuropsychologists do believe it is important to understand cultural issues, especially when dealing with Spanish speakers. Clearly, one way to resolve this is to increase the number of individuals who are bilingual and bicultural. Unfortunately, there is limited evidence that this is occurring. The Hispanic Neuropsychological Society is comprised of about 50 members and the organization, at this point, is not very active. Also, a review of all the members of Division 40 revealed only one Hispanic is a fellow of the division and the total number of individuals with Hispanic surnames (one way to estimate Hispanic membership) approximately 1% of the close to 4,000 members. While the senior author of this chapter helped organize a Division 40 committee on ethnic minority affairs, its impact has been highly limited. The situation needs quick remedy. At present, there is little to suggest that the pipeline of Hispanic students is being reversed.

Another possible alternative, as the responders of the Echemendia et al. (1996) survey suggested, is to increase awareness of the issue in question. APA Ethical Guidelines emphasize the need for multicultural understanding and, presumably, this would obviously translate into neuropsychology as well. The authors of this chapter have presented two workshops at NAN, with the first one occurring during the early 1990s. Also, the Hispanic Neuropsychological Society has met irregularly at NAN, APA, and INS meetings. However, in almost all instances the number of non-Hispanics attending these meetings is always very, very small, in large part due to the lack of a regularly published newsletter or a very active group of officers.

Tests for Spanish speakers need to be developed and made widely available to neuropsychologists. Outside the work by Ardila (e.g., Ardila, Rosselli, & Puente, 1994), the few things that are published are research reports with minimal normative data (except for Ponton et al, 1997). The major test publishing house in Spain (TEA) has made several tests (e.g., Stroop) available but almost none of the tests have norms. The first neuropsychological test development project the company sponsored, the Luria–Nebraska Neuropsychological Battery, will be published in the early part of 2000 (with an N of over 300). During the past decade, the Psychological Corporation has been interested in developing Spanish translations of the Wechsler scales (already described in this chapter). Under the direction of the senior author, a workgroup eventually was convened which included several of the prominent researchers both in neuropsychology and school psychology (including one of the authors of the Puerto Rican adaptation of the WISC). After a number of years of preliminary planning, a translation was eventually developed. After the painstaking work on developing the translation, a tryout phase was initiated. Due to the low number of responses and potential budgetary reasons, the project has been placed on hold for the foreseeable future. The commercially available tests that are currently available with norms (e.g., WAIS and WISC) are very outdated and included norms essentially only from Puerto Rico. Recently, the Psychological Corporation has begun to distribute in the United States a brief neuropsychological test battery known as NEUROPSI (Ostrosky-Solís, Ardila & Rosselli, 1997) developed in Spanish and normalized in Mexico.

What about the present? Considering the ever-increasing number of Spanish speakers in the United States, there is no question that serious problems are being faced by neuropsychologists wishing to evaluate Hispanics. Some practical suggestions include: 1) whenever possible, refer to a bilingual and bicultural neuropsychologist; 2) if possible, use appropriately translated tests; 3) if possible, use applicable norms; 4) if necessary, use a translator and preferably a trained and unbiased one; 5) understand the limitations of the evaluation procedure; and 6) identify perceived limitations in the context of the report and contextualize the overall findings within the limitations of the evaluation procedure.

At this point, the situation does not appear to have many potential remedies in the immediate future. Whereas there is clearly a demonstrated need and the field considers this a critical issue, there is little to suggest that the traditional approaches to testing Spanish speakers will be changed. Hence, translators, idiosyncratic translations, and no norms will continue for the foreseeable future unless the field begins to address more aggressively the issues in question.

Conclusion

Two issues should be evident from reading this chapter. One, there is an increasing need to understand the uniqueness associated with the neuropsychological evaluation of the Spanish speaker. Demographic characteristics indicate that the largest ethnic minority in the United States by the early part of the twenty-first century will be Hispanics. In some populous states, such as California, Texas, and Florida, Hispanics will be the majority very soon. The second issue is that there is no evidence to suggest that neuropsychology is prepared to meet that pressing need. In fact, using Division 40 membership and published tests with norms as rough guidelines, the field is nowhere near adequately addressing this problem. Whether the assumption is that culture is not important to brain function or whether it is that culture could be easily held constant with idiosyncratically translated tests with no norms is not clear. Regardless, the resolution of this problem would also further the generalizability of neuropsychology beyond the clinical realm. Such knowledge would go a long way in helping address the possibility of a neuropsychological "g" and in the development of a neuropsychology that is usable to more than just majority individuals from well-developed nations. Majority individuals of well-developed countries represent no more than 10% of the world population. In this global context, neuropsychology has been almost exclusively directed to the study of world minorities.

References

Anderson, R. M. (1994). *Practitioner's guide to clinical neuropsychology.* New York: Plenum.

Ardila, A. (1998a). A note of caution: Normative neuropsychological test performance: Effects of age, education, gender and ethnicity: A comment on Saykin et al. (1995). *Applied Neuropsychology, 5,* 51–53.

Ardila, A. (1998b). Bilingualism: A neglected and chaotic area. *Aphasiology, 12,* 131–134.

Ardila, A., Ardila, O., Bryden, M. P., & Ostrosky, F. (1989). Effects of cultural background and education on handedness. *Neuropsychologia, 27,* 893–897.

Ardila, A., & Rosselli, M. (1989). Neuropsychological characteristics of normal aging. *Developmental Neuropsychology, 5,* 307–320.

Ardila, A. Rosselli, M., & Puente, A. E. (1994). *Neuropsychological evaluation of the Spanish speaker.* New York: Plenum.

Ardila, A., Rosselli, M., Ostrosky-Solfís, F., Marcos, J., Granda, G. & Soto, M. (in press). Memory abilities and syntactic comprehension in Spanish–English bilinguals. *Applied Neuropsychology.*

Arnold, B. R., Montgomery, G. T., Castaneda, I., Longoria, R. (1994). Acculturaltion and performance of Hispanics on selected Halstead–Reitan neuropsychological tests. *Assessment, 1*(3), 239–448.

Bernard, L. C. (1989). Halstead–Reitan Neuropsychology Test performance of Black, Hispanic, and White young adult males from poor academic backgrounds. *Archives of Clinical Neuropsychology, 4,* 267–274.

Berry, J. W. (1997). Immigration, acculturation and adaption. *Applied Psychology, 46,* 5–68.

Brislin, R. W. (1983). Translation and content analysis of oral and written material. In H. C. Triandis and J. W. Berry (Eds.) *Handbook of cross-cultural psychology methodology.* Boston: Allyn & Bacon.

Camara, W., Nathan, J., & Puente, A. E. (in press). Professional usage of psychological tests. *Professional Psychology.*

Dergan, J. J. (1987). La bateria neuropsicologica Luria–Nebraska. *Avances en Psicological Clinica Latinoamericana, 5,* 2–36.

Diccionario de la lengua Española (1984). (Vigésima Ed., Tomo II). Madrid: Real Academia Española.

Echemendia, R. J., Harris, J.C. Congett, S. M., Diaz, M. L., & Puente, A. E. (1997). Neuropsychological training and practices with Hispanics: A national survey. *The Clinical Neuropsychologist, 11,* 229–243.

Golden, C. J., Purisch, A,D., & Hammeke, T. A. (1979) *The Luria–Nebraska Neuropsychological Battery: A manual for clinical and experimental uses.* Lincoln: University of Nebraska Press.

Grosjean, F. (1989). Neurolinguistics beware! The bilingual is not two monolinguals in one person. *Brain and Language, 36,* 3–15.

Harris, J., Cullum, M., & Puente, A. E. (1995). Effects of bilingualism on verbal learning and memory in Hispanics adults. *Journal of the International Neuropsychological Society, 1,* 10–16.

Heaton, R., Grant, I., & Matthews C. (1991). Comprehensive norms for an expanded Halstead–Reitan Neuropsychological Battery. Demographic corrections, research findings, and clinical applications. Odessa, FL: Psychological Assessment Resources.

Kempler, D., Teng, E. L., Dick, M., Taussig, I. M., & Davis, S. (1998). The effects of age, education, and ethnicity on verbal fluency. *Journal of the International Neuropsychological Society, 4,* 531–538.

Kilborn, K. (1994). Learning a language late: Second language acquisition in adults. In M. A. Gernsbacher (Ed.), *Handbook of psycholinguistics* (pp. 917–944). New York: Academic Press.

Lezak, M.D. (1995). *Neuropsychological assessment* (3rd ed.). New York: Oxford University Press.

Loewenstein, D. A., Arguelles, T., Arguelles, S., & Linn-Fuentes, P. (1994). Potential cultural bias in the neuropsychological assessment of the older adult. *Journal of Clinical and Experimental Neuropsychology, 16,* 623–629.

Loewenstein, D. A., Duara, R., Arguelles, T., & Arguelles, S. (1995a). Use of the Fuld Object Memory Evaluation in the detection of mild dementia among Spanish and English speakers. *American Journal of Geriatric Psychiatry, 3,* 300–307.

Loewenstein, S. A., Rubert, M. P., Arguelles, T., & Duara, T. (1995b). Neuropsychological test performance and prediction of functional capacities among Spanish-speaking and English-speaking patients with dementia. *Archives of Clinical Neuropsychology, 10,* 75–88.

Manuel-Dupont, S., Ardila, A., Rosselli, M., & Puente, A. E. (1992) Bilingualism. In A. E. Puente and R. J. McCaffrey (Eds.), *Handbook of neuropsychological assessment* (pp. 193–212). New York: Plenum.

Merriam-Webster's Collegiate Dictionary (1996). (6th ed.) Springfield, MA: Merriam-Webster.

Mitrushina, M. N., Boone, K. B., & D'Elia, L. F. D. (1999). *Handbook of normative data for neuropsychological assessment.* New York: Oxford University Press.

Munges, D. (1996). The process of development of valid and reliable neuropsychological assessment measures for English- and Spanish-speaking elderly persons. In G. Yeo & D. Gallagher-Thompson (Eds.), *Ethnicity and the dementias* (pp. 33–46). Washington, D.C.: Taylor & Francis.

Muniz, J., & Hambleton, R. K. (1996). Directrices para la traducion y adaption de los tests. *Papeles del Psicologo, 66,* 63–70.

Olazaran J., Jacobs, D. M., & Stern, Y. (1996). Comparative study of visual and verbal short-term memory in English and Spanish speakers: Testing a linguistic hypothesis. *Journal of the International Neuropsychological Society,* 2, 105–110.

Ostrosky, F., Ardila, A., Rosselli, M., López-Arango, G., & Uriel-Mendoza, V. (1998). Neuropsychological test performance in illiterates. *Archives of Clinical Neuropsychology, 13,* 645–660.

Ostrosky-Solís, F., Ardila, A., & Rosselli, M. (1997). *NEUROPSI: Evaluación neuropsicológica breve en español. Manual, instructivo y protocolo de aplicación* [NEUROPSI: A brief neuropsychological evaluation in Spanish. Manual, instructions, and application protocol]. México: Bayer de México.

Ostrosky, F., Canseco, E., Quintanar, L., Navarro, E., & Ardila, A. (1985). Sociocultural effects in neuropsychological assessment. *International Journal of Neuroscience, 27,* 53–66.

Perez-Arce, P., & Puente, A. E. (1996). Neuropsychological assessment of ethnic-minorities: The case for assessing Hispanics living in North America. In R. J. Sbordone & C. J. Long (Eds.), *Ecological validity of neuropsychological testing.* Delray Beach, FL: St. Lucie.

Perri, B. M, Naplin, N. A., & Carpenter, G. A. (1995) A Spanish auditory verbal learning and memory test. *Assessment, 2,* 245–253.

Ponton, M. O., Satz, P., Herrera, L., & Ortiz, F. (1998). Normative data stratified by age and education for the Neuropsychological Screening Battery for Hispanics (NeSBHIS): Initial report. *Journal of the International Neuropsychological Society, 2,* 96–104.

Puente, A. E., Cespedes, J. M., Iruarrizaga, I., Tobal, J. M., & Vindel, A. C. (2000). The Luria–Nebraska Neuropsychological Battery and culturally dissimilar individuals. In C. J. Golden & L. Warren (Eds.), *The LNNB 20th anniversary handbook. Volume I: A guide to clinical interpretation and use in special settings.* Los Angeles: Western Psychological Services.

Puente, A. E., & McCaffrey, R. J. (Eds.) (1992). *Handbook of neuropsychological assessment.* New York: Plenum.

Puente, A. E. & Perez, M. (2000). Psychological assessment of ethnic-minorities. In G. Goldstein & M. Hersen (Eds.), *Handbook of psychological assessment* (pp. 527–551). Boston: Allyn & Bacon.

Puente, A. E., & Salazar, G. (1998). Assessment of minority and culturally diverse children. In A. Prifetera & D. Saklokske (Eds.) *WISC-III: Clinical use and interpretation* (pp. 227–248). New York: Academic Press.

Reitan, R. & Wolfson, D. (1984). *The Halstead–Reitan Neuropsychological Battery.* Tucson, AZ: Neuropsychology Press.

Rosselli, M., Ardila, A., Florez, A., & Castro, C. (1990). Normative data on the Boston Diagnostic Aphasia Examination in a Spanish-speaking population. *Journal of Clinical and Experimental Neuropsychology, 12,* 313–322.

Rosselli, M. & Ardila, A. Verbal fluency in Spanish and English. Unpublished manuscript.

Shorris, E. (1992). *Latinos.* New York: Norton.

Sperry, R. W. (1994). Holding course amid shifting paradigms. In W. Hartman and J. Clark (Eds.), *The metaphysical foundations of modern science: Issues of causality* (pp. 99–123). San Francisco: Institute of Noetic Sciences.

Spreen, O. & Strauss, E. (1998). *A compendium of neuropsychological tests* (2nd ed.). New York: Oxford University Press.

Stricks, L., Pittman, J., Jacobs, D. M., Sano, M., & Stern, Y (1998). Normativa data for a brief neuropsychological battery administered to English- and Spanish-speaking community-dwelling elders. *Journal of the International Neuropsychological Society, 4,* 311–318.

Taussig, M. I., Mack, W., & Henderson, V. W. (1996) Concurrent validity of Spanish-language versions of the Mini-Mental State Examination, Mental Status Questionnaire, Information-Memory-Concentration Test, and Presentation-Memory-Concentration Test: Alzheimer's disease patients and non-demented elderly comparison. *Journal of the International Neuropsychological Society, 2,* 286–298.

Taussig, M. I., & Ponton, M. (1996). Issues in neuropsychological assessment for Hispanic older adults: Cultural and linguistic factors. In G. Yeo and D. Gallagher-Thompson (Eds.), *Ethnicity and the dementias.* Washington, D.C.: Taylor & Francis.

U.S. Bureau of the Census (1999). *United States population.* Washington, D.C.: Author.

Wilson, Z. O. (1995). *Naturalist.* New York: Warner Books.

Neuropsychological Assessment and Intervention with Native Americans

JEFF KING AND ELAINE FLETCHER-JANZEN

Introduction

Much of the attention given to significant Native American issues in the neuropsychology research literature is minimal (Dauphinais & King, 1992). In the past 30 years there has been a disappointing number of neuropsychological studies with this population. Studies began in the 1970s on subjects such as culture patterns of speech (Philipsen, 1972), cerebral speech lateralization (Scott, Hynd, Hunt, & Weed, 1979), addressing performance on the Bender-Gestalt (Taylor & Thweatt, 1972), and intellectual assessment in general (Hynd & Garcia, 1979). In the early 1980s studies focused mostly on performance differences on the Wechsler scales and hemispheric specialization of language (McKeever & Hunt, 1984; Mishra, 1982; Mishra, Lord, & Sabers, 1989; Zarske, & Moore, 1982). The 1990s have produced studies that are more reflective of bioethics (Carrese, & Rhodes, 1995), Native American elderly health status (Ferraro, Bercier, & Chelmiinski, 1997; Mercer, 1994), and access to health care (Anderson, Bastida, Kramer, Williams, & Wong, 1995; Bagley, Angel, Dilworth-Anderson, Liu, & Schinke, 1995; Myers, Kagawa-Singer, Kumanyika, Lex, & Markides, 1995; Norton & Manson, 1995).

Native Americans are not typically included in major national health surveys because although well over one-half of the American Indian population resides in urban areas their numbers are comparatively small and adequate health surveys would require local oversampling (Myers, Kagawa-Singer, Kumanyika, Lex, & Markides, 1995). Therefore, little information is available about the health issues of Native Americans, and what is available represents the 60% of American Indians that are served by the Indian Health Service. There is no data about how the other 40% of Native Americans are served (Johnson et al., 1995). The gaps and limitations of data gathering are starting to be addressed, and collaboration has begun among

JEFF KING • Native American Counseling Center, Denver Colorado, 80222; and University of Denver, Denver, Colorado 80208.   ELAINE FLETCHER-JANZEN • University of Northern Colorado, Colorado Springs, Colorado 80921.

Handbook of Cross-Cultural Neuropsychology, edited by Fletcher-Janzen, Strickland, and Reynolds. Kluwer Academic/Plenum Publishers, New York, 2000.

the Indian Health Service, other federal agencies, and tribal authorities (Myers et al., 1995). This is no easy task because, as with other ethnic minority groups, American Indians are a heterogeneous and diverse population.

Health beliefs and practices for Native Americans are generally holistic, promote wellness, and are philosophically integrated with religion (Johnson et al., 1995). Factors that interfere with appropriate health care are access to health care systems, institutionalized racism, and poverty. In addition, distance from health facilities, available technologies, and environmental health hazards affect treatment and prevention (Johnson et al., 1995).

The field of psychology has paid much attention to ethnic variables in the delivery of effective assessment and therapy for diverse patient populations. However, evidence of multicultural competence requirements for neuropsychology is lagging. Hence the paucity of research studies that address brain–behavior relationships and psychopharmacology for this population. This chapter will describe the Native American population characteristics in the United States, address historical and sociopolitical factors of Native American culture, present an overview of neuropsychological data in the research literature, present cultural aspects of neuropsychological assessment instruments, and suggest adaptations that clinicians can make to reflect sensitivity to Native American culture and enhance neuropsychological treatment outcome. For the purposes of this chapter, the terms Native American and American Indian are used interchangeably and the terms European American and Anglo-American refer to white Americans or Americans of European descent.

Demographics

There are over 500 federally recognized American Indian tribes and over 250 distinct languages among these tribes. Census data report that there are approximately two million American Indian, Eskimo, and Aleut people in the United States (U.S. Bureau of the Census, 1991). The Native population is young, approximately half are 18 years of age or younger (Nelson, McCoy, Stetter, & Vanderwagen, 1992). The median ages range from 18.8 years to 26.3 years on reservation lands, with those living within tribal jurisdictional areas ranging from 22.7 to 27.2 years of age, and Alaska Native villagers ranging from 16.8 to 25.0 years of age (U.S. Bureau of the Census, 1991).

There are areas within the United States that have greater numbers of tribes and population density. Alaskan Natives comprise over 15% of Alaska's population, and American Indians comprise close to 9% of New Mexico's population, 8% of Oklahoma's population, and 6% of Arizona's population. Cities with large American Indian populations are Los Angeles (87,487), Tulsa, Oklahoma (48,196), New York City (46,191), Oklahoma City (45,720), and San Francisco (40,847). Approximately one-fifth of American Indians reside on over 300 reservation and trust lands, while another 15% live within tribal jurisdiction, Alaska Native villages, or other tribal designated areas.

It is estimated that over 50% live in urban areas. Regardless of location, Native people face higher poverty levels and lower educational achievement than any other ethnic minority group in the United States (U.S. Bureau of the Census, 1991).

Historical Perspectives

The impact of colonization on American Indian people and the corresponding issues of mental health (Duran & Duran, 1995; Brave Heart & DeBruyn, 1998) are important factors in the contextural understanding of modern day health issues. Modern science has described

American Indian people as having come to the Americas across the Bering Strait during a recent ice age. However, those notions have been recently disputed (Deloria, 1997).

Although some early contacts between American Indians and Europeans were positive, most were not. At first contact there were several million native peoples. Diseases foreign to native people brought by European settlers wiped out over half of the American Indian population. The diseases also killed many tribal leaders and elders, thus cutting off tribal leadership, as well as the oral sources for knowledge and tradition central to Native culture.

Forced relocation was another factor that caused many deaths and cultural disturbance as well as numerous other problems, many of which were mental health related. Dealing with the reality of being conquered and the forced dependency upon the U.S. government affected tribes for centuries. Other impacts of forced relocation include: broken treaties by the U.S. Government, restrictions made upon reservations (in the not-so-distant past, an Indian had to have a permit in order to leave the reservation), poverty conditions, and the consequences of not relocating oftentimes meant severe suffering or death for many Native Americans (O'Sullivan & Handal, 1988; Vogel, 1972).

Forced education in boarding schools caused considerable damage to the structure and function of tribal societies as well as to the mental health of American Indians. The early charters for American Indian education were the same: To remove the child from the influence of his or her "savage" parents (Joe, 1994). Historically, American Indian children were taken from their tribal homes to attend boarding schools sometimes hundreds or thousands of miles away. Although boarding schools had been used by Europeans since the early 1600s as a means to civilize American Indians, the full-fledged efforts did not begin until after the Civil War when Richard Henry Pratt, an army lieutenant and Civil War veteran, began a government-approved experiment to save the American Indians. After working with American Indian prisoners of war, he founded the Carlisle Indian School. This institution was the beginning of a movement that soon became the primary method for educating American Indian children across the United States. Pratt believed that this education should combine military discipline with hard work and strong cultural immersion. Every moment of every day was structured for these children. With military regimen, they were awakened by bugles, ate in stages according to the ringing of bells, and marched to and from each activity. They were forbidden to speak their tribal languages, given new names, made to wear uniforms (oftentimes a military one), their hair was shorn (hair is very sacred to most tribes), and they were taught the ways of European American society. Rebellious children were incarcerated in cells and/or whipped, and oftentimes this "rebellion" was defined as speaking their tribal languages. The main objective for the boarding schools was to separate these children from their tribal life and to eradicate all identification with American Indian culture.

The effects of boarding schools on tribes resulted in the long-term undermining of tribal ways of parenting, traditional childrearing, use of language, and natural resistance to the forced assimilation of European American culture. Today, there are counseling groups specifically designed to address the posttraumatic effects of boarding school experiences.

Acculturation Process

American Indians cannot be understood without knowledge of their unique acculturation processes. As mentioned previously, the goal of the United States government was total assimilation of the American Indians. The assimilation process meant the abandoning of cultural traditions and values and adopting the values of the dominant culture. Many American Indians did assimilate, and many did not.

The Social Science Research Council (1954) has defined acculturation as:

> culture change that is initiated by the conjunction of two or more autonomous cultural systems. Acculturative change may be the consequence of direct cultural transmission; it may be derived from noncultural causes, such as ecological or demographic modification induced by imping-ing culture; it may be delayed as with internal adjustments following upon the acceptance of alien traits or patterns; or it may be a reactive adaptation of traditional modes of life. The dynamics of acculturation can be seen as the selective adaptation of value systems, the processes of integration and differentiation, the generation of developmental sequences, and the operation of role determinants and personality factors. (p. 974)

Acculturation refers both to the processes and products of change. Psychological accul-turation has been added to this definition (Graves, 1967). It refers to acculturative changes that occur at the individual level. Cultural and psychological acculturation are dynamically related. Cultural change requires psychological acculturation of individuals within the culture, but an individual may undergo psychological acculturation without the culture in which they are a part of changing, or vice versa.

The acculturation process highlights four primary dimensions: assimilation, bicultural, traditional, and rejection. These are dynamic, ongoing process/outcomes for Native people in response to contact with European American culture. The bicultural dimension is one in which the person (or tribe) is able to move fairly comfortably within both cultures. One holds on to one's own culture, but has also adapted to or adopted some of the majority culture as well. The traditional dimension is where the person or tribe maintains the culture and does not adopt European American values and customs. The fourth dimension, rejection or deculturation, relates to a process in which the person does not identify with either culture (Berry, 1980; Smither, 1982).

Recent research on acculturative effects for Native Americans have demonstrated that retention of some form of Native culture appears to have a psychological strengthening component. Both traditional and bicultural groups tended to have less psychological distress than the assimilated and deculturated groups (King, 1994). Acculturation outcomes have been researched for their role in well-being and psychological distress. Acculturative stress has been linked to numerous negative psychological and emotional effects (Berry, Kim, Minde, & Mok, 1987; Boyce & Boyce, 1983).

Current Health Issues

Recent decades have shown remarkable improvements in the health of American Indians and Alaska Natives who qualify for treaty-based services (Penn, Kar, Kramer, Skinner, & Zambrana, 1995). However, on reservations poverty, lack of opportunities, and high morbidity and mortality rates witness high risk conditions for stress-related psychological conditions such as depression (Manson, Shore, & Bloom, 1985), and homicide and suicide rates (Young, 1990). Physical conditions that support high morbidity and mortality rates are diabetes, hepatitis, anemia, poor nutrition, tuberculosis, cancer (lung), cardiovascular diseases, obesity-related problems, and alcohol-related diseases, and seizure disorders related to alcohol abuse (Bagley et al., 1995; Johnson et al., 1995). Common problems for adults include lack of prenatal care, lack of access to substance abuse or diabetes treatment, and excess deaths from cigarette smoking and alcohol abuse. Problems for adolescents also include lack of access to alcohol and substance abuse prevention and treatment, and excess deaths from suicide (Myers et al., 1995). Indeed, the Native American adolescent death rate is more than twice as high as that of youths from other ethnic groups. Bagley et al. (1995) report that:

> The death rate of Native American boys 10–19 years old is nearly three times higher than that of all other racial and ethnic groups. For older teens, the ethnic disparity only increases. Native American adolescents 15–24 years old have a death rate three times the frequency from unintentional injuries compared with all other ethnic-racial groups. A large percentage of these deaths are associated with substance use. Unintentional injuries and suicide account for nearly three fourths of the total death rate. (p. 636)

Again, because of nonuniform health reporting, morbidity and mortality rates may vary greatly from one tribe to another. For example, Myers et al. (1995) analyzed data on the incidence of fetal alcohol syndrome (FAS) and found that "the lowest FAS rates (1.3 per 1,000) among Navajo women. A much higher rate occurred among Plains Indian women (10.3 per 1,000) and 25% of all Plains women with one child with FAS also gave birth to others with FAS" (p. 617). Apart from FAS, many of the other medical conditions cited previously have neuropsychological sequelae (Kodituwakku, Handmaker, Cutler, Weathersby & Handmaker, 1995; Kodituwakku et al., 1997). Poor prenatal care and nutrition create many subtle developmental and learning issues for children that may require differential diagnosis and treatment from neuropsychologists. Otitis media (inner ear infection) affects American Indian children in greater proportions than any other ethnic group (McShane & Plas, 1984). Accidents many times mean traumatic brain injury and long-term brain injury rehabiltiation, as do cardiovascular disease sequelae.

Long-term and serious health issues usually require ongoing evaluation, treatment, and intervention by the clinician, and treatment compliance on the part of the patient. Given that Native American health practices are closely tied to religion, failure to incorporate those beliefs may influence self-care and treatment compliance (Johnson et al., 1995). Carrese and Rhodes (1995) have recently studied the Navajo concept of *hozho* (a concept that combines the concepts of beauty, goodness, order, harmony, and everything that is positive or ideal) in relation to European American bioethics. Standard healthcare policies adhering to the Patient Self-Determination Act intend to expose all hospitalized Navajo patients to advance care planning. This is in direct conflict with *hozho* because Navajo patients believe that providers should only plan and speak in positive terms and should avoid speaking about negative outcomes and so forth. Carrese and Rhodes (1995) consider advance care planning with this population "a dangerous violation of traditional Navajo values" (p. 826). Kazal (1996) concurs with the Carrese and Rhodes findings and suggests that health care providers can use the third person plural approach in communicating sensitive information, an approach that has been received by Navajo patients positively. The relationship between the Native American patient and the health care provider is therefore extremely important for treatment access, planning, and compliance. Johnson et al. (1995) suggest that American Indians do not expect to be treated fairly by non-Indian health care providers and prefer treatment by culturally sensitive providers who are also usually American Indian. This statement paves the way for understanding cultural aspects of successful treatment outcome.

Neuropsychological Assessment with Native Americans

Professional ethics mandates that psychologists recognize differences among people that "may be associated with age, sex, socioeconomic, and ethnic backgrounds. When necessary, they obtain training, experience, or counsel to assure competent service or research relating to such persons" (American Psychological Association [APA], 1990, p. 391). In addition, when reporting assessment results, "psychologists indicate any reservations that exist regarding validity or reliability because of the circumstances of the assessment or the inappropriateness of the norms for the person tested" (APA, 1990, p. 394). Given the lack of assessment data on Native Americans in the research literature, and the diversity of the Native American population, these ethical mandates may be more difficult to carry out than expected. However, there are some general considerations that can be presented about American Indian culture that may assist in the assessment process.

Cognitive Processes

Research suggests that Native American people think differently than European American people (Deyhle & Swisher, 1997; Tafoya, 1989). Native Americans' reasoning process tends to be less linear–sequential–analytical and more global or holistic (Cattey, 1980; Tharp, 1994). Some researchers suggest significant differences in cerebral lateralization (Scott et al., 1979). Communication styles (Berlin, 1987), decision making strategies (King & Draguns, 1988), and learning styles (Tafoya, 1989; Tharp, 1994) have been shown to differ significantly from European Americans. Tharp (1994) links holistic thought to differences in cognitive processing. He further links these with multilevel, interconnected aspects of (a) perceptual, (b) problem-solving, (c) semiotic, (d) neurological, (e) representational, (f) sociological, and (g) interpersonal processing.

Researchers are beginning to investigate the following cultural variables: They fall within the categories of world-view and relational styles that may well contribute to test taking approaches and strategies used by American Indians. Cooperation versus competition, time orientation, bodily movement and proximity, touching, eye contact, gender relationship/ interactions, individuality versus family, verbal versus nonverbal/modeling, issues of fate versus individual responses, perceptual style, and cognitive style (Chamberlain & Medinos-Landurand, 1991; Deyhle & Swisher, 1997; Tharp, 1994).

American Indians will reflect some of these differences within tribes, between tribes, and interactionally with examiners when presenting for assessment. These relational differences, symbolized in American Indian values, behaviors, or culture will place those persons on an acculturational continuum that may, in fact, color the assessment process and outcomes (McShane & Plas, 1984; Sack, Beiser, Clarke, & Red Shirt, 1987). Many factors present problems for both American Indians and for the clinicians that attempt to assess them. There are environmental factors unique to American Indian communities; physical problems that are common to many American Indian adults and children; language differences and deficits exist; there are sociopolitical determinants, cultural differences, and social/personal domains—all of which may influence the assessment process and outcome (Dana, 1984; Dauphinais & King, 1992; Lonner & Ibrahim, 1996; McShane, 1980).

Language

Most standardized tests are believed to underestimate the abilities and aptitudes of linguistically diverse students (Hamayan & Damico, 1991). While many American Indian children are not bilingual, many are limited English proficient (LEP). Cooley (1979) has demonstrated specific American Indian speech and language patterns different from those of Anglos, even though English was the common language.

Two independent studies (Dauphinais L., 1981; Dauphinais, P., 1981) have examined language styles and language interpretive systems, and found significant differences between European American and American Indian language systems. These differences may be partially explained by Heath (1983) who reported that "fundamental genres that occur in recurrent situations ... is so patterned ... that listeners can anticipate by the prosody or a recounting of shared past experiences" (p. 166). O'Conner (1989) also reports:

> a collaborative, cooperative, group motivated child may evince reluctance or lack of interest in the individualistic, competitive context of test taking. In the domain of language, the mismatch between culturally determined patterns of language use, and the decontextualized genres of test items is a promising area of study for those interested in understanding in detail the interaction of test taker and test. (p. 173)

The question then for a psychological examiner is: To what degree does facility with the culturally based language of an instrument affect performance? While language problems are demonstrated more explicitly during cognitive, language, and academic assessment, both receptive and expressive language differences may affect responses on personality and projective assessments because language and thought are likely to be inextricable (Vygotsky, 1962). Without an understanding of the effect of subtle language differences, and without cognizance of how a child is understanding the process, the nuances of the examiner–respondent interface can potentially result in inaccurate conclusions. O'Conner (1989) goes even further to say that fair, equitable test policy, and obviously test development, are lacking if we do not attempt to understand how at least "macrolevel factors" impact the interaction of test taker and test.

Sociopolitical/Interpersonal

Individuals react differently when there is an unequal power base. When an American Indian attends an interview with a neuropsychologist, the nature of the interaction may be different if the clinician goes to the home or another neutral setting to test, rather than conducting it in an (non-Indian) institutional setting. The power base may shift and the behavior of each person change, according to the setting. "Noninterference" (Goodtracks, 1973; Sage, 1991), an American Indian value, denotes the deference of one person to another while minimizing the power base influences. This style may be misunderstood in a non-Indian setting. Trust is another sociopolitical variable in which American Indian people appear to differ from others. Mistrust of European Americans and agencies can be traced to the long history of mistrust engendered by missionaries and the federal government. Hence, initial feelings for an American Indian person may be quite different than those of an Anglo person when entering an institutional setting.

Personality/Sociality

Many behaviors are obviously related to their social context, i.e., family, community, and so forth. The desired level of independence in personality development is one such example. However, independence is viewed quite differently in middle-class Anglo versus Indian communities. The latter has traditionally been more group-oriented than Anglo society, which tends to be more individualistic. Among American Indians "individualization of responsibility is emphasized as a means for achieving community solidarity rather than a mechanism for personal achievement" (LaFromboise, 1988, p. 392).

American Indian family members also teach and model certain ways to interact with others, such as when to have eye contact, when it is appropriate to talk openly in groups, and when and how to initiate social interaction. These behaviors may, in subtle but real ways, affect the assessment process. Thus, neuropsychological assessment should take place with an awareness of the varieties of cultural dimensions that might interact within the testing milieu.

Neuropsychological Test Instruments and Native Americans

There are only a few studies within the last decade that addressed the variety of instruments utilized with American Indian children. Most studies have recommended caution in the use of these instruments with American Indian populations.

Wechsler Intelligence Scales

The Wechsler scales are the most frequently used instruments for the assessment of intelligence among American Indians (McShane & Plas, 1984; Mishra, 1982). Naglieri (1982) has suggested that the Verbal Scale is an estimate of English-language ability, not intelligence, for American Indians. Tanner-Halverson and Burden (1995) hypothesize that the test measures acculturation into American middle-class society rather than intelligence. No doubt, the Wechsler tests will continue to be used to assess Native Americans until a better assessment instrument is developed. The question for the examiner is to what extent can the information derived be used to portray actual cognitive processes.

Tanner-Halverson and Burden (1995) report that although the WISC-III contains many improvements over the WISC-R, which had at least 15 Verbal Scale items that were biased against American Indians (Mishra, 1982), some items still appear to be irrelevant or biased against minority children. Tanner-Halverson and Burden's (1995) research with the Tohono O'odham found the average student's Verbal and Full Scale score to be one standard deviation below the national norm, similar to many previous studies. However, Verbal and Performance Scores were closer together than the 8–19 point Verbal–Performance split often found with the WISC-R and American Indian children.

McShane has followed the testing of American Indian children with the WISC-R for over a decade (McShane, 1980, 1988; McShane & Plas, 1982, 1984). American Indian samples have generally demonstrated an 8–19 point difference between the Verbal and Performance subsections, with the Performance scores typically falling at or above the national mean. The intellectual abilities of American Indian referred samples on the WISC-R have also shown subtest recategorization patterns of Spatial–Sequential–Conceptual–Acquired Knowledge. This pattern is unlike Bannatyne's (1968, 1974) and Smith, Coleman, Dokecki, & Davis's (1977) demonstrated WISC and WISC-R patterns of Spatial–Conceptual–Sequential–Acquired Knowledge in the general population learning disabled (LD) samples. These patterns reflect, in order, the students' preferred intellectual style. McShane and Plas (1982) conclude that these intellectual styles are not invariant across cultural groups. In addition, Kaufman's (1975) Freedom of Distractibility factor generally failed to be substantiated for American Indian samples. After a review of studies in this area, McShane and Plas (1982) describe an "Indian intellectual style" against which they recommend that American Indians be measured. Unfortunately, to date, such a "style" remains too imprecise a concept to be employed universally.

Kaufman Assessment Battery for Children (K-ABC)

The K-ABC has been recommended by some (e.g., Sattler, 1982) as the instrument of choice for assessing cognitive abilities with American Indian children, primarily because of its ability to isolate hemispheric-based strengths that are thought to be characteristic of American Indian children. Davidson (1992) found that Native American children tended to score higher on the Simultaneous rather than Sequential Scales of the K-ABC; a premise that supports previous research on holistic thinking styles. However, relatively few studies have been published with the K-ABC, and the few published reports have not always substantiated the claims of the test's developers. For example, Scaldwell (cited in Common & Frost, 1988) reported that his sample of Canadian Indian children ($N = 47$) scored significantly lower than the norm group on all subtests. He went on to question the usefulness of the Kaufman test. At this stage, insufficient data exists to make reliable judgements concerning the K-ABC's unique applicability and validity with American Indian populations.

Other Cognitive Tests

Sacuzzo and Johnson (1995) conducted an extensive research study concerning the use of traditional psychometric tests and proportionate representation. They supported the view of test bias being most appropriate from a qualified individualism perspective, where gender and ethnic background is considered in the selection/clinical process. Their study involved the use and comparison of the WISC-R and Raven's Progressive Matrices performance in the selection of children for gifted programs. Over 16,000 students were tested. The Raven's was used because of previous data indicating that the test was found to be predictive of success in a program for gifted students of Hispanic and Native American origin; it was not known, however, if the Raven's could be used to achieve proportionate representation for selection purposes. The results of the study, with regard to the Raven's, was confounded by other factors entering into the qualifying process. It did seem, however, that the Raven's as a measure represented cognitive processes across ethnicities.

The Test of Nonverbal Intelligence (TONI)'s effectiveness in assessment of cognitive ability with American Indian youth is discussed by Whorton and Morgan (1990). They reported correlations of .68, .42, and .48 between the TONI and the WISC-R Verbal, Performance, Full Scale scores respectively. No differences were found in the Verbal, Performance, and Full Scale IQs of a modest sample of European American ($N = 29$) and American Indian ($N = 17$) children. Scaldwell (1986) reports mean scores of 97.27 ($N = 47$) on the TONI for an American Indian sample.

It seems clear that, as suggested by Braden (1990), tests that can appropriately assess the unique intellectual abilities of the American Indian child and that avoid the burden of cultural bias are still at the beginning stages of experimental refinement. While the TONI is recommended as unbiased by some, it still requires a linear–sequential logical style that is not the American Indian preferred learning style. Therefore, it is probably best that local ethnic norms are developed for selection purposes (Raven 1989), or traditional tests are used in qualitative and creative ways (Sacuzzo & Johnson, 1995).

Achievement Tests

Very little research has been reported in the psychological literature concerning diagnostic achievement testing with American Indian children. Dauphinais (1990) has obtained achievement data from a norming project with 267 American Indian children, ages 6–16. The WISC-R, the Woodcock–Johnson Psychoeducational Battery—Part II, the Wide Range Achievement Test-Revised (WRAT-R), the Test of Language Development-Intermediate and Primary (TOLD-I & P), and the Clinical Evaluation of Language Fundamentals-Revised (CELF-R) were utilized. His sample's performance on the Woodcock–Johnson Battery ranged from four to eight points below the national mean depending on the knowledge area. Female subjects averaged three to five points higher than males on the various knowledge areas on the

Woodcock–Johnson. Females also scored five to six points higher on the WRAT-R. Compared to national WRAT-R norms, scores were five to six points lower for females and 10–12 points lower for males. TOLD-2-I&P scores were five to seven points lower than the national norms on the Primary test for children aged six through eight. The scores for children aged 9–12 were 10–12 points below the national mean.

The CELF-R was used in the Dauphinais project for children aged 13–16. This American Indian sample scored 13 points lower than the national mean for the Receptive component and 11 points lower for the Expressive component.

Examination of the Dauphinais' preliminary findings indicates that American Indian children score lower than the national mean on tests of acquired knowledge. However, as O'Conner (1989) notes: "both tests and schools stress the use of English and incorporate the assumptions of mainstream American society; a test can appear to be psychometrically valid while still overlooking the student's learning potential" (p. 261).

A review of the existing literature on assessment of American Indian children allows us to examine the assumptions of validity and reliability of the instruments of general use today. Those who are responsible for the assessment of American Indian children need to be quite cognizant of the dangers in assuming that established measures reflect the learning potential of the American Indian child. Although the WISC-III is the instrument of choice with American Indian students, local norming is recommended by researchers. Performance scale scores exceed verbal scores among non-handicapped American Indian samples, with seven points as the minimum average difference found in a single sample, and a 33-point difference as the maximum. Performance scale scores may be the better indicators of the Native person's cognitive ability.

Personality and Adjustment Instruments

Personality test validation studies among American Indians, especially American Indian youth, have been neglected (Dana, 1986; Davis, Hoffman, & Nelson, 1990; Manson, Walker, & Kivlahan, 1987). A review of literature by Greene (1987) identified only seven Minnesota Multiphasic Personality Inventory (MMPI) studies comparing American Indian test results with those of Anglos. Likewise, Dahlstrom (1986) found only six MMPI studies using nonpsychiatric American Indian samples. Most of the Thematic Apperception Test (TAT) and Rorschach studies among Indian people were conducted over 40 years ago (Dana, 1986).

A study by Lonner and Ibrahim (1989) revealed that graduate programs in counseling, school, and clinical psychology generally failed to consider cross-cultural issues. Such failure could potentially lead to numerous problems in the provision of adequate and appropriate mental health services to ethnic minority people. The following is a brief review of the small cluster of data-based studies on personality assessment with American Indian samples.

Minnesota Multiphasic Psychological Inventory (MMPI and MMPI-2)

MMPI-2 developers included 77 American Indians as part of its field sample (Butcher, Graham, Dahlstrom, Tellegen, & Kraemmer, 1989). However, for a test containing ten major clinical subscales and numerous other subscales, 77 Indians is clearly too small a number for the MMPI-2's validation on this population (Lawley & Maxwell, 1971). Furthermore, tribal diversity has been overlooked with only one tribe used to represent Indian people in general.

To our knowledge, there have been no validation studies on the MMPI-2 and American Indian youth (or adults), in spite of the fact that the MMPI has been the most frequently used psychological measure with American Indians (Manson et al., 1987).

MMPI research with American Indian populations has yielded mixed results. Greene (1987) in his review of that literature found that most studies noted differences among Indian and Anglo groups, but was unable to identify distinct patterns for these differences. Pollack and Shore (1980) found significant cultural influences on MMPI responses of American Indian psychiatric inpatients who belonged to a Pacific Northwest tribe. They noted elevated scores on the validity (F), psychopathic deviate (Pd), and schizophrenia (Sc) scales. The MMPI profiles among this sample remained remarkably similar across diagnostic categories, which led them to question the MMPI's diagnostic specificity among American Indian people. Uecker, Boutilier, and Richardson (1980) compared European American and American Indian veterans' scores on the MMPI alcoholic profile and after close examination of the results found them to be dissimilar across groups. Vesely (1990) likewise found significant differences between American Indian and European American MMPI alcoholic profiles. In a study that compared MMPI responses among American Indian and European American adolescents, Bryde (1970) identified 26 significant differences between the American Indian and European American samples on 28 personality variables. An MMPI study that compared American Indian, Black, and European American psychiatric inpatients (Butcher, Braswell, & Raney, 1983) found that MMPI differences between groups were related to actual symptoms and not to ethnicity. They also noted that within-group norms would have to be developed before the effects due to ethnicity versus those due to symptom tendencies could be clarified.

Several authors have referred to subjects' degree of acculturation or traditionality as a variable that could impact on MMPI-measured psychopathology (Dana, 1986; Hoffman, Dana, & Bolton, 1985). The culturally based responses of normal individuals may appear as pathological on the MMPI. Until the MMPI-2 is better understood in light of its appropriateness across American Indian tribes, its results must be considered cautiously.

Thematic Apperception Test (TAT).   Most TAT studies among American Indians were conducted over 40 years ago. They include Henry (1951), Leighton and Kluckhohn (1947), MacGregor (1946), and Thompson and Joseph (1951). These early studies appear to demonstrate very clear differences in responses for American Indian people. Granzberg (1972) noted that Hopi boys would not be able to understand the situations depicted in most of the TAT cards. In fact, many of the examiners began to develop modified TAT cards to individual tribes (Alexander & Anderson, 1957; Dana, 1984; Henry, 1947; Hunt & Smith, 1966; Lindzey, 1961). Most of these findings conclude with the notion that local norms and an in-depth knowledge of the culture is a prerequisite for interpretation (Dana, 1986; Lonner & Ibrahim, 1989). Validity of the TAT with European American samples has been poorly demonstrated, yet its use continues to be widespread. The use of the TAT with Indian clients remains questionable.

Rorschach.   Most Rorschach studies conducted among American Indian children, adolescents, and adults do not question the validity of the instrument for its cultural sensitivity. However, Day, Boyer, & DeVos (1975) reported specific differences between Apache and European American children in their Rorschach responses. These differences were interpreted as reflecting the two groups contrasting modes of perception of external reality. The authors concluded that there were culturally determined differences in the style of cognitive approach to the cards. A more recent study (Boyer et al., 1989) which included field observations, as well as personality testing, reported Rorschach scores among two related Alaska native tribes to be consonant with the observations of fieldworkers. However, the interpretations and observations were made from a psychoanalytic perspective and cultural views of the meanings of the

Rorschach responses were not explored. Day et al. (1975) have reported that an American Indian adolescent sample gave significantly more animal movement responses than a comparable European American sample. Dauphinais and King (1992) suggest that cultural differences cause American Indian clients to provide more content responses of anthropology, art, food, animal, and animal detail. Studies by Hallowell (1950), Henry (1947), Henry and Spiro (1951), and Schachtel, Henry, and Henry (1942), provide a logical rationale for how cultural diversity could impact the responses of American Indian children and adolescents to projective stimuli. These works are recommended reading for both researchers and practitioners in this area.

California Psychological Inventory (CPI).   Like other personality tests, very little has been reported concerning the effectiveness of the CPI with American Indian clients. Davis et al., (1990) note that most studies using the CPI find more psychopathology among Indians than European Americans. However, their own study of 70 Indian adults and 100 European American adults, matched across age, education, and socioeconomic status, suggested that cultural variables significantly influence test results. They conclude that: "Careful consideration of the ethnic background of respondents may be warranted in situations in which the CPI is used as a screening measure" (p. 242).

Recommendations for Clinicians

The first and most basic of recommendations for working with Native Americans (as with any patient) is that the clincian should make an assessment as to whether he or she is culturally competent to work with the patient. This self-assessment may be conducted on many levels during initial contact. There are issues of language, gender, age, ethnicity, and personality congruence between neuropsychologist and the client that need to be resolved before continuing with treatment. As stated previously, the American Indian population is very diverse, and having competence with one tribe does not presuppose competence with another tribe.

Second, any potential cultural conflicts between the clincian and client need to be resolved either by discussion, training, consultation, or withdrawal from the case.

Third, any potential bias in assessment instruments, service delivery, access to healthcare, and so forth must be documented and thoroughly explained to the client and in reports/progress notes. This requires that the neuropsychologist place the assessment and treatment in a cultural context.

Fourth, the clincian should become aware of and familiar with instruments that assist in the determination of the client's level of acculturation. Many of these instruments with American Indians were developed in the 1940s, were developed by anthropologists, and may not be applicable. However, Brown (1982) developed an informal process using the case history to document level of acculturation. Brown's method assesses four areas of behaviors that focus on family/self relationships, spiritual/religious, social/recreational, and training/education. These four areas assess, essentially, the client's *worldview* and are very intimate in nature. Of course, the entire acculturation interview is based on the premise that the American Indian client and family have a trusting and positive rapport with the examiner. Dana (1993) recommends that when conducting an assessment with reservation residents, tribe-specific measures are preferable because they will provide greater detail and demonstrate awareness and competence of the clinician to the examinee.

The following are general recommendations for the assessment and treatment process.

Rapport

American Indians are less likely to be task-oriented and/or eager for assessment to occur. Thus, the initial meeting between American Indian client and examiner may be critical. American Indians tend more than European Americans to respond on the basis of the client–examiner relationship rather than initial intrinsic interest (Dana, 1985; Gibbs, 1980; Roll, Millen, & Martinez, 1980). The manner in which the assessor identifies him or herself to an American Indian individual sets the tone for the session. American Indians are more comfortable with introductions that are less formal and prefer to talk more about where you are from geographically than noting professional credentials (which some state laws require). Many times, Indian people will not begin to participate until the proper introduction has occurred. Also, they may be skeptical about the particular test they are about to take, knowing that historically test results have cast American Indian people in a negative light. It is generally helpful and comforting if the examiner explains both the purpose and the process of testing. In addition it is probably better, for rapport purposes, for the clinician to be informally dressed. Formal dress is not customary and may provide a visual barrier to a comfortable rapport with the neurospycholgist.

Setting

As mentioned previously, the assessment setting can have an impact on the outcome of testing. Thus, it is important for the clinician to assess the comfort level of the native person (or family) among nonnatives. If there appears to be a high level of distrust, suspicion, or discomfort, then perhaps a neutral setting would be helpful. Obviously, this is not possible in a number of settings, and when not, at least the clinician can be aware of the influence of setting.

Introducing the Testing

Many native people are suspicious of testing. Again, knowing the history of native people and the countless times testing, evaluation, and other analyses have portrayed American Indians as less than capable can allow the clinician to address their fears. Acknowledging that much of the testing has been developed on European American norms, yet cultural factors will be accounted for while scoring and interpreting, will work towards reducing suspicion. Asking the client if they have any questions about the tests themselves or what the test results will be used for is also helpful.

Testing Procedures

As rigorous as neuropsychological testing is, it is helpful to keep the procedure as informal as possible. Joking about the testing, asking questions about brothers, sisters, and so forth are means to keep the client engaged, trusting, and motivated. Ways one can show respect is quite beneficial. To address elders with respect, perhaps using a more formal title (Mr. or Mrs.) is cultural and welcomed.

In addition, as the Report of the National Commission on Testing and Public Policy (1990) has stated: No testing should lead to nowhere. Treatment and discharge planning must be as culturally competent as the testing and evaluation. Discharge planning may be particularly difficult with Native Americans because of instances of lack of access to appropriate health care, poverty, geographic locality, and other issues that contribute to underutilization of facilites. As American Indian clients leave the neuropsychologist's care, they will engage with systems and individuals that may not be culturally competent. Therefore, followup requires awareness of the referral competencies and funding sources.

Research Directions and Conclusions

Research studies attempting to define and codify cultural information about Native American tribes are sparse and have traditionally had major setbacks because of lack of cultural awareness on the part of the researchers (Darou, Hum, & Kurtness, 1993). For example, the Crees of northern Quebec have had eight psychological studies conducted in their territory and have rejected all the researchers except one. The reasons for rejection were specifically related to lack of respect for the culture and authority of the tribe (Darou et al., 1993). The National Institutes of Health (NIH) also support a history of researchers not being aware of tribal authority systems (Norton & Manson, 1996). The NIH have published guidelines for recruiting ethnic minorities and women into clinical research that include:

> Defining the population of American Indians and Alaska Natives for inclusion in a study, participation of the tribes in research and approval by the Institutional Review Board, issues of confidentiality and anonymity of individuals and tribes, identifying potential benefits to American Indian and Alaska Native Communities, and the importance of evaluating the scientific merit of a proposed study. (Norton & Manson, 1995, p. 1)

Therefore, the first direction for research in the field of neuropsychology and American Indians, is that researchers receive training in how to conduct culturally competent studies with this population. This training is left up to the doctoral training and postdoctoral training sites around the country, or the motivation of individual researchers to obtain ongoing training.

In terms of test construction and assessment instruments, for decades researchers and practitioners have called for research on the validity of psychological measures for American Indians. Once again this need is highlighted. Until further test validation research is accomplished, it must be assumed that most tests, when used cross-culturally, are biased (Frijda & Jahoda, 1966; Lonner & Ibrahim, 1989). Assessment devices are merely tools with inherent limitations, especially when applied in a cross-cultural situation. It is the responsibility of the assessor to weigh the risks against the benefits in this endeavor. An assumption that any psychological examiner, without special training and supervision, can adequately assess American Indian people is extremely hazardous. The time has come to require at least some instruction in the area of ethnic minority assessment in all accredited training programs in neuropsychology. However, the greatest need appears to be awareness of the diversity that exists for American Indians, because of both social conditions and factors that are distinctly cultural. More scientific data is needed, but more awareness and cultural competence must occur for data gathering to be facilitated. As Lonner and Ibrahim (1996) suggest: "Nothing will ever replace ... careful consideration of what is best for the client" (p. 324).

Clearly, the need for neuropsychological research is paramount. Norms developed both within and across tribes are necessary if we are to be competent in our assessments. Establishing the links between cultural differences in cognitive processes and neuropsychological domains may further our knowledge of thought and culture, culture and cognitive development, and culture and brain physiology. However, when we look at the broad scope of the field of neuropsychology, the overall neglect of American Indians in our attention and studies invites, hopefully, a moral response that will effect significant change in the future.

References

Alexander, T., & Anderson, R. (1957). Children in a society under stress. *Behavioral Science, 2*, 46–55.

American Psychological Association (1990). Ethical principles of psychologists (Amended). *American Psychologist, 45*, 390–395.

Bagley, S. P., Angel, R., Dilworth-Anderson, P., Liu, W., & Schinke, S. (1995). Adaptive health behaviors among ethnic minorities. *American Psychologist, 14*, 632–640.

Bannatyne, A. (1968). Diagnosing learning disabilities and writing medical prescriptions. *Journal of Learning Disabilities, 1*, 242–249.

Bannatyne, A. (1974). Diagnosis: A note on recategorization of the WISC scales scores. *Journal of Learning Disabilities, 7*, 272–273.

Berkhofer, R. F. (1978). *The white man's Indian: Images of the American Indian from Columbus to the present.* New York: Knopf.

Berlin, I. N. (1987). Current status and future directions of research on the American Indian child. *American Journal of Psychiatry, 144*, 1135–1142.

Berry, J. W. (1980). Acculturation as varieties of adaptation. In A. M. Padilla (Ed.), *Acculturation: Theory, models and some new findings* (pp. 9–25). Boulder, CO: Westview.

Berry, J. W., Kim, U., Minde, T., & Mok, D. (1987). Comparative studies of acculturative stress. *International Migration Review, 21*, 491–511.

Boyce, W. T., & Boyce, J. C. (1983). Acculturation and changes in health among Navajo boarding school students. *Social Science and Medicine, 17*, 219–226.

Boyer, L. B., Boyer, R. M., Dithrich, C. W., Harned, H., Hippler, A. E., Stone, J. S., & Walt, A. (1989). The relation between psychological states and acculturation among the Tanaina and Upper Tanana Indians of Alaska: An ethnographic Rorschach study. *Ethos, 17*, 450–479.

Braden, J. P. (1990). Guest editors' comments: Experimental methods for assessing intelligence. *School Psychology Review, 19*, 397–398.

Brave Heart, M. Y. H., & DeBruyn, L. M. (1998) The American Indian holocaust: Healing historical unresolved grief. *American Indian and Alaska Native Mental Health Research, 8*(2), 56–78.

Brown, S. (1982). *Native generations diagnosis and placement on the conflict/resolution chart.* Paper presented at the annual meeting of the School of Addiction Studies, University of Alaska, Anchorage.

Bryde, J. F. (1970). *The Indian student—A study of scholastic failure and personality conflict.* Vermillion: University of South Dakota Press.

Butcher, J. N., Braswell, L., & Raney, D. (1983). A cross-cultural comparison of American Indian, black, and white inpatients on the MMPI and presenting symptoms. *Journal of Consulting and Clinical Psychology, 51*, 587–594.

Butcher, J. N., Graham, J. R., Dahlstrom, W. G., Tellegen, A. M., & Kraemmer, B. (1989). *MMPI-2 manual for administration and scoring.* Minneapolis: University of Minnesota Press.

Carrese, J. A., & Rhodes, L. A. (1995). Western bioethics on the Navajo reservation: Benefit or harm? *Journal of the American Medical Association, 274*, 826–829.

Cattey, M. (1980). Cultural differences in processing information. *Journal of American Indian Education, 20*(1), 23–28.

Chamberlain, P. & Medinos-Landurand, P. (1991). Practical considerations for the assessment of limited English proficient students with special needs. In E. V. Hamayan & J. S. Damico (Eds.), *Limiting bias in the assessment of bilingual students* (pp. 111–156). Austin, TX: ProED.

Common, R. W., & Frost, L. G. (1988). The implications of the mismeasurement of native students' intelligence through the use of standardized intelligence tests. *Canadian Journal of Native Education, 15*, 18–30.

Cooley, R. (1979). *Spokes in a wheel: A rhetorical and linguistic analysis of Native American public speeches.* A paper presented at the Cross-Cultural Communication Symposium, University of California, Berkeley.

Dana, R. H. (1984). Intelligence testing of American Indian children: Sidesteps in quest of ethical practice. *White Cloud Journal, 3*, 35–43.

Dana, R. H. (1985). The Thematic Apperception Test (TAT). In C. S. Newmark (Ed.), *Major psychological assessment instruments* (pp. 89–134). Newton, MA: Allyn & Bacon.

Dana, R. H. (1986). Personality assessment and Native Americans. *Journal of Personality Assessment, 50*, 480–500.

Dana, R. H. (1993). Multicultural assessment perspectives for professional psychology. Boston: Allyn & Bacon.

Darou, W. G., Hum, A., & Kurtness, J. (1993). An investigation of the impact of psychosocial research on a native population. *American Psychologist, 24*, 325–329.

Dauphinais, L. (1981). *American Indian and Anglo perceptions of speaker, message structure, and message orientation.* Unpublished doctoral dissertation, University of Oklahoma, Norman, OK.

Dauphinais, P. (1981). *American Indian college student preference of counselor communication style.* Unpublished dissertation, University of Oklahoma, Norman, OK.

Dauphinais, P. (1990). [Local norming data: averages, standard deviations, archival data]. Unpublished raw data.

Dauphinais, P., & King, J. (1992). Psychological assessment with American Indian children. *Applied & Preventive Psychology: Current Scientific Perspectives, 1,* 97–110.

Davidson, K. L. (1992). A comparison of Native American and white student's cognitive strengths as measured by the Kaufman Assessment Battery for Children. *Roeper Review, 14,* 111–115.

Davis, G. L., Hoffman, R. G., Nelson, K. S. (1990). Differences between Native Americans and whites on the California Psychological Inventory. *Journal of Consulting and Clinical Psychology, 2,* 238–242.

Day, R., Boyer, L. B., & DeVos, G. A. (1975). Two styles of ego development: A cross-cultural, longitudinal comparison of Apache and Anglo school children. *Ethos, 3,* 345–380.

Deloria, V. (1997). *Red earth, white lies: Native Americans and the myth of scientific fact.* Golden, CO: Fulcrum.

Deyhle, D., & Swisher, K. (1997). Research in American Indian and Alaska Native education: From assimilation to self-determination. In M. W. Apple (Ed.), *Review of research in education* (vol. 22, pp. 113–194). Washington, D.C.: American Educational Research Association.

Duran, E., & Duran, B. (1995). *Native American postcolonial psychology.* New York: State University of New York Press.

Ferraro, F. R., Bercier, B., & Chelminski, I. (1997). Geriatric Depression Scale-Short Form (GDS-SF) performance in Native American elderly adults. *Clinical Gerontologist, 18,* 52–55.

Frijda, N., & Jahoda, G. (1966). On the scope and methods of cross-cultural research. *International Journal of Psychology, 1,* 109–127.

Gibbs, J. T. (1980). The interpersonal orientation in mental health consultation: Toward a model of ethnic variations in consultation. *Journal of Community Psychology, 8,* 195–207.

Goodtracks, J. G. (1973). Native American non-interference. *Social Work, 18,* 30–34.

Granzberg, G. (1972). Hopi initiation rites: A case study of the validity of the Freudian theory of culture. *Journal of Social Psychology, 87,* 189–195.

Graves, T. D. (1967). Psychological acculturation in a tri-ethnic community. *Southwestern Journal of Anthropology, 23,* 337–350.

Greene, R. L. (1987). Ethnicity and MMPI performance: A review. *Journal of Consulting and Clinical Psychology, 55,* 497–512.

Hallowell, A. I. (1950). Acculturation processes and personality changes. In C. Kluckhohn & H. A. Murray (Eds.), *Personality in nature, society, and culture* (pp. 340–346). New York: Knopf.

Hamayan, E. V., & Damico, J. S. (1991). Developing and using a second language. In E. V. Hamayan & J. S. Damico (Eds.), *Limiting bias in the assessment of bilingual students* (pp. 248–279). Austin, TX: ProEd.

Heath, S. B. (1983). *Ways with words: Language, life and work in communities and classrooms.* Cambridge, UK: Cambridge University Press.

Henry, W. E. (1947). The thematic apperception technique in the study of culture-personality relations. *Genetic Psychology Monographs, 35,* 3–135.

Henry, W. E. (1951). The Thematic Apperception Test in the study group and cultural problems. In H. H. Anderson & G. L. Anderson (Eds.), *An introduction to projective techniques* (pp. 230–278). New York: Prentice-Hall.

Henry, W. E., & Spiro, M. E. (1951). Psychological techniques: Projective techniques in field work. In A. L. Kroeber (Ed.), *Anthropology today* (pp. 417–429). Chicago: University of Chicago Press.

Hoffman, T., Dana, R., & Bolton, B. (1985). Measured acculturation and MMPI-168 performance of Native American adults. *Journal of Cross-Cultural Psychology, 16,* 243–246.

Hunt, R. G., & Smith, M. E. (1966). Cultural symbols and response to thematic test materials. *Journal of Projective Techniques and Personality Assessment, 30,* 587–590.

Hynd, G. W., & Garcia, W. I. (1979). Intellectual assessment of the Native American student. *School Psychology Review, 8,* 446–454.

Joe, J. (1994). Revaluing Native American concepts of development and education. In P. Greenfield & R. Cocking (Eds.) *Cross-cultural roots of minority child development* (pp. 107–113). Hillsdale, NJ: Erlbaum.

Johnson, K. W., Anderson, N. B., Bastida, E., Kramer, B. J., Williams, D., & Wong, M. (1995). Macrosocial and environmental influences in minority health. *American Psychologist, 14,* 601–612.

Kaufman, A. S. (1975). Factor analysis of the WISC-R at 11 age levels between 6.5 and 16.5 years. *Journal of Consulting and Clinical Psychology, 43,* 135–147.

Kazal, L. A. (1996). Western bioethics on the Navajo reservation: Benefit or harm? *Journal of the American Medical Association, 275,* 108.

King, J. (1994). Ethnic identity and mental health among urban Indians. Seventh Annual Convention of American Indian Psychologists and Psychology Graduate Students, Sponsored by Utah State University and Indian Health Service, June 27–28, Logan, Utah.

King, J. J., & Draguns, J. G. (1988). Decision making strategies among Cherokee Indians in eastern Oklahoma. Poster presented at the 9th International Congress on Cross-Cultural Psychology, August 21–26, Newcastle, Australia.

Kodituwakku, P. W., Handmaker, N. S., Cutler, S. K., Weathersby, E. K., & Handmaker, S. D. (1995). Specific impairments in self-regulation in children exposed to alcohol prenatally. *Alcoholism: Clinical and Experimental Research, 19,* 1558–1564.

Kodituwakku, P. W., May, P., Ballinger, L., Harris, M., Aase, J., & Aragon, A. (1997). Executive control functioning and theory of mind in children prenatally exposed to alcohol. Poster presented at the 1997 FAS Conference, Breckenridge, Colorado, September 25–27, 1997.

LaFramboise, T. (1988). American Indian mental health policy. *American Psychologist, 43,* 388–397.

Lawley, D. N., & Maxwell, A. E. (1971). *Factor analysis as a statistical method* (2nd ed.). London: Butterworth.

Leighton, D. C., & Kluckhohn, C. (1947). *Children of the people.* Cambridge, MA: Harvard University Press.

Lindzey, G. (1961). *Projective techniques and cross-cultural research.* New York: Appleton-Century-Crofts.

Lonner, W. J., & Ibrahim, F. A. (1989). Assessment in cross-cultural counseling. In P. B. Pedersen, J. G. Draguns, W. J. Lonner, and J. E. Trimble (Eds.), *Counseling across cultures* (3rd ed., pp. 299–333). Honolulu: University of Hawaii Press.

Lonner, W. J. & Ibrahim, F. A. (1996). Appraisal and assessment in cross-cultural counseling. In P. B. Pedersen, J. G. Draguns, W. J. Lonner, & J. E. Trimble (Eds.), *Counseling across cultures* (3rd ed., pp. 293–322). Thousand Oaks, CA: Sage.

MacGregor, G. (1946). *Warriors without weapons.* Chicago: University of Chicago Press.

Manson, S. M., Shore, J. H., & Bloom, J. D. (1985). The depressive experience in American Indian communities: A challenge for psychiatric theory and diagnosis. In A. Kleinman & B. Good, (Eds.), *Culture and depression* (pp. 331–368). Berkeley: University of California Press.

Manson, S. M., Walker, R. D., & Kivlahan, D. R. (1987). Psychiatric assessment and treatment of American Indians and Alaska Natives. *Hospital and Community Psychiatry, 38,* 165–173.

McKeever, W. F., & Hunt, L. J. (1984). Failure to replicate the Scott et al. findings of reversed ear dominance in the Native American Navajo. *Neuropsychologia, 22,* 539–541.

McShane, D. (1980). A review of scores of American Indian children on the Wechsler Intelligence Scales. *White Cloud Journal, 1,* 3–9.

McShane, D. (1988). The relationship of intellectual and psycholinguistic abilities to the achievement gains of American Indian children. *Canadian Journal of Native Education, 15,* 66–86.

McShane, D., & Plas, J. M. (1982). WISC-R factor structures of the Ojibwa Indian children. *White Cloud Journal, 2,* 18–22.

McShane, D., & Plas, J. M. (1984). The cognitive functioning of American Indian children: Moving from the WISC to the WISC-R. *School Psychology Review, 13,* 61–73.

Mercer, S. (1994). Navajo elders in a reservation nursing home: Health status profile. *Journal of Gerontological Social Work, 23,* 3–29.

Mishra, S. P. (1982). The WISC-R and evidence of item bias for Native American Navajos. *Psychology in the Schools, 19,* 458–464.

Mishra, S. P., Lord, J., & Sabers, D. L. (1989). Cognitive processes underlying WISC-R performance of gifted and learning disabled Navajos. *Psychology in the Schools, 26,* 31–36.

Myers, H. F., Kagawa-Singer, M., Kumanyika, S. K., Lex, B. W., & Markides, K. S. (1995). Behavioral risk factors related to chronic diseases in ethnic minorities. *American Psychologist, 14,* 613–621.

Naglieri, J. A. (1982). Does the WISC-R measure intelligence for non-English speaking children? *Psychology in the Schools, 19,* 478–479.

National Commission on Testing and Public Policy (1990). *From gatekeeper to gateway: Transforming testing in America.* Chestnut Hill, MA: Boston College.

Nelson, S., McCoy, G., Stetter, M., & Vanderwagen, W. C. (1992). An overview of mental health services for American Indians and Alaska Natives in the 1990s. *Hospital and Community Psychiatry, 43,* 257–261.

Norton, I. M., & Manson, S. M. (1996). Research in American Indian and Alaska Native communities: Navigating the cultural universe of values and process. *American Psychologist, 64,* 856–860.

O'Conner, M. C. (1989). Aspects of differential performance by minorities on standardized tests: Linguistic and sociocultural factors. In B. R. Gifford (Ed.), *Test policy and test performance: Education, language, and culture* (pp. 129–181). Boston: Kluwer Academic.

O'Sullivan, M.H., & Handal, P.J. (1988). Medical and psychological effects of the threat of compulsory relocation for an American Indian tribe. *Indian and Alaska Native Mental Health Research, 2*(1), 3–20.

Penn, N. E., Kar, S., Kramer, J., Skinner, J., & Zambrana, R. E. (1995). Ethnic minorities, health care systems, and behvaior. *American Psychologist, 14,* 641–646.

Philipsen, G. (1972). Navajo world view and cultural patterns of speech: A case study in ethnorhetoric. *Speech Monographs, 39*, 132–139.

Pollack, D., & Shore, J. H. (1980). Validity of the MMPI with Native Americans. *American Journal of Psychiatry, 137*, 946–950.

Raven, J. (1989). The Raven Progressive Matrices: A review of national norming studies and ethnic and socio-economic variation within the United States. *Journal of Educational Measurement, 26*, 1–16.

Roll, S., Millen, L., & Martinez, R. (1980). Common errors in psychotherapy with Chicanos: Extrapolations from research and clinical experience. *Psychotherapy: Theory, Research, and Practice, 17*, 158–168.

Saccuzzo, D. P., & Johnson, N. E. (1995). Traditional psychometric tests and proportionate representation: An intervention and program evaluation study. *American Psychologist, 7*, 183–194.

Sack, W. H., Beiser, M., Clarke, G., & Red Shirt, R. (1987). The high achieving Sioux Indian child: Some preliminary findings from the Flower of Two Soils project. *The Journal of the National Center, 1*, 41–56.

Sage, G. P. (1991). Counseling American Indian adults. In C. Lee, & B. Richardson (Eds.), *Multicultural issues in counseling: New approaches to diversity* (pp. 23–35). Alexandria, VA: American Counseling Association.

Sattler, J. M. (1982). Assessment of ethnic minority group children. In J. M. Sattler (Ed.), *Assessment of children's intelligence and special abilities* (pp. 354–388). Boston: Allyn & Bacon.

Scaldwell, W. A. (1986). *WISC-R, Kaufman-ABC, and TONI results, Wikwemikong, 1985–1986*. Government of Canada: Department of Indian Affairs and Northern Development.

Schachtel, A. H., Henry, J., & Henry, Z. (1942). Rorschach analysis of Pilagra Indian children. *American Journal of Orthopsychiatry, 12*, 679–712.

Scott, S., Hynd, G., Hunt, L., & Weed, W. (1979). Cerebral speech lateralization in the Native American Navajo. *Neuropsychologia, 17*, 89–92.

Smith, M. D., Coleman, M. C., Dokecki, P. R., & Davis, E. E. (1977). Recategorization of WISC-R scores of learning disabled children. *Journal of Learning Disabilities, 10*, 48–54.

Smither, R. (1982). Human migration and the acculturation of minorities. *Human Relations, 35*(1), 57–68.

Social Science Research Council (1954). Acculturation: An exploratory formulation. *American Anthropologist, 56*, 973–1002.

Tafoya, T. (1982). Coyote's eyes: Native cognition styles. *Journal of American Indian Education, 21*, 21–33.

Tanner-Halverson, P. & Burden, T. (1995). WISC-III normative data for Tohono O'odham Native American Children. *Journal of Psychoeducational Assessment*, WISC-III Monograph, pp. 124–133.

Taylor, H. D., & Thweatt, R. C. (1972). Cross-cultural developmental performance of Navajo children on the Bender-Gestalt Test. *Perceptual and Motor Skills, 35*, 307–309.

Tharp, R. (1994). Intergroup differences among Native Americans in socialization and child cognition: An ethnographic analysis. In P. Greenfield & R. Cocking (Eds.), *Cross-cultural roots of minority child development* (pp. 87–105). Hillsdale, NJ: Erlbaum.

Thompson, L., & Joseph, A. (1951). White pressures on Indian personality and culture. *American Journal of Sociology, 53*, 17–22.

Uecker, A. E., Boutilier, L. R., & Richardson, E. H. (1980). "Indianism" and MMPI scores of men alcoholics. *Journal of Studies on Alcohol, 41*, 357–362.

U.S. Bureau of the Census. (1991). *1990 census count of American Indians, Eskimos, or Aleuts and American Indian and Alaska Native areas*. Washington, D.C.: Bureau of the Census, Racial Statistics Branch, Population Division.

U.S. Congress. (1990). *Indian adolescent mental health* (OTA-H-446). Washington, D.C.: U.S. Government Printing Office, Office of Technology Assessment.

Vesely, B. N. (1990). *Representative MMPI profiles in Native American and White alcoholics*. Paper presented at the 98th Annual Convention of the American Psychological Association, Boston, MA, August, 1990.

Vogel, V. J. (1972). *This country was ours: A documentary history of the American Indian*. New York: Harper & Row.

Vygotsky, L. S. (1962). *Thought and language*. Cambridge, MA: MIT Press.

Whorton, J. E., & Morgan, R. L. (1990). Comparison of the Test of Nonverbal Intelligence and Wechsler Intelligence Scale for Children-Revised in rural Native American and white children. *Perceptual and Motor Skills, 70*, 12–14.

Young, T. J. (1990). Poverty, suicide, and homicide among Native Americans. *Psychology Reports, 67*, 1153–1154.

Zarske, J. A., & Moore, C. L. (1982). Recategorized WISC-R scores for non-handicapped, leraning disabled, educationally disadvantaged and regular classroom Navajo children. *School Psychology Review, 11*, 319–323.

9

Multicultural Perspectives on the Neuropsychological and Neuropsychiatric Assessment and Treatment of the Elderly

PAUL G. LONGOBARDI, JEFFREY L. CUMMINGS, AND CAY ANDERSON-HANLEY

Introduction

Overview of Dementia

Dementia is a clinical syndrome evidenced by the presence of memory impairment and disturbances in at least one additional cognitive domain (language, visuospatial skills, executive function). The symptoms must be acquired, disabling, and not attributable to a co-occurring delirium (American Psychiatric Association, 1994). Dementia is an etiologically nonspecific disorder and may occur as a consequence of a large number of conditions adversely affecting brain function. Table 1 presents a list of the most commonly encountered dementias affecting elderly individuals.

In majority culture studies, Alzheimer's disease (AD) is the most common cause of dementia, followed by vascular dementia, depression, iatrogenic drug-induced disorders, and chronic medical conditions.

Epidemiological Trends in Aging and Ethnicity

Projections for the coming decades indicate that older people will increasingly comprise a larger portion of the population. By 2030, one in three Americans is expected to be 55 years

PAUL G. LONGOBARDI • Charles R. Drew University of Medicine and Science, Los Angeles, California 90059; and UCLA School of Medicine, Los Angeles, California 90095.   **JEFFREY L. CUMMINGS** • UCLA School of Medicine, Los Angeles, California 90095; and Charles R. Drew University of Medicine and Science, Los Angeles, California 90059.   **CAY ANDERSON-HANLEY** • Glens Falls Hospital, Glens Falls, New York 12801.
Handbook of Cross-Cultural Neuropsychology, edited by Fletcher-Janzen, Strickland, and Reynolds. Kluwer Academic/Plenum Publishers, New York, 2000.

TABLE 1. Most Common Etiologies of Dementia in the Elderly

Degenerative brain disorders	Toxic–metabolic disturbances
Alzheimer's disease	Iatrogenic drug-induced dementia
Dementia with Lewy Bodies	Alcoholism
Frontotemporal dementia	Cardiopulmonary disease
Dementia with Parkinson's disease	B_{12} deficiency
Dementia with other late onset	Hypothyroidism
extrapyramidal symptoms	Central nervous system infections
Cerebrovascular dementia	Chronic meningitis
Multiinfarct dementia (cortical and	Central nervous system syphilis
subcortical infarctions)	Creutzfeldt–Jakob disease
Binswanger's disease (lacunar state)	Miscellaneous
Cerebral hemorrhage	Traumatic brain injury
	Brain tumors
	Hydrocephalus
	Depression

or older and one in five to be at least 65 years old (U.S. Senate Special Committee on Aging, 1987–1988). Very old people (85 years old and older) currently constitute one of the fastest growing groups in the country. Older African American populations are growing even faster than the increasing population of older adults in general. According to the 1990 U.S. census (U.S. Bureau of the Census, 1992), African Americans aged 65 years and older number 2.5 million (8%) while those 85 years and older constitute almost one-quarter million (7.5% of that grouping nationally). Data from the U.S. Bureau of the Census have indicated that the U.S. population of Hispanics aged 65 and older grew to a total of more than one million between 1980 and 1990, a growth rate double that of older non-Hispanics. Larson and Imai (1996) have noted that in the United States, racially diverse elderly populations are growing twice as fast as the general population.

Interaction of Ethnicity and Dementia

While estimates of prevalence of dementia vary for different samples and diagnostic procedures, there is a range of studies with findings consistent with estimates of rates of probable Alzheimer's disease of 3–5% for 65- to 74-year-olds to 18–20% for 75- to 84-year-olds, and 47% for those aged 85 years or older (Evans et al., 1989; Hofman et al., 1991; Rocca et al., 1990). Compared to older Caucasians, older African Americans have lower incomes, poorer health, less access to health care, higher death rates for a host of diseases, and lower life expectancies (Manuel, 1988; Reed, 1990; Watson, 1990). Reed (1990) observed that for several of the leading causes of death African American elderly are at greater risk than Caucasian elderly. Thus, many of these poor health factors place minority elderly at greater risk both for disability and for the development of dementing illness at earlier stages in the life cycle as well as greater severity of illness. In a study of patients evaluated at nine California Alzheimer's Disease Diagnostic and Treatment Centers, Hargrave, Stoeklin, Haan, and Reed (1998) found that African American patients, when compared with Caucasian patients, had fewer years of education and more often had hypertension, reported shorter durations of illness at the time of initial diagnosis, and had lower Mini-Mental State Examination (MMSE) scores and higher Blessed Roth Dementia Rating Scale scores at the time of initial diagnosis. The authors noted that issues of social class and education are seen as independent risk factors for dementia that affect cross-cultural dementia research. Gorelick et al. (1994) compared demographic and other epidemiologic factors among African Americans with AD and those with vascular dementia. Alzheimer's patients were likely to be older than those with vascular dementia; to have a family history of AD, Parkinson's disease, and dementia; to have a history of head injury with loss of consciousness and hip fracture; and to have more severe cognitive impairment and difficulty with instrumental activities of daily living. In a study of differences in physical and cognitive functioning among chronically ill African American and Caucasian elderly in home care following hospital discharge, Proctor et al. (1997) found that African Americans went home more physically sick, dependent, and cognitively impaired. Issues of differential access of minorities to health care, lower education and socioeconomic class, and tendencies to enter the health care system at later stages of disease, all were raised by the findings of these studies.

There have been few studies of the prevalence of dementia or of the specific types of dementia in minority populations. The few existing studies sometimes have produced conflicting results. Schoenberg, Anderson, and Haerer (1985) conducted a community-based study of dementia among Caucasians and African Americans in Copiah County, Mississippi. They found that approximately 1% of individuals over age 40 had severe dementia and this increased to 7% of individuals over age 80. The prevalence ratios for severe dementia and clinically-diagnosed AD were similar in the two ethnic groups. Heyman et al. (1991), however, examined a stratified random sample of Caucasian and African American community residents in the Piedmont region of North Carolina and found the estimated prevalence of dementia to be 16% for African Americans and 3.05% for Caucasians. In this group there was a distinctly higher prevalence rate of dementia among African American women (19.9%). Hendrie et al. (1995) examined the prevalence of dementia and AD among Yorubas living in Ibadan, Nigeria and African Americans living in Indianapolis, Indiana. The percent with dementia in Ibadan for those over age 65 was 2.29, whereas the percentage among community-dwelling Indianapolis residents was 4.82. When the prevalence of AD was determined, 1.41% of those residing in Ibadan had AD whereas 3.69% of those community-residing elderly in Indianapolis had AD. These studies indicate that there is still much to learn about the relative prevalence of dementia and AD among Caucasians and African Americans. Differences in selection criteria, sampling methodology, survivorship, and educational and socioeconomic factors all may contribute to the discrepancies among existing studies.

A consistent finding among studies of minority elderly is the high prevalence of mixed dementia, particularly the co-occurrence of AD and cerebrovascular disease. Heyman et al. (1991) found mixed or vascular dementia to be more common among African American than Caucasian patients. Auchus (1997) noted that among patients with possible AD, a diagnosis applied when two conditions exist but AD is thought to be the predominant cause of the dementing disorder, 73% had hypertension, 27% had diabetes, and 15% had coronary artery disease. Mulrow et al. (1996) similarly noted that cerebrovascular disease, diabetes, and hypertension were all more common among Mexican American nursing home residents than among comparable Caucasian residents. In an autopsy-based study of dementia, De la Monte, Hutchins, and Moore (1989) found the frequency of AD to be 2.6 times higher among Caucasians, dementia due to Parkinson's disease more frequent among Caucasians, and the frequencies of vascular dementia and dementia due to chronic alcohol use higher among African Americans. Alzheimer-type lesions also were more common among Caucasian normal controls than among African American controls. Overall, these studies indicate that cerebrovascular disease is more common among ethnic minorities than among Caucasians and that this difference manifests itself in higher prevalence rates of vascular dementia and mixed AD/cerebrovascular disease in demented minority groups.

Genetic differences may substantially influence the etiologies of dementia in different ethnic minorities. Apolipoprotein e4 (APOE e4) has been found to be a risk factor for AD among Caucasian elderly. When this association was examined among different ethnic populations, variable associations emerged (Maestre et al., 1995). The e4 homozygotes were at increased risk for AD in all ethnic populations examined (African Americans, Hispanics, and Caucasians). APOE e4 heterozygosity was more weakly associated with AD among African Americans than among Hispanics and Caucasians. In contrast, an e2/e3 genotype was associated with an eightfold increase in risk for AD in African Americans but was associated with a decreased risk in Caucasians. These results suggest that AD may be a product of different genetic and environmental mechanisms in different ethnic minority populations.

Sociodemographic Factors and Aging

There is substantial evidence and general consensus that socioeconomic status (SES) is a major contributor to differential morbidity and mortality resulting from a variety of physical and psychiatric disorders. Data consistently indicate that persons with low SES have higher rates of morbidity and mortality than those with higher SES. Williams and Collins (1995) reviewed evidence of the SES gradient in health and the basis for consistent racial differences in health and in most epidemiologic reports. They noted that there is unequivocal evidence of disproportionate risk for morbidity and mortality among the lower SES groups and that race/ethnicity conditions increase this relationship such that low SES minority populations suffer a greater burden of morbidity and mortality than Caucasians. Several factors have been implicated in this inverse SES–health relationship, including greater exposure to pathogenic social environmental conditions, greater life stress burden, more negative health behavior profiles, and less access to and utilization of quality health care. These factors may help explain phenomena such as the greater number of bed days of disability at earlier ages seen for African Americans, for example, by age 55 and above, than for other groups, as documented and described by Reed (1990) and Watson (1990). In fact, Gibson (1988) agrued that retirement should be added to a list of events that occurs earlier for African Americans. The implication is that age-based policies tied to the life course and experiences of the majority population may have limited relevance and applicability to minority elders. In a recent review of race, SES, and health, Schoenbaum and Waidmann (1997) noted that while African American males and females have higher overall mortality than Caucasians, much of the gap disappears when some measure of SES is controlled. They suggested strongly that health is a variable that should be related to the status and course of cognitive functioning in older minority groups. In the MacArthur Study of Successful Aging, Whitfield et al. (1997) studied associations between cognition and measures of health in 224 generally health elderly African Americans 70–79 years of age at initial interview. Greater peak expiratory flow was predictive of better cognitive performance at the first interview with lower levels of average peak expiratory flow and low education predictive of decline at reexamination 24–32 months after initial interview. Whitfield and colleagues stressed the importance of both current and self-rated health as well as education as related to the maintenance of cognitive function among African Americans in later life.

Tennstedt and Chang (1998) examined the relative contribution of ethnicity and SES variables to explaining differences in the need for and receipt of informal care in a population of African American, Puerto Rican, and Caucasian people age 60 years and older. SES had no direct effect on disability when controlling for ethnicity although both minority elder groups were more disabled than the Caucasian group. However, ethnicity did explain between-group differences in the amount of informal care received. Elders in the two minority groups received more informal care than did older Caucasians, even when controlling for levels of disability. The authors stressed the importance of the findings to the role played by ethnicity in explaining an older person's need for and receipt of long-term care. Taylor's (1988) review of the literature regarding aging and supportive relationships among African American elders clearly supported the general conclusion that family, nonkin, and church involvement all are of critical importance to subjective well-being. Idler and Kasl (1997), in a recent study of religion among disabled and nondisabled people using Caucasians and African American elders from the New Haven site of the Established Populations for the Epidemiologic Study of the Elderly, found that religious involvement is tied to a broad array of behavioral and psychosocial resources.

Thus, in evaluating possible cognitive deterioration in minority elderly, examiners are advised to include assessment/consideration of the effects of SES, current and self-rated health, level and quality of education attained, cultural/familial involvement in the care process, and religious involvement.

Neuropsychiatric Assessment/Multicultural Issues

There has been little attention to the occurrence and assessment of neuropsychiatric symptoms in different ethnic populations with dementia. Based on observations of Caucasian patients, Mega, Cummings, Fiorello, and Gornbein (1996) found that neuropsychiatric symptoms were present in nearly all AD patients. Apathy was the most common symptom, occurring in 70%; agitation was present in 60%; irritability, anxiety, and depression were present in nearly 50% of patients; and delusions, hallucinations, disinhibition, and euphoria occurred in a smaller number of individuals. A similar pattern of neuropsychiatric symptoms was identified in Italian patients with AD and among Mexican AD patients using similar methodologies (Cummings, Diaz, Levy, Binetti, & Litvan, 1996). In both non-U.S. samples, the frequency of neuropsychiatric symptoms tended to be higher although the relative prevalence of the varying neuropsychiatric disorders was similar across populations.

Assessment of neuropsychiatric symptoms in different ethnic groups poses substantial methodologic challenges. Patients often lack sufficient insight to provide a basis for self-report questionnaires, and caregivers across different ethnic groups may vary according to educational level, intensity of the caring relationship, concern about the attitude of the interviewer, shame regarding neuropsychiatric symptoms, and attitudes regarding behavioral disturbances. Psychiatric symptom complexes also may differ among ethnic populations. For example, Baker and Espino (1997) found that the Geriatric Depression Scale appeared to be less valid for Hispanic elderly since they frequently have neurovegetative and somatic symptoms which are underemphasized in this commonly used depression screening inventory. Such differences in disease presentation must be considered when attempting to compare neuropsychiatric symptoms among ethnic groups.

Neuropsychological Assessment/Multicultural Issues

Issues in Cognitive Assessment of Dementia

Investigators working with a variety of minority populations have raised issues regarding the use of neuropsychological tests with minority populations (Ardila, 1995; Ardila, Rosselli, & Ostrosky-Solís, 1992; Baker, 1996; Taussig & Ponton, 1996; Teng, 1996). Depending on whether the investigator is working with Hispanic or non-Hispanic minority groups, the issues identified have included the influence of education, language, cultural appropriateness and relevance of test items (ecological validity), the context of assessment, and cultural influences in the development of cognitive abilities.

Ardila and colleagues have pointed out the criticality of the influence of education on neuropsychological test performance. Less educated individuals or those who are functionally illiterate tend to score on neuropsychological measures much like brain-injured individuals. However, as Taussig and Ponton (1996) have discussed, even the classification of education can be difficult based on differences in the types and quality of education received by individuals in different locations. For example, they recommended dichotomies based on urban/rural background, private/public education, and country of education. For African American elders with limited education, the state in which their education was received will help clarify the quality of the education.

Ardila and colleagues have noted that language usage differs according to cultural background and is strongly correlated with educational level. The test instructions and language used in testing often are a formal language difficult for the individual with limited education to understand. While this is particularly true for non-English speakers, it also is true for English-speaking minority elders with limited educational background and testing experience. In fact, Ardila and colleagues noted that the expression of aphasias are not the same in different language systems. For example, patients with aphasias in Spanish will not have problems with grammatical construction, as the Spanish language is more flexible than English, but will present with significant difficulties in the semantic aspects of language.

Teng (1996) noted that cognitive tests generally are designed by academicians for individuals who probably have had limited experience with test taking and have emphasized different skills in life than those assessed on most cognitive tests, for example, nurturing, social relatedness, carpentry, and so forth. These individuals are at risk to appear impaired on many neuropsychological tests. This is why Baker's (1996) recommendation, given in the context of assessment of elderly African Americans, to include culturally appropriate measures of activities of daily living (ADL) and instrumental activities of daily living (IADL), is important to help reduce the risk of a false positive conclusion of a dementing disorder in minority elders. Baker (1996) recommended consideration of decreased economic resources, limited access to health care, multiple medical problems, and possible nutritional deficiencies because of poor diet related to limited economic resources. The importance of providing a meaningful context also will help elicit the older African American's cooperation and provide more meaningful/valid results.

Finally, it is critical to note that cognitive activity is culturally dependent. Ardila and colleagues (1992) have provided cross-cultural data consistent with the conclusion that cognitive performances of a wide range, including memory and visuospatial abilities, are influenced by educational variations as well as by differences in cultural background that emphasize certain types and strategies of learning.

Selective Review of Studies of Neuropsychological Assessment in Culturally Diverse Elderly Populations

Heaton, Grant, and Matthews (1986), using data for the Halstead–Reitan Battery, have demonstrated that older, less-educated people of diverse races more frequently are misclassified as brain damaged compared to younger, more highly educated persons. Marcopulos, McLain, and Giuliano (1997), in a study to establish preliminary norms for nine commonly administered neuropsychological tests for a rural community sample of Caucasian and African American nondemented elders with 10 or fewer years of education, found that the use of previously existent test norms with lower-educated, rural-dwelling, older adults resulted in overestimation of cognitive impairment. Consistent with other research using the commonly employed MMSE (Folstein, Folstein, & McHugh, 1975), these investigators noted that persons with fewer than 8 years of education often scored below the cutoff originally suggested for indicating cognitive impairment. This also was true for the Mattis Dementia Rating Scale. Important *exceptions* for the education effect were noted on indices of the Fuld Object Memory Evaluation (FOME) (Fuld, 1981) and on savings scores derived from the Wechsler Memory Scale-Revised. In studies of dementia in African American elders employing instrumentation, many investigators exclusively have used screening instruments such as the MMSE. Investigators have noted both limitations of the MMSE in screening for dementia in nonmajority populations as well as the importance of the performance of subjects on measures of ADL and IADL, education, and age (Baker, Johnson, Velli, & Wiley, 1996; Ford, Haley, Thrower, West, & Harrell, 1996). Teresi et al. (1995) found that out of 50 cognitive items examined from six widely used cognitive screening measures to include the MMSE, 16 items were identified as biased for either high or low education groups or ethnic/racial group membership among African American, Hispanic, and non-Hispanic white elderly subjects. Bohnstedt, Fox, and Kohatsu (1994) used MMSE data from a large sample of 1888 patients seen at Alzheimer's disease diagnostic and treatment centers to examine differences in results for different racial–ethnic groups. The authors suggested that clinicians consider MMSE scores for African American and Hispanic patients an underestimate of their cognitive capabilities relative to that of Caucasian patients. Baker (1996) recommended use of the MMSE in combination with another screening instrument for cognitive impairment with adjustments for age and education. Also, he further recommended inclusion of an instrument assessing ADL and IADL performance as well as assessment of work history and current economic resources as an indicator of the risk of African American elders for psychosocial stress and nutritional deficiencies. Stern et al. (1992) used education corrections to reclassify part of their sample of diverse elders on a brief diagnostic neuropsychological test. They noted that subjects reclassified as demented were significantly more impaired in activities of daily living than nondemented subjects who were not reclassified. The authors, consistent with many others, concluded that corrections for demographic influences and activities of daily living may be needed in epidemiological studies when assessing older and less educated persons.

The Neurobehavioral Cognitive Status Examination (NCSE, now Cognistat) (Kiernan, Mueller, Langston, & Van Dyke, 1987) increasingly has been used with elderly populations to assess cognition in a brief but quantitative manner. The NCSE purportedly independently assesses multiple domains of cognitive functioning and thus provides the clinician with a differentiated profile of the patient's status. This is in contrast to the MMSE where only one summary score is obtained. The NCSE also uses a screen and metric approach that allows unimpaired individuals to complete the examination in shorter time. In work with elderly populations, Starratt, Fields, & Fishman (1992) found the NCSE, in comparison with the MMSE, to be similarly sensitive in the detection of dementia, although it was more sensitive to known neuropathology in stroke and traumatic brain-injured nonelderly groups. They concluded that the NCSE had promise as a screening instrument particularly among patients with focal lesions. Osato and colleagues (Osato, Yang, & La Rue, 1993; Osato, La Rue, & Yang, 1994) compared the psychometric properties of the NCSE and the MMSE in an elderly psychiatric sample. They found the NCSE to provide greater sensitivity than the MMSE using a cutoff of two or more subtests in the impaired range as providing the maximal discrimination between depressed patients and those with organic mental disorders. Specificity was lower than that for the MMSE. Engelhart, Eisenstein, & Meininger (1994) used the NCSE to examine 109 geriatric subjects who were classified as neurologically impaired only, psychiatrically impaired only, neither, or both. They found that with advancing age the mean number of NCSE scales falling into the impaired range increased irrespective of clinical presence of neurological impairment. However, the mean number of impaired scores was higher for people with neurological impairment. Suggestions were made as to using different numbers of scales impaired to distinguish organicity from monogenicity in geriatric populations. Marcotte, van Gorp, Hinkin, & Osato (1997) examined the concurrent validity of the NCSE subtests using a predominantly white male veteran group averaging 62 years of age. Their subjects completed both the NCSE and common neuropsychological tests. Most NCSE subtest screens exhibited low false negative rates but high false positive rates. Using the neuropsychological tests as a criterion on which to base judgments of impairment, NCSE subtests classified impaired and unimpaired patients at a much lower than expected rate. The authors raised questions about the efficacy of the NCSE subtests in delineating domain specific cognitive functioning. Drane and Osato (1997) evaluated the ability of the NCSE to distinguish between healthy older adults and geriatric patients suffering from dementia. They found a high rate of false positives among the healthy elderly (70%) although the test was efficient in identifying correctly all dementia patients. Suggestions were made for calculating a percentage of subscales passed that may be helpful in group differentiation. Strickland et al. (1996) compared the NCSE to the MMSE in a generally healthy community dwelling group of African American seniors. All 95 subjects were given the MMSE and NCSE. The predominantly female group (78 females, 17 males) averaged 70 years of age and 12 years of education. Correlational and inferential analyses indicated that current NCSE published norms generally were consistent with findings in this study. Subjects who complained of memory and other cognitive problems, as well as deficits in functional behaviors, performed significantly poorer than those without such problems. The authors judged the NCSE as more sensitive in detecting mild cognitive impairment than the MMSE.

Other studies of dementia have emerged from the Consortium to Establish a Registry for Alzheimer's Disease (CERAD) (Welsh et al., 1995; Unverzagt et al., 1996). Welsh et al. (1995) compared performance on the CERAD battery between 830 Caucasian and 158 African American elders all diagnosed with AD. African American seniors scored lower than Caucasians on tests of visual naming and constructional praxis and on the MMSE. There were no statistical differences in performance on measures of fluency and word list memory. The authors suggested that cultural or experiential differences may modify performance on specific neuropsychological tests. Unverzagt et al. (1996) examined 83 normal, healthy African American men and women aged 65 years and older with the neuropsychological battery of the CERAD. Regression analyses indicated powerful education and less marked age and gender influences on test performance. Education-stratified normative data were also presented. Fillenbaum, Huber, and Taussig (1997), using the abbreviated CERAD Boston Naming Test, found that after controlling for gender, years of education, and age, Caucasian elders performed significantly better than African American elders. Also, the ordering of item difficulties for both racial groups did not show the expected gradation based on development of the test, indicating less familiarity for the groups with some items resulting in poorer performance. The authors questioned whether, in some cases, low scores actually are indicative of cognitive impairment.

Teng (1996) has made a noteworthy effort to develop an instrument useful for cross-cultural dementia assessment. The Cognitive Abilities Screening Instrument (CASI) covers 10 cognitive domains commonly assessed in dementia research. Most of the CASI items have been taken or modified from the MMSE, the Modified Mini-Mental State Examination (Teng & Chui, 1987), and the Hasegawa Dementia Screening Scale (Hasegawa, 1983). Teng (1996) reported that the four CASI items of repeating three words, temporal orientation, list-generating fluency, and recalling three words have been found as good as or better than the MMSE in screening for dementia for American, Japanese, and Chinese participants. It is noted that these items do not involve reading, writing, calculations, the use of a pen or pencil, and may well be suited to cross-cultural epidemiological studies.

Lichtenberg (1998) and colleagues (Ross & Lichtenberg, 1997) designed the Normative Studies Research Project Test Battery (NSRP) to develop normative data and examine the clinical utility of particular neuropsychological tests. This was done in an older urban medical population which included more people with less than a high school education and more minority subjects. Six tests were studied in depth over a series of studies including the Mattis Dementia Rating Scale, the Logical Memory subtest of the Wechsler Memory Scale-Revised (WMS-R), the FOME, the Boston Naming Test, the Visual Form Discrimination Test, and the Hooper Visual Organization Test. Lichtenberg and colleagues have provided a new source of normative data with these tests for populations previously studied in less depth. Also, the test battery appears clinically useful for older adult urban medical patients. There was good discrimination between cognitively unimpaired and impaired participants. However, in contrast to previous factor analyses indicating two or three factors, all of the tests loaded on a single factor. Lichtenberg (1998) contended that in an urban population with a majority of less educated and African American patients, the tests all are measuring the same construct: cognition. Means and standard deviations were lower overall on all tests except the FOME and the Mattis Dementia Rating Scale. However, race as a variable was not explanatory. Some test scores, for example, the Boston Naming Test, were influenced more by demographic variables than others, for example, FOME. These last several efforts (Teng, Lichtenberg) represent fruitful directions for better understanding how to interpret performances on neuropsychological measures in minority populations. Careful attention must be paid to acquisition of larger subject-samples and more careful sample description on relevant dimensions including SES, health status, education, acculturation, functionality on ADL and IADL dimensions, and psychiatric symptomatology (particularly depression).

Neuropsychological Prediction Studies

Given the increasing population of older minority individuals, the accurate distinction of older persons with normal cognitive functioning for their age from those with early dementia of whatever cause is of considerable clinical and public health importance. The ability to identify early dementia in its preclinical stages will increase in importance as additional pharmacologic treatments of dementia are developed.

A handful of studies have attempted long-term prediction of dementia using neuropsychological test instruments (Bondi, Monsch, & Galasko, 1994; Fuld, Masur, Blau, Crystal, & Aronson, 1990; La Rue & Jarvik, 1987; La Rue, Matsuyama, McPherson, Sherman, & Jarvik, 1992; Masur, Sliwinski, Lipton, Blau, & Crystal, 1994; Persson, Berg, Nilsson, & Svanborg, 1991; Smith et al., 1996; Tierney et al., 1996; Zonderman, Giambra, Arenberg, Resnick, & Costa, 1995). In one of the earliest studies, La Rue and Jarvik (1987) found that demented individuals had poorer cognitive test performance twenty years before diagnosis than those surviving to similar ages without dementia. Fuld et al. (1990) found that a brief version of the

FOME was a moderately sensitive predictor of dementia and a fairly specific predictor when administered one year prior to diagnosis. In a study using a wide range of levels of educational background, Masur et al. (1994) administered four measures of cognitive function to 317 initially nondemented elders between 75 and 85 years of age and followed them for at least four years. The four measures achieved significant positive predictive rates for development of dementia. There were no gender differences but this study, like most in this area, employed no African American elders as participants. Zonderman et al. (1995) found that six-year changes in immediate visual memory performance assessed by the Benton Visual Retention test predicted AD prior to its onset in a longitudinal study of 371 community-dwelling Caucasian males and females. In an important study combining both cognitive tests and genotyping, Tierney et al. (1996) followed prospectively for two years 107 males and females undescribed by race and referred by physicians for memory problems. While most participants did not develop dementia, the presence of the APOE e4 allele was a reliable prognostic indicator of who developed AD but *only* when memory test performance on the Rey Auditory Verbal Learning Test was included in the predictive model. In a recent study in Sweden, Small, Basun, and Backman (1998) examined whether baseline cognitive performance and 3-year longitudinal changes were influenced by APOE e4 allele. Participants were 20 APOE e4 and 54 non-e4 very old people without dementia. Results indicated that at 3-year follow-up the APOE e4 group experienced greater negative change in recognition memory for faces and words. No other differences on other measures were significant at 3-year follow-up. They suggested that when the effects of APOE status do occur, they may be related to impending dementia or conditions other than normal aging, such as depression, rather than to the effect of specific gene types on cognitive performance. However, their APOE e4 group was small and heterozygous, with only one of 20 subjects being homozygous for the e4 allele. Also, it has been reported that the potency of the e4 allele as a risk factor for AD decreases with increasing age, and this was a sample of very old adults, averaging 81 years.

Thus, except for the recent Small et al. (1998) study, results are consistent with the impression that tests of both verbal and visual memory, verbal ability, and speeded psychomotor performance have been successful in discriminating healthy elder persons from those with dementia of the Alzheimer's type. Baseline measures of cognitive functioning, often obtained 2–4 years before the actual diagnosis of dementia, have provided important information about dementia risk. However, in the existent studies, African Americans and other minority groups either have not been included or not described as participants. Predictive rates using cognitive tests and/or genotyping are unknown in these populations. It also may be that in many cases the presence of mild cognitive impairment, described by Smith et al. (1996) as a boundary area between dementia and normal aging, combined with genotyping, may help differentiate those elders who proceed to develop dementia from those who do not. Furthermore, the general health status of the participants often has been left uncontrolled or poorly described, causes of dementia other than AD have not been examined, and depression and/or other psychiatric conditions have not been ruled out as influencing the results.

Apolipoprotein E and Neuropsychological Assessment of Alzheimer's Disease

Another recent direction in studying the risk of individuals to develop dementia has been to examine genetic factors. In many studies of Caucasian populations, the frequency of the e4 allele of APOE has been found to be increased among patients with either sporadic or familial late-onset AD compared with control subjects and patients with early-onset familial AD (Pericak-Vance, Bebout, & Gaskell, 1991; Saunders et al., 1996; Strittmatter, Saunders, & Schmechel, 1993). Saunders et al. (1996) noted that the inheritance of the e4/e4 genotype (about 2% of the general population) is associated with a mean age of onset of AD of 60 to 70 years in most clinic populations. Few homozygous e4/e4 persons reach the age of 90 without developing AD (Rebeck, Perls, & West, 1994). Additionally, there is some indication that presence of APOE e2 is underrepresented in AD populations and may protect against AD (Corder, Saunders, & Risch, 1994). In some families with early onset of AD before age 60 years, particularly in those with a positive family history, the presence of the e4 allele also may be increased in patients with multiinfarct dementia and it is suggested that e4 is a marker of both AD and vascular dementia (Noguchi, Murakami, & Yamada, 1993).

Data for minority populations are limited, vary in results by sample, and indicate a possibly weaker association between increased risk of AD and the presence of at least one APOE e4 allele (Hendrie et al., 1995; Maestre et al., 1995; Osuntokun et al., 1995; Saunders et al., 1996). Results of several of these studies raise a question whether the strength of association between AD and genotype frequencies is similar for African Americans as compared to other racial/ethnic groups. A weakened association between APOE e4 and AD among African Americans and Hispanics, relative to Caucasians and Japanese, was noted in a report of results from a multi-site study described by Farrer and colleagues (1997). The authors noted that the co-occurrence of other factors with APOE status may be necessary to establish strongly the relationship between APOE e4 and AD. One such factor is family history of dementia, examined by Duara and colleagues (1996). They studied late-onset AD in Hispanic, African American, Jewish Ashkenazi, non-Jewish, and non-Hispanic Caucasian groups. The combination of positive family history of dementia and e4+ status, but not gender or education, were significant in that they were both associated with an earlier age of onset of AD. As in most studies in this area, no neuropsychological tests were included as possible correlative measures of genotype status and/or family history of dementia. Only Tierney et al. (1996), as described earlier, have combined genotyping and neurocognitive testing in reporting results in a sample not described by racial/ethnic identity. Thus, further research with larger, well-described minority populations including neuropsychological measurements will help clarify the nature of the relationship between genotype status and AD onset.

Neuropsychiatric Treatment Issues

Pharmacologic Management of Dementia

There has been marked progress in developing treatments for dementing disorders, particularly AD. Vitamin E has been shown to slow the progress of AD (Sano et al., 1997), and cholinesterase inhibitors improve cognition or slow the rate of cognitive decline in a majority of patients (Morris et al., 1998; Rogers et al., 1998). The effect of these agents in different ethnic groups has not been examined. In general, the number of ethnic minorities enrolled in the pivotal trials which led to the approval of these agents has been small. Preliminary data indicate that Chinese subjects are more sensitive to the effect of atropine (an anticholinergic agent) than Caucasian subjects (Zhou, Adedoyin, & Wood, 1992). This suggests that the cholinergic system is subject to ethnic variations that might translate into differences in treatment responsiveness with cholinesterase inhibitors.

Pharmacologic Management of Behavioral Disorders in Dementing Diseases

Behavioral disturbances in patients with dementia generally are treated with the same psychopharmacologic agents used in nondemented patients. Thus, antidepressants, antipsychotics, anxiolytics, and sedative hypnotics are used to treat depression, psychosis, anxiety, and insomnia, respectively, in demented as well as nondemented individuals (Wright & Cummings, 1996). Dementia patients appear to be more susceptible to adverse side effects and the response rate tends to be lower among demented than non-demented individuals.

There is substantial inter-ethnic variation in the pharmacokinetics and pharmacodynamics of psychotropic medications. African Americans, Hispanics, and Asians all appear to exhibit clinical benefit and adverse side effects at lower dosages of tricyclic antidepressants than Caucasians (Silver, Poland, & Lin, 1993). Benzodiazepines have been found to be metabolized more slowly among Asian than Caucasian individuals (Lin, Poland, Fleishaker, & Phillips, 1993). Chinese Americans tend to have higher plasma haloperidol concentrations after oral administration of the drug than African American or Caucasian patients, with Hispanic individuals having intermediate levels (Jann, Kam, & Chang, 1993).

Cholinesterase inhibitors may exert beneficial effects on behavioral disturbances in patients with AD (Kaufer, Cummings, & Christine, 1998), and these effects may be impacted by differences in metabolism or sensitivity to cholinergic compounds.

Consideration of Ethnicity in Caregiving

Introduction to Caregiver Issues

As we enter the twenty-first century, concern for meeting the needs of the growing older-adult population is on the rise. Of particular concern is the expected difficulty of meeting the needs of elders with dementias such as Alzheimer's disease. While the number of nursing homes has been rapidly increasing to meet growing demands, most older adults with dementia (an estimated 80%) are still cared for at home by family members (Henderson, Gutierrez-Mayka, Garcia, & Boyd, 1993; Scott et al., 1997; Young & Montgomery, 1998)). Thus, consideration of the stress felt by family caregivers has come more into focus.

Investigations have aimed to clarify the roles played by a number of variables in the caregiving process. Of particular concern has been the caregiver's experience of "burden," which has been described as the caregiver's subjective sense of distress that is related to their caregiving role (Lawton, Kleban, Moss, Rovine, & Glicksman, 1989). Burden can encompass such experiences as anxiety and depression, or guilt and fatigue (Lawton et al., 1989). Recently, an emphasis has been made to examine the positive end of the spectrum of experiences of caregiving to include such experiences as sense of satisfaction or mastery in caregiving, as well as finding meaning (Miller & Lawton, 1997).

A myriad of other variables have been examined for their possible impact on the caregiving process, including age, relationship to care recipient (e.g., spouse or adult child), SES, impairment of the patient, social support, and health of the caregiver (Talamantes, Cornell, Espino, Lichtenstein, & Hazuda, 1996).

Consideration of Ethnicity in Caregiving

While research on the caregiving process has been intensive in the past few decades, samples have naturally reflected the majority, or Caucasian, culture in composition, leaving knowledge of minority-ethnic caregiving lagging behind. A growing number of studies now exist that compare and contrast the nature of caregiving among different ethnic groups (Anderson-Hanley et al., 1997; Anetzberger, Korbin, & Tomita, 1996; Connell & Gibson, 1997; Gonzales, Gitlin, & Lyons, 1995; Lee & Sung, 1997).

Recent reviews of the literature reveal approximately a dozen studies on the caregiving process in which ethnic variability was examined (Connell & Gibson, 1997; Gonzales et al., 1995). Most of these studies compare Caucasians and African Americans, and a few studies compare Hispanics with another ethnic group (Cox, 1993, 1996; Cox & Monk, 1993, 1996). There is a continued dearth of comparative research on the caregiving process in Asian American, Native American, or other ethnic groups.

Studies of Negative and Positive Outcomes

Table 2 displays the results of 28 comparative studies, simplified to show whether or not there were significant differences on either negative or positive outcomes between the ethnic groups compared. If a significant difference was reported, the direction of the difference is noted. The evidence seems strong, though not necessarily definitive, that there is a significant difference between African American and Caucasian caregivers' experiences of negative outcomes such as burden or depression. Nine findings of significantly different levels of negative outcomes were reported (with Caucasians showing more negative outcomes in each) in contrast with five reports of equivocal or nonsignificant differences. Furthermore, there were no studies finding the reverse difference (i.e., Caucasians reporting fewer negative outcomes than African American caregivers in general). However, when Bowman and colleagues (1998) took the relationship between the caregiver and care recipient into consideration, an interaction effect was found. African American spouses reported more negative outcomes than their Caucasian counterparts, while African American adult-children reported fewer negative outcomes than Caucasian adult children caregivers (Miller & Kaufman, 1996; Mintzer et al., 1992). Thus, it seems important for the nature of the relationship between the caregiver and the care recipient be taken into consideration in future research.

Studies involving other ethnic groups are fewer and even less definitive. Three studies show Hispanic caregivers as having more negative outcomes than African Americans. No nonsignificant results were reported, nor were any results in the opposite direction. One study suggests that Caucasians have more negative outcomes than Hispanics, but two studies found no significant differences between the two ethnic groups. Only one study compared African American and Asian American caregivers and the former had significantly fewer negative outcomes than the latter. In a study of Canadians (of English and French descent) and other minorities (specific ethnic backgrounds not specified in the study), the minority caregivers were found to have significantly more negative outcomes than Canadians (Meshefedjian, McCusker, Bellavance, & Baumgarten, 1998).

As noted above, fewer studies have examined the positive outcomes for caregivers. Four studies found African Americans reported more positive outcomes than Caucasians (Hinrichsen & Ramirez, 1992; Lawton, Rajagopal, Brody, & Kleban, 1992; Macera et al., 1992; Morycz, Malloy, Bozich, & Martz, 1987). Similarly, two studies revealed that African Americans reported more positive outcomes than either Hispanics or Asians; no equivocal or reverse outcomes were reported for these ethnic groups.

In sum, it appears fairly consistent that African Americans report fewer negative and more positive outcomes than Caucasian, Hispanic, or Asian caregivers.

Explanations for Differences

Attempts to explain the differences observed between ethnic groups have included the possibility that the variability is secondary to a response bias due to ethnicity. More research is needed on the hypothesis that certain ethnic groups may have more comfort endorsing items

TABLE 2. Significance of Variables in Models Comparing Ethnic Groups of Primarily Dementia Caregivers

First author	Yr	AF	CA	HI	AS	Negative outcomes[1]	Positive outcomes[2]	Other variables
Morycz	87	44	329			AF < CA		AF < CA in desire to institutionalize
Cox	90	31		19		AF < HI		
Wood	90	36	49			AF ≈ CA		AF < CA in use of support groups; CA < AF in use of cognitive reframing
Wykle	91	20	20					AF prob#1: respite, CA prob#1: guilt, both prob#2: behav; CA < AF in use of religious coping
Hinrichsen	92	33	119			AF < CA		AF < CA in desire to institutionalize
Lawton	92	157	472			AF < CA	CA < AF	AF vs CA: > cognitive reappraisal, > mastery
Macera	92	20	62			AF < CA		
Mintzer	92		15	13		CA ≈ HI		
Mui	92	117	464			AF < CA		
Cox	93	76	88			AF ≈ CA		AF > CA in belief in filial responsibility
Valle	94		52	38		CA ≈ HI		CA < HI in use of religious coping
Cox	95	76	88			AF ≈ CA		
Haley	95	70	105			AF < CA	CA < AF	
Anetzberger	96	16	18	12	16			Differing perceptions of elder abuse
Cox	96	76		86		AF < HI		
Cox	96	99	80					Majority of AF and CA are discharged home

Author	Year					Depends on coping style	Depends on coping style	
Haley	96	74	123			AF < CA		AF ≈ CA in social supports
Miller	96	77	138					HI widows were less likely to have a caregiver
Talamantes	96		340	158				
Anderson-Hanley	97	55	257	35	13	Burden: AF < HI and AF < AS, AF ≈ CA; depression: AF < HI and CA < HI, AF ≈ CA	AS < AF and CA < AF and HI < AF	No differences on mastery; cognitive reappraisal: CA < AF/HI; guilt: AF/CA < AS and AF < HI
Farran	97	77	138			AF < CA		Finding meaning related to less depression
Gonzalez	97	25	25					CA < AF: resourcefulness, and benign appraisals of problem behaviors
Lee & Sung	97	47	60[3]					CA < K in sense of filial responsibility
Picot	97	136	255				CA < AF	CA < AF in use of religious coping
Scott	97	492	294					AF < CA for risk of institutionalization
Bowman	98	176	194			AF < CA[4] child: CA < AF spouse: AF < CA		
Meshefedjian	98	X[5]	1816[6] 85[7]	X[5]	X[5]	Minorities < CC		
Young	98	178	392					AF less receptive to institutionalization, but similar admission rates

[1](e.g., depression, burden, strain, etc.); [2](e.g., well-being, rewards, etc.); [3](native Koreans, not Korean Americans); [4](until relationship to care-recipient is factored in); [5](total "minorities" = 55, no breakdown provided); [6](European Canadians); [7](French Canadians); AF = African American; AS = Asian American; CA = Caucasian American; CC = Caucasian Canadian; HI = Hispanic American; K = native Korean; ≈ = groups were similar/not statistically significant.

that acknowledge psychological difficulties, such as experiences of burden or depression. However, one study evaluating response bias relating to caregiver's ratings of *patient* variables revealed few differences between African Americans, Caucasians, and Hispanics (Lawrence, Tennstedt, & Almy, 1997).

African American caregivers possibly are especially resilient to the stresses of dementia caregiving because of the unfortunate reality that many are familiar with significant stressors in American society. Thus, African American caregivers may have developed certain coping strategies for dealing with significant stressors, of which dementia caregiving may be just one more.

Consideration of the caregiver's relationship with the patient could also explain some variability in outcomes as it may serve as a "third variable," described below. Bowman and colleagues (1998) discuss additional possible explanations.

Research on Other Variables

Samples tend to reveal that Caucasian caregivers are older with higher SES, more years of education, and are more likely to be caring for a spouse than African American caregivers (e.g., Haley, Hand, & Henderson, 1998; Haley et al., 1996; Haley, West, Wadley, & Ford, 1995; Mui, 1992; Wood & Parham, 1990). This last fact alone could account for some of the differences seen in outcomes of Caucasian and African American caregivers, since those caregiving for a spouse tend to report more stress than those caring for a parent or other relative (Wood & Parham, 1990). Similarly, in one of the few studies reporting no significant difference in negative outcomes between Caucasian and African American caregivers, the proportion of daughter caregivers was almost equal, perhaps having an equilibrating effect (Cox, 1995). Interestingly however, when just daughters were examined (Mui, 1992), the African American advantage appears again, a finding in contrast with Bowman and colleagues (1998). Future research should be careful to quantify the nature of the caregiving relationship. A number of additional studies have been reported that are primarily descriptive in nature or provide further details or comparisons of subgroups within larger ethnic categories (e.g., Puerto Ricans and Cuban Americans). Many of their descriptions can be found in Yeo & Gallagher-Thompson's (1996) book.

Interventions and Practice

Specific interventions to address the needs of ethnic-minority caregivers have been pursued since underutilization of services has often been noted. Reports on interventions can be found for African Americans and Hispanics (Henderson et al., 1993), Asians (Braun, Takamura, Forman, Sasaki, & Meininger, 1995), and Hispanics alone (Gallagher-Thompson et al., 1997). These authors suggest that meaningful interventions for caregivers may need to be designed with an understanding of the ethnic and cultural background of participants in mind. Informed awareness of variability in caregiver perceptions, attitudes, and the like, should lead to improved interventions that most directly address the relevant needs of the caregivers. Literature also is available that reviews the importance of understanding ethnic variability in clinical practice with older adults and caregivers (Farran, Miller, Kaufman, & Davis, 1997; Gonzalez, 1997; Picot, Debanne, Namazi, & Wykle, 1997; Valle, 1994).

Future Directions in Caregiving

While exploring group differences is a necessary first step in describing a phenomenon, future studies should strive to examine variability within groups that may cut across groups. It is expected that several major patterns of adjustment related to coping with the stress of dementia caregiving will be identified, perhaps similar to those which have been found with individuals coping with a serious illness. Also, future research should aim to examine the individual's level of acculturation to a given ethnic group or to the majority culture, thus providing a more realistic picture of individuals falling along a continuum rather than into discrete categories.

Understanding the apparent resilience of African American caregivers may lead to development of techniques or philosophies that could be incorporated into caregiver interventions and taught to caregivers of different ethnic backgrounds. For instance, African Americans use cognitive strategies to reframe situations in positive terms, express determination to survive, and find support in a deity (e.g., Picot, 1995). Some of these strategies, if not all, may be teachable to caregivers through structured support groups, written materials, and the like. Certainly, there is the potential for much to be gained by studying variability in the caregiver process. The hope is that this will be translated into meaningful interventions to help a rapidly growing population of caregivers to meet the daunting challenge, and to meet it well.

Conclusions and Recommendations

The studies reviewed in this chapter indicate that there has been a paucity of studies regarding ethnic variations in the frequency, etiology, clinical manifestations of dementia syndromes, and caregiving dimensions among different ethnic populations. Existing studies suggest that there are differences in the frequency, causes, clinical phenomenology, treatment responsiveness, and caregiving factors across ethnic groups. The existence of these differences makes it imperative that there be greater attention to ethnic differences in studies of dementia, that there be more research including or focused on ethnic minorities with dementia, and that a solid data base be developed that will allow practitioners to adjust diagnostic and therapeutic behaviors according to the ethnicity of the patients.

References

American Psychiatric Association (1994). *Diagnostic and Statistical Manual of Mental Disorders* (4th ed.). Washington, D.C.: Author.

Anderson-Hanley, C., Dunkin, J., Cummings, J. L., Rosenberg-Thompson, R., Strickland, T. L., Miller, B. L., & Fitten, J. L. (1997, November). *Ethnic variability in caregiver appraisal and depression.* Paper presented at the annual meeting of the Gerontological Society of America, Cincinnati, OH.

Anetzberger, G. J., Korbin, J. E., & Tomita, S. K. (1996). Defining elder mistreatment in four ethnic groups across two generations. *Journal of Cross Cultural Gerontology, 11*(2), 187–212.

Ardila, A. (1995). Directions of research in cross-cultural neuropsychology. *Journal of Clinical and Experimental Neuropsychology, 17*, 143–150.

Ardila, A., Rosselli, M., & Ostrosky-Solís, F. (1992). Socioeducational. In A. E. Puente & R. J. McCaffrey (Eds.), *Handbook of neuropsychological assessment: A biopsychosocial perspective* (pp. 181–193). New York: Plenum.

Auchus, A. P. (1997). Demographic and clinical features of Alzheimer disease in black Americans: Preliminary observations on an outpatient sample in Atlanta, Georgia. *Alzheimer Disease and Associated Disorders, 11*, 38–46.

Baker, F. M. (1996). Issues in assessing dementia in African American elders. In G. Yeo & D. Gallagher-Thompson (Eds.), *Ethnicity and the dementias* (pp. 59–77). Washington, D.C.: Taylor & Francis.

Baker, F. M., & Espino, D. V. (1997). A Spanish version of the Geriatric Depression Scale in Mexican-American elders. *International Journal of Geriatric Psychiatry, 12*(21), 21–25.

Baker, F. M., Johnson, J. T., Velli, S. A., & Wiley, C. (1996). Congruence between education and reading levels of older persons. *Psychiatric Services, 47*, 194–196.

Bohnstedt, M., Fox, P. J., & Kohatsu, N. D. (1994). Correlates of Mini-Mental Status Examination scores among elderly demented patients: The influence of race-ethnicity. *Journal of Clinical Epidemiology, 47*, 1381–1387.

Bondi, M., Monsch, A., & Galasko, E. (1994). Preclinical cognitive markers of dementia of the Alzheimer's type. *Neuropsychology, 8*, 374–384.

Bowman, K. F., Landefeld, C. S., Quinn, L. M., Palmer, R. M., Kowal, J., & Fortinsky, R. H. (1998). Strain in African American and white American caregivers of hospitalized elderly: Implications for discharge planning. *Research on Aging, 20*, 547–568.

Braun, K. L., Takamura, J. C., Forman, S. M., Sasaki, P. A., & Meininger, L. (1995). Developing and testing outreach materials on Alzheimer's disease for Asian and Pacific Islander Americans. *The Gerontologist, 35*, 122–126.

Connell, C. M., & Gibson, G. D. (1997). Racial, ethnic, and cultural differences in dementia caregiving: Review and analysis. *The Gerontologist, 37*, 355–364.

Corder, E. H., Saunders, A. M., & Risch, N. J. (1994). Protective effect of apolipoprotein E type 2 allele for late onset Alzheimer disease. *Nature Genetics, 7*, 180–194.

Cox, C., & Monk, A. (1990). Minority caregivers of dementia victims: A comparison of black and Hispanic families. *The Journal of Applied Gerontology, 9*, 340–354.

Cox, C. (1993). Service needs and interests: A comparison of African American and white caregivers seeking Alzheimer assistance. *American Journal of Alzheimer's Disease* (May/June), 33–40.

Cox, C. (1995). Comparing the experiences of black and white caregivers of dementia patients. *Social Work, 40*, 343–349.

Cox, C. (1996). Outcomes of hospitalization: Factors influencing the discharges of African American and white dementia patients. *Social Work in Health Care, 23*(1), 23–38.

Cox, C., & Monk, A. (1993). Hispanic culture and family care of Alzheimer's patients. *Health and Social Work, 18*(2), 92–100.

Cox, C., & Monk, A. (1996). Strain among caregivers: Comparing the experiences of African American and Hispanic caregivers of Alzheimer's relatives. *International Journal of Aging and Human Development, 43*(2), 93–106.

Cummings, J. L., Diaz, C., Levy, M., Binetti, G., & Litvan, I. (1996). Neuropsychiatric syndrome in neurodegenerative diseases: Frequency and significance. *Seminars in Clinical Neuropsychiatry, 1*, 241–247.

De la Monte, S. M., Hutchins, G. M., & Moore, G. W. (1989). Racial differences in the etiology of dementia and frequency of Alzheimer lesions in the brain. *Journal of the National Medical Association, 81*, 644–652.

Drane, D. L., & Osato, S. S. (1997). Using the Neurobehavioral Cognitive Status Examination as a screening measure for older adults. *Archives of Clinical Neuropsychology, 12*, 139–143.

Duara, E., Barker, W. W., Lopez-Alberola, R., Loewenstein, D. A., Grau, L. B., Gilchrist, D., Sevush, S., & St. George-Hyslop, P. H. (1996). Interaction of apolipoprotein E genotype, family history of dementia, gender, education, ethnicity, and age of onset. *Neurology, 46*, 1575–1579.

Engelhart, C., Eisenstein, N., & Meininger, J. (1994). Psychometric properties of the Neurobehavioral Cognitive Status Exam. *The Clinical Neuropsychologist, 8*, 405–415.

Evans, D. A., Funkenstein, H. H., Albert, M. S., Scherr, P. A., Cook, N. R., Chown, M. J., Hebert, L. E., Hennekens, C. H., & Taylor, J. O. (1989). Prevalence of Alzheimer's disease in a community population of older persons. *Journal of the American Medical Association, 262*, 2551–2556.

Farran, C. J., Miller, B. H., Kaufman, J. E., & Davis, L. (1997). Race, finding meaning and caregiver distress. *Journal of Aging and Health, 9*, 316–333.

Farrer, L. A., Cupples, L. A., Haines, J. L., Hyman, B., Kukull, W. A., Mayeux, R., Myers, R. H., Pericak-Vance, M. A., Risch, N., & van Duijn, C. M. (1997). Effects of age, sex, and ethnicity on the association between apolipoprotein E genotype and Alzheimer disease. *Journal of the American Medical Association, 278*, 1349–1356.

Fillenbaum, G. G., Huber, M., & Taussig, I. M. (1997). Performance of elderly white and African American community residents on the Abbreviated CERAD Boston Naming Test. *Journal of Clinical and Experimental Neuropsychology, 19*, 204–210.

Folstein, M. F., Folstein, S. E., & McHugh, P. R. (1975). Mini-Mental State: A practical method for grading the cognitive state of patients for the clinician. *Journal of Psychiatric Research, 12*, 189–198.

Ford, G. R., Haley, W. E., Thrower, S. L., West, C. A. C., & Harrell, L. E. (1996). Utility of Mini-Mental State Exam scores in predicting functional impairment among white and African American dementia patients. *Journal of Gerontology: Medical Sciences, 51A*(4), M185-M188.

Fuld, P. A. (1981). *Fuld Object Memory Evaluation*. New York: Albert Einstein College of Medicine.

Fuld, P. A., Masur, D. M., Blau, A. D., Crystal, H., & Aronson, M. K. (1990). Object Memory Evaluation for prospective detection of dementia in normal functioning elderly: Predictive and normative date. *Journal of Clinical and Experimental Neuropsychology, 12*, 520–528.

Gallagher-Thompson, D., Leary, M. C., Ossinalde, C., Romero, J. J., Wald, M. J., & Fernandez-Gamarra, E. (1997). Hispanic caregivers of older adults with dementia: Cultural issues in outreach and intervention. *Group, 21*, 211–232.

Gibson, R. C. (1988). The work, retirement, and disability of older black Americans. In J. S. Jackson, P. Newton, A.

Ostfield, D. Savage, & E. L. Schneider (Eds.), *The black American elderly: Research on physical and psychosocial health* (pp. 304–327). New York: Springer.

Gonzales, E., Gitlin, L. N., & Lyons, K. J. (1995). Review of the literature on African American caregivers of individuals with dementia. *Journal of Cultural Diversity, 2*(2), 40–48.

Gonzalez, E. W. (1997). Resourcefulness, appraisals, and coping efforts of family caregivers. *Residential Group Care and Treatment, 18,* 209–227.

Gorelick, P. B., Freels, S., Harris, Y., Dollear, T., Billingsley, M., & Brown, N. (1994). Epidemiology of vascular and Alzheimer's dementia among African Americans in Chicago, IL: Baseline frequency and comparison of risk factors. *Neurology, 44,* 1391–1395.

Haley, W. E., Han, B., & Henderson, J. N. (1998). Aging and ethnicity: Issues for clinical practice. *Journal of Clinical Psychology in Medical Settings, 5,* 393–409.

Haley, W. E., Roth, D. L., Coleton, M. I., Ford, G. R., West, C. A., Collins, R. P., & Isobe, T. L. (1996). Appraisal, coping, and social support as mediators of well-being in black and white family caregivers of patients with Alzheimer's disease. *Journal of Consulting and Clinical Psychology, 64,* 121–129.

Haley, W. E., West, C. A. C., Wadley, V. G., & Ford, G. R. (1995). Psychological, social, and health impact of caregiving: A comparison of black and white dementia family caregivers and noncaregivers. *Psychology and Aging, 10,* 540–552.

Hargrave, R., Stoeklin, M., Haan, M., & Reed, B. (1998). Clinical aspects of Alzheimer's disease in black and white patients. *Journal of the National Medical Association, 90,* 78–84.

Hasegawa, K. (1983). The clinical assessment of dementia in the aged: A dementia screening scale for psychogeriatric patients. In M. Bergener, U. Lehr, E. Lang, & R. Schmitz-Scherzer (Eds.), *Aging in the eighties and beyond* (pp. 207–218). New York: Springer.

Heaton, R. K., Grant, I., & Matthews, C. G. (1986). Differences in neuropsychological test performance associated with age, education, and sex. In I. Grant & K. M. Adams (Eds.), *Neuropsychological assessment in neuropsychiatric disorders: Clinical methods and empirical findings* (pp. 100–120). New York: Oxford University Press.

Henderson, J. N., Gutierrez-Mayka, M., Garcia, J., & Boyd, S. (1993). A model for Alzheimer's disease support group development in African-American and Hispanic populations. *The Gerontologist, 33,* 409–414.

Hendrie, H. C., Osuntokun, B. O., Hall, K. S., Ogunniyi, A. O., Hui, S. L., Unverzagt, F. W., Gureje, O., Rodenberg, C. A., Baiyewu, O., Musick, B. S., Adeyinka, A., Farlow, M. R., Oluwode, S. O., Calss, C. A., Komolafe, O., Brashear, A., & Burdine, V. (1995). Prevalence of Alzheimer's disease and dementia in two communities: Nigerian Africans and African Americans. *American Journal of Psychiatry, 152,* 1485–1492.

Heyman, A., Fillenbaum, G., Prosnitz, B., Raiford, K., Burchett, B., & Clark, C. (1991). Estimated prevalence of dementia among elderly black and white residents. *Archives of Neurology, 48,* 594–598.

Hinrichsen, G. A., & Ramirez, M. (1992). Black and white dementia caregivers: A comparison of their adaptation, adjustment, and service utilization. *The Gerontologist, 32,* 375–381.

Hofman, A., Rocca, W. A., Brayne, C., Breteler, M. M., Clarke, M., Cooper, B., Copeland, J. R., Dartigues, J. F., da Silva-Droux, A., & Hagnell, O. (1991). The prevalence of dementia in Europe: A collaborative study of 1980–1990 findings: EURODEM Prevalence Research Group. *International Journal of Epidemiology, 20,* 736–748.

Idler, E. L., & Kasl, S. V. (1997). Religion among disabled and nondisabled persons: I. Cross-sectional patterns in health practices, social activities, and well-being. *Journal of Gerontology: Social Sciences, 52B,* S294–S306.

Jann, M. W., Kam, Y. W., & Chang, W-H. (1993). Haloperidol and reduced haloperidol plasma concentrations in different ethnic populations and interindividual variabilities in haloperidol metabolism. In K-M. Lin, R. E. Poland, & G. Nakasaki (Eds.), *Psychopharmacology and psychobiology of ethnicity* (pp. 133–152). Washington, D.C.: American Psychiatric Press.

Kaufer, D., Cummings, J. L., & Christine, D. (1998). Differential neuropsychiatric symptom responses to tacrine in Alzheimer's disease: Relationship to dementia severity. *The Journal of Neuropsychiatry and Clinical Neurosciences, 10,* 55–63.

Kiernan, R. J., Mueller, J., Langston, J. W., & Van Dyke, C. (1987). The Neurobehavioral Cognitive Status Examination: A brief but quantitative approach to cognitive assessment. *Annals of Internal Medicine, 107,* 481–485.

Larson, E. B., & Imai, Y. (1996). An overview of dementia and ethnicity with special emphasis on the epidemiology of dementia. In G. Yeo & D. Gallagher-Thompson (Eds.), *Ethnicity and the dementias* (pp. 9–21). Washington, D.C.: Taylor & Francis.

La Rue, A., & Jarvik, L. F. (1987). Cognitive function and prediction of dementia in old age. *International Journal of Aging and Human Development, 25,* 79–89.

La Rue, A., Matsuyama, S. S., McPherson, S., Sherman, J., & Jarvik, L. F. (1992). Cognitive performance in relatives of patients with probable Alzheimer disease: An age at onset effect? *Journal of Clinical and Experimental Neuropsychology, 14,* 533–538.

Lawrence, R. H., Tennstedt, S. L., & Almy, S. L. (1997). Subject-caregiver response comparability on global health and functional status measures for African American, Puerto Rican, and Caucasian elders and their primary caregivers. *Journals of Gerontology: Series B, Psychological Sciences and Social Sciences, 52,* S103–S111.

Lawton, M. P., Kleban, M. H., Moss, M., Rovine, M., & Glicksman, A. (1989). Measuring caregiving appraisal. *Journal of Gerontology: Psychological Sciences, 44,* P61–P71.

Lawton, M. P., Rajagopal, D., Brody, E., & Kleban, M. H. (1992). The dynamics of caregiving for a demented elder among black and white families. *Journal of Gerontology, 47,* S156–S164.

Lee, Y. R., & Sung, K. T. (1997). Cultural differences in caregiving motivations for demented parents: Korean caregivers versus American caregivers. *International Journal of Aging and Human Development, 44,* 115–127.

Lichtenberg, P. A. (1998). *Mental health practice in geriatric health care settings.* New York: Haworth.

Lin, K.-M., Poland, R. E., Fleishaker, J. C., & Phillips, J. P. (1993). Ethnicity and differential responses to benzodiazepines. In K-M. Lin, R. E. Poland, & G. Nakasaki (Eds.), *Psychopharmacology and psychobiology of ethnicity* (pp. 91–105). Washington, D.C.: American Psychiatric Press.

Macera, C. A., Eaker, E. D., Goslar, P. W., Deandrade, S. J., Williamson, J. S., Cornman, C., & Jannarone, R. J. (1992). Ethnic differences in the burden of caregiving. *American Journal of Alzheimer's Disease,* (September/October), 4–7.

Maestre, G., Ottman, R., Stern, Y., Gurland, B., Chun, M., Tang, M.-X., Shelanski, M., Tycko, B., & Mayeux, R. (1995). Apolipoprotein E and Alzheimer's disease: Ethnic variation in genotypic risks. *Annals of Neurology, 37,* 254–259.

Manuel, R. C. (1988). The demography of older blacks in the United States. In J. S. Jackson, P. Newton, A. Ostfield, D. Savage, & E. L. Schneider (Eds.), *The black American elderly: Research on physical and psychosocial health* (pp. 25-43). New York: Springer.

Marcopulos, B. A., McLain, C. A., & Giuliano, A. J. (1997). Cognitive impairment or inadequate norms? A study of healthy, rural, older adults with limited education. *The Clinical Neuropsychologist, 11,* 111–131.

Marcotte, T. D., van Gorp, W., Hinkin, C. H., & Osato, S. (1997). Concurrent validity of the Neurobehavioral Cognitive Status Exam subtests. *Journal of Clinical and Experimental Neuropsychology, 19,* 386–395.

Masur, D. M., Sliwinski, M., Lipton, R. B., Blau, A. D., & Crystal, H. A. (1994). Neuropsychological prediction of dementia and the absence of dementia in healthy elderly persons. *Neurology, 44,* 1427–1432.

Mega, M., Cummings, J. L., Fiorello, T., & Gornbein, J. (1996). The spectrum of behavioral changes in Alzheimer's disease. *Neurology, 46,* 130–135.

Meshefedjian, G., McCusker, J., Bellavance, F., & Baumgarten, M. (1998). Factors associated with symptoms of depression among informal caregivers of demented elders in the community. *The Gerontologist, 38,* 247–253.

Miller, B., & Kaufman, J. E. (1996). Beyond gender stereotypes: Spouse caregivers of persons with dementia. *Journal of Aging Studies, 10,* 189–204.

Miller, B., & Lawton, M. P. (1997). Introduction: Finding balance in caregiver research. *The Gerontologist, 37,* 216–217.

Mintzer, J. E., Rubert, M. P., Loewenstein, D., Gamez, E., Millor, A., Quinteros, R., Flores, L., Miller, M., Rainerman, A., & Eisdorfer, C. (1992). Daughters caregiving for Hispanic and non-Hispanic Alzheimer patients: Does ethnicity make a difference? *Community Mental Health Journal, 28,* 293–303.

Morris, J. C., Cyrus, P. A., Orazem, J., Mas, J., Bieber, F., Ruzicka, B. B., & Gulanski, B. (1998). Metrifonate benefits cognitive, behavioral, and global function in patients with Alzheimer's disease. *Neurology, 50,* 1222–1230.

Morycz, R. K., Malloy, J., Bozich, M., & Martz, P. (1987). Racial differences in family burden: Clinical implications for social work. *Gerontological Social Work with Families, 10,* 133–154.

Mui, A. C. (1992). Caregiver strain among black and white daughter caregivers: A role theory perspective. *The Gerontologist, 32,* 203–212.

Mulrow, C. D., Chiodo, L. K., Gerety, M. B., Lee, S., Basu, S., & Nelson, D. (1996). Function and medical comorbidity South Texas nursing home residents: Variations by ethnic group. *Journal of the American Geriatric Society, 44,* 279–284.

Noguchi, S., Murakami, K., & Yamada, N. (1993). Apolipoprotein E genotype and Alzheimer's disease. *The Lancet, 342,* 737.

Osato, S. S., La Rue, A., & Yang, J. (1994). Validity of the Neurobehavioral Cognitive Status Examination (NCSE) subtests in older psychiatric patients. *Journal of the International Neuropsychological Society, 1,* 356.

Osato, S. S., Yang, J., & La Rue, A. (1993). The Neurobehavioral Cognitive Status Examination in an older psychiatric population: An exploratory study of validity. *Neuropsychiatry, Neuropsychology, and Behavioral Neurology, 6,* 103–110.

Osuntokun, B. O., Sahota, A., Ogunniyi, A. O., Gureje, O., Baiyewu, O., Adeyinka, A., Oluwoke, S. O., Komolafe, O., Hall, K. S., Unverzagt, F. W., Hui, S. L., Yang, M., & Hendrie, H. C. (1995). Lack of an association between Apoliprotein E e4 and Alzheimer's disease in elderly Nigerians. *Annals of Neurology, 38,* 463–465.

Pericak-Vance, M. A., Bebout, J. L., & Gaskell, P. C. (1991). Linkage studies in familial Alzheimer disease: Evidence for chromosome 19 linkage. *American Journal of Human Genetics, 48,* 1034–1050.

Persson, G., Berg, S., Nilsson, L., & Svanborg, A. (1991). Subclinical dementia: Relation to cognition, personality and psychopathology: A nine-year prospective study. *International Journal of Geriatric Psychiatry, 6,* 239–247.

Picot, S. J. (1995). Rewards, costs, and coping of African American caregivers. *Nursing Research, 44,* 147–152.

Picot, S. J., Debanne, S. M., Namazi, K. H., & Wykle, M. L. (1997). Religiosity and perceived rewards of black and white caregivers. *The Gerontologist, 37,* 89–101.

Proctor, E. K., Morrow-Howell, N., Chadiha, L., Braverman, A. C., Darkwa, O., & Dore, P. (1997). Physical and cognitive functioning among chronically ill African-American and white elderly in home care following hospital discharge. *Medical Care, 35,* 782–791.

Rebeck, G. W., Perls, T. T., & West, H. L. (1994). Reduced apolipoprotein epsilon 4 allele frequency in the oldest old Alzheimer's patients and cognitively normal individuals. *Neurology, 44,* 1513–1516.

Reed, W. L. (1990). Health care needs and services. In Z. Harel, E. A. McKinney, & M. Williams (Eds.), *Black aged: Understanding diversity and service needs* (pp. 183–205). London: Sage.

Rocca, W. A., Bonaiuto, S., Lippi, A., Luciani, P., Turtu, F., Cavarzeran, F., & Amaducci, L. (1990). Prevalence of clinically diagnosed Alzheimer's disease and other dementing disorders: A door-to-door survey in Appignano, Macerata province, Italy. *Neurology, 40,* 626–631.

Ross, T. P., & Lichtenberg, P. A. (1997). Effects of age and education on neuropsychological test performance: A comparison of normal versus cognitively impaired geriatric medical patients. *Aging, Neuropsychology, and Cognition, 4*(1), 74–79.

Rogers, S. L., Farlow, M. R., Doody, R. S., Mohs, R., Friedhoff, L. T., & the Donepezil Study Group. (1998). A 24-week, double-blind, placebo-controlled trial of donepezil in patients with Alzheimer's disease. *Neurology, 50,* 136–145.

Sano, M., Ernesto, C., Thomas, R. G., Klauber, M. R., Schafer, K., Grundman, M., Woodbury, P., Growdon, J., Cotman, C. W., Pfeiffer, E., Schneider, L. S., & Thal, L. J., for the Members of the Alzheimer's Disease Cooperative Study (1997). A controlled trial of selegiline, alpha-tocopherol, or both as treatment for Alzheimer's disease. *New England Journal of Medicine, 336,* 1216–1222.

Saunders, A. M., Hulette, C., Welsh-Bohmer, K. A., Schmechel, D. E., Crain, B., Burke, J. R., Alberts, M. J., Strittmatter, W. J., Breitner, J. C. S., Rosenberg, C., Scott, S. V., Gaskell, P. C., Pericak-Vance, M. A., & Roses, A. D. (1996). Specificity, sensitivity, and predictive value of apolipoprotein-E genotyping for sporadic Alzheimer's disease. *The Lancet, 348,* 90–93.

Schoenbaum, M., & Waidmann, T. (1997). Race, socioeconomic status, and health: Accounting for race differences in health. *Journal of Gerontology Series B, 52B* (special issue), 61–73.

Schoenberg, B. S., Anderson, D. W., & Haerer, A. F. (1985). Severe dementia: Prevalence and clinical features in a biracial US population. *Archives of Neurology, 42,* 740–743.

Scott, W. K., Edwards, K. B., Davis, D. R., Cornman, C. B., & Macera, C. A. (1997). Risk of institutionalization among community long-term care clients with dementia. *The Gerontologist, 37,* 46–51.

Silver, B., Poland, R. E., & Lin, K.-M. (1993). Ethnicity and the pharmacology of tricyclic antidepressants. In K.-M. Lin, R. E. Poland, & G. Nakasaki (Eds.), *Psychopharmacology and psychobiology of ethnicity* (pp. 61–89). Washington, D.C.: American Psychiatric Press.

Small, B. J., Basun, H., & Backman, L. (1998). Three-year changes in cognitive performance as a function of apoliprotein E genotype: Evidence from very old adults without dementia. *Psychology and Aging, 13,* 80–87.

Smith, G. E., Petersen, R. C., Parisi, J. E., Ivnik, R. J., Kokmen, E., Tangalos, E. G., & Waring, S. (1996). Definition, course, and outcome of mild cognitive impairment. *Aging, Neuropsychology, and Cognition, 3,* 141–147.

Starratt, C., Fields, R. B., & Fishman, E. (1992). Differential utility of the NCSE and MMSE with neuropsychiatric patients. *The Clinical Neuropsychologist, 6,* 331.

Stern, Y., Andrews, H., Pittman, J., Sano, M., Tatemichi, T., Lantigua, R., & Mayeux, R. (1992). Diagnosis of dementia in a heterogeneous population: Development of a neuropsychological paradigm-based diagnosis of dementia and quantified correction for the effects of education. *Archives of Neurology, 49,* 453–460.

Strittmatter, W. J., Saunders, A. M., & Schmechel, D. (1993). Apolipoprotein E: high affinity binding to beta-amyloid and increased frequency of type 4 allele in late-onset familial Alzheimer's disease. *Proceedings of the National Academy of Science USA, 90,* 1977–1981.

Strickland, T. L., Longobardi, P. G., Kington, R., Cummings, J., Louis, A., & Smith, L. (1996). Comparison of two cognitive screening measures in differentiating functioning among community dwelling African American seniors (Abstract). National Academy of Neuropsychology 1996 meeting.

Talamantes, M. A., Cornell, J., Espino, D. V., Lichtenstein, M. J., & Hazuda, H. P. (1996). SES and ethnic differences in perceived caregiver availability among young-old Mexican Americans and non-Hispanic whites. *The Gerontologist, 36,* 88–99.

Taussig, I. M., & Ponton, M. (1996). Issues in neuropsychological assessment for Hispanic older adults: Cultural and linguistic factors. In G. Yeo & D. Gallagher-Thompson (Eds.), *Ethnicity and the dementias* (pp. 47–58). Washington, D.C.: Taylor & Francis.

Taylor, R. J. (1988). Aging and supportive relationships among black Americans. In J. S. Jackson, P. Newton, A. Ostfield, D. Savage, & E. L. Schneider (Eds.), *The black American elderly: Research on physical and psychosocial health* (pp. 259–282). New York: Springer.

Teng, E. L. (1996). Cross-cultural testing and the Cognitive Abilities Screening Instrument. In G. Yeo & D. Gallagher-Thompson (Eds.), *Ethnicity and the dementias.* (pp. 77–85). Washington, D.C.: Taylor & Francis.

Teng, E. L., & Chui, H. C. (1987). The Modified Mini-Mental State (3MS) Examination. *Journal of Clinical Psychiatry, 48*, 314–318.

Tennstedt, S., & Chang, B.-H. (1998). The relative contribution of ethnicity versus socioeconomic status in explaining differences in disability and receipt of informal care. *Journal of Gerontology: Social Sciences, 53B*, S61–S70.

Teresi, J. A., Golden, R. R., Cross, P., Gurland, B., Kleinman, M., & Wilder, D. (1995). Item bias in cognitive screening measures: Comparisons of elderly white, Afro-American, Hispanic and high and low education subgroups. *Journal of Clinical Epidemiology, 48*, 473–483.

Tierney, M. C., Szalai, J. P., Snow, W. G., Fisher, R. H., Tsuda, T., Chi, H., McLachlan, D. R., & St. George-Hyslop, P. H. (1996). A prospective study of the clinical utility of ApoE genotype in the prediction of outcome in patients with memory impairment. *Neurology, 46*, 149–154.

Unverzagt, F. W., Hall, K. S., Torke, A. M., Rediger, J. D., Mercado, N., Gureje, O., Osuntokun, B. O., & Hendrie, H. C. (1996). Effects of age, education, gender on CERAD neuropsychological test performance in an African American sample. *The Clinical Neuropsychologist, 10*, 180–190.

U. S. Bureau of the Census. (1992). *1990 Census of population: General population characteristics* (United States, 1990 CP-1-1). Washington, D.C.: Author.

U.S. Senate Special Committee on Aging. (1987-1988). *Aging America: Trends and projections.* Washington, D.C.: Department of Health and Human Services.

Valle, R. (1994). Culture-fair behavioral symptom differential assessment and intervention in dementing illness. *Alzheimer Disease and Associated Disorders, 8 Suppl 3*, 21–45.

Watson, W. H. (1990). Family care, economics, and health. In Z. Harel, E. A. McKinney, & M. Williams (Eds.), *Black aged: Understanding diversity and service needs* (pp. 50-69). London: Sage.

Welsh, K. A., Fillenbaum, G., Wilkinson, W., Heyman, A., Mohs, R. C., Stern, Y., Harrell, L., Edland, S. D., & Beekly, D. (1995). Neuropsychological test performance in African-American and white patients with Alzheimer's disease. *Neurology, 45*, 2207–2211.

Whitfield, K. E., Seeman, T. E., Miles, T. P., Albert, M. S., Berkman, L. F., Blazer, D. G., & Rowe, J. W. (1997). Health indices as predictors of cognition among older African Americans: MacArthur studies of successful aging. *Ethnicity and Disease, 7*, 127–136.

Williams, D. R., & Collins, C. (1995). US socioeconomic and racial differences in health: Patterns and explanations. *Annual Review of Sociology, 21*, 349–386.

Wood, J. B., & Parham, I. A. (1990). Coping with perceived burden: Ethnic and cultural issues in Alzheimer's family caregiving. *Journal of Applied Gerontology, 9*, 325–339.

Wright, M. T., & Cummings, J. L. (1996). Neuropsychiatric disturbances in Alzheimer's disease and other dementias: Recognition and management. *Neurologist, 2*, 207–218.

Wykle, M., & Segall, M. (1991). A comparison of black and white family caregivers experience with dementia. *Journal of the National Black Nurses Association, 5*, 29–41.

Yeo, G., & Gallagher-Thompson, D. (Eds.), *Ethnicity and the dementias.* Washington, D.C.: Taylor & Francis.

Young, R. F. K., & Montgomery, R. J. (1998). Psychosocial factors in institutionalization of Alzheimer's patients. *Journal of Clinical Geropsychology, 4*, 241–251.

Zhou, H-H., Adedoyin, A., & Wood, A. J. J. (1992). Differing effect of atropine on heart rate in Chinese and white subjects. *Clinical Pharmacological Therapy, 52*, 120–124.

Zonderman, A. B., Giambra, L. M., Arenberg, D., Resnick, S. M., & Costa, P. T. (1995). Changes in immediate visual memory predict cognitive impairment. *Archives of Clinical Neuropsychology, 10*, 111–123.

10

Multicultural Perspectives on the Neuropsychological Assessment of Children and Adolescents

WENDY B. MARLOWE

Introduction

Childhood is a syndrome that has become the subject of serious investigation by neuropsychologists. However, the syndrome is not new. In 1983 Dr. Seuss estimated that over half of the Americans alive had experienced childhood directly. The U.S. Bureau of the Census (1997) reported that 28.8% of the current population were children and that 100% had experienced childhood at some point in the past.

Childhood has a congenital onset: It is always present at birth. Cross-cultural studies have revealed an increased incidence of childhood in many parts of Asia.

U.S. demographics are changing regarding the cultural composition of those experiencing childhood as well. In 1995 the U.S. Census Bureau predicted that one-third of the population would be people of color by the year 2000 and that one-half of the population would be people of color by the year 2050. Among school children, so-called cultural minorities represent the majority in all but two of the 25 largest cities in the United States (Delpit, 1995). By the year 2000 almost 40% of school-age children will come from African American, Hispanic American, Asian American or Native American homes (Delpit, 1995). Thus, the impact of culture on the practice of child and adolescent neuropsychology will increase in the future.

The process of neuropsychological assessment in children and adolescents differs from the process of assessment in adults. Because evaluation can occur at any stage of development, from birth onward, the child/adolescent neuropsychologist must understand ontogenetic environmental factors (Chelune & Edwards, 1981; Fletcher & Taylor, 1984; Risser & Edgell, 1988) as well as the body of knowledge common to neuropsychology. Although the initial assessment procedures in child and adolescent neuropsychology were largely a downward extension of adult neuropsychological models and methods (Reitan & Davidson, 1974) without any

WENDY B. MARLOWE • Seattle, Washington 98104.

Handbook of Cross-Cultural Neuropsychology, edited by Fletcher-Janzen, Strickland, and Reynolds. Kluwer Academic/Plenum Publishers, New York, 2000.

relation to the development of brain and cognition, newer approaches have enabled the assessment of infants, toddlers, and preschoolers as well (Chapman, 1995; Ewing-Cobbs, Fletcher, & Levin, 1985; Fletcher, Ewing-Cobbs, Miner, Levine, & Eisenberg, 1990; Korkman, Kirk, & Kemp, 1998, Pennington, 1994).

There are a number of general concerns in child and adolescent neuropsychology addressed by all clinicians and researchers in one fashion or another. The issues of multiculturalism have a much greater impact on these general concerns than is ordinarily recognized by institutional neuropsychology, which tends to think primarily in terms of white, European American children. In many respects, neuropsychology addresses culture in a manner similar to that of cognitive psychology in the early 1980s (Bentancourt & Lopez, 1993), considering it in respect to literacy levels (Lave, 1977; Olson, 1976; Roselli, Ardila, & Rosas, 1990; Scribner & Cole, 1981) or a "difference" model rather than the impact on cognition per se.

Neuropsychologists tend to be more aware of how test performance is influenced by social class, educational opportunity, parental educational attainment, cultural orientation at home, English proficiency, motivation (Babcock & Ross, 1992; Perez-Arce & Puente, 1996; Suzuki, Meller, & Ponterotto, 1996), and so forth, than we are about how our own linguistic, social class, cultural, and educational experiences influence our constructs of knowledge, selection of particular tests, and interpretations of these tests. Differences in worldviews or culturally specific cognitions (Dana, 1993; Heath, 1991) have a profound effect on nonverbal behaviors, language, and assumptions regarding causality. The worldviews of both the neuropsychologist and the child or adolescent client interact in the assessment process. It is important that neuropsychologists who study the neurocognitive, neurobehavioral, academic, and emotional functions of children develop an understanding of how our institutional culture has impacted our procedures and results, and to develop more appropriate approaches in order to increase the validity and reliability of our methods.

Institutional neuropsychology is composed primarily of white, middle-class (general American) practitioners. Most senior neuropsychologists were raised and educated in a de facto or de jure segregated society. Even today the majority of children attend school and play primarily with peers from a similar cultural and ethnic background. Most of the research subjects in psychology and neuropsychology have been from a homogenous, white community until very recently (Graham, 1992). Relatively few white neuropsychologists have social networks that include the active membership of ethnic minorities. Relatively few neuropsychologists have actively explored the relationship between culture and cognition. Many have not given it a passing thought. Only as more neuropsychologists from diverse cultural and linguistic backgrounds have been trained and have begun practicing has there been consideration of the roles these factors play in assessment.

Most mainstream neuropsychologists, like other citizens, have little understanding about the insidious effects of racism in America in general and within psychology in particular (Hall, 1997; Jackson, 1992; Lee, Jussim, & McCarthy, 1995; Sue, 1998; Suinn, 1992; Valencia & Guardarrama, 1996). Most do not recognize differences between cultural groups regarding family structures, values, and belief systems (Bennett, 1986a,b; Dana, 1993; Rubin, 1998; Saarni, 1998; Schneider, 1998; Stevenson-Hinde, 1998; Suzuki et al., 1996). There has been little investigation of the role of cultural and educational variables in the neuropsychologist who selects the test instruments, performs the assessment, builds the inferences, and writes the reports. Neuropsychologists rarely consider how our own linguistic, social class, cultural, and educational experiences influence our constructs of knowledge and bias, selection of particular tests, and the interpretation of those tests. Our worldviews and assumptions impact our approach to the science of neuropsychology, understanding of human behavior, and manner in which we approach the children or adolescents we assess. Although an extended discussion of these issues is beyond the scope of this chapter, recognition that our prior absence of social and academic exposure to multicultural concepts has created a vacuum in which to begin is essential (Hall, 1997; Jackson, 1992; Suinn, 1992). (See Hall, 1997; Keitel, Copala, & Adamson, 1996; Posner et al., 1994; Rankin, 1996; Resnick et al., 1991; Sattler, 1998; Suzuki et al., 1996 for an extended discussion regarding the issues of multiculturalism on assessment in general psychology.)

Culture is reflected in the terminology one uses to describe concepts. The culture of neuropsychology as it relates to children and adolescents is in a developmental stage. There is no consensus regarding terminology. Some neuropsychologists want to use the term "pediatric neuropsychology" to reflect the medical roots of our field. Others want to use "child neuropsychology," and still others feel that "developmental neuropsychology" best describes the process. Some neuropsychologists believe that child or pediatric neuropsychology includes adolescents, whereas others feel that the developmental issues and problems of adolescents are sufficiently different from those of younger children that they should be included in a more specific fashion. The Federal Office of Adolescent Health, a part of the Department of Health and Human Services, has defined adolescence as a period encompassing ages 10 to 21 years. The American Psychological Association has recognized the unique biopsychosocial tasks of adolescents and is participating in the Healthy Adolescents Project through the Office of Adolescent Health. The consistent inclusion of adolescents as distinct from children in this chapter is a reflection of the author's recognition of the importance of these issues.

In order to understand these multicultural issues in the neuropsychological assessment of children and adolescents, it is helpful to consider some of the primary concerns of child/ adolescent or developmental neuropsychology.

Issues in Developmental Neuropsychology

Morbidity/Mortality

Advances in medical care have resulted in the survival of infants and children with conditions and/or who received treatments that may have a potentially adverse affect on brain development (Taylor et al., 1992). Factors such as low birth weight associated with prematurity (Barsky & Siegel, 1992; Breslau, 1995; Breslau et al., 1996; Taylor, Hack & Klein, 1998), iatrogenic effects of cancer treatment (Taylor, Albo, Phoebus, Sachs, & Bierl, 1987), and the effects of traumatic brain injury (Broman & Michel, 1995; Ewing-Cobbs et al., 1985, 1989; Levin, Ewing-Cobbs, & Eisenberg, 1995) have resulted in reduced mortality, but an increase in morbidity in the childhood survivors.

Malnutrition, inadequate medical care, and other conditions associated with poverty (inadequate education, exposure to toxins, etc.) affect large numbers of children in the United States (Mirsky, 1995). These conditions "reduce the individual's capacity to learn and to cope effectively with the environment" (Mirsky, 1995, p. 482) and are perpetuated to succeeding generations (Cravioto, DeLicardie & Birch, 1966). The incidence of poverty and its negative effects are rampant in communities of ethnic minorities. Minorities are overrepresented in groups of low-income working individuals who lack medical insurance (Bazzoli, 1986) and therefore access to adequate healthcare (Aday & Andersen, 1981; Burstin, Lipsitz, & Brennan, 1992). The problems of limited healthcare and nutritional access have been recently compounded by the reduction in benefits to recipients of public assistance, both native-born and immigrant.

Inadequate health care during the preschool years may result in untreated conditions such as chronic otitis media, associated with lifelong developmental consequences including auditory processing, language, reading, and behavioral problems (Chalmers, Stewart, Silva, & Mulvena, 1989; Teele et al., 1990).

Education

Education has a profound impact on the neuropsychological assessment issues in children. The increased representation of multicultural children in the classroom is not mirrored by a similar increase in multicultural educators. Teachers are still most likely to be European American despite the increasing number of children from diverse cultural backgrounds. Many of these teachers have little understanding of the cultures from which the learners come and the impact of these cultures on the educational process (Delpit, 1995). Many teachers do not understand the language spoken by their students. Thus, the diversity of the population is not mirrored in our educational or psychological institutions (Hale, 1982; Hall, 1997; Suzuki et al., 1996).

Public Law 94-142, the Education for All Handicapped Children Act of 1975 (U.S. Congress, 1975) granted the right of education for all persons, including children with disabilities. The law recognized the neurological basis for a number of developmental disorders, including learning disabilities and health impairments such as epilepsy. The law has been amended a number of times with expansions and modifications including the Family Educational Rights and Privacy Act of 1974 and Public Law 99-457, amended in 1986 (U.S. Congress, 1986), which authorized early intervention programs for infants and toddlers and extended the rights of children from ages three to five. The current law, the Individuals with Disabilities Education Act (IDEA) has included specific criteria for children with traumatic brain injury and children with autism as neurological conditions. Children with attention deficit disorder have not been specifically included as an individual category, but continue to qualify as health-impaired if the evaluating psychologist understands both the disorder and special education law. Public Law 94-142 stipulated that the tests and other evaluation materials be provided and administered in the child's native language if at all feasible and that the materials used for evaluation and placement be selected and administered "so as not to be racially or culturally discriminatory" (U.S. Congress, 1975, pp. 42.496, 121a.530).

Some of the greatest weaknesses in the law were and continue to be in the assessment (Reynolds, 1982) and placement of children from culturally diverse backgrounds. Numerous lawsuits and hearings have addressed issues related to disproportionality in assessment (see Sattler, 1992, 1998, for a review).

Children who are not part of the majority culture tend to be referred for psychoeducational or special educational evaluations at rates much higher than their overall enrollment would indicate. There is a high probability (estimated at $P = 0.73$) of eligibility for special education once referred (Mahady, Towne, Algozzine, Mercer & Ysseldyke, 1990). Thus, it is likely that more minority children will be placed in special education due to the greater percentage of children referred and tested. If special education were a place of skill acquisition followed by transition back into the mainstream with the requisite skills to compete successfully with peers, the qualification for special education would not be problematic. However, since placement in special education tends to be associated with reduction in life skills and vocational options (Wagner, Blackorby, Cameto, Hebbler, & Newman, 1993; Wagner, D'Amico, Marder, Newman, & Blackorby, 1992; Wagner et al., 1991), the problems associated with the overrepresentation of minority children in special education are of great concern.

In 1991 the U.S. Department of Education Office of Civil Rights investigated the incidence of minority placements in special education. The report studied 40,020 schools nationwide located in 4,556 districts that represented 75% of African American public school enrollment. The data indicated that African American students constituted 21% of total school enrollment, but a far higher incidence of enrollment in special education. Within special education African American students represented 42% of those students classified as educable mentally retarded, 38% of those classified as trainable mentally retarded, and 22% of those classified as learning disabled. They represented only 11% of those enrolled in gifted and talented programs. Hispanic American students constituted 13% of the overall enrollment and 10% of the educable mentally retarded, 22% of the trainable mentally retarded, and 12% of the learning disabled. They represented 7% of those qualified as gifted and talented. Thus, these figures indicate that African American and Hispanic American students were classified as mentally retarded and learning disabled at much higher percentages than their overall enrollment and classified at lower percentages in gifted and talented programs. In contrast, Asian American students were classified as mentally retarded and learning disabled at lower percentages in relation to their overall enrollment. They were classified at higher percentages than their overall enrollment in gifted and talented programs. The majority of Asian American students who were qualified for special education were qualified for speech and language disorders.

The problems inherent in the assessment of children from diverse cultural backgrounds for special education are the same problems inherent in the assessment of these children for other purposes.

Ontogenetic–Environmental Factors

The differences between a developing brain of a child and the fully developed brain of an adult are profound, especially when disruption occurs. Children generally differ from adults in the kinds of brain insults sustained (Chelune & Edwards, 1981; Tramontana & Hooper, 1988). Childhood neurological disorders may involve hereditary or chromosomal abnormalities (such as Turner's or Down's syndrome), structural abnormalities (such as hydrocephalus or agenesis of the corpus callosum), anoxia (frequently in the prenatal and perinatal period), toxicity (lead, alcohol, or cocaine exposure in utero), nutritional disorders, brain infections (meningitis and encephalitis), as well as the disorders seen in all age groups, including stroke, metabolic disorders, tumors, seizures, traumatic brain injury and/or systemic illnesses. An extended discussion of the impact of each of these disorders is beyond the scope of this chapter. However, a few summary statements are clearly in order.

The type and degree of deficits in brain function and behavior vary with the level of ontogenetic development at the time of insult (Ewing-Cobbs, Miner, Fletcher, & Levin, 1989; Fletcher, 1996). Early brain damage interferes with the normal acquisition of skills during the developmental years (Fischer & Rose, 1994; Fletcher, Ewing-Cobbs, Frances, & Levin, 1995), whereas brain damage in adults results in a loss of previously acquired skills (Reitan & Davidson, 1974). Lesions that occur in the perinatal or neonatal periods tend to be associated with very poor outcomes (Chelune & Edwards, 1981; Clarren & Smith, 1978; Mirsky, 1995; Salamy, Mendelson, Tooley, & Chaplin, 1980). Widespread alterations in the morphologic and functional growth of the brain are commonly associated with mental retardation. Animal studies (Goldman-Rakic, Isserhoff, Schwartz, & Bugbee, 1983) have demonstrated that damage to the functionally uncommitted brain differs significantly from damage to the already committed brain. Older children and adolescents who sustain brain damage tend to have more discrete areas of impairment, more like adults, whereas infants and young children will have more diffuse impairment (Levin et al., 1995). The full impact of early brain lesions may not become apparent until the child has failed to acquire a wide range of developmental skills over the course of childhood or adolescence (Levin et al., 1995). Although often the presence of impairment is clear, "an insult early in life may never be overcome, since the neuroanatomical scaffolding upon which to build the next cognitive level is defective" (Mirsky, 1995, p. 494). Similar findings are present in the animal literature (Goldman, 1975). Despite new advances in the understanding of functional brain reorganization, our knowledge of mechanisms of reorganization is inhibited by our assessment tools and models.

We tend to address primarily one cognitive aspect of brain impairment in terms of measures of psychometric intelligence (Fletcher et al., 1996) although "central nervous system damage or abnormality is probably the single most powerful of risk factors for psychiatric disorder. Behavioral complications are probably the most prevalent complications of head injury" (Shaffer, 1995, p. 67) in both children and adults. For children and adolescents, the psychosocial environment (Rivera et al., 1993; Taylor et al., 1995) has been demonstrated to be a major predictor of the degree of recovery and adjustment. Similar results have been demonstrated in the animal literature (Suomi, 1997).

Problems of Assessment

Most test instruments used in the neuropsychological assessment of children or adolescents are atheoretical and mainly reflect a downward extension of tests developed for adults. They do not reflect ontogeny and the development of functional skills, the issues of sensitivity and specificity for childhood brain disorders, or discriminate between brain abnormalities and the absence of experience. Some tests may assess different functions at different ages or stages because of the developmental changes in strategies employed for the same task at different ages.

There are few tests currently available that satisfy the scientific criteria established by developmental neuropsychologists (Baron, Fennell, & Voeller, 1995; Hynd & Willis, 1988; Taylor & Schatschneider, 1992; Tramontana & Hooper, 1988). The problems relate to both theoretical constructs and normative issues. Many of the tests developed contain subtests that are labeled by function that bears no relationship to results obtained on factor analytic studies. Often visual or verbal analogues of memory developed in the course of publication of a new test do not appear to measure what they say they measure. For example, the design memory subtest for the Wide Range Assessment of Memory and Learning (Sheslow & Adams, 1990) has a 5-second exposure duration followed by a 10-second delay before the testee has the opportunity to reproduce the design. The test does not appear to measure any useful ability, based on methodological or clinical utility.

Although normative data on a single test can reflect performance differences across age-groups, the scores cannot identify developmental trends. Individual tests do not enable the neuropsychologist to evaluate the way in which emerging competencies in one functional domain may affect developing competencies in other functional domains (Fischer & Rose, 1994). Use of isolated tests prevents evaluation of the way in which a dysfunction in multiple domains may contribute to learning problems. Of greatest concern, normative data from single tests tend to be based on a relatively small number of children drawn from different age, ethnic, and/or socioeconomic groups that are not comparable. Thus, these results become difficult to interpret. Comparability between one test population and another is often limited. There are frequently confounding effects of the test results. One cannot differentiate whether performance discrepancies represent differences in the child's patterns of abilities/disabilities or variation in the test norms themselves.

An adequate neuropsychological assessment of a child includes assessment of a broad spectrum of behaviors including measures of attention and vigilance, executive functioning, and problem solving, learning and memory, language, sensory processing, motor performance, social skills, affective behavior, and academic performance. In children and adolescents we test for purposes of intervention because we have some reason to believe, either from history or observation or both, that the child being assessed has a problem which will impact future development or performance, often in school. We make inferences based upon an assessment during one or more static periods in the history of a developing and changing organism. Tests that assess loss of acquired skills in adults are not adequate to assess ongoing skill acquisition or strategies in children (Baron et al., 1995; Hynd & Willis, 1988; Kirk, 1985). More recent practice has involved serial assessments of children and adolescents in order to utilize more data points to study the developmental course and benefits of treatment.

Professional concern regarding the psychometric or methodologic limitations of many of the popular neuropsychological measures have been discussed at length (Franzen, 1989; Russell, 1986, 1987; Spreen & Strauss, 1991). Russell (1987) reported that many of the neuropsychological tests failed to meet the criteria set forth in the APA manual, *Standards for Educational and Psychological Testing*, published in 1985. Many more fail to meet the new standards for educational and psychological testing (American Education Research Association et al., 1999). Issues related to reliability, validity, standard error of measurement estimates, and demographic characteristics of the normative reference group are often not readily available. Although some efforts to correct this have been forthcoming recently, the problems remain. Ardila, Rosselli, and Puente (1994), report that most neuropsychological tests designed for adults generate their normative data by comparing neurologically normal and brain-damaged subjects from middle-class, English-speaking populations. There is limited applicability of these norms to multicultural populations (Padilla & Medina, 1996; Simonian, Tarnowski, Stancin, Friman, & Atkins, 1991). Spreen & Strauss (1991) report that many instruments provide explicit warnings concerning the inappropriateness of their norms for persons with ethnic differences. There are very few such caveats available in child or adolescent neuropsychological batteries.

Validity and Predictability

Wedding & Faust (1989) argued for the development of an actuarial basis for predicting future behavior. Actuarial models have been demonstrated to have consistently higher probabilities of accurate diagnosis than do clinical models, presumably due to the differences and methods of data integration (see Willis, 1988, for an extended discussion of neurological diagnosis in children using actuarial and clinical models). Wedding and Faust recommended a number of corrective procedures in order to increase the predictability of neuropsychological assessment. They recommend the use of appropriate norms, valid information, an extensive history, and a knowledge of the literature. Following these recommendations is problematic for the assessment of children and adolescents in the majority culture. The problems are exacerbated in diverse cultural groups.

For many years we have relied on an assumption that our test procedures provide reliable and valid information regardless of cultural origins. This assumption has not been investigated and is not likely to be true. What little information exists on normative data in multicultural populations exists in the adult literature. Attempts to control for cultural factors has led to the use of moderator variables such as measures of acculturation, educational background, linguistic functions, SES, and so forth, when assessing adults. We have no similar procedures for children and probably have little if any idea as to what moderator variables we would utilize and how.

Regarding the use of norms, cultural variables have been shown to significantly impact performance on measures of intelligence. Some of the most widely used measures of intelligence in children and adolescents, the WPPSI-R, WISC-III, WAIS-III, and Stanford-Binet-IV, included some cultural and linguistic minorities in the standardization samples (Wechsler, 1974, 1991). However, factor structure patterns differ across cultural groups (Dana, 1993). The absence of construct equivalents for all groups, that is, cross-cultural construct validity, increases the likelihood that test taking variables such as rapport or the use of gender or race-balanced examiners will have a greater impact (Hanley & Barclay, 1979; Terrell & Terrell, 1983) for children and adolescents from diverse cultures than they do for children or adolescents in the European American culture, who have a much higher probability of being assessed by someone from their own culture. The Kaufman Assessment Battery for Children (Kaufman & Kaufman, 1983), used much less frequently by neuropsychologists who evaluate children and early adolescents than the Wechsler tests, was developed with the intention for use with multicultural populations. As a result, the test was developed and constructed to insure comparability in measurement of multicultural populations with earlier standardized intelligence tests, but used scores with different origins. The scores use a process dichotomy, sequential versus simultaneous. The test also included a measure based on nonverbal administration and response. The test construction methodology involved more sophisticated selection and sampling of demographic variables, which probably reduced IQ differences between the groups as well. The construct validation studies included a variety of methods for cross-cultural validation in addition to factor analysis. Ethnic differences between Hispanic American and African American children, as compared with European American children, were less than on the WISC-R. Level of parental education contributed to more group differences than did ethnicity per se. However, the KABC is less sensitive to cerebral dysfunction in comparison with the WISC-R and probably the WISC-III (Donders, 1992).

Unfortunately, the Kaufmans did not consider multicultural issues when they developed the Kaufman Adolescent and Adult Intelligence Test (Kaufman & Kaufman, 1993). Although the standardization sample was consistent with the U.S. population proportions in 1990, there were some problems with ethnicity by parental education level at the upper educational levels for the "other" minority groups which included Asian Americans, Native Americans, Alaskan Natives, and Pacific Islanders. Further, there are no comparative analyses by ethnicity in the KAIT.

None of the traditional neuropsychological measures have been formally investigated for the role of ethnicity in performance. Although there have been restandardizations of a number of neuropsychological measures for adults in various cultural populations (Ardila et al., 1994; Donias, Vassilopoulou, Golden, & Lovell, 1989; Taussig, Henderson, & Mack, 1992; Tsushima, Boyar, Shimizu, & Harada, 1995; Xu, Gong, & Matthews, 1987; Yun, Yao-Xion, & Matthews, 1987), methodological problems abound (Hall, 1997; Peng, Nesbett, & Wong, 1997; Simonian et al., 1991; Xu, 1995; Sue, Fujino, Hu, Takeuchi, & Zane, 1991).

Although one's performance on neuropsychological tests should be theoretically indicative of the integrity of the person's cerebral functions, demographic factors such as age, educational attainment, intelligence, and gender have been found to impact performance on basic measures of sensory and motor functions, as well as on cognitive functions including attention, memory, language, and executive functions in adults (Finlayson, Johnson, & Reitan,

1977; Heaton, Grant, & Matthews, 1986, 1991; Hudson, 1960; Leckliter & Mattarazzo, 1989; Reitan & Wolfson, 1992). These statistical relationships have affected the accuracy of diagnostic classification resulting in differential misclassification rates (Heaton et al., 1991).

Education plays a critical role in cognitive development. This concept is not new (D'Andrade, 1969). Luria began his career as a cognitive psychologist (Cole, 1990). In his collaborations with Vygotsky (Vygotsky & Luria, 1993) in the early 1930s he studied the impact of education on cognitive functions in remote regions of Uzbekistan and Kirghizia (Luria, 1976). As the peasants were exposed to literacy and different work contexts they began to approach intellectual puzzles in a totally different manner, utilizing new strategies and engaging in new forms of abstract, categorical relationships and the ability to conceptualize beyond their own experiences. Luria reported changes in self-awareness and personality as well. Although some of Luria's interpretations fell into disfavor, causing him to switch to the field of neuropsychology, his methodology and conclusions are worthy of contemporary review.

Mirsky found the same relationship in his San Pablo studies. The strongest variable was level of parental education, which correlated with all of the poverty variables including malnutrition, disease, toxic exposure, and so forth, (1995). He commented that cultural/educational factors are either not addressed by neuropsychologists or are dealt with by covariance analysis. His Irish family studies and other studies emphasized "the powerful affect of the quality of the familial milieu on the development of cognition" (Mirsky, 1995, p. 490).

In adult neuropsychology educational achievement is an important predictor variable for premorbid intelligence. More than 50% of the variance is accounted for by parental education (Kaufman, 1990). Parental educational attainment is highly correlated with SES (Suzuki, Vraniak, & Kugler, 1996), and SES is a strong predictor of metacognitive functioning (Wang, 1991), presumably due to the quality of home life experiences. Tests involving verbal memory are more highly associated with educational attainment (Ardila & Rosselli, 1988; Cornelius & Caspi, 1987; Ostrosky et al., 1985). The variable of parental education is particularly important because of the disproportionately high educational drop-out rates for particular racial or ethnic groups.

Educational achievement of the child cannot be used as a predictor of cognitive abilities because much of the time the evaluation is for purposes of assessing educational performance (Kirk, 1983). Thus, the issue becomes a circular one. In addition to the problems related to educational opportunities and environments, cultural values related to education also play a significant role (Howell & Reuda, 1996; Perez-Arce & Puente, 1996; Sattler, 1998; Suzuki et al., 1996).

The valid history deemed essential by Wedding and Faust (1989) may be difficult to obtain. Because young children are unable to provide reliable subjective reports, information from parents and teachers regarding the child's behavior and abilities outside of the testing session is crucial in order to determine the ecological validity of the test findings. Teachers and other school personnel may be the most common referral source as well, particularly for special education evaluation. Thus, it is essential that both the teacher and evaluator understand the values, assumptions, culture, and language of the student and his/her family. Expectations and attitudes determine who is referred, for what reason, and the outcome. Cooperation with the family is critical in developing a meaningful understanding of the child.

In adolescents it is also the family who provides the history. Adolescents rarely have sufficient insight into who they have been over the course of time in order to provide a history or determine if they have changed as a result of an event, such as a traumatic brain injury. They often remember themselves as different from how they were, rendering them poor historians.

The history obtained is an integral part of the neuropsychological assessment. During the interview, pertinent information concerning both the family and the child or adolescent's medical, educational, and psychosocial history must be obtained (Lezak, 1995). Although background information should be confirmed and supplemented by medical records, prior school records, and prior test results if available (Matarazzo, 1990), the most basic information generally comes from the family. The accuracy of the information obtained clearly affects the validity of the assessment. History taking is a complex process under the best of circumstances.

One of the primary sources of bias in the history taking is failure to disclose relevant information related to the problem. Sources of interview bias may result from problems in communication between the interviewer and family member, discomfort regarding the sharing of sensitive information, or lack of understanding about the relevance of such issues. Problems in communications can result from simply speaking different languages (Artiola & Mullaney, 1997).

Most commonly, interviews are conducted in English. Much has been written about the problem of using interpreters when communicating with clients who are not fluent in English (Artiola & Mullaney, 1998; Dana, 1993; Friedman & Clayton, 1996; Perez-Arce & Puente, 1996; Sattler, 1998; Yansen & Shulman, 1996). Translators and interpreters may facilitate the communication (Manuel-Dupont, Ardila, Rosselli, & Puente, 1992; Vasquez & Javier, 1991). However, they may also add to, substitute, alter, or omit statements made by the interviewer or family member. Either exaggeration or minimization may occur (Friedman & Clayton, 1996; Sattler, 1998). In adults, symptom severity is judged to be greater when the client and clinician speak the same language (Malgady & Constantino, 1998). We do not have similar research available on children or adolescents.

Beyond the basic issues of language, interview bias or misinformation may come from more subtle disruptions in the communication process. Gender roles may be an important factor in determining who provides the history and how it is provided. In Asian and Hispanic families male leadership and obedience to parents is the norm (Conoley & Bryant, 1996; Sattler, 1998). Thus, it is common for a father or older brother to provide the history. Asking questions of the mother (who may be more aware of the details because she is the primary caretaker) may offend family members and interfere with the acquisition of information. In African American households the mother and other female relatives are the repository of knowledge about the family and its individual members. The neuropsychologist should therefore interview the woman designated by the family as knowledgeable about the child or adolescent, whether that woman is a biological relative or not. Family may be defined beyond biological borders in African American families. The child's primary caretaker may be a parent, aunt, cousin, or "sister." Regardless of how the person is related to the child, family members may be better informed as to who should provide the information than is the neuropsychologist.

Misinformation regarding history which results in bias may be due to very different worldviews between the neuropsychologist and the family. Some questions regarding current cognitive and emotional status may not be perceived as appropriate to communicate either with a stranger or an authority figure such as the neuropsychologist (Conoley & Bryant, 1996; Sue, 1977). How issues related to emotional distress are communicated differs across ethnic groups (Perez-Arce & Puente, 1996; Rubin, 1998; Saarni, 1998; Wilson & MacCarthy, 1994; Xu et al., 1987). Child-rearing practices vary across cultures (Stevenson-Hinde, 1998), as do parameters of acceptable behavior (Arnett & Balle-Jensen, 1993; Bornstein et al., 1998; Chen et al., 1998; Greenburg & Chen, 1996). Behavioral issues important to the neuropsychologist may be deemed too personal or embarrassing (Sue, 1977, 1992) to the parent. Questions may be phrased in a manner that is misunderstood. The importance of symptoms or developmental patterns may be interpreted differently by family members and by the neuropsychologist. Parents may be uncomfortable about sharing the details of the child or adolescent's history (Simonian et al., 1991). Parents may also feel defensive about answering certain kinds of questions related to discipline, maternal drug use during pregnancy, or other highly sensitive issues (Friedman & Clayton, 1996; Sattler, 1998).

Sometimes it is the complex interaction between socioeconomic and educational issues that may make it difficult for parents from diverse cultural and linguistic backgrounds to be willing to share information and to be able to do so. In general, it is the responsibility of the neuropsychologist to enable the family member to provide information in a manner that is comfortable as well as informative. The better a parent understands the purpose of the evaluation and the rationale for acquiring highly personal information, the better the parent is able to participate in the evaluation process and provide that information. Often parents have a different understanding of historical facts and their significance, which may interfere with the ability to communicate information to the neuropsychologist in the way in which the neuropsychologist is accustomed to receiving it. Sensitivity to the courtesies and customs of different cultures will enable the neuropsychologist to obtain more accurate information. Looking directly at the historian may facilitate information gathering in some cultures and inhibit it in others (Conoley & Bryant, 1996; Dana, 1993; Friedman & Clayton, 1996; Kohatsu & Richardson, 1996; Meller & Ohr, 1996; Sattler, 1998). Body language, facial expression, and vocal intonation may communicate more than words in many cultures. The responses of the neuropsychologist to the historical information may also alter the information sharing process. When assessing someone from a different linguistic background, more is needed than simply a translator of the language. Cultural factors play a profound role in information gathering. Asking questions directly versus engaging in a more gradual series of open-ended questions or perhaps observations about the child may provide greater or lesser information, depending upon the culture of the historian. In some cultures, it will be more useful to make a home visit and observe the child in a home setting, particularly if the child is a preschooler. For other cultures the notion of a home visit would be considered an invasion of privacy and highly inappropriate.

How a specific culture views disability issues may also impact the communication process in taking a history. Beliefs about illness and disability (Conoley & Bryant, 1996) have a significant impact on what information is communicated as well as how it is communicated. Cultures in which there is a belief that illness or disability is a manifestation of a life out of balance due to evil forces in an individual or family member will be far less willing to share information about illness or disability than family from a culture that believes the illness or disability is a biological phenomenon. How a parent reacts to disability in a child is also highly dependent on cultural variables. It is not only the worldview, but also the extent to which the historian feels alienated or a part of the process as well as the dominant culture. For example, African Americans may feel so alienated from institutions such as the school and the medical (also neuropsychological) community due to problems with access and institutional racism, that they have difficulty participating in the assessment process unless the neuropsychologist has a good understanding of the issues and can enable the parent or other family member to feel comfortable about participating in the process. This is particularly important because African American adolescents are "one of the most vulnerable and victimized groups in American society. As the largest group of minority youth, they frequently have been misdiagnosed by the mental health system, mislabeled by the educational system, mishandled by the juvenile justice system, and mistreated by the social welfare system" (Gibbs, 1990, p. 21).

In addition to the cultural expectations, the degree of acculturation and success in coping and adapting to the procedures involved in the interaction process with the dominant culture all have a profound impact on the communication process and the success of history taking (Chelune, 1978; Conoley & Bryant, 1996; Dana, 1993; Friedman & Clayton, 1996; Meller & Ohr, 1996; Moreland, 1996; Perez-Arce & Puente, 1996).

Knowledge of the literature, the last recommendation of Wedding & Faust (1989), is becoming an increasingly viable undertaking. Since the early 1990s the role of culture in psychological development and assessment has been addressed by numerous psychologists. Although the literature relates primarily to adults, there is a growing body of literature related to children which has been referenced herein. The culture-dependent nature of cognitive activity has been summarized (Ardila, Rosselli, & Ostrosky-Solís, 1992; Meller & Ohr, 1996; Perez-Arce & Puente, 1996; Sattler, 1998). Research reported from the Laboratory of Comparative Human Cognition (1983a,b) demonstrated that culture had a profound affect on language, perception, memory, and logical reasoning. Perceptual abilities, elements investigated routinely on neuropsychological tests, vary according to cultural experiences (Brislin, 1983; Modiano, Maldonado & Villasana, 1982; Segall, 1986). Hudson (1960) found a significant difference in depth perception in 12-year-old European children as compared with Bantu or Ghanaian children. European laborers and nonliterate Bantu adults without perceptual training also had difficulty in three-dimensional perception. Culture and education have also been found to have a strong influence on the ability to copy geometric figures and patterns (Amante, VanHouton, Grieve, Bader, & Margules, 1997; Deregowski, 1980; Osuji, 1982). Although much of this literature is older than many practicing neuropsychologists, the implications are quite contemporary.

For many psychologists who serve children, their earliest exposure to multiculturalism may date back to theories of cultural disadvantage developed in the 1960s which resulted in the establishment of the Head Start program (U.S. Congress, 1964). The original Head Start program was designed to decrease the likelihood of school failure by giving low-income students the skills to succeed in elementary school. It is not surprising to note that economically disadvantaged children tended to include a large percentage of children from diverse cultural backgrounds.

The cultural disadvantage theory maintains that children from diverse cultural backgrounds are not provided with the requisite cognitive, preacademic, and social skills necessary for school success. The "disadvantage" occurs in the preschool years so that children enter school already behind in their development. The cultural disadvantage theory tended to be highly biased against multicultural families. The theory failed to recognize that children from culturally diverse backgrounds differed in a number of dimensions including race, linguistic background, ethnicity, parental education, SES, and frequently level of acculturation. Their backgrounds were highly dissimilar from the mainstream of American culture at the time. The theory also ignored the findings of general psychology that there is more variability of functioning within ethnic groups as compared with across them (Kaufman, 1990; Meller & Ohr, 1996; Stevenson-Hinde, 1998).

Psychologists from culturally diverse backgrounds such as Piaget (1983), Luria (1961, 1979, 1982), Vygotsky (1962, 1978), and Feuerstein (1980), recognized the social context of early learning in child development. Although much of Piaget's early research focused on the issues of maturation and experience, his later work dealt with social transmission and its impact on development. According to Piaget, children first grow and develop using culturally bound tools such as language, alphabets, math symbols, and so forth, which are both the vehicles and the catalysts for their development. Social transmission also involves the process by which significant individuals in the child's life act as social mediators for that development. Feuerstein (1980) discussed mediation of learning experiences, indicating that the agent of such mediation was the parent or teacher. This mediator was strongly influenced by cultural values and expectations and basically organized the world for the child. Feuerstein developed a strategy for cognitive remediation involving the restructuring of that environment. Luria (1961), who was strongly influenced by Vygotsky, developed a theory that speech and language are mediated by experience and that there is a dynamic interactive relationship between cultural experiences and child development via the vehicle of language. These researchers provided perspectives that have had contemporary reconfirmation by Mirsky (1995) regarding the critical nature of the social milieu in which the child develops. Further discussion regarding these issues as they relate to child development can be found in Ardila, Roselli, & Ostrosky-Solís (1992) and Meller & Ohr (1996).

The Future of Developmental Neuropsychology

"The focus of any assessment is the person being assessed, not the test" (Kaufman, 1990, p. 24). "The most indirect method of obtaining information regarding the real world is via psychometric tests; yet they represent the major source of information for many neuropsychological evaluations" (Long, 1996, p. 9). Neuropsychologists have become preoccupied with quantification rather than focusing on the goal of understanding the development and behavior of the child or adolescent under investigation. Executive functions mediated by the frontal brain (Benton, 1991; Dennis, 1991; Eslinger & Gratten, 1991; Fletcher, 1996; Gratten & Eslinger, 1991; Roberts & Pennington, 1996; Stuss & Benson, 1986) involve not only metacognitive activities such as planning, problem solving, and cognitive flexibility (Fletcher et al., 1996; Gratten & Eslinger, 1991; Stuss & Benson, 1986). Executive functions also include frustration tolerance, self-regulatory functions, and environmental judgments (Gratten & Eslinger, 1991). Eslinger & Gratten (1991, p. 257) reported "frontal neural systems are the pivotal mediators of acculturation and social conduct, flexibility of thought and action, adaptive behavior, and goal attainment." Although little if anything has been written specifically about how the frontal brain mediates cultural experience with the exception of attention (Mirsky, 1995; Posner, 1992), there is an interaction effect because these behaviors are mediated by both psychobiological and cultural factors.

The tests used by neuropsychologists as well as clinical psychologists are strategies for sampling behavior. The tests and tasks were not meant to be exhaustive. As neuropsychologists learn more about neuropsychological functions, it is clear that we need to expand and modify the types of samples we collect in order to understand and assess those functions.

In order for the neuropsychologist to attain the goal stated by Kaufman (1990) "to be better than the test he or she uses" (p. 25), the neuropsychologist must actively consider the impact of the assessment process on the acquisition of information. Given our knowledge of the impact of the investigation on the function studied (see Webb, Campbell, Schwartz, & Sechrest, 1972, *Unobtrusive Measures*), the neuropsychologist must assess the extent to which the neuropsychological procedures alter and/or distort rather than clarify the neuropsychological functions of the child or adolescent being assessed. McShane (1989) recommended a number of modifications or sociolinguistic adaptations in his assessment of Native American children. These modifications involved allowing additional time during untimed tests, avoiding eye contact during certain subtests such as digit span, avoiding touching behaviors, and adjusting to generally lower levels of speech since Native American children tend to speak softly. (Speaking louder could be interpreted as indicating anger.) Additional accommodations included learning to listen and observe effectively since Native-American children reportedly tend to use short, rapid responses and facial or other gestures rather than pointing. Although the extent to which accommodations may be necessary may be dependent upon perhaps both the culture and the degree of acculturation of the child or adolescent being assessed, normative studies are clearly required in order to understand how these accommodations alter the results obtained. The absence of careful investigation of the impact of any accommodations on the scores obtained and the meaning of those scores is poor science. It also further discriminates against children and adolescents from diverse cultural backgrounds.

Part of the paradigm shift in neuropsychology has been to address the ecological validity of neuropsychological testing. Ecological validity as a term was first used by Egon Brunswick (1955). The term referred to the conditions under which one could generalize from controlled experiments to the naturalistic environment. Problems in generalizability from neuropsychological test data to daily life situations have hampered the ability of clients, families, and rehabilitationists to understand and cope with the impact of neuropsychological and neurobehavioral disorders. The need for contemporary neuropsychology to address predictions to daily life functions was introduced by Tupper & Cicerone (1990).

Sbordone & Long (1996) and their collaborators recommended rethinking many of our beliefs and assumptions in neuropsychology in order to establish and utilize more meaningful methodology in the assessment process. They define ecological validity as "the functional and predictive relationship between the patient's performance on a set of neuropsychological tests and the patient's behavior in a variety of real world settings (e.g., at home, work, school, community)" (p. 16). Implicit in the definition is the notion that the neuropsychologist's choice of tests will assess the cognitive, emotional, and behavioral functions that are germane to the demand characteristics of the various real world settings of the person being assessed. These principles are particularly relevant to the assessment of children and adolescents, where the demand characteristics change over the course of development, as well as to children and adolescents from diverse cultures.

Hartlage & Templer (1996) opined that ecological validity in child neuropsychology involved attention to two special issues. One issue they described as "the developmental diversity of child neuropsychological functions" (p. 301), referring to the alterations in neural organization that occur over the course of development from infancy through adolescence. The second issue they addressed was the problem of neuropsychological test instruments available for assessing children and the measurement problems involved therein. Their suggestion that achievement test scores might provide greater ecological validity failed to consider the confounding of issues related to learning disabilities and the impact of culture on educational access and opportunity. However, they began the discussion regarding one way in which developmental neuropsychology could address the issues of ecological validity.

Developmental neuropsychology is faced with a number of exciting challenges as we move into the next century. The opportunity to study the interaction of culture and behavior is greater and more critical than ever. Although the issue of "cultural loading" has been discussed for many years with recognition that all tests are a reflection of some of the unique aspects of the culture in which they were developed (Reynolds, 1982), the importance of addressing these issues is far more apparent today.

References

Aday, L. A., & Anderson, R. (1978). Insurance coverage and access: Implications for health policy. *Health Services Research, 13*, 369–377.

Amante, D., VanHouton, V. W., Grieve, J. H., Bader, C. A., & Margules, P. H. (1977). Neuropsychological deficit, ethnicity, and socioeconomic status. *Journal of Consulting and Clinical Psychology, 45*, 524–535.

American Education Research Association, American Psychological Association, & Natioanl Council on Measurement in Education (1999). *Standards for educational and psychological testing*. Washington, DC: American Educational Research Association.

Ardila, A., & Rosselli, M. (1988). *Sociocultural effects on language abilities*. Orlando, FL: National Academy of Neuropsychologists.

Ardila, A., Rosselli, M., & Ostrosky-Solís, F. (1992). Socioeducational. In A. E. Puente & R. J. McCaffrey (Eds.), *Handbook of neuropsychological assessment*, (pp. 181–192). New York: Plenum.

Ardila, A., Rosselli, M., & Puente, A. (1994). *Neuropsychological evaluation of the Spanish speaker*. New York: Plenum.

Arnett, J., & Balle-Jensen, L. (1993). Cultural basis of risk behavior: Danish adolescents. *Child Development, 64*, 1842–1855.

Artiola, L., & Mullaney, H. A. (1997). Neuropsychology with Spanish-speakers: Language use and proficiency issues for test development. *Journal of Clinical and Experimental Neuropsychology, 19*, 615–622).

Artiola, L., & Mullaney, H. A. (1998). Assessing patients whose language you do not know: Can the absurd be ethical? *The Clinical Neuropsychologist, 12*, 113–126.

Babcock, K. A., & Ross, M. W. (1982). Neuropsychological testing with Australian Aborigines. *Australian Psychologist, 17*, 297–299.

Baron, D. S., Fennell, E. B., & Voeller, K. K. S. (1995). *Pediatric neuropsychology in the medical setting*. New York: Oxford University Press.

Barsky, V. E., & Siegel, L. S. (1992). Predicting future cognitive, academic, and behavioral outcomes for very low birth-weight (1500-grams) infants. In S. L. Friedman, & M. D. Sigman (Eds.), *The psychological development of low birth-weight children* (pp. 275–289). Norwood, NJ: Ablex.

Bazzoli, G. J. (1986). Healthcare for the indigent: Overview of critical issues. *Health Services Research, 21*, 353–393.

Bennett, J. M. (1986a). A developmental approach to training for intercultural sensitivity. *International Journal of Intercultural Relations, 10*, 179–196.

Bennett, J. M. (1986b). Modes of cross-cultural training. *International Journal of Intercultural Relations, 10*, 117–134.

Bentancourt, H., & Lopez, S. R. (1993). The study of culture, ethnicity, and race in American psychology. *American Psychologist, 48*, 629–637.

Benton, A. (1991). Prefrontal injury and behavior in children. *Developmental Neuropsychology, 7*, 275–281.

Bornstein, M., Hayes, O. M., Azuma, H., Galperin, C., Maital, S., Ogino, M., Painter, K., Pascual, L., Pecheux, M., Rohn, C., Toda, S., Venuti, P., Vyt, A., & Wright, B. (1998). A cross-national study of self-evaluators and attributions in parenting: Argentina, Belgium, France, Israel, Italy, Japan and the United States. *Developmental Psychology, 34*, 662–666.

Breslau, N. (1995). Psychiatric sequelæ of low birth-weight. *Epidemiologic Reviews, 17*, 96–106.

Breslau, N., Chilcoat, H., DelDotto, J., Andreski, P., & Brown, G. (1996). Low birth-weight and neurocognitive status at 6 years of age. *Biological Psychiatry, 40*, 389–397.

Brislin, R. W. (1983). Cross-cultural research in psychology. *Annual Review of Psychology, 34*, 363–400.

Broman, S. H. & Michel, M. E. (Eds.) (1995). *Traumatic head injury in children*. New York: Oxford University Press.

Brown, R. (1976). In memorial tribute to Eric Lenneberg. *Cognition, 4*, 125–153.

Brunswick, E. (1955). Representative design and probabilistic theory in a functional psychology. *Psychology Review, 62*, 193–217.

Burstin, H. R., Lipsitz, S. R., & Brennan, T. A. (1992). Socioeconomic status and risk for substandard medical care. *Journal of the American Medical Association, 268*, 2383–2387.

Chalmers, D., Stewart, D., Silva, P., & Mulvena, A. (1989). *Otitis media with effusion in children: The Dunedin study*. Philadelphia: Lippincott.

Chapman, S. B. (1995). Discourse as an outcome measure in pediatric head-injured populations. In S. H. Broman & M. E. Michel (Eds.), *Traumatic head injury in children* (pp. 95–116). New York: Oxford University Press.

Chelune, G. J. (1978). Nature and assessment of self-disclosing behavior. In P. McReynolds (Ed.), *Advances in psychological assessment* (vol. 4; pp. 278–320). San Francisco: Jossey-Bass.

Chelune, G. J., & Edwards, P. (1981). Early brain lesions: Ontogenetic–environmental considerations. *Journal of Consulting and Clinical Psychology, 49*, 777–790.

Chen, X., Hastings, P., Rubin, K., Chen, H., Cen, G., & Stewart, S. (1998). Child-rearing attitudes and behavioral inhibitions in Chinese and Canadian toddlers: A cross-cultural study. *Developmental Psychology, 34,* 677–686.

Clarren, S. K., & Smith, D. W. (1978). The fetal alcohol syndrome. *New England Journal of Medicine, 298,* 1063–1067.

Cole, M. (1990). Alexandr Romanovich Luria: Cultural psychologist. In E. Goldberg (Ed.), *Contemporary neuropsychology and the legacy of Luria* (pp. 11–28). Hillsdale, NJ: Erlbaum.

Conoley, J. C., & Bryant, L. E. (1996). Assessing diverse family systems. In L. A. Suzuki, P. J. Meller, & J. G. Ponterotto (Eds.), *Handbook of multicultural assessment* (pp. 395–428). San Francisco: Jossey-Bass.

Cornelius, S. W., & Caspi, A. (1987). Everyday problem solving in adulthood and old age. *Psychology and Aging, 2,* 144–153.

Cravioto, J., DeLicardie, E. R., & Birch, H. G. (1966). Nutrition, growth and neurointegrative development: An experimental and ecological study. *Pediatrics, 38,* 319–320.

Dana, R. (1993). *Multicultural assessment perspectives for professional psychology.* Needham Heights, MA: Allyn & Bacon.

D'Andrade, R. (1969). Cultural cognition. In M. I. Posner (Ed.), *Foundations of cognitive science* (pp. 795–830). Cambridge MA: Bradford Books, MIT Press.

Delpit, L. (1995). *Other people's children: cultural conflict in the classroom.* New York: Norton.

Dennis, M. (1991). Frontal lobe function in childhood and adolescence: A heuristic for assessing attention regulation, executive control, and the intentional states important for social discourse. *Developmental Neuropsychology, 7,* 327–358.

Deregowski, J. B. (1980). *Illusions, patterns and pictures: A cross-cultural perspective.* New York: Academic Press.

Donders, J. (1992). Validity of the Kaufman Battery for Children when employed with children with traumatic brain injury. *Journal of Clinical Neuropsychology, 48,* 225–230.

Donias, S. H., Vassilopoulou, E. O., Golden, C. J., & Lovell, M. R. (1989). Reliability and clinical effectiveness of the standardized Greek version of the Luria–Nebraska Neuropsychological Battery. *International Journal of Clinical Neuropsychology, 11*(13), 129–133.

Eslinger, P. J., & Gratten, L. M. (1991). Perspectives on the developmental consequences of early frontal lobe damage: Introduction. *Developmental Neuropsychology, 7,* 257–260.

Ewing-Cobbs, L., Fletcher, J. M., & Levin, H. S. (1985). Neuropsychological sequelæ following pediatric head injury. In M. Ylvisaker (Ed.), *Head injury rehabilitation: Children and adolescents* (pp. 71–89). Philadelphia: Taylor & Francis.

Ewing-Cobbs, L., Miner, M. E., Fletcher, J. M., & Levin, H. S. (1989). Intellectual, motor, and language sequelæ following closed head injury in infants and pre-schoolers. *Journal of Pediatric Psychology, 14,* 531–547.

Feuerstein, R. (1980). *Instrumental enrichment: An intervention for cognitive modifiability.* Baltimore, MD: University Park Press.

Finlayson, M. A., Johnson, K. A., & Reitan, R. (1977). Relationship of level of education to neuropsychological measures in brain-damaged and non-brain-damaged adults. *Journal of Consulting Clinical Neuropsychology, 45,* 536–542.

Fischer, K. W., & Rose, S. P. (1994). Dynamic development of coordination of components in brain and behavior: A framework for theory and research. In G. Dawson & K. W. Fischer (Eds.), *Human behavior and the developing brain* (pp. 3–66). New York: Guilford.

Fletcher, J. M. (1996). Executive functions in children: Introduction to the special senses. *Developmental Neuropsychology, 12,* 1–3.

Fletcher, J. M., & Taylor, H. G. (1984). Neuropsychological approaches to children: Towards a developmental neuropsychology. *Journal of Clinical Neuropsychology, 6,* 39–56.

Fletcher, J. M., Ewing-Cobbs, L., Frances, D., & Levin, H. (1995). Variability in outcomes after traumatic brain injury in children: A developmental perspective. S. H. Broman & M. E. Michel (Eds.), *Traumatic head injury in children* (pp. 3–21). New York: Oxford University Press.

Fletcher, J. M., Ewing-Cobbs, L., Miner, M. E., Levin, H. S., & Eisenberg, H. M. (1990). Behavioral changes after closed head injury in children. *Journal of Consulting and Clinical Psychology, 58,* 93–98.

Fletcher, J. M., Brookshire, B. L., Landry, S. H., Bohan, T. P., Davidson, K. C., Frances, D. J., Levin, H. S., Brandt, M. E., Kramer, L. A., & Morris, R. D. (1996). Attentional skills and executive functions in children with early hydrocephalus. *Developmental Neuropsychology, 12,* 53–76.

Franzen, M. D. (1989). *Reliability and validity in neuropsychological assessment.* New York: Plenum.

Friedman, C. A., & Clayton, R. J. (1996). Multiculturalism and neuropsychological assessment. In L. A. Suzuki, P. J. Meller, & J. G. Ponterotto (Eds.), *Handbook of multicultural assessment* (pp. 291–318). San Francisco: Jossey-Bass.

Gibbs, J. T. (1990). Mental health issues of Black adolescents: Implications for policy and practice. In A. R. Stiffman & L. E. Doris (Eds.), *Ethnic issues in adolescent mental health* (pp. 21–52). Newbury Park, CA: Sage.

Goldman, P. S. (1975). Age, sex, and experience as related to the neural bases of cognitive development. In N. A. Buchwald & M. A. B. Brazier (Eds.), *Brain mechanisms in mental retardation* (pp. 379–399). New York: Academic Press.

Goldman-Rakic, P., Isserhoff, A., Schwartz, M. L., & Bugbee, N. M. (1983). The neurobiology of cognitive development. In P. H. Mussen (Series Ed.), M. M. Haifth & J. J. Campos (Volume Eds.), *Handbook of child psychology* (4th ed): *Vol. 2: Infancy and Developmental Psychobiology* (pp. 281–344). New York: Wiley.

Graham, S. (1992). Most of the subjects were white and middle-class: Trends in published research on African-Americans. In selected American Psychological Association Journals, 1970–89. *American Psychologist, 47*, 629–639.

Gratten, L. M., & Eslinger, P. J. (1991). Frontal lobe damage in children and adolescents: A comparative review. *Developmental Neuropsychology, 7*, 283–326.

Greenberg, E., & Chen, C. (1996). Perceived family relationships and depressed mood in early and late adolescence: A comparison of European and Asian Americans. *Developmental Psychology, 32*, 707–716.

Hale, J. (1982). *Black children their roots, culture and learning styles*. Provo, UT: Brigham Young University Press.

Hall, C. (1997). Cultural malpractice: The growing obsolescence of psychology with the changing U.S. population. *American Psychologist, 52*, 642–651.

Hanley, J. H., & Barclay, A. J. (1979). Sensitivity of the WISC and WISC-R to subject and examiner variables. *Journal of Black Psychology, 5*, 79–84.

Hartlage, L., & Templer, D. (1996). Ecological issues and child neuropsychological assessment. In R. J. Sbordone & C. J. Long (Eds.), *Ecological validity of neuropsychological testing* (pp. 301–314). Delray Beach, FL: St. Lucie.

Heath, S. B. (1991). "It's about winning!" The language of knowledge in baseball. In L. B. Resnick, J. M. Levine, & S. D. Teasley (Eds), *Perspectives on socially shared cognition* (pp. 101–124). Washington, D.C.: American Psychological Association.

Heaton, R. K., Grant, I. G., & Matthews, C. G. (1986). Differences in neuropsychological test performance associated with age, education, and sex. In I. G. Grant & K. M. Adams (Eds.) *Neuropsychological assessment of neuropsychiatric disorders* (pp. 100–120). New York: Oxford University Press.

Heaton, R. K., Grant, I. G., & Matthews, C. G. (1991). *Comprehensive norms for an expanded Halstead–Reitan Battery: Demographic corrections, research findings, and clinical applications*. Odessa, FL: Psychological Assessment Resources.

Howell, K. W., & Reuda, R. (1996). Achievement testing with culturally and linguistically diverse students. In L. A. Suzuki, P. J. Meller, & J. G. Ponterotto (Eds.), *Handbook of multicultural assessment* (pp. 253–290). San Francisco: Jossey-Bass.

Hudson, W. (1960). Pictorial depth perception in subcultural groups in Africa. *Journal of Social Psychology, 52*, 183–208.

Hynd, G. W., & Willis, W. G. (1988). *Pediatric neuropsychology*. New York: Grune & Stratton.

Jackson, J. H. (1992). Trials, tribulations, and triumphs of minorities in psychology: Reflections at century's end. *Professional Psychology: Research & Practice, 23*, 80–86.

Kaufman, A. S. (1990). *Assessing adolescent and adult intelligence*. Needham Heights, MA: Allyn & Bacon.

Kaufman, A. S., & Kaufman, N. L. (1983). *Kaufman Assessment Battery for Children: Administration and scoring manual*. Circle Pines, MN: American Guidance Service.

Kaufman, A. S., & Kaufman, N. L. (1993). *Manual for the Kaufman Adolescent and Adult Intelligence Test*. Circle Pines, MN: American Guidance Service.

Keitel, M. A., Copala, M., & Adamson, W. S. (1996). Ethical issues in multicultural assessment. In L. A. Suzuki, P. J. Meller, & J. G. Ponterotto (Eds.), *Handbook of multicultural assessment* (pp. 29–48). San Francisco: Jossey-Bass.

Kirk U. (1983). Language and the brain: Implications for education. In U. Kirk (Ed.), *Neuropsychology of language, reading and spelling* (pp. 257–272). New York: Academic Press.

Kirk, U. (1985). Hemisphere contributions to the development of graphic skills. In C. T. Best (Ed.), *Hemispheric function and collaboration in the child* (pp. 193–228). Orlando, FL: Academic Press.

Kohatsu, E. L., & Richardson, T. Q. (1996). Racial and ethnic identity assessment. In L. A. Suzuki, P. J. Meller, & J. G. Ponterotto (Eds.), *Handbook of multicultural assessment* (pp. 611–650). San Francisco: Jossey-Bass.

Korkman, M., Kirk, V., & Kemp, S. (1998). *NEPSY: A developmental neuropsychological assessment*. San Antonio: The Psychological Corporation.

Laboratory of Comparative Human Cognition (1983a). Culture and cognitive development. In P. Mussen (Ed.), *Handbook on child development: Vol. 1: History, therapy and methods* (pp. 295–356). New York: Wiley.

Laboratory of Comparative Human Cognition (1983b). Culture and cognitive development. In P. Mussen (Ed.) *Handbook of child psychology* (Vol. 1; pp. 342–397). New York: Wiley.

Lave, J. (1977). Tailor-made experiments in evaluating the intellectual consequences of apprenticeship training. *The Quarterly Newsletter of the Institute for Comparative Human Development, 1,* 1–3.

Leckliter, I. N., & Matarazzo, J. D. (1989). The influence of age, education, IQ, gender, and alcohol abuse on Halstead–Reitan Neuropsychological Test Battery performance. *Journal of Clinical Neuropsychology, 45,* 484–512.

Lee, Y., Jussim, L., & McCauley, C. (1995). *Stereotype accuracy.* Washington D.C.: American Psychological Association.

Levin, H. S., Ewing-Cobbs, L., & Eisenberg, H. M. (1995). Neurobehavioral outcome of pediatric closed head injury. In S. H. Broman & M. E. Michel (Eds.), *Traumatic head injury in children* (pp. 70–94). New York: Oxford University Press

Lezak, M. D. (1995). *Neuropsychological assessment* (3rd ed.). New York: Oxford University Press.

Long, C. J. (1996). Neuropsychological tests: A look at our past and the impact that ecological issues may have on our future. In R. J. Sbordone & C. J. Long (Eds.), *Ecological validity of neuropsychological testing* (pp. 1–14). Delray Beach, FL: St. Lucie.

Luria, A. R. (1961). *The role of speech in the regulation of normal and abnormal behavior.* New York: Liveright.

Luria, A. R. (1976). *Cognitive development: Its cultural and social foundations.* Cambridge, MA: Harvard University Press.

Luria, A. R. (1979). *The making of mind.* Cambridge MA: Harvard University Press.

Luria, A. R. (1982). *Language and cognition.* New York: Wiley.

Mahady, L., Towne, R., Algozzine, B., Mercer, J., & Ysseldyke, J. (1990). Minority overrepresentation: A case for alternative practice prior to referral. In S. Sigmon (Ed.), *Critical voices on special education: Problems and progress concerning the mildly handicapped* (pp. 89–102). Albany: State University of New York Press.

Malgady, R., & Constantino, C. (1998). Symptom severity in bilingual Hispanics as a function of ethnicity and language of interview. *Psychological Assessment, 10,* 120–127.

Manuel-Dupont, S., Ardila, A., Rosselli, M., & Puente, A. E. (1992). Bilingualism. In A. E. Puente & R. J. McCaffrey (Eds.), *Handbook of neuropsychological assessment* (pp. 193–212). New York: Plenum.

Matarazzo, J. D. (1990). Psychological assessment versus psychological testing. *American Psychologist, 45,* 999–1017.

McShane, D. (1989, April). *Testing and American Indians, Alaska natives.* Sponsored by the National Commission on Testing Public Policy. Symposium concerning the effects of testing on American Indians and Alaska natives. Albuquerque, NM.

Meller, P. J., & Ohr, P. S. (1996). The assessment of culturally diverse infants and pre-school children. In L. A. Suzuki, P. J. Meller, & J. G. Ponterotto (Eds.), *Handbook of multicultural assessment* (pp. 509–560). San Francisco: Jossey-Bass.

Mirsky, A. (1995). Perils and pitfalls on the path to normal potential: The role of impaired attention. *Journal of Clinical and Experimental Neuropsychology, 17,* 481–498.

Modiano, N., Maldonado, L. M., & Villasana, L. (1982). Accurate perception of color illustrations: Rates of comprehension in Mexican–Indian children. *Journal of Cross-Cultural Psychology, 13,* 490–495.

Moreland, K. L. (1996). Persistent issues in multicultural assessment of social and emotional functioning. In L. A. Suzuki, P. J. Meller, & J. G. Ponterotto (Eds.), *Handbook of multicultural assessment* (pp. 51–76). San Francisco: Jossey-Bass.

Olson, D. R. (1976). Culture, technology and intellect. In L. B. Resnick (Ed.), *The nature of intelligence.* Hillsdale, NJ: Erlbaum.

Ostrosky, F., Canseco, E., Quintonar, L., Navarro, E., Menses, S., & Ardila, A. (1985). Sociocultural effects in neuropsychological assessment. *International Journal of Neuroscience, 27,* 53–66.

Osuji, O. N. (1982). Constructing complex geometric patterns: A study of age and ability among Igbo children in Eastern Nigeria. *Journal of Cross-Cultural Psychology, 13,* 481–499.

Padilla, A. M., & Medina, A. (1996). Cross-cultural sensitivity in assessment: Using tests in culturally appropriate ways. In L. A. Suzuki, P. J. Meller, & J. G. Ponterotto (Eds.), *Handbook of multicultural assessment* (pp. 3–28). San Francisco: Jossey-Bass.

Peng, K., Nesbett, R. E., Wong, N. Y. C. (1997). Validity problems comparing values across cultures and possible solutions. *Psychological Methods, 2,* 329–344.

Pennington, B. F. (1994). The working memory functions of the prefrontal cortices: Implications for developmental and individual differences in cognition. M. Harth, J. Benson, R. Roberts, & B. F. Pennington (Eds.), *Future orientation processes in development* (pp. 243–289). Chicago: University of Chicago Press.

Perez-Arce, P., & Puente, A. E. (1996). Neuropsychological assessment of ethnic minorities. The case of assessing

Hispanics living in North America. In R. J. Sbordone & C. J. Long (Eds.), *Ecological validity of neuropsychological tests* (pp. 283–300). Delray Beach, FL: St. Lucie.

Piaget, J. (1983). Piaget's theory. In P. H. Mussen (Ed.) *Handbook of child psychology* (vol. 1, 4th ed.). New York: Wiley.

Posner, M. I. (1992). Attention as a cognitive and neural system. *Current Directions in Psychological Science, 1*, 11–14.

Posner, M. I., Rothbart, M. K., & Harman, C. (1994). Cognitive sciences contribution to culture and emotion. In F. Kitayama & H. R. Markus (Eds.), *Emotion and culture: Empirical studies of mutual influence* (pp. 197–216). Washington, DC: American Psychological Association.

Rankin, J. R. (1996). A historical perspective of cognitive and educational assessment. In L. A. Suzuki, P. J. Meller, & J. G. Ponterotto (Eds.), *Handbook of multicultural assessment* (pp. 139–140). San Francisco: Jossey-Bass.

Reitan, R., & Wolfson, D. (1992). Conventional intelligence measures and neuropsychological concepts of adaptive abilities. *Journal of Clinical Psychology, 48*, 521–529.

Reitan, R. M., & Davidson, L. (Eds.) (1974). *Clinical neuropsychology: Current status and applications*. Washington D.C.: Winston.

Resnick, L., Levine, J., & Teasley, S. (1991). *Perspectives on socially shared cognition*. Washington, D.C.: American Psychological Association.

Reynolds, C. (1982). The problem of bias in psychological assessment. In C. Reynolds & T. B. Gutkin (Eds.), *The handbook of school psychology* (pp. 178–208). New York: Wiley.

Risser, A. H., & Edgell, D. (1988). Neuropsychology of the developing brain: Implications for neuropsychological assessment. In M. G. Tramontana & S. R. Hooper (Eds.), *Assessment issues in child neuropsychology* (pp. 41–66). New York: Plenum.

Rivera, J. B., Jaffe, K., Fay, G. C., Polissor, N. L., Martin, K. M., Shurtleff, H. A., & Liao, S. (1993). Family functioning and injury severity as predictors of child functioning one year following traumatic brain injury. *Archives of Physical Medicine & Rehabilitation, 74*, 1047–1055.

Roberts, R. J., & Pennington, B. F. (1996). An interactive framework for examining prefrontal cognitive processes. *Developmental Neuropsychology, 12*, 105–126.

Rosselli, M., Ardila, A., & Rosas, P. (1990). Neuropsychological assessment in illiterates: II: Language and praxic abilities. *Brain & Cognition, 12*, 281–296.

Rubin, K. H. (1998). Social and emotional development from a cultural perspective. *Developmental Psychology, 34*, 611–615.

Russell, E. W. (1986). The psychometric foundation of clinical neuropsychology. In D. Weiner (Series ed.), S. B. Filskov, & T. Boll (Vol. eds.), *Handbook of clinical neuropsychology, 2*, (pp. 45–80). New York: Wiley.

Russell, E. W. (1987). A reference scale method of constructing neuropsychological test batteries. *Journal of Clinical and Experimental Neuropsychology, 9*, 376–392.

Saarni, C. (1998). Issues of cultural meaningfulness in emotional development. *Developmental Psychology, 34*, 647–652.

Salamy, A., Mendelson, T., Tooley, W. H., & Chaplin, E. R. (1980). Differential development of brain stem potential in healthy and high-risk infants. *Science, 210*, 553–555.

Sattler, J. M. (1992). *Assessment of children* (Revised and updated 3rd ed.). San Diego, CA: Sattler.

Sattler, J. M. (1998). *Clinical and forensic interviewing of children and families*. San Diego: Sattler.

Sbordone, R. J., & Long, C. J. (Eds.) (1996). *Ecological validity of neuropsychological testing*. Delray Beach, FL: St. Lucie.

Schneider, B. (1998). Cross-cultural comparison as doorkeeper in research on the social and emotional adjustment in children and adolescents. *Developmental Psychology, 34*, 793–797.

Scribner, S., & Cole, M. (1981). *The psychology of literacy*. Cambridge, MA: Harvard University Press.

Segall, M. H. (1986). Culture and behavior: Psychology in global perspective. *Annual Review of Psychology, 37* 523–564.

Shaffer, D. (1995). Behavioral sequelæ of serious head injury in children and adolescents: The British studies. In S. H. Broman & M. E. Michel (Eds.), *Traumatic head injury in children* (pp. 55–69). New York: Oxford University Press.

Sheslow, D., & Adams, W. (1990). *Wide range assessment of memory and learning*. Wilmington, DE: Jastak Assessment Systems.

Simonian, S. J., Tarnowski, K. J., Stancin, T., Friman, P. C., & Atkins, M. S. (1991). Disadvantaged children & families in pediatric primary care settings: III. Screening for behavioral disturbance. *Journal of Clinical Child Psychology, 20*, 360–371.

Spreen, O., & Strauss, E. (1991). *A compendium of neuropsychological tests*. New York: Oxford University Press.

Stevenson-Hinde, J. (1998). Parenting in different cultures: Time to focus. *Developmental Psychology, 34*, 698–700.

Stuss, D. T., & Benson, D. F. (1986). *The frontal lobes*. New York: Raven.

Sue, S. (1977). Community mental health services to minority groups: Some optimism, some pessimism. *American Psychologist, 32*, 616–624.

Sue, S. (1992). Ethnicity and mental health: Research and policy issues. *Journal of Social Issues, 48*, 187–205.

Sue, S. (1998). In search of cultural competence in psychotherapy and counseling. *American Psychologist, 53*, 440–448.

Sue, S., Fujino, D., Hu, L., Takeuchi, D., & Zane, N. (1991). Community mental health services for ethnic minority groups: A test of cultural responsiveness hypothesis. *Journal of Clinical and Consulting Psychology, 59*, 533–540.

Suinn, R. M. (1992). Reflections on minority developments: An Asian-American perspective. *Professional Psychology: Research & Practice, 23*, 14–17.

Suomi, S. (1997). Long-term effects of different early rearing experiences on social, emotional, and physiological development in non-human primates. In M. Keshavan & R. M. Murray (Eds.), *Neurodevelopment and adult psychopathology*, (pp. 104–116). Cambridge, MA: Harvard University Press.

Suzuki, L. A., Vraniak, D. A., & Kugler, J. F. (1996). Intellectual assessment across cultures. In L. A. Suzuki, P. J. Meller, & J. G. Ponterotto (Eds.), *Handbook of multicultural assessment* (pp. 141–178). San Francisco: Jossey-Bass.

Suzuki, L. A., Meller, P. J., & Ponterotto, J. G. (Eds.) (1996). *Handbook of multicultural assessment: Present trends and future directions* (pp. 673–684). San Francisco: Jossey-Bass.

Taussig, F. M., Henderson, V. W., & Mack, W. (1992). Spanish translation and validation of a neuropsychological battery: Performance of Spanish and English-speaking Alzheimer's disease patients and normal comparison subjects. *Clinical Gerontologist, 11*, 95–107.

Taylor, H., Albo, V., Phoebus, C., Sachs, B., & Bierl, P. (1987). Post irradiation treatment outcomes for children with acute lymphocytic leukemia: Clarification of risks. *Journal of Pediatric Psychology, 12*, 395–411.

Taylor, H., Drotar, D., Wade, S., Yates, K., Stancin, T., & Klein, S. (1995). Recovery from traumatic brain injury in children: The importance of the family. In S. H. Broman & M. E. Michel (Eds.), *Traumatic head injury in children* (pp. 188–216). New York: Oxford University Press.

Taylor, H., Hack, M., & Klein, N. K. (1998). Attention deficits in children < 750-gram birth-weight child. *Neuropsychology, 4*(1), 21–34.

Taylor, H., & Schatschneider, C. (1992). Child neuropsychological assessment: A test of basic assumptions. *Clinical Neuropsychology, 6*, 259–275.

Taylor, H., Schatschneider, C., & Rich, D. (1992). Sequelæ of *Hemophilus influenzae* meningitis: Implications for the study of brain disease and development. In M. Tramontana & S. Cooper (Eds.), *Advances in child neuropsychology* (vol. 1, pp. 50–108). New York: Springer-Verlag.

Teele, D. W., Klein, J. O., Chase, C., Menyuk, P., Rosner, B., & The Greater Boston Otitis Media Study Group (1990). Otitis media in infancy and intellectual ability, school achievement, speech and language at age 7-years. *Journal of Infectious Diseases, 162*, 685–694.

Terrell, F., & Terrell, S. L. (1983). The relationship between race of examiner, cultural mistrust, and the intelligence test performance of Black children. *Psychology in the Schools, 20*, 367–369.

Tramontana, M. G., & Hooper, S. R. (1988). Child neuropsychological assessment: Overview of current status. In M. G. Tramontana & S. R. Hooper (Eds.), *Assessment issues in child neuropsychology*, (pp. 3–38). New York: Plenum.

Tsushima, W. T., Boyar, J. I., Shimizu, A. A., & Harada, A. S. M. (1995). Applicability of the Luria–Nebraska Neuropsychological Battery with Asian and Pacific Islander Americans. *Advances in Medical Psychotherapy, 8*, 137–144.

Tupper, D. E., & Cicerone, K. D. (Eds.) (1990). *The neuropsychology of everyday life: Assessment and basic competencies*. Boston: Kluwer Academic.

U.S. Bureau of the Census (1995). *Statistical abstracts of the U.S.* (115th ed.), Washington D.C.: Author.

U.S. Bureau of the Census (1997). *Statistical abstracts of the U.S.* (117th ed.), Washington D.C.: Author.

U.S. Congress (1964). *Economic Opportunity Act of 1964*, PL 89-16. Stat. 108, as amended in scattered sections of 42 USC.

U.S. Congress (1975). *Education for All Handicapped Children Act of 1975*. PL 94-142, Stat. 773, as amended in scattered sections of 42 USC.

U.S. Congress (1986). *Education of the Handicapped Act of 1986*. PL 99-457, Stat. 1145-1177, as amended in scattered sections of 20 USC.

U.S. Department of Commerce and Bureau of the Census (1997). *Statistical abstracts of the United States* (117 ed., p. 15). Washington, D.C.: Economic Statistics Administration.

Valencia, R. R., & Guadarrama, I. (1996). High-stakes testing and its impact on racial and ethnic minority students. In

L. A. Suzuki, P. J. Meller, & J. G. Ponterotto (Eds.), *Handbook of multicultural assessment* (pp. 561–610). San Francisco: Jossey-Bass.

Vasquez, C., & Javier, R. A. (1991). The problem with interpreters: Communicating with Spanish-speaking patients. *Hospital and Community Psychiatry, 42,* 163–165.

Vygotsky, L. S. (1962). *Thought and language.* Cambridge, MA: MIT Press.

Vygotsky, L. S. (1978). *Mind in society: The development of higher psychological processes.* Cambridge, MA: Harvard University Press.

Vygotsky, L. S., & Luria, A. R. (1993). Studies on the history of behavior: Ape, primate, and child. In V. I. Golod & J. E. Knox (Eds.), *Collected works of Vygotsky.* Hillsdale, NJ: Erlbaum.

Wagner, M., Blackorby, J., Cameto, R., Hebbler, K., & Newman, L. (1993, December). *The transition experiences of young people with disabilities.* A summary of findings from the National Longitudinal Transition Study of Special Education Students. Prepared for the Office of Special Education Programs, U.S. Department of Education, Menlo Park, CA: SRI International.

Wagner, M., D'Amico, R., Marder, C., Newman, L., & Blackorby, J. (1992, December). *What happens next? Trends in post school outcomes of youth with disabilities.* Second comprehensive report form the National Longitudinal Transition Study of Special Education Students. Prepared for the Office of Special Education Programs, U.S. Department of Education, Menlo Park, CA: SRI International.

Wagner, M., Newman, L., D'Amico, R., Jay, E., Butler-Nalin, P., Marder, C., & Cox, R. (1991, September). *Youth with disabilities: How are they doing?* The first comprehensive report from the National Longitudinal Transition Study of Special Education Students. Prepared for the Office of Special Education Programs, U.S. Department of Education, Menlo Park, CA: SRI International.

Wang, A. (1991). *Cultural–familial predictors of children's metacognitive and academic performance.* San Francisco: American Psychological Association.

Webb, E. J., Campbell, D. T., Schwartz, R. D., & Sechrest, L. (1972). *Unobtrusive measures: Nonreactive research in the social sciences.* Chicago: Rand McNally.

Wechsler, D. (1974). *Manual for the Wechsler Intelligence Scale for Children-Revised.* San Antonio, TX: The Psychological Corporation.

Wechsler, D. (1991). *Manual for the Wechsler Intelligence Scale for Children-Third Edition.* San Antonio, TX: The Psychological Corporation.

Wedding, D., & Faust, D. (1989). Clinical judgment and decision making in neuropsychology. *Archives of Clinical Neuropsychology, 4,* 233–265.

Willis, W. G. (1988). Neuropsychological diagnosis with children: Actuarial and clinical models. In M. G. Tramontana & S. R. Hooper (Eds.), *Assessment issues in child neuropsychology* (pp. 93–111). New York: Plenum.

Wilson, M., & MacCarthy, B. (1994). GP consultation as a factor in the low rate of mental health service used by Asians. *Psychological Medicine, 24,* 113–119.

Xu, S. (1995). The implications of diversity for scientific standards of practice. In S. C. Hayes, V. M. Follette, R. M. Dawes, & K. E. Grady (Eds.), *Scientific standards for psychological practice: Issues and recommendations* (pp. 265–279). Reno, NV: Content.

Xu, Y., Gong, Y. X., & Matthews, J. R. (1987). The Luria–Nebraska Neuropsychological Battery revised in China. *International Journal of Clinical Neuropsychology, 9*(3), 97–101.

Yansen, E. A., & Shulman, E. L. (1996). Language assessment: Multicultural considerations. In L. A. Suzuki, P. J. Meller, & J. G. Ponterotto (Eds.), *Handbook of multicultural assessment* (pp. 353–396). San Francisco: Jossey-Bass.

Yun, X., Yao-Xion, C., & Matthews, J. R. (1987). The Luria–Nebraska Neuropsychological Battery Revised. In *Chinese International Journal of Clinical Neuropsychology, 9,* 97–101.

III

Multicultural Aspects of Neuropsychological Assessment and Treatment of Special Populations

11

Multicultural Perspectives on the Neuropsychology of Brain Injury Assessment and Rehabilitation

JAY M. UOMOTO AND TONY M. WONG

Each year it is estimated that 500,000 new cases of traumatic brain injury occur in the United States resulting in an estimated incidence rate of approximately 200 per 100,000 in the population when they are accounted for in epidemiological studies of hospitalized patients. Further, it is estimated that more than 200,000 people per year suffer continuous symptoms of functional disability as a result of brain injury (Jennett, Snoek, Bond, & Brooks, 1981; Kalsbeek, McLauren, Harris, & Miller, 1981; Kraus, 1978). In data collected from 46,761 households in the 1991 National Health Interview Survey, Sosin, Sniezek, and Thurman (1996) found an estimated 1.5 million individuals who reportedly sustained mild to moderate brain injury and were not hospitalized. The economic drain on families is tremendous. This was demonstrated by Jacobs (1988) who found that 62% of families of those with brain injury who were surveyed in the Los Angeles area reported anywhere between mild financial drain and a situation where all family resources were used to pay for the costs of care. These statistics in combination highlight the vast numbers of individuals who have acquired a brain injury with resultant disability, and who can therefore benefit from services to improve functional abilities and quality of life.

Ethnic differences appear to exist in mortality rates. DeJong and Sutton (1995) present findings that show African Americans have a higher mortality rate for strokes and unintentional injuries than Caucasians, and that these mortality rates are decreasing. They also comment that there is often a corresponding increased rate of disability in the population as a result. Individuals from culturally diverse backgrounds have also been suggested to be in a high-risk category for traumatic brain injury. For example, in an epidemiological study by Cooper and colleagues (1993) conducted in Bronx, New York, it was found that rates of brain injury were highest among African American males, where a high prevalence of violent causes of brain injury occurred. The Cooper et al. study also estimated the national incidence rate of

JAY M. UOMOTO • Seattle Pacific University, Seattle, Washington 98119.   TONY M. WONG • St. Mary's Hospital/University of Rochester, Rochester, New York 14611.

Handbook of Cross-Cultural Neuropsychology, edited by Fletcher-Janzen, Strickland, and Reynolds. Kluwer Academic/Plenum Publishers, New York, 2000.

brain injury to be 262 and 278 per 100,000 for Hispanics and African Americans, respectively. Cavallo and Saucedo (1995) suggest that there may be differential etiologies of brain injuries among ethnic minority individuals compared to majority group populations.

These epidemiological findings underscore some unique characteristics of brain injury in ethnic minorities. Not only are there high incidence and prevalence rates for brain injuries in the United States, but the causes of brain injuries differ significantly as well. These findings have clear implications for the delivery of culturally appropriate and sensitive rehabilitation services to those from diverse multicultural backgrounds. There is a trend toward an increasing number of medical rehabilitation facilities appearing across the country (Wolk & Blair, 1994). Further, in a health care environment where brain injury rehabilitation programming is held accountable to cost effectiveness within the context of a payor-driven system with shorter lengths of stay, it is a particular challenge to also provide these services in a way that meets the culturally diverse needs of patients with acquired brain injury. The focus of this chapter, therefore, is to (1) provide a framework and practical recommendations for multicultural brain injury assessment, and (2) delineate culturally relevant aspects of care conceptualization that bear upon the rehabilitation process.

Multicultural Perspectives on the Neuropsychological Assessment of Brain Injury

In recent years clinical neuropsychologists have become increasingly aware of and frustrated with the limitations of their standard tests and instruments when used with patients from different ethnic backgrounds or culturally dissimilar environments. The effects of the shortage of cross-culturally valid test instruments, the paucity of cross-cultural investigations into brain–behavior relationships, and the lack of a coherent strategy for solving these limitations have become even more pronounced as our society becomes increasingly more diverse. For example, the U.S. Bureau of the Census (1996) projects that the Hispanic-origin population will increase rapidly from 1995 to 2025, accounting for 44% of the growth in the nation's population (32 million Hispanics out of a total of 72 million added to the population). Similarly, the Asian population is projected to the have the greatest gains in the West with an increase of 7 million people over the same period. The rapidly increasing ethnic-minority population in our country has resulted in the increased likelihood that the clinical neuropsychologist will be asked to do that for which they have little training or knowledge: to perform neuropsychological evaluations on patients of sufficiently different sociocultural background that typical procedures and interpretations would not apply.

Although the challenges of cross-cultural neuropsychological assessment are present for neuropsychologists working in all settings, the situation may be even more acute for those employed in inpatient brain-injury rehabilitation programs. Rehabilitation neuropsychologists are not only interested in determining the current cognitive/behavioral status and sequelae of the patient's brain injury, but are also invested in providing information that is of assistance to the patient's recovery and rehabilitation from a neuropsychological perspective. Answers to questions regarding return to work and school, return to driving, and other issues directly related to the patient's potential quality of life are often sought from neuropsychological consultations in rehabilitation. Unlike neuropsychologists in other settings, where diagnosis may be the primary focus of the evaluation, those in rehabilitation programs are more likely to be involved in ongoing treatment and intervention with the patient in addition to initial diagnostic services. In this section, the impact of cross-cultural factors upon neuropsychological assessment of brain injury will be examined, with particular emphasis on the rehabilitation context.

The Impact of Cultural Differences on Brain Injury Assessment

"Culture" refers to a body of customary beliefs and social norms that are shared by a particular group of people. It is a complex entity that may have ethnic, geographic, generational, linguistic, and social determinants. Culture influences our social norms and expectations. As such, no one is culture free, and everyone has a cultural background. It is this fact that is often ignored or forgotten by neuropsychologists who behave as if the accurate assessment of brain function depends entirely on the well-trained professional and good neuropsychological tests (Ardila, Rosselli, & Puente, 1994). Neuropsychological assessment is both an art and a science. Not only does it involve the accurate use of tests and instruments validated for their ability to indirectly measure brain function (science), but also the ability and skill to facilitate the individual's performance through sensitive, thorough professional interaction so that meaningful data can be obtained (art). Cultural factors may influence any part of the neuropsychological assessment process, and they need to be considered carefully in order that appropriate conclusions are made. In other words, cultural issues may impinge upon the overarching context within which the assessment occurs, the neuropsychological assessment process itself, the validity of the tests, instruments, and procedures used in the assessment, and the results or recommendations of the assessment.

Cross-Cultural Context for Neuropsychological Assessment

Before the actual formal neuropsychological assessment occurs, it is important to examine how cultural factors or differences may already be operating to influence the patient's (and the neuropsychologist's) behavior, cognition, and attitude. First, consider the stimulus value of the rehabilitation unit and milieu to the patient of nonmajority culture or ethnicity. For most of the professional rehabilitation staff, who are likely from a cultural and ethnic majority background, the hospital unit is viewed as a benignly clean and safe environment, where dedicated, committed professionals are there for the welfare of the patient and to optimally promote their rehabilitation from what can be a most devastating injury. Patients who are from majority backgrounds, the effects of the brain injury itself notwithstanding, may also view the milieu similarly. However, the culturally dissimilar patient may not feel as comfortable with the environment. A person of lower socioeconomic status, for instance, may feel out of place in what is essentially a white-collar setting, with its somewhat different norms and expectations in terms of language, social behavior, and mores. A patient who is a recent immigrant from Korea and does not speak English may not only be bewildered by her inability to communicate effectively with the staff, but the hospital food may be even more disagreeable than it is to the average patient. For patients from some cultural backgrounds, especially those for whom the family is the dominant social unit, the very fact of being in an institution for any duration of time beyond what is generally perceived as an acute hospital stay may provoke intense feelings of fear, anxiety, and concerns regarding abandonment. These examples illustrate instances in which behaviors are situationally provoked secondary to cultural issues, and staff may innocently, but erroneously attribute those behaviors to internal or brain-injury related factors.

A second manner in which the cross-cultural context needs to be considered relates to expectations regarding assessment and treatment. The neuropsychological assessment process may be somewhat mysterious and intimidating to a patient from a culturally dissimilar background. Shepherd and Leathem (1999) administered a service satisfaction questionnaire to Maori and non-Maori traumatic brain injury (TBI) patients in New Zealand who were referred for a neuropsychological evaluation. The results indicated that the Maori clients were less satisfied overall than the non-Maori respondents. The authors suggested that preparing the clients for the assessment experience, providing a rationale for the tests, and adequate feedback would be especially helpful to the Maori clients in minimizing some of their anxiety and discomfort with the evaluation experience. The cost of not considering the possible impact of cultural factors on expectations is clear: The patient may not be optimally motivated or cooperative during the evaluation. This can lead to either an underestimation of the patient's true cognitive capacities or an attribution of reduced effort to internal, dispositional factors on the patient's part. A related problem or issue, especially in instances where there is a cultural–linguistic difference, is that due to difficulties in accurately translating the term "neuropsychologist" in some cases, the stimulus value of the examiner to the patient is underestimated. That is, the patient's understanding may be that the examiner is a "psychologist," and that psychopathology or mental illness is the focus of the evaluation. Of course, this may lead the patient to experience unnecessary anxiety or defensiveness, or result in a reluctance to participate in rehabilitation.

Another factor to consider is that of potentially skewed historical and behavioral information provided by rehabilitation staff who may not be cross-culturally sensitive or who may have problems with ethnic or other forms of social prejudice. While in most cases the multi- or interdisciplinary nature of most rehabilitation units provides a rich resource of background information and observations for the neuropsychologist, the influence of cross-cultural factors here cannot be ignored. For example, it is both unsettling and unfortunate, in the experience of these authors, to have experienced multiple occasions in which an African American male patient from a lower socioeconomic status background was described to them as having a drug abuse history by other staff, only to find later that this was unverified. Similarly, patients from certain ethnic or cultural backgrounds who may be exhibiting common behavioral/cognitive sequelae of certain types of brain injuries, such as restlessness, agitation, or disinhibition following frontal lobe damage, may be suspected of having premorbid personality problems.

Cross-Cultural Interaction and Neuropsychological Assessment

There is no question that cross-cultural dynamics can negatively affect a valid neuropsychological assessment, despite the otherwise impeccable skills and training of the clinical neuropsychologist. Within the more general clinical assessment literature, there is ample research and discussion on the impact of a cultural or ethnic mismatch between professional and client on assessment results. Westermeyer (1987) provides examples of misdiagnosis and overestimation or underestimation of psychopathology that are based on cross-cultural misunderstanding. Consistent with this, Russell, Fujino, Sue, Cheung, and Snowden (1996), investigating the effects of therapist–client ethnic match upon assessment of mental health functioning, obtained results suggesting that ethnically matched therapists tended to assign less severe ratings of psychopathology in comparison to non-matched therapist–client dyads. Sue and Sue (1987) describe the complexities of assessment when there is not only a cultural mismatch, but when the patient cannot speak the language and interpretive distortions occur due to mistranslation. These and similar studies suggest that, unless cross-cultural factors are taken into account, the neuropsychologist who is culturally mismatched with the patient may unwittingly have a difficult time diagnosing and understanding the patient.

That problems may occur simply because of a cultural mismatch between the professional and the client is not surprising given the history of social-psychological research on intergroup behavior. Pettigrew (1979) coined the notion of an ultimate attribution error to describe the tendency to grant the benefit of the doubt to members of one's own group and not to members of another group. Thus, while socially undesirable behaviors of one's own group are attributed to external, situational factors, those same behaviors of members of other groups are explained by internal dispositional factors. Thus, as Meyers (1990) noted, the shove that is perceived by Caucasians as mere "horsing around" when done by a fellow Caucasian becomes a "violent gesture" when done by an African American. Similarly, in the brain injury rehabilitation setting, the prominent physician with a stroke who does not want to get up in time to attend his therapy is described as being "overly fatigued from his unfortunate injury," and is left to get more rest. By comparison the Cuban American homeless man who sustained a TBI and wants to sleep in is characterized as "lazy and unmotivated," and is compelled to comply with his scheduled therapies.

To overcome the difficulties that may be inherent in a cultural mismatch, it is especially important for the neuropsychologist to take the time to establish rapport with patients and to understand their cultural identity, heritage, and perspectives. This is especially helpful in a rehabilitation setting, where the patient may already feel alienated or misunderstood. Understanding cultural nuances and culture-specific preferences may go a long way in increasing the patient's comfort and compliance with the neuropsychological assessment. Likewise, spending the extra time in describing the nature and goals of the assessment would be profitable in engendering respect and cooperation.

Cross-Cultural Validity of Neuropsychological Assessment

That most neuropsychological tests and procedures available to the clinician currently were developed and normed for use with English-speaking, European American examinees and are essentially inappropriate for use with patients from other cultural backgrounds has been well established (Ardila, Rosselli, & Puente, 1994; Ardila, 1995). An even more difficult situation arises when the patient does not speak English and the neuropsychologist is not fluent in the patient's native language (Artiola i Fortuny & Mullaney, 1998). This problem may be even more vexing for the neuropsychologist who is employed in a rehabilitation setting, and may have a more difficult time referring the patient elsewhere relative to colleagues who are in private practice or who work in outpatient settings. Moreover, the language issue notwithstanding, the neuropsychologist in the rehabilitation setting is often asked to assist in making decisions regarding discharge placement, competency, vocational reentry, educational reentry, driving, and other issues that directly affect the patient's quality of life.

Given that the cross-cultural validity of neuropsychological assessment has essentially not been established, and given the challenge of the other cross-cultural issues mentioned that impinge upon the assessment process, how does one obtain a meaningful assessment of the culturally dissimilar patient within this context? Some practical suggestions are offered in the next section.

Practical Suggestions for Neuropsychological Assessment of Brain Injury in Rehabilitation Settings

In Chapter 1 of this volume, Wong et al. (2000) offered some general guidelines to help neuropsychologists who are confronted with a request to conduct a neuropsychological evaluation with a culturally dissimilar patient. In this section, similar guidelines will be offered with revisions and comments aimed toward the rehabilitation context. Readers are encouraged to read the Wong et al. chapter first, where there is more extensive discussion of the guidelines, and then follow through with the current section to "round out" the discussion.

1. *Recognize and train for cross-cultural diversity and sensitivity.* In addition to being personally trained in this area, it would be beneficial to encourage such awareness and training for staff in other disciplines also, so that the unit can be a "culture-friendly" environment.

2. *Be aware of cultural nuances, consider sociocultural influences on the patient's behavior, and try your best to naturally offer a culturally sensitive environment.* As with the first principle, the neuropsychologist can also take the lead in educating fellow staff regarding cultural nuances and influences on behavior. In case conferences and discussions, a practice could be made of considering sociocultural influences and explanations of the patients' behavior, preferences, or both.

3. *A thorough clinical interview is of paramount importance.* As in the general case, this will communicate respect and sensitivity to the patient, and will provide information that may be culture-specific of which the professional is not aware. Thorough collateral interviews with family members and others could also be very helpful in determining what may be normative behavior within a certain culture.

4. *If the primary language of the patient is unfamiliar to the neuropsychologist, an earnest attempt should be made to ameliorate this situation.* Although the recommendation in the more general case is to refer to another neuropsychologist who is competent in the patient's primary language, as mentioned earlier, this may not be possible in the inpatient rehabilitation setting. An alternative would be to obtain consultation or supervision from a neuropsychologist who is familiar with the patient's language and culture.

5. *Even when language is not an issue, other cultural issues may be a hindrance to a competent evaluation.* Even though this may be especially inconvenient or personally threatening for a neuropsychologist in an institutional setting, it is nevertheless our obligation to deal with personal problems that may affect our work with patients, and this would include cultural or ethnic bias. Thus, assigning the patient at issue to another neuropsychologist, if available, would be a reasonable short-term solution. If the problem is more pervasive (general ethnic/racial prejudice, for example), it is consistent with the ethical standards of the American Psychological Association (1992) to seek professional help.

6. *If at all possible, the use of translators or interpreters should be avoided.* Again, in the inpatient rehabilitation setting, this may not be an alternative, as it may not be feasible to refer out to a neuropsychologist who speaks the same language. The careful and judicious selection and preparation of interpreters/translators should then occur.

7. *Avoid the use of translated tests or instruments unless they are validated in the translated form.* The caveats here are the same as in the general situation. Tests may not always be easily and smoothly translated. More importantly, reliability and construct validity cannot be assumed for the group for which the test is translated.

8. *A set of tests chosen judiciously with cross-cultural considerations in mind should be used.* Although this principle should certainly be followed if tests are to be used, in the rehabilitation setting the neuropsychologist has the opportunity to observe the patient's cognitive/behavioral repertoire in a functional setting and context. Thus, a good argument could be made that, especially for culturally dissimilar patients for whom standardized tests have questionable validity, the neuropsychologist might be better off merely observing the patient's functional behavior and cognition, and keeping the conclusions and recommenda-

tions at that level. That way, the dangerous temptation to make precise statements regarding underlying capacity based on procedures of questionable validity for that group would be avoided.

9. *Cross-cultural issues should be elucidated clearly in the evaluation report.* As in the general case, honesty is the best policy. Readers of the report should be keenly aware of the limitations of neuropsychological assessment with patients from different cultures so that the information contained in the report would not be misused.

Multicultural Care Conceptualization in Neurorehabilitation

In conceptualizing the process of care in the rehabilitation of those with brain injury, integrating multicultural perspectives involves considering such variables as ethnicity, age, socioeconomic status, gender, and religiosity. Each alone, and in combination with each other, defines a range of diversity for patients in the brain-injury rehabilitation setting. It is the interaction of these cultural variables with the fact of acquired disability that challenges rehabilitation professionals to provide efficacious and culturally sensitive services.

System Delivery Considerations

There are several lessons to be learned from the literature on the delivery of mental health services to multicultural populations that can be applied to the rehabilitation setting. Dating back to the 1950s, concern has been raised regarding the inequity of service delivery to minorities as exemplified by the landmark midtown Manhattan study of Hollingshead and Redlich (1958) which found that African American hospitalized mental health patients were more likely than Caucasian patients to be treated "custodially" rather than being offered psychotherapy. This and other studies (e.g., Acosta, Yamamoto, & Evans, 1982; Evans, Acosta, Yamamoto, & Skilbeck, 1984; Sue, 1977, 1983) set in motion a movement for services to respond to the unique mental health needs in diverse cultural populations. The same can be applied in the rehabilitation setting, where those nonmajority group patients may not benefit as well as their majority group peers if services are not responsive to the specific cultural variations that are presented by such individuals.

Schofield (1964) suggested in a somewhat tongue-in-cheek manner that there existed inequities in the delivery of psychotherapeutic services to those clients from ethnic minority groups. He described the enterprise of psychotherapy as serving YAVIS clients: young, attractive, verbal, intelligent, and successful. By contrast, it is thought that those who do not possess these characteristics may be underserved or poorly served. This situation may represent the current status concerning the need for brain-injury programs to better serve non-YAVIS patients. Few models, if any, exist with regard to the tailoring of rehabilitation services to address the needs of patients from diverse cultural backgrounds. This may be due, in part, to the fact that if a model should exist, it probably would not generalize across cultures. Cross-cultural models of neuropsychological rehabilitation have emphasized elements of such programs that seem very similar to those found in the United States. For example, neuro-rehabilitation programming in Denmark (Christensen & Danielsen, 1987), Finland (Laaksonen, 1987), and European French-language countries (Seron, 1987) draw from Luria's (Christensen, 1979) investigational method of assessment and rehabilitation. Generalization of this rehabilitation methodology capitalizes upon concepts that are common in human neurophysiology and neuropsychology. Universal elements of human functioning are *necessary* to consider in organizing rehabilitation goals and therapies, yet *may not be sufficient* to benefit the patient or optimize treatment outcomes in the multicultural patient. It is posited here that in developing neurorehabilitation services, the spectrum of diverse cultural differences that specific patients and their families bring to the rehabilitation setting must be addressed.

Clinical Outcomes and Multicultural Implications

There is a spectrum of services which a patient follows from the moment of acquired brain injury to the time of community reentry. A continuum of health care (Uomoto & McLean, 1989) exists for many with brain injury, particularly if the patient resides in urban areas of the United States. The care continuum includes neurosurgical intensive care units (ICU), early recovery and coma care programs, acute and postacute rehabilitation programs, transitional care units, residential transition programs, neurobehavioral programs, day treatment, outpatient rehabilitation clinics and programs, and educational/vocational/community reentry programs and services. Cope and Sundance (1995) present a model that distinguishes five outcome levels throughout the continuum of care that ranges from medical instability to productive activity. Table 1 presents the essential elements of their outcome model and describes the proposed level of multicultural sensitivity and programming necessary at each level. Family and significant members of the patient's social network are also included in this model since, from a cultural sensitivity perspective, this can be an essential element that determines patient outcomes. As can be seen in the table, in the early phases of recovery and treatment (e.g., ICU and acute rehabilitation), less specific emphasis upon culturally tailored interventions may be necessary to achieve good clinical outcomes. This is due to the main task of medical rehabilitation, which at this phase of recovery is focused on neurophysiological stabilization and enhancement of basic functional skills. As the patient becomes more engaged in the process of rehabilitation and efforts are translated from healthcare providers applying treatment to the patient's efforts at self-management and independence, there comes a need for being more sensitive to cultural variations in worldviews and cultural practices. Here, rehabilitation goals need to be tailored to the particular cultural context to which the patient will likely return postrehabilitation. Once a patient begins the process of community reintegration, consideration of the patient's cultural practices is paramount and, in fact, may comprise a majority of therapy activities *in vivo*. For example, in some Asian and Pacific Islander cultures, there may be a high value attached to academic achievement or career advancement as evidence of achievement. Acquired brain injury may impose limits on the extent to which such academic or vocational goals may be attained. This potentially raises a conflict within the Asian/Pacific patient with brain injury that goes beyond the disappointment of not being on the same trajectory of career path after brain injury. It may also involve aspects of shame (e.g., Kim, 1997) for that individual within the context of family kinship systems. Thus, sensitivity to cultural values and beliefs is critical to the way community reintegration services are delivered. Finding a way for such a patient to accept an alternative career path and "save face" within the family system would be an appropriate rehabilitation goal at the community-reintegration phase of rehabilitation.

Sensitivity to cultural values in the delivery of rehabilitation services begins early postinjury with regard to working with family members and those in the social network. Education of family members is commonly conducted from the time of injury forward. It should be assumed that family members of different cultures will comprehend such information from their own worldview perspective. Conceptions of illness and recovery may have cultural overtones (e.g., Culhane-Pera & Vawter, 1998). What may appear as a neurobehav-

TABLE 1. Rehabilitation Outcome Levels and Multicultural Considerations

Outcome level	Outcome description	Level of multicultural specificity for patient services	Level of multicultural specificity for family and support network services
Physiological instability	Medical and physiological conditions have not been completely assessed, diagnosed, and managed. Describes patients at the onset of an illness or injury.	Patient's neurophysiological needs are addressed. *Low* emphasis on culturally specific services.	Family and social network interventions require *high* sensitivity to cultural practices and worldview conceptualization of illness and injury.
Physiological stability	All major medical and physiological problems are stabilized and managed.	Depending on condition of patient, cultural practices and worldviews can be introduced into the health care provision setting. *Low* to *moderate* culturally specific elements to treatment may be needed.	Family and social network are enlisted in support of the patient. *High* cultural specificity of approach to enlist support may be needed.
Physiological maintenance	Basic rehabilitation outcomes are achieved. Preservation of immediate and long-term health needs is addressed. Functional goals are limited to basic activities of daily living, most often achieved in the acute rehabilitation phase in the care continuum.	*Moderate* elements of culturally tailored elements of rehabilitation may need to be addressed, though emphasis remains on achievement of basic daily needs that may be more universal across cultures.	*High* sensitivity to cultural practices and perceptions of recovery and prognosis may need to be addressed in interactions with family and members of the social network.
Primary functional goals—home and/or residential integration	Achievement of contextually relevant and acceptable level of functioning is sought in the anticipated long-term residence of the patient.	*High* degree of culturally sensitive treatment and goals are needed for the patient to achieve relevant long-term goals.	*High* cultural specificity needed to continue family and social network support to be of optimal assistance to the patient.
Advanced functional goals—community reintegration	Focus on advance community reintegration goals. Achievement of self-management competencies and independent community functioning is targeted.	*High* level of culturally tailored elements of rehabilitation may be needed to reintegrate the patient to his or her community of choice. May need to take into account the mores of the culture to which the patient returns.	*High* sensitivity to cultural practices and mores of family and social network resources. The rehabilitation team may need significant direction from the family/social network of the patient to develop appropriate goals for the patient.
Productive activity	Achievement of vocational, avocational, or educational pursuits are targeted.	*High* level of culturally specific interventions may be necessary to achieve this level of outcome. Conflicts may arise between cultural expectations and the degree to which the patient may be able to achieve a particular goal.	*High* cultural specificity may be needed to align expectations of rehabilitation and family views. This may be balanced by the limitations imposed by recovery from brain injury.

ioral outcome of acquired brain injury (e.g., agitation during Ranchos Los Amigos Level IV), may be interpreted as volitional behavior, where folk beliefs explain its appearance and amelioration. Substituted judgment and surrogate decisionmaking cannot be assumed to follow Western values and beliefs. This may be particularly relevant in severe brain injury where ethical decisions about maintaining life support and end-of-life decisions are being made (Bedolla, 1994; Gallagher, 1998; Hepburn & Reed, 1995; Hern, Koenig, Moore, & Marshall, 1998; Jecker, Carrese, & Pearlman, 1995; Orr, Marshall, & Osborn, 1995).

Several methods exist to evaluate the outcome of rehabilitation services, both on an individual basis and from a programmatic point of view. These evaluations provide feedback to the individual brain-injury facility for purposes of continuous quality improvement, accreditation, and program evaluation. Ratings scales such as the Disability Rating Scale, Glasgow Outcome Scale, Functional Independence Measure, and the Functional Assessment Measure are traditional means of evaluating the patient's functional ability after acute and postacute rehabilitation. Such measures are global in nature and are potentially biased against those of different cultures in evaluating the benefits of rehabilitation. Changes in mobility, safety, and transfers, for example, are less open to misinterpretation in gauging a patient's progress. Changes in neurobehavioral status, speech, language, communication, and adjustment to disability variables, however, may need to be reinterpreted in terms of appropriate cultural morays and expectations. Newer measures, such as the Brain Injury Community Rehabilitation Outcome Scale (Powell, Beckers, & Greenwood, 1998) that assesses community integration variables, or the Craig Handicap Assessment and Reporting Technique (Boake & High, 1996), show promise in terms of being more specifically functional in orientation and multidimensional in nature. Such measures, therefore, allow for a range of dimensions that can be assessed rather than relying upon singular omnibus indices for determining improvement and outcome.

Determinants of outcomes after rehabilitation have been found to be affected by the degree to which a working alliance exists between the patient, family members, and professional staff (Klonoff, Lamb, Henderson, & Shepherd, 1998). This underscores the need for staff to be acutely aware of salient cultural variables that may play a part in developing such alliances. Here, some of the scientific literature on the development of trust and distrust in the multicultural psychotherapeutic context is relevant. Sue and Zane (1987) state that therapist behaviors during therapy can affect a therapist's credibility and attractiveness. If both credibility and attractiveness are enhanced in the treating relationship, this leads to the elicitation of trust, incentive for engagement in treatment, and investment in change, as well as in increased self-disclosure. Although the goals of therapy are different in the rehabilitation setting, it is likely that the same provisos hold true. Therapists in brain-injury rehabilitation settings can enhance effectiveness by the nonverbal and verbal behavior they exhibit during treatment sessions. Respect for the interpersonal style of the multicultural client, though it may be altered by brain injury, does not obviate the fact of long-term preferences for particular kinds of social interactions, assuming that long-term memory abilities remain somewhat intact. The particular kinds of interpersonal styles that are characteristic for a given patient vary widely. Resources such as McGoldrick, Giordano, and Pearce (1996), and Sue and Sue (1999) are good starting points for understanding some of the unique social and psychological preferences of specific ethnic groups. Group-oriented comprehensive postacute rehabilitation practices (Malec, Smigielski, DePompolo, & Thompson, 1993), reduced latency-to-rehabilitation after brain injury (Ashley, Persel, Clark, & Krych, 1997), and combined neuropsychological data with standard variables of brain injury severity (Karzmark, 1992) have all been implicated as predictors of outcome after rehabilitation. Each of these variables can interact with the individual cultural practices of the patient. Many Asian Americans, for example, may be uncomfortable in group-oriented rehabilitation settings particularly if other group members are not Asian American. This may result in a barrier to obtaining maximum benefit from a postacute rehabilitation stay. Referral patterns and time delays in seeking treatment may be more characteristic of Asian and Hispanic American populations, again reducing the benefit of rehabilitation services. Neuropsychological data can be of assistance in developing appropriate rehabilitation targets, and as mentioned earlier in this chapter, such evaluations need to take into account language and culture in the interpretation of findings.

Emic and Etic Distinctions in Care Conceptualization

An appreciation of cultural differences in the patient with brain injury requires that the rehabilitation professional understand distinctions between those aspects of functioning that are enhanced or changed due to brain injury, those aspects that are unique to the patient's culture, and those that are common across many different cultures. The *emic* perspective refers to those dimensions of human functioning that are specific to a culture, whereas *etic* dimensions are those aspects of human functioning that are more universal across cultures. The emic–etic distinction is important in organizing effective rehabilitation services for the multicultural patient with brain injury. Western modes of therapy, assuming an etic position, may be inappropriate for members of certain ethnic minority groups. A similar error can be made by assuming an emic position that runs the risk of stereotyping a particular patient's behavior as arising strictly out of cultural norms. For example, in a study on alexithymia on students in Toronto, Canada, native Chinese language speakers scored consistently higher than native English and native European language speakers on the Toronto Alexithymia Scale (Dion, 1996). This suggests that there may exist ethnolinguistic differences between these ethnic groups: Chinese students are less apt to be psychologically minded regarding their emotions, thus possibly demonstrating that alexithymia, in Chinese or Chinese American populations, may be an emic construct. A possible implication of these findings for brain injury rehabilitation may be that some who may be more apt to present with a clinical picture of alexithymia after brain injury would be those whose native cultures have few verbal expressions for concepts of emotions. It may therefore be inappropriate to judge a patient's lack of emotional engagement in the process of adjustment to disability as abnormal if that patient's culture tended not to have such words for the expression of dysphoria and grief. Rather, it would be wise to evaluate the extent to which symptoms of alexithymia may appear or decrease as the patient becomes accustomed to changes that have occurred as a result of brain injury.

Conversely, self-efficacy as a cognitive process has been debated as to whether or not it is an emic or etic construct. Earley and Randel (1995), after reviewing cross-cultural empirical studies on self-efficacy, argue that the concept is more universal across cultures and has significance as an etic construct. In the context of rehabilitation, therefore, capitalizing upon and building into a brain-injury rehabilitation program concepts of self-efficacy are likely to be relevant across individuals from many different cultural backgrounds. How the construct of self-efficacy is concretely applied will likely need to integrate emic dimensions.

Conceptualizations of Illness and Disability

Acquired brain injury and its sequelae are often foreign concepts to the patient and his or her family. Due to its sudden onset, all involved have little time to consider its impact or implications. Many may impose their own worldviews and organizing systems so as to make sense of the changes that have occurred. What may appear to the ethnic patient or family as a culture-bound syndrome, may in fact be sequelae of brain injury. For example, *susto*, or "soul loss" is a folk illness found among some Latinos residing in the United States where symptoms of decreased appetite, restlessness, fatigue, weakness, withdrawal, and somatic complaints are presented (Sue & Sue, 1999). The folk explanation is that *susto* is caused by fright or a traumatic experience with healing occurring through rituals that encourage the soul to return to the body, often with the assistance of folk healers. These symptoms have a remarkable resemblance to the postconcussion syndrome with consequent elements of post-traumatic stress disorder. The Hispanic folk illness of *mal ojo* has similarities to acute brain injury with symptoms of headaches, crying, irritability, restlessness, vomiting, diarrhea, and fever. *Mal ojo* is brought about by having been looked upon by a person with the "evil eye." *Nervios* among Latinos is a condition characterized by headaches, "brain aches," sleep difficulties, nervousness, easy tearfulness, dizziness, and sensations of tingling (Sue & Sue, 1999). These syndromes also bear resemblance to common sequelae after brain injury.

Ethnocultural differences have been found in the perception of pain. For example, Lee and Essoka (1998) compared the experience of pain between Korean American and European American obstetric patients, from the perspective of gate-control theory. They found differences in the reported quality of pain between the two groups: Korean Americans reported fewer affective descriptors of pain than European Americans. There were no significant differences between the groups on the intensity of pain. This study illustrates both emic (the experience of pain lacking affective labels in Korean Americans) and etic (neurophysiological perception of pain intensity) dimensions. Acute and chronic pain experiences are prevalent among those with brain injury, and cultural differences in the pain experience are likely to be expected among different ethnic groups.

Psychological and Neurobehavioral Differences

Emic and etic distinctions are also critical to understand with regard to the assessment and treatment of concomitant neurobehavioral conditions in the patient with brain injury. Much has been written on personality, mood, and behavioral changes that occur after brain injury (e.g., Prigatano, 1987). However, personality and alterations in personality after brain injury occur within a cultural context. That is to say, it is not so much an etic dimension, but rather personality constructs have strong emic influence: The cultural context will determine, in part, the nature of personality and delimit its boundaries as far as what is normal and abnormal (Alarcon & Foulks, 1995a,b). Different expressions of depression have also been demonstrated in the literature. In a study comparing moderately depressed African American outpatients to a matched sample of Caucasian outpatients, Wohl, Lesser, and Smith (1997) found that Caucasian patients endorsed significantly more articulated and observed mood and anxiety symptoms than African Americans. By comparison, African American patients showed more diurnal variation in their depression. There were no differences between the groups on other vegetative symptoms. The suggestion of emic and etic dimensions to depression is presented in this study. In the rehabilitation setting, cultural sensitivity to the evaluation of mood is necessary to fairly evaluate the efficacy of interventions for depression in the multicultural patient.

Immigration Status and Issues

In evaluating the clinical presentation of the patient during brain injury rehabilitation activities it may be important to understand the emigration history of the patient. The following case illustrates this point:

Dimitri is a 35-year-old Russian male who was working in a large city as a maintenance worker in a high-rise office building when he took a 12-foot-fall off a ladder, striking his head on concrete pavement, resulting in a moderate level of traumatic brain injury. His initial Glasgow Coma Scale score was a 9 and an initial head computed tomography scan found small bifrontal contusions. He spent two days in the neurosurgical intensive care unit, then transferred to an acute acquired brain injury unit where he spent one week, and was then discharged to a postacute day treatment program. Dimitri is monolingual in Russian, although he can understand some English. He came to the United States on a visa to work, and he wished to emigrate eventually. Dimitri presented to the day treatment rehabilitation staff as quite guarded in his self-disclosures through his interpreter. He wished only to work on physical rehabilitation activities and did not see the need for developing compensatory memory strategies, though given his difficulty in pathfinding and need for numerous repetitions in his physical therapy exercise program it was apparent he had significant cognitive impairments. The patient complained of marked headaches throughout his stay in the program, and on some days he would not show for treatment due to headaches. When asked how he was doing emotionally, he stated that "everything was fine and he was coping extremely well" and was "enjoying life." This raised the question among team members about the patient presenting with anosognosia, particularly in light of the neuroimaging findings. Dimitri refused to meet with the neuropsychologist on the team but would not give any reason why he did not wish to do so. After repeated invitations to meet with the neuropsychologist, Dimitri agreed to a "short meeting" to "satisfy the needs of the team." Dimitri did allow the neuropsychologist to assist the occupational therapist in working on biofeedback strategies for coordinated gait training and for reduction of tension levels in the frontalis muscle group because it was there that headaches were frequently located. The patient had gained the trust of the interpreter who was of Russian descent but born in America. Shortly before discharge from the day treatment program he revealed that the main reason he did not wish to meet with the neuropsychologist was his fear of being reported to the KGB, and he told the case manager of the team that psychologists in Russia had been used as an arm of the KGB. Upon hearing this disclosure, some of the rehabilitation team members wondered about whether or not Dimitri was presenting also with paranoid ideation. Up to this time, the team had only known that Dimitri held a job at a printing business in Moscow immediately before coming to the United States. However, the interpreter disclosed to the team after discharge, with Dimitri's permission, that he actually had been a writer in Russia. He had written in underground publications and newspapers criticizing the government, and that he was working on a book at the time of his temporary move to the United States.

This case illustrates several cultural issues that affected the process and outcome of rehabilitative therapies. Dimitri's entrance to the health care system in America was likely confusing. In fact, due to posttraumatic amnesia, his first memory after the injury was being on the acute acquired brain injury rehabilitation unit. He presented with significant headaches that are common after brain injury, however, the team had learned later that his headaches correlated well with requests from the team for the neuropsychologist to be involved in his care. Stress and tension were likely significant contributors to the magnitude of his headache difficulties. Further, having been raised in the culture of Russia, it would have been a sign of weakness to have admitted that he was "stressed" which would have connoted a sense of personal weakness. Dimitri may have had anosognosia though his presentation of himself as doing well may have also been a face-saving strategy as may have been his refusal to work on compensatory cognitive strategies. The ban on emigration was lifted in Russian in 1991 and Dimitri was one of thousands who wished to move to the United States to seek a better life. Althausen (1996) notes that members of the intelligentsia, professionals, and the more highly educated were among the first wave to emigrate after the ban was lifted. Dimitri was well-educated and apparently an accomplished writer. Due to his monolingual status, however, he could not find a more professional job and settled upon a manual labor position. This is common for immigrants who were professionals in their own country, but are only able to find jobs below their capability in the United States. His refusal to work with the neuropsychologist could have easily been taken as a manifestation of paranoia, a function of a limited self-awareness of his deficits, or both. However, his view of protecting himself by not meeting the neuropsychologist for fear of being reported to the KGB may have been a realistic fear based upon his personal experiences in Russia, and therefore a good coping strategy. Many components of brain-injury rehabilitation were delivered as they would have been to other patients. The importance of having a knowledgable and trained interpreter included as a member of the rehabilitation team was critical in Dimitri's situation to enable the team to continue to work with him effectively. Many of the emic dimensions of the case allowed for an expansion of the care conceptualization to better understand Dimitri's dilemmas from a cultural perspective and therefore deliver more culturally relevant services.

Conclusion

Challenges are raised when delivering brain-injury rehabilitation services to diverse cultural populations. Culturally relevant assessment techniques and strategies set the stage for the development of appropriate treatment goals and to accurately track recovery of functions across time and as a result of interventions. With training, clinicians can be more aware of those cultural differences that make a difference in outcomes of rehabilitation. Awareness of salient cultural differences in worldviews, values, beliefs, and practices in the multicultural patient rests largely upon making the relevant distinctions between emic and etic dimensions of the patient's presentation, and integrating these perspectives with knowledge about the specific sequelae of brain injury that the patient presents. The task of delivering effective services to multicultural patients will likely require the enlistment and assistance of family members, significant members of the patient's social network, interpreters who are trained with a knowledge base in brain injury, as well as indigenous healers and other complimentary therapies that respect the worldview of the patient. Taken together, these strategies will enhance functional recovery and quality of life for those who have suffered an acquired brain injury.

References

Acosta, F. X., Yamamoto, J., & Evans, L. A. (1982). *Effective psychotherapy for low-income and minority patients.* New York: Plenum.

Alarcon, R. D., & Foulks, E. F. (1995a). Personality disorders and culture: Contemporary clinical views (Part A). *Cultural Diversity and Mental Health, 1,* 3–17.

Alarcon, R. D., & Foulks, E. F. (1995b). Personality disorders and culture: Contemporary clinical views (Part B). *Cultural Diversity and Mental Health, 1,* 79–91.

Althausen, L. (1996). Russian families. In M. McGoldrick, J. Giordano, & J. K. Pearce (Eds.), *Ethnicity and family therapy* (2nd ed.; pp. 680–687). New York: Guilford.

American Psychological Association (1992). Ethical principles of psychologists and code of conduct. *American Psychologist, 47,* 1597–1611.

Ardila, A. (1995). Directions of research in cross-cultural neuropsychology. *Journal of Clinical and Experimental Neuropsychology, 17,* 143–150.

Ardila, A., Rosselli, M., & Puente, A. (1994). *Neuropsychological evaluation of the Spanish speaker*. New York: Plenum.

Artiola i Fortuny, L., & Mullaney, H. (1998) Assessing patients whose language you do not know: Can the absurd be ethical? *The Clinical Neuropsychologist, 12*, 113–126.

Ashley, M. J., Persel, C. S., Clark, M. C., & Krych, D. K. (1997). Long-term follow-up of post-acute traumatic brain injury rehabilitation: A statistical analysis to test for stability and predictability of outcome. *Brain Injury, 11*, 677–690.

Bedolla, M. (1994). Patient Self-Determination Act: A Hispanic perspective. *Cambridge Quarterly of Healthcare Ethics, 3*, 413–417.

Boake, C., & High, W. M. (1996). Functional outcome from traumatic brain injury: Unidimensional or multidimensional? *American Journal of Physical Medicine and Rehabilitation, 75*, 105–113.

Cavallo, M. M., & Saucedo, C. (1995). Traumatic brain injury in families from culturally diverse populations. *Journal of Head Trauma Rehabilitation, 10*, 66–77.

Christensen, A.-L. (1979). A practical application of the Luria methodology. *Journal of Clinical Neuropsychology, 1*, 241–247.

Christensen, A.-L., & Danielsen, U. T. (1987). Neuropsychological rehabilitation in Denmark. In M. Meier, A. Benton, & L. Diller (Eds.), *Neuropsychological rehabilitation* (pp. 381–386). New York: Guilford.

Cooper, K. D., Tabaddor, K., Hauser, W. A., Shulman, K., Feiner, C., & Factor, P. R. (1993). The epidemiology of head injury in the Bronx. *Neuroepidemiology, 2*, 70–78.

Cope, D. N., & Sundance, P. (1995). Conceptualizing clinical outcomes. In P. K. Landrum, N. D. Schmidt, & A. McLean (Eds.), *Outcome-oriented rehabilitation: Principles, strategies, and tools for effective program management* (pp. 43–56). Gaithersburg, MD: Aspen.

Culhane-Pera, K. A., & Vawter, D. E. (1998). A study of healthcare professionals' perspectives about a cross-cultural ethical conflict involving a Hmong patient and her family. *Journal of Clinical Ethics, 9*, 179–190.

DeJong, G., & Sutton, J. P. (1995). Rehab 2000: The evolution of medical rehabilitation in American health care. In P. K. Landrum, N. D. Schmidt, & A. McLean (Eds.), *Outcome-oriented rehabilitation: Principles, strategies, and tools for effective program management* (pp. 3–42). Gaithersburg, MD: Aspen.

Dion, K. L. (1996). Ethnolinguistic correlates of alexithymia: Toward a cultural perspective. *Journal of Psychosomatic Research, 41*, 531–539.

Earley, P. C., & Randel, A. (1995). Cognitive causal mechanisms in human agency: Etic and emic considerations. *Journal of Behaviour Therapy and Experimental Psychiatry, 26*, 221–227.

Evans, L. A., Acosta, F. X., Yamamoto, J., & Skilbeck, W. M. (1984). Orienting psychotherapists to better serve low income and minority patients. *Journal of Clinical Psychology, 40*, 90–96.

Gallagher, S. M. (1998). Cultural influences on medical disclosure. *Ostomy Wound Management, 44*, 16–18.

Hepburn, K., & Reed, R. (1995). Ethical and clinical issues with Native-American elders. End-of-life decision making. *Clinical Geriatric Medicine, 11*, 97–111.

Hern, H. E., Koenig, B. A., Moore, L. J., & Marshall, P. A. (1998). The difference that culture can make in end-of-life decision making. *Cambridge Quarterly of Healthcare Ethics, 7*, 27–40.

Hollingshead, A. B., & Redlich, F. C. (1958). *Social class and mental illness*. New York: Wiley.

Jacobs, H. E. (1988). The Los Angeles Head Injury Survey: Procedures and initial findings. *Archives of Physical Medicine and Rehabilitation, 69*, 425–431.

Jecker, N. S., Carrese, J. A., & Pearlman, R. A. (1995). Caring for patients in cross-cultural settings. *Hastings Center Report, 25*, 6–14.

Jennett, B., Snoek, J., Bond, M., & Brooks, N. (1981). Disability after severe head injury: Observations on use of the Glasgow Outcome Scale. *Journal of Neurology, Neurosurgery, and Psychiatry, 4*, 285–293.

Kalsbeek, W., McLauren, R., Harris, B., & Miller, J. (1981). The national head and spinal cord injury survey: Major findings. *Journal of Neurosurgery, 53*, S19–S31.

Karzmark, P. (1992). Prediction of long-term cognitive outcome of brain injury with neuropsychological, severity of injury, and demographic data. *Brain Injury, 6*, 213–217.

Kim, S. C. (1997). Korean American families. In E. Lee (Ed.), *Working with Asian Americans: A guide for clinicians* (pp. 125–135). New York: Guilford.

Klonoff, P. S., Lamb, D. G., Henderson, S. W., & Shepherd, J. (1998). Outcome assessment after milieu-oriented rehabilitation: New considerations. *Archives of Physical Medicine and Rehabilitation, 79*, 684–690.

Kraus, J. (1978). Epidemiological features of head and spinal cord injury. *Advances in Neurology, 19*, 261–279.

Laaksonen, R. (1987). Neuropsychological rehabilitation in Finland. In M. Meier, A. Benton, & L. Diller (Eds.), *Neuropsychological rehabilitation* (pp. 387–395). New York: Guilford.

Lee, M. C., & Essoka, G. (1998). Patient's perceptions of pain: Comparison between Korean-American and Euro-American obstetric patients. *Journal of Cultural Diversity, 5*, 29–37.

Malec, J. F., Smigielski, J. S., DePompolo, R. W., & Thompson, J. M. (1993). Outcome evaluation and prediction in a comprehensive-integrated post-acute outpatient brain injury rehabilitation programme. *Brain Injury, 7*, 15–29.

McGoldrick, M., Giordano, J., & Pearce, J. K. (Eds.) (1996). *Ethnicity and family therapy* (2nd ed.). New York: Guilford.

Meyers, D. G. (1990). *Social psychology* (3rd ed.). New York: McGraw-Hill.

Orr, R. D., Marshall, P. A., & Osborn, J. (1995). Cross-cultural considerations in clinical ethics consultations. *Archives of Family Medicine, 4*, 159–164.

Pettigrew, T.F. (1979). The ultimate attribution error: Extending Allport's cognitive analysis of prejudice. *Personality and Social Psychology Bulletin, 5*, 461–476.

Powell, J. H., Beckers, K., & Greenwood, R. J. (1998). Measuring progress and outcome in community rehabilitation after brain injury with a new assessment instrument: The BICRO-39 scales. *Archives of Physical Medicine and Rehabilitation, 79*, 1213–1225.

Prigatano, G. (1987). Personality and psychosocial consequences after brain injury. In M. Meier, A. Benton, & L. Diller (Eds.), *Neuropsychological rehabilitation* (pp. 355–378). New York: Guilford.

Russell, G. L., Fujino, D. C., Sue, S., Cheung, M., & Snowden, L. R. (1996). The effects of therapist–client ethnic match in the assessment of mental health functioning. *Journal of Cross-Cultural Psychology, 27*, 598–615.

Schofield, W. (1964). *Psychotherapy: The purchase of friendship*. Englewood Cliffs, NJ: Prentice-Hall.

Seron, X. (1987). Neuropsychological rehabilitation in European French-language countries. In M. Meier, A. Benton, & L. Diller (Eds.), *Neuropsychological rehabilitation* (pp. 396–405). New York: Guilford.

Shepherd, I. & Leathem, J. (1999). Factors affecting performance in cross-cultural neuropsychology: From a New Zealand bicultural perspective. *Journal of the International Neuropsychological Society, 5*, 83–84.

Sosin, D. M., Sniezek, J. E., & Thurman, D. J. (1996). Incidence of mild and moderate brain injury in the United States, 1991. *Brain Injury, 10*, 47–54.

Sue, D., & Sue, S. (1987). Cultural factors in the clinical assessment of Asian Americans. *Journal of Consulting and Clinical Psychology, 55*, 479–487.

Sue, D. W., & Sue, D. (1999). *Counseling the culturally different: Theory and practice* (3rd ed.). New York: Wiley.

Sue, S. (1977). Community mental health services to minority groups: Some optimism, some pessimism. *American Psychologist, 32*, 616–624.

Sue, S. (1983). Ethnic minority issues in psychology: A reexamination. *American Psychologist, 38*, 583–592.

Sue, S., & Zane, N. (1987). The role of culture and cultural techniques in psychotherapy: A reformulation. *American Psychologist, 42*, 37–45.

Uomoto, J. M., & McLean, A. (1989). The care continuum in traumatic brain injury rehabilitation. *Rehabilitation Psychology, 34*, 71–79.

U.S. Bureau of the Census. (1996). *Population projections for states by age, sex, race, & Hispanic origin*. Washington, D.C.: Author.

Westermeyer, J. (1987). Cultural factors in clinical assessment. *Journal of Consulting and Clinical Psychology, 55*, 471–478.

Wohl, M., Lesser, I., & Smith, M. (1997). Clinical presentations of depression in African American and white outpatients. *Cultural Diversity and Mental Health, 3*, 279–284.

Wolk, S., & Blair, T. (1994). *Trends in medical rehabilitation*. Reston, VA: American Rehabilitation Association.

12

Multicultural Perspectives on the Neuropsychological Assessment and Treatment of Epilepsy

ELAINE FLETCHER-JANZEN

Introduction

Rajendra Kale (1997) states that, "The history of epilepsy can be summarized as 4000 years of ignorance, superstition, and stigma followed by 100 years of knowledge, superstition, and stigma" (p. 1). Epilepsy was first recorded in Babylonian times, as far back as 2000 BC. The recordings of that time describe many of the different seizure types that we see today and treatments that were essentially spiritual in manner (WHO, 1997a). In the 5th century Hippocrates believed that epilepsy was not a "sacred disease" but rather a disorder of the brain. The word "epilepsia" is of Greek origin and means to "seize" or "take hold of." The stigma and superstition associated with this condition was pervasive. It was not until the 19th century, when the field of neurology appeared, that the concept of epilepsy being a disorder of the brain became widespread and the idea of it being a medical condition started to counter the magical thinking to date (WHO, 1997b). However, Rajendra Kale is correct: After 100 years of medical knowledge and learning about epilepsy, most of the world continues to shroud the disorder in mystical and spiritual terms. This means that many who suffer from the disorder do not receive help, those that do receive help are many times discriminated against, and epilepsy stays "in the shadows" (WHO, 1997c).

Dodrill and Matthews (1992) suggest that the role of neuropsychology in the diagnosis, assessment, and treatment of epilepsy is evident from the nature of the disorder. During epileptic attacks, and in between the attacks, brain dysfunction occurs. Adequate brain functioning for the demands of everyday living is critical and therefore the neuropsychological study of individuals with epilepsy is of great importance. On the other hand, Robert Novelly (1992) suggests that neuropsychology owes a debt to the epilepsies because a significant body of neuropsychological concepts originated or were confirmed through epilepsy-based treatment and research. These concepts include:

ELAINE FLETCHER-JANZEN • University of Northern Colorado, Colorado Springs, Colorado 80921.
Handbook of Cross-Cultural Neuropsychology, edited by Fletcher-Janzen, Strickland, and Reynolds. Kluwer Academic/Plenum Publishers, New York, 2000.

The peri-Rolandic homunculus, the role of the hippocampal–temporal lobe complex in cognitive memory, hemisphere plasticity for speech in childhood, the intracarotid amytal procedure for determining hemisphere memory patency, and hemisphere-based models of cognition confirmed through human commissurotomy. (p. 1)

As the evolution of neuropsychology continues, the population of study has changed in the United States. The epidemiology of epilepsy has shifted as immigration and socioeconomic patterns have shifted. The practice of neuropsychology now incorporates the demands of a more diverse population than ever before. As diversity increases in America, so does the need for clinicians who are culturally competent.

This chapter primarily focuses on the multicultural aspects of neuropsychological diagnosis, assessment, and treatment of individuals with epilepsy in the United States. It is, however, beneficial to understand the domestic management of epilepsy in context: Compared to most of the world, which is underdeveloped, the average person with epilepsy in the United States receives excellent medical care. We must keep this in mind when we are evaluating domestic services because a global perspective is critical to our understanding of epilepsy in a contextual and culturally competent way.

Epidemiology

Global Context of Epilepsy

Forty million people in the world have epilepsy at any one time and the lifetime prevalence of this disorder is approximately 100 million people worldwide (WHO, 1997b). It is medically possible for up to 70% of people with epilepsy to have their disorder brought under reasonable control. However, because of many cultural and financial conditions, three-quarters (approximately 30 million people) of the population with epilepsy do not receive any treatment at all (WHO, 1997c). In 1995 the World Health Organization tabulated epidemiologic data on epilepsy and found that the highest incidence was found in the western Pacific region followed by southeast Asia; the highest age group was in the 20–64 years group; that males and females were equally distributed; and that developing countries have triple the cases that developed countries have (WHO, 1995).

Epilepsy is seldom a hereditary condition (Epilepsy Ontario, 1999). In terms of etiology, in developing countries, no cause can be found in over 50% of cases. Known causes are attributed to infections such as bacterial meningitis, focal lesions, fungal infections, parasitic infections, protozoa, and helminthes (cysticercosis, paragonimiasis, schistosomiasis, and echinococcosis) (Bharucha & Shorvon, 1997). In addition, a Mexican study found that neurocysticercosis accounted for 50% of cases of late-onset epilepsy (Medina, Rosa, Rubio-Donnadieu, & Sotelo, 1990). Tuberculomas are a common cause in India (Bharuch & Shorvon, 1997). Of course, seizures associated with mental retardation and related conditions are also common in developing and developed countries (McLin, 1992).

Superstition about epilepsy is rampant in nearly every country in the world, and there is little evidence that prejudice is disappearing (Baumann, Wilson, & Wiese, 1995). The World Health Organization reports the following facts about developing and developed countries:

- In Cameroon it is still believed that people with epilepsy are inhabited by the devil. This does not mean that they are seen as evil—just that the devil invades them and causes them to convulse from time to time.
- In Liberia as in many others parts of Africa, the cause of epilepsy is related to witchcraft or evil spirits.
- Most traditional healers in Swaziland mention sorcery as the cause of epilepsy.

- In contrast to surrounding countries, the people of Senegal have particular beliefs about spirit possession and seem to hold people with epilepsy in esteem.
- In Indonesia, epilepsy is often considered either as karma or as a punishment from unknown dark forces.
- There are rural areas of India where attempts are made to exorcise evil spirits from people with epilepsy by tying them to trees, beating them, cutting a portion of hair from the scalp, squeezing lemon and other juices on the head, and starving them.
- In Nepal, epilepsy is associated with weakness, possession by an evil spirit, or the reflection of a red color. Bystanders who witness a seizure will often spray water on the forehead of the victim or make him or her smell a leather shoe.
- Epilepsy is often thought to be contagious, and this prevents other people from helping, or even touching the person having a seizure—even if this person is in a dangerous place and is threatened by fire or water. In Uganda, as well as many other African countries, people with epilepsy are not allowed to join the communal foodpot for the fear that epilepsy is spread through saliva.
- A survey carried out in Germany in 1996 revealed that 20% of respondents believed that epilepsy was a form of mental disease and 21% objected to their child marrying someone with epilepsy.
- In the Netherlands, as recently as 1996, there was an example of a person being whipped and put into isolation because of seizures.
- Epilepsy is still commonly viewed as a reason for prohibiting or annulling marriages in India and China.
- Epilepsy often diminishes the prospect of marriage, especially for women. In China, a survey of public awareness in 1992 revealed that 72% of parents objected to their children marrying someone with epilepsy.
- Epilepsy and violent behavior have long been associated in peoples' beliefs. It has now been largely accepted that crimes of violence are unlikely to be committed in association with seizures (WHO, 1997d, pp. 2–3).

Lack of education and prevention for populations in underdeveloped or developing countries keeps the incidence of epilepsy constant. It is estimated that most of the individuals in these countries could be treated with phenytoin at a cost of $5.00 per year and yet the majority go untreated (WHO, 1997d). However, economics are not the only reason why these individuals do not receive treatment. The mystical perception of the disorder creates underreporting and cultural obstructions to treatment and maintenance.

The World Health Organization has joined with the International League Against Epilepsy and the International Bureau Against Epilepsy to launch a global campaign to help individuals with this disorder called "Out of the Shadows—A Global Campaign Against Epilepsy." The campaign has two main goals: 1) the raising of general awareness and understanding of epilepsy, and 2) the rendering of assistance to departments of health in identifying epilepsy, and promoting education, training, services, research, and prevention (WHO, 1997c).

Epilepsy in the United States

Approximately 2.3 million Americans have some form of epilepsy, with an estimated annual cost of $12.5 billion in direct and indirect costs (Epilepsy Foundation of America [EFA], 1999a). Between 125,000 and 181,000 new cases of seizures and epilepsy are diagnosed each year (EFA, 1999b). With reported prevalence rates of 4–9 cases per 1,000 children, childhood epilepsy is a major public health concern (Murphy, Trevathan, & Yeargin-Allsopp,

1995). Of course, prevalence rates data depend on how the information is collected, and how the researcher defines the disorder (Hauser, 1997; Murphy et al., 1995). Centers for Disease Control and Prevention (CDC) surveys of epilepsy rely on household self-report surveys that are admittedly unreliable (CDC, 1995). However, CDC trends over a period of years indicate that the number of people with epilepsy tabulated by age, race, and geographic region indicate significantly higher rates for African Americans in nearly every age group, and for people living in the South (CDC, 1994, 1995). Indeed, until recently, epidemiologic studies have concentrated on white and black American vital statistics (Hauser, 1997; Shamansky & Glaser, 1979) and have left out other ethnic minorities who compose an ever-increasing proportion of the U.S. population (Flack et al., 1995). Many support the view that "ethnicity should be viewed as a measure of lifestyle and social influences such as diet, economic status, psychosocial stressors, societal acceptance, and interactions and risk taking behaviors" (Flack et al., p. 1). Studies are now looking into areas of health care that are culture bound and not researched to date, such as: "health care utilization; health care seeking behaviors; health care provider behavior; research on doctor–patient relationships; adherence to medical regimes; self-care practices; and the underutilization of health care services by different ethnic groups" (Penn Kar, Kramer, Skinner, & Zambrana, 1995, p. 1). A further confounding factor in the collection of data about epilepsy is that very few studies either worldwide or in the United States define epilepsy in the same way. Therefore, some studies define epilepsy as a condition characterized by two or more unprovoked seizures and others may include febrile seizures (Hauser, 1997).

Reports that epilepsy rates are essentially somewhat higher for males than females, and occur at specific age periods in life in the United States is supported across the research literature (Hauser, 1997; Hauser & Hesdorffer, 1990). In terms of race/ethnicity and socioeconomic status, however, there is great variability in prevalence rates (Hauser, 1997). The general theme for ethnicity and epilepsy is that individuals who are Black American, Hispanic American, and Native American are at much higher risk for developing epilepsy than Anglo-Americans. This risk is mainly due to socioeconomic factors and not so much as biologic/ genetic differences (Shamansky & Glaser, 1979).

Demographics are new areas of study in epilepsy. A study conducted by Serge in 1996 at Cook County Hospital in Chicago of 300 adult seizure patients found the following clinical profiles of that epileptic population: The average age was 39.5 years, the gender ratio was slightly higher for males, and African Americans and Hispanics represented 85% of the population. The most common etiology for the African Americans was head trauma, and neurocysticercosis was the most common for Hispanics. Substance abuse, language barriers, and noncompliance to treatment were the most common reasons for poor outcome. Serge concluded from this analysis that the epilepsies seen in this inner city population were largely preventable and therefore cultural in a socioeconomic sense. Another study conducted in an urban hospital emergency room (Krumholz, Grufferman, Orr, & Stern, 1989) found similar results and also found that associated psychosocial problems of no medical insurance, indigence, and alcohol abuse contributed to the population picture. This study suggested that although a disproportionate number of individuals with seizure disorders use emergency rooms as a primary care source, the emergency rooms did not have the capabilities for long-term followup and maintenance that people with epilepsy need. In general, poor people are at higher risk for developing seizures from socioenvironmental sources and are at high risk for not getting the medical attention and support that the disorder requires (CDC, 1994; EFA, 1999; Simpson, Bloom, Cohen, & Parsons, 1993). Twenty to thirty percent of people with epilepsy are unable to work or are unemployed (Hauser & Hesdorffer, 1990), and employment status of individuals with epilepsy also is related to ethnicity (Minh-Thu & Rausch, 1996). Hopefully, some of these figures may change with further developments in the Americans with Disabilities Act.

Epidemiological studies that include cultural factors other than ethnicity will provide rich data that will become the basis for sound public health policies. Unfortunately, incidence studies are expensive and difficult to do. Many studies include self-reports: a method that is fraught with the confounding aspects of the stigma and fear surrounding epilepsy (CDC, 1994). Therefore there are relatively few reports dealing with total populations (Hauser, 1997). This means that information from ad hoc research studies and indirect sources must be used to create an objective picture of how culturally complex epilepsy is, and how a clinician can use this information to assist the patient's diagnosis, treatment, and maintenance. In addition, in terms of research funding, Pedley's (1995) statements are particularly relevant:

> Current research dollars which have grown minimally in the aggregate are now being spread increasingly thin to find high quality applications that include not only traditional clinical and laboratory research, but epidemiological, psychosocial, quality of life issues, and ethics studies as well. These "new" areas of research and, ultimately, of education are vitally important for a chronic, mulitdimensional illness such as epilepsy. (p. S18)

Diagnosis

The diagnosis of epilepsy has never been easy. The increasing diversity of the patient population further complicates diagnosis and treatment notwithstanding technological advances in brain wave monitoring, brain imaging such as positron emission tomography (PET) and magnetoencephalography (National Institute of Neurological Disorders and Stroke, 1999), brain function, and blood drug levels measurement (EFA, 1999a). These technological advances have redefined focal epilepsy because neuroimaging may show the presence of a lesion not suspected on clinical or EEG grounds, detects mesial temporal sclerosis accurately, detects neuronal migration abnormalities, delineates abnormal areas of cortical dysplasia invisible to magnetic resonance imaging and detects dual pathology (International Epilepsy Commission, 1989). Notwithstanding these technologies, lower socioeconomic groups having limited access to health care or to the expensive procedures mentioned above suggests that individuals in the highest incidence groups may go undiagnosed or with delayed diagnosis and treatment (CDC, 1995). Evidence suggests that the sooner seizure disorders are diagnosed and effective treatment started, the better the chances of a positive longterm outcome, especially in children (EFA, 1999a). Therefore, it may be reasonable to assume that many instances of epilepsy are underdiagnosed in groups that have limited access to healthcare and the delay in diagnosis may have far reaching neuropsychological and psychosocial effects for those individuals.

A further complication of diagnosis in epilepsy is the fact that diagnosis is essentially ongoing and closely tied to patient treatment compliance and self-report of quality of life. The latter is, by definition, culture bound and proper assessment is dependent on the cultural competence of the practitioner. Indeed, a study conducted by (Carrazana et al., 1999) suggests that the doctor–patient relationship has a significant impact on the patient's perception of accuracy of diagnosis and treatment compliance.

For the most part, diagnosis of epilepsy is based on the clinical history of the patient. The clinical history of the patient is many times based on self- and family report. These reports are dependent on patient perceptions of events and their cultural approach to medical complaints. The information given in the clinical history can dramatically affect diagnosis. Therefore, a study finding that about one-fifth of patients referred to specialist units with "intractable epilepsy" were found, on further assessment, not to have epilepsy is not surprising (Lesser, 1996).

Ethnic variances in response to antiepileptic medications can effect ongoing diagnosis (Lin, Anderson, & Poland, 1995; Stein & Strickland, 1998; Strickland, Ranganath, Lin, & Poland, 1991). Studies suggesting differences such as phenytoin metabolism between Japanese and white epileptic patients (Watanabe, Iwahashi, Kugoh, & Suwaki, 1998) and differences in leukocyte presence in black American and white American children (Dhanak, 1996; Tohen, 1996) are seen more and more in the research literature.

Many alternative diagnoses to epilepsy are culture bound and difficult to assess. These alternative diagnoses are usually syncope, cerebrovascular disorders, migraine, sleep and movement disorders, endocrine dysfunction, delirium, hyperventilation, dizziness, vertigo, hysteria (Fisher, 1994), and postconcussion convulsions that are incorrectly assigned to seizure disorders (Sander & O'Donoghue, 1997). In addition, malingering, episodic dyscontrol, pseudoseizures, and psychogenic seizures may also be present (Fisher, 1994). The distinguishing of seizures and pseudoseizures is very difficult in some cases and psychogenic seizures have been found to be much more prevalent in individuals who have experienced childhood sexual abuse (Alper, Devinsky, Perrine, Vazquez, & Luciano, 1993) or psychiatric disorders (Jones, Duncan, Mirsky, Post, & Thodore, 1993; Tucker, 1998). Cross-cultural manifestations of the psychogenic components of seizures are vividly portrayed in the "ataque de nervios" syndrome, a culturally condoned expression of distress most frequently seen in Hispanic women (Oquendo, 1995) and in certain religious experiences such as voodoo possession (Carrazana et al., 1999). Carrazana et al. (1999) suggest that:

> When treating patients, the physician must take into account the patient's cultural background and system of beliefs, an important point particularly in areas with a high percentage of new immigrants. Regardless of faith, epileptic seizures should be considered in the differential diagnosis of atypical and episodic religious experiences. (p. 241)

The diagnosis and ongoing evaluation and treatment of seizures, then, are based on the clinical history of the patient, treatment compliance, and the self-report of the patient's quality of life. All of these aspects are culture bound and cultural awareness on the part of the practitioner can assist in differential diagnosis and long-term evaluation and treatment.

Neuropsychological Assessment

Cognitive Impairment

The research literature suggests that seizure disorders are associated with cognitive impairment (Bennett & Maile, 1997; Strauss, Hunter, & Wada, 1995). Studies have paid much attention to variables such as age of onset, duration of disorder, etiology, location, and laterality of function (Strauss et al., 1995). Dodrill (1992) and Strauss and colleagues (1995) found that later age of onset is correlated with better cognitive abilities. In addition, the number of seizures as opposed to the duration of the disorder is also related to impairment in mental abilities; at least for those who have tonic-clonic seizures. In terms of seizure type, Dodrill (1992) found that generalized tonic-clonic seizures were associated with diminished mental abilities in comparison with those with partial seizures. However, there is much variability within subjects, especially in light of more recent evidence that interictal or subclinical activity is often present and affects neuropsychological functioning (Dodrill & Matthews, 1992).

Strauss, Hunter, and Wada (1995) have concluded that in patients with medically refractory seizures:

> the location of dysfunction, age of seizure onset, and handedness are the single best predictors of overall cognitive status (FSIQ, VIQ, and PIQ). The unique contribution of speech dominance, gender, etiology, seizure duration, and laterality of seizure to general intellectual status appear negligible. (p. 8)

It is unfortunate that Strauss et al. do not mention or examine the role of ethnicity, socioeconomic status, or level of acculturation in their examination of cognitive abilities and seizures in particular. This etic perspective is, according to Boivin and colleagues (1996) one of the difficult barriers to adequate neuropsychological assessment.

Many researchers are arguing that abilities measured by the Wechsler scales, for instance, are only part of the universal picture of intelligent behavior (Chen & Gardner, 1997) and are highly dependent on achievement, and are not necessarily sensitive to cognitive impairment with brain injury or seizures (Bennett & Maile, 1997). Boivin et al. (1996) refer to Vygotskian concepts of analyzing the day-to-day social functions and activities in which thinking occurs as more appropriate approaches to cognitive assessment. Dodrill's (1978) modification and extension of the Halstead–Reitan Battery for assessment of seizure disorders significantly improved assessment of individuals with epilepsy. The cultural competence of neuropsychological batteries is addressed elsewhere in this volume and will not be reiterated here. It is important to note that the need for neuropsychological assessment in the diagnosis and treatment of seizure disorders is not in question: The universality of results of these measures, however, should be examined. For example, a study performed by Hempel, Risse, Frost, and Ritter (1994) examined the utility of neuropsychological testing for identifying lateralization of the epileptogenic region in children. The study concludes that the impairment on measures of verbal reasoning may be useful in identifying pediatric patients with left-hemisphere seizure onset. On the surface, it may seem reasonable to assume that several measures of reading and language accurately identify verbal ability. However, without a marked effort to correlate cultural aspects of verbal ability with test performance, groups of subjects could be identified as having left-hemisphere seizure onset, when in reality, the verbal deficits are reflective of educational experience and/or linguistic issues. In this particular study, it is impossible to extrapolate cultural considerations because cultural factors were not studied or reported; a circumstance common in the research literature. Boivin et al. (1996) summarize the central issue of current neuropsychological assessment as: "what is essentially at issue for developmental neuropsychology is the extent to which universal features of brain–behavior development and cognitive ability can be assessed in a similar manner in a variety of cultural contexts. Is the cultural context of daily social interactions and adaptations paramount to interpreting cognitive ability or development at any level?" (p. 2).

Quality of Life

Recently, the focus of quality of life for seizure patients has been studied in much more depth than ever before. Hermann, Whitman, and Anton (1992) have proposed a multietiological model of psychological and social dysfunction in epilepsy because of their awareness of their own limitations in understanding the causes of psychosocial problems in epilepsy (p. 40). Hermann et al. introduce their model by way of an example of a fictitious patient and the "multiplicity of forces" that are impinging on that patient:

> For instance, consider an individual, perhaps a 22-year-old man with a high school education, who presents with the following: a history of a significant neurological insult (e.g., perinatal

stroke), extremely overprotective parents, associated neuropsychological deficits, poor academic achievement, less than optimal medical management characterized by polytherapy and
the use of barbiturate anticonvulsant medications, poor seizure control, and (as a child) a
history of considerable teasing and abuse by his peers because of his seizure disorder. (p. 39)

Herman and colleagues ask the following questions about this patient: "What are the important etiological variables, and where should intervention be aimed if the patient is profoundly
depressed? If he is unemployed, what are the likely causes of his joblessness, and how should
rehabilitation and intervention proceed?" (p. 39). They then go on to list the multietiological
risk factors for psychosocial problems in individuals with epilepsy.

It is important to notice that at no time do the authors initiate speculation about the
contribution of the above subject's ethnicity, level of acculturation, socioeconomic status, or
gender. If we change this scenario and add that the subject is a single-mother, nonwhite ethnicity, indigent, who has limited English-speaking ability, can we speculate that the psychosocial
adjustment or treatment outcome for this patient would be worse or better? Obviously the
answer is: We do not know if we do not study those variables.

Herman, Whitman, and Anton's establishment of a multietiological model of psychosocial variables and risk factors in epilepsy is seminal. However, it needs to be updated and
expanded to real life reflections of diverse individuals. In America today, the reality of life for
some individuals with epilepsy is that they do not have equal access to health care, treatment,
jobs, income, support, education, and other variables that affect adjustment.

Carl Dodrill was one of the first to establish a movement toward the objective analysis of
quality of life with his development of the Washington Psychosocial Seizure Inventory.
(Dodrill, Batzel, Queisser, & Temkin, 1980). This instrument was developed specifically to
evaluate psychosocial concerns in adults with epilepsy. A list of psychosocial concerns were
complied as: family background, emotional adjustment, interpersonal problems, vocational
adjustment, financial status, adjustment to seizures, medicine and medical management, and
overall psychosocial functioning (Dodrill & Batzel, 1994). Many of these areas pertaining to
(nonseizure) adjustment and nonwhite populations are examined in a multicultural perspective
by Derald Wing Sue and David Sue in their pioneering work: *Counseling the Culturally
Different* (1981, 1990). They and others began to illuminate the experiences of ethnic minorities in the mental and medical health systems. By examining data on the underutilization of
health care centers and cultural responses to illness and mental disorders, a specific and
powerful statement was made about how many persons of minority status were not receiving
the health care and followup needed to successfully ameliorate their health problems. The
progression for Sue and Sue's work to be understood, accepted, and adopted in the mental
health field started in the mid-1980s and continues today. Trostle, Hauser, and Sharbrough
(1989) completed a study on the psychological and social adjustment to epilepsy in Rochester,
Minnesota, using the Washington Psychosocial Seizure Inventory. The study is unique in that
the researchers delineated the ethnicity of their subjects and generalized results only to that
group. Unfortunately, and for various reasons known and unknown, multicultural perspectives
on psychosocial issues with seizures since the Trostle et al. study has gone unmarked. Apart
from attempts to translate the Washington Psychosocial Seizure Inventory into other languages, the cultural aspects of psychosocial adjustment in epilepsy is still research territory yet
to be explored.

Devinksy and colleagues (1995) and others have continued the movement to develop
instruments that assist in the measurement of quality of life for individuals with epilepsy. In
1995, Devinsky et al. described the development of the Quality of Life in Epilepsy Inventory, a
99-item inventory that shows "a four factor solution to quality of life: mental health, physical

health, cognitive, and epilepsy targeted" (p. 1097). The inventory targets aspects of quality of life through open-ended questions about role limitations, social isolation, health perceptions, emotional wellbeing, health discouragement, work, driving, language, attention/concentration, and so on. Unfortunately, in the validity study for this instrument Devinsky and his colleagues do not mention any investigation of the subjects in some important aspects of culture. The subjects were delineated in terms of gender, age, seizure frequency, marital status, and education, however no mention was made of ethnicity, level of acculturation, or socio-economic status. Given the impact of economics on etiology of seizure disorders (access to health care, utilization of health care, treatment compliance, and followup) it is of concern that these influences were not examined in a quality-of-life study. In addition, given the abundant literature on diverse ethnic responses to healthcare personnel, ethnic differences in etiology of seizures, social and economic constraints, and level of acculturation, again, it is difficult to accept the results of the validation study as universal. It is of great concern for clinicians to see instruments purporting to have construct validity for assessing quality of life that completely ignore confounding variables of socioeconomic status and ethnicity in the ever-increasing diverse population in the United States. Many Native Americans, African Americans, Asian Americans, and Hispanic Americans tend to hold different concepts of what constitutes mental health, mental illness, and adjustment than do Anglo/European Americans (Sue & Sue 1990). Asking some individuals in these groups the second question on the Quality of Life in Epilepsy Inventory: "Overall, how would you rate your quality of life (10–0)? 10 = Best Possible Quality of Life—0 = Worst Possible Quality of Life (as bad as or worse than being dead)" is a test construction mine-field. Each of the above groups view quality of life in very different ways and the presumption that a bad quality of life is as bad as being dead or near to it tells more about the person asking the question than the person answering the question. Different ethnic groups view death in different ways and some may view being close to death (as a way of life) as a positive concept. For example, a Lakota Sioux prayer ends with the phrase "it is a good day to die." This is a positive statement about life and the individual's relationship with the quality of his or her life. How would this individual give a reliable and valid response to question two on the inventory? Another example is question 81 which asks the patient how satisfied the patient is with the "amount of togetherness" he or she has with family or friends. Many minority groups in the United States come from cultures where collective thinking and functioning is central. In fact, it is only in white American culture that the individual is seen as separate from family and community: Only in this culture would this question make sense. The test item is therefore culturally valid and reliable for Anglo/European Americans, and the wisdom of applying this item in the same manner to Asian, Black, and Hispanic Americans is questionable. In addition, it is important to note that the differences within these groups exist in terms of "individualistic" thinking and that within-group levels of acculturation may change the patient's response.

Devinsky and colleagues went on to further validate the Quality of Life in Epilepsy Inventory in 1998 (Cramer et al., 1997). Thirty-one items from the original inventory were translated into nine languages as an abbreviated questionnaire through a forward–backward–forward system. The authors report reliability and validity support for the questionnaire in a cross-cultural context. It would be more accurate to describe this activity as cross-linguistic rather than cross-cultural.

Research literature distinguishing complex definitions of culture is common and has specific adaptations of issues other than just translation. Hays (1997) suggests that for a test to "travel freely" there must be universal agreement on the value of particular responses to questions, and the same items must mean the same things in different cultures, given an appropriate translation of the instrument. The validation of questionnaires in different countries may be problematic if the countries are as diverse as Nigeria, for example, which has over 75 languages and just as many differences in cultural mores. However, the quest to provide multinational trials for evaluation of psychosocial functioning in individuals with epilepsy has obvious merit. For example, a cross-cultural study of psychosocial functioning in epilepsy subjects in England and Sweden was conducted by Chaplin and Malmgren (1999). The Epilepsy Psycho-Social Effects Scale (EPSES) was given to a sample of 57 matched subjects. Statistically significant differences were found in 4 of 42 statements on the scale. Although the patient responses were largely similar, attitudes to employment, to the future, and to fear of seizures were significantly more a problem for patients in England. Treatment for patients in England, therefore, may focus on different aspects of adjustment than in Sweden.

It is not possible to develop a test that is absolutely culture-free—nor is this desirable. Being aware of cultural differences increases the likelihood of good treatment outcome. However, it is essential that test developers at least make an attempt to create items that accurately reflect everyday experiences of as many populations as possible, and that validation studies reflect cultural competence on the part of the test items, a process that is addressed by identification of unique cultural response patterns by means of item response theory (Ellis & Kimmel, 1992). In this way, for individuals with seizure disorders, it would not be assumed that the quality-of-life inventories measure universal concepts for this medically and culturally diverse population. Multinational studies are emerging and are wrestling with ways to determine cultural differences; we can learn from these studies in the United States.

General Considerations for Special Populations

Patricia Shafer (1998) states in her article, "Counseling Women with Epilepsy," that: "All persons with epilepsy have a right to timely, accurate, culturally sensitive information that will help them manage their seizures and their lives successfully" (p. S38). This statement, and many like it, are becoming more and more familiar in the research literature because successful treatment outcomes are dependent on treatment compliance and patient reports of quality of life. Epilepsy research is beginning to report enough data on specific populations that general considerations can be suggested for working with certain groups of individuals with seizures. The following considerations are general summaries of research focusing on diverse populations.

Gender

Males

The highest incidence of seizure disorders in the United States is found with middle-aged black American males. The research literature is only just beginning to define the etiology of this number. Research studies are indicating that the reason for elevated numbers with this group is because of increased risk of trauma and cerebrovascular disease (CDC, 1994).

In terms of special considerations regarding quality of life for males with epilepsy, unfortunately there is little written in the research literature. Organizations such as EFA (1999c) are beginning to establish initiatives for special populations with epilepsy, such as women, but the impetus for special initiatives is still relatively new and has not yet examined issues specific to men.

Females

More than one million women in the United States are living with seizure disorders (EFA, 1999c). Recent research studies have shed new light on seizure disorders in the various phases of a woman's life from puberty to menopause. Stories of women being told they should never have children because of their epilepsy or medications are common and such advice is unfounded (American Academy of Neurology, 1999; EFA, 1999c). Indeed, most women with epilepsy who become pregnant will have successful pregnancies and healthy babies (American Academy of Neurology, 1999). It is important to keep in mind that women's issues in epilepsy care pertain to more than just pregnancy. Lifelong issues are present and should be taken into consideration (Shafer, 1998).

Menstruation.   The relationship between seizures and menstruation has been examined for many years. Studies have shown that the changes in hormones throughout the monthly cycle can stimulate seizures (catamenial seizures) in some women not only in terms of frequency but in type of seizure as well (American Academy of Neurology, 1999; Epilepsy Ontario, 1996). Amenorrhea and oligomenorrhea and cycles of irregular length may be associated with complex partial seizures. In addition, the mood swings associated with the period prior to and during menstruation may be aggravated by anticonvulsant medications (Epilepsy Ontario, 1996).

Psychologists who are assisting female patients with epilepsy can help the patient and physician monitor seizure frequency to the patient's monthly cycle and help establish or eliminate predictable ictal activity and/or necessary medication adjustments. Patients and clinicians can chart seizures, determine when to complete more detailed evaluations, and assist in the determination of the use of adjunctive medications or hormonal therapy to assist in seizure control (Klein & Herzog, 1997). In addition, when conducting neuropsychological assessments with women, the menstrual history and the presence of cyclical seizure activity should be considered when the actual testing is taking place. The examiner must determine if there are any confounding effects on testing due to the menstrual cycle. Repeated neuropsychological testing may also help establish cyclical aspects of ictal activity, and cognitive and psychosocial functioning.

Pregnancy.   The effects of birth control pills may be impaired when women take certain types of anticonvulsants, and fertility rates, monitored over the past 50 years, have been found to be lower in women and men who have epilepsy.

Approximately 50% of all women with epilepsy have increased seizure frequency during pregnancy and many are naturally worried about the effect on the fetus. Lack of sleep during the last trimester and postnatal months also often stimulates seizure frequency (Epilepsy Ontario, 1996). Neuropsychological assessments of pregnant women and new mothers must monitor sleep deprivation as a part of the presenting and ongoing clinical history. Women with epilepsy are considered to have high-risk pregnancies because of eclampsia, which can result in brain hemorrhage, coma, and death, and placental problems such as vaginal hemorrhage and spontaneous rupture of membranes (Epilepsy Ontario, 1996).

Menopause.   As in other areas of life for the woman with epilepsy, the hormonal changes during menopause can initiate seizures, or upset a stable treatment regime and quality of life (Epilepsy Ontario, 1996). The use of hormone replacement therapy (HRT) is more complex for the menopausal woman with epilepsy (Shafer, 1998) and should be given careful consideration. Often, seizure frequency decreases during menopause, especially if seizures have been linked to menstruation cycles in the past. Sometimes, epilepsy completely disappears in menopausal years. Neuropsychological assessment, again, should be sensitive to where women patients are in the menopausal process, and neuropsychological clinicians should contribute to the ongoing evaluation of this change in life.

Safety Issues for Women.   There are two main areas of safety concern for women with epilepsy. The first concerns the responsibilities of mothering. Women who have an aura before a seizure can prepare themselves and their older children for the seizure. However, those women who experience irregular occurrences and seizures without warning are at considerable disadvantage in terms of making sure that the children's welfare is protected. The quality of life issues for mothers of young children are serious and require a great deal of planning and support on the part of the clinician and family to insure that mechanisms are in place to prevent adverse events. Provisions for patients who have young children should be a regular part of the treatment plan and followup.

The second area of safety concern for women is that of potential sexual assault or abuse during or after a seizure. Shafer (1998) advocates that all women who have epilepsy should be counseled about the potential for assault because anecdotal reports of such abuse are not uncommon, especially for those who have partial seizures who may wander or be confused during or after a seizure. Again, the support of neighbors, friends, family, and clinicians, and sometimes especially trained service dogs, is necessary for successful protection of some women and mothers of young children.

Age

Children

The National Center for Health Statistics reports 422,000 cases of epilepsy in children 18 years old and younger. Of these children, 65.5% have special needs that are defined as "condition caused problems during past year, such as missing school, staying in bed, or feeling upset most of the time" (EFA, 1996). Many epidemiologic studies report prevalence for active epilepsy of 4–9 cases per 1,000 children. However, there is a great deal of variance in prevalence rates due mainly to studies missing anywhere from 7% to 27% of children with epilepsy (Murphy et al., 1995). Children who come to be noticed in epidemiologic studies many times are those that have severe enough conditions that they come to the attention of school districts or require hospitalization, and those mechanisms for treatment involve having access to health care. Although it is imperative that seizure disorders be diagnosed early, millions of children do not receive needed health care services in the United States. Uninsured children and those in families with low incomes are at the greatest risk of having unmet health needs (Simpson et al., 1994). CDC studies have repeatedly recognized that children of low-income families are at much higher risk for undiagnosed and untreated chronic health conditions (Penn et al., 1995).

For those children who do have access to adequate medical care, the differential diagnosis of epilepsy is still very difficult. Murphy and Dehkharghani (1994) have identified many recurrent events that can mimic or cause seizures, such as: paroxysmal vertigo, breath-holding spells, cardiogenic syncope, shuddering attacks, night terrors, rages, and learning disorders. They suggest also that subtle seizures are difficult to detect in infants and are not necessarily associated with electrical changes on the accompanying EEG. Subtle seizures in infants can consist of: repetitive, stereotyped, unusual, and involuntary movements, such as sustained eye opening or blinking; bicycling movements of either upper or lower extremities; forced eye deviation; and oral buccal movements such as chewing or sucking (p. S7).

In terms of diagnosis for older children and teenagers, Smith (1998) suggests that three aspects of adolescent epilepsy must be taken into account:

> Firstly, some epilepsies, such as juvenile myoclonic epilepsy, present in adolescence and carry specific implications for management. Secondly, some childhood onset epilepsies, such as benign childhood epilepsy with centrotemporal spikes, consistently remit in adolescence. Thirdly, common conditions such a vasovagal syncope, psychogenic non-epileptic attack disorder, and migraine often present first in teenagers and may mimic epilepsy. (p. 1)

Much about the neuropsychological assessment of children has been written elsewhere in this volume; however, some considerations specific to seizure disorders should be noted. The research literature generally supports the idea that children with seizure disorders are at high risk for cognitive and/or adaptive problems because of multifocal or diffuse brain insult (Black & Hynd, 1995; Bourgeois, 1998; Hubert, 1992; Murphy & Dehkharghani, 1994) and long-term sequelae of anticonvulsant medications (Bourgeois, 1998; Williams, Roscoe, Griebal, Lange, & Bates, 1996). In some cases, as exemplified by a Tennessee Medicaid study conducted by Cooper, Federspiel, Griffin, and Hickson (1997), negative outcome may be due to prescriptions for antiepileptic drugs not being filled by the family in the year postdiagnosis—an example of cultural factors confounding treatment compliance. Another study supporting the latter study was conducted by Griebel, Roscoe, Dykman, and Williams (1997) who found similar circumstances where families from certain ethnic groups were not complying with medication regimes. They concluded that, "although the reasons for differences in compliance among ethnic groups in this study are unclear, findings would suggest the importance of addressing sociocultural factors in the treatment of epilepsy" (p. 1). The neuropsychological evaluation of children with seizure disorders is complicated with the cultural factors associated with neuropsychological instruments (documented elsewhere in this book), and the fact that quality-of-life issues are dependent on the appropriate financial and social functioning of the family system (Mitchell, Scheier, & Baker, 1994).

The adjustment issues of incorporating epilepsy into identity formation in the teenage years are difficult. Issues of cognitive and cosmetic side effects of anticonvulsant medications need to be addressed, as well as medication effects with birth control and unplanned pregnancies. Advice on regular sleep is very important in teenagers with generalized epilepsy, and the use of alcohol/substance–medication interactions must be addressed (Smith, 1998). Teenagers with epilepsy must also face career choices that are restricted by their medical condition, and may require specialized vocational counseling. The psychosocial adjustment of teenagers with epilepsy mirrors many of the issues of normal identity formation; however, issues of independence and responsibility can be particularly difficult.

Elderly

The diagnosis and treatment of elderly individuals with epilepsy is written about elsewhere in this volume and is well documented in the research literature (Snyder & McConnell, (1997). However, some general considerations for this population should be noted. Recent evidence suggests that because we are now living longer and pediatric medical care has significantly improved, the incidence of epilepsy in the elderly has surpassed that of children (Everitt & Sander, 1998). It is suggested that cerebrovascular disease is the commonest cause of seizures in this age group, and that it is possible that small vessel cerebrovascular disease in newly diagnosed seizure patients is responsible for onset as opposed to overt cerebrovascular disease (Everitt & Sander, 1998).

Hauser, Morris, Heston, and Anderson (1986) also began studies in the incidence of seizures with Alzheimer's disease and found that the incidence of seizures was 10 times higher than they expected. The question of the use of long-term treatment with antiepileptic drugs has been questioned with this population (Hauser, 1994).

Studies looking at ethnic differences on neuropsychological test performance of elderly subjects are few in number, and with elderly seizure patients are nonexistent. However, Manly and colleagues (1998) conducted a study of nondemented African Americans and whites and found significant ethnic group differences on measures of figure memory, verbal abstraction, category fluency, and visuospatial skills even after matching subjects for years of education. The researchers could not account for the discrepancies in test performance by occupational attainment or history of chronic medical conditions. These results, if duplicated in further research, could confound neuropsychological test interpretation of elderly seizure patients.

Ethnicity

Race is a biologic concept denoting a single breeding population that varies in definable ways from other subpopulations (CDC, 1993), or it could be a "societally constructed taxonomy that reflects the intersection of biological, cultural, socioeconomic, political, and legal determinants, as well as racism" (CDC, 1993). No one has proved to date that race has a biological correlate relevant to seizures (McKenzie, 1996). For the most part, there is no agreed upon operational definition of race among humans at the present time and therefore the concept of race in this study is essentially irrelevant. However ethnicity, at least, does recognize social arrangements on health and perhaps is a preferred descriptor over race for the examination of epilepsy. Ethnicity, then, is operationally defined here as a dynamic category determined by genes, culture, and social class, and is a product of social evolution (CDC, 1993). The following are general considerations applicable to individuals with epilepsy and of ethnicity different than European American culture in the United States.

African Americans

The general health status of African Americans compared with Anglo/European Americans is well documented. Twenty-one percent of African Americans report no usual source of medical care and many times conditions are first seen by the health care system when they are acute and in outpatient settings (Flack et al., 1995). Diagnostic testing and high-cost interventions are used less frequently with African Americans even when insurance is present. Often there is a degree of distrust of the health-care system and its professionals who are predominantly of nonminority status. For example, Flack et al. (1995) suggest that in African American culture, it shows a lack of respect to call an older person by his or her first name. Many health professionals and staff consistently use the patient's first name, regardless of age. For African Americans to feel receptive and comfortable it would be helpful to have health professionals who are cognizant of the lifestyle of the community. Treatment compliance is often based on the patient's relationship with the professional. The success of this relationship can be based on social customs that initiate demarcations of the patient's status, and the interest of the professional in the welfare of the patient.

Asian and Pacific Islander Americans

Asian/Pacific Islanders are not a homogeneous group in America. Chinese and Filipinos are the two largest populations followed by Japanese, Asian Indians, and Koreans. The five largest Pacific Islander populations are Hawaiians, Samoans, Guamanians, Tongans, and Fijians (Flack et al., 1995). The diversity of language, family customs, nonverbal and verbal mannerisms, diet, religion, and so forth is vast. It is important to note that about two-thirds of the current Asian American population are foreign-born and their acculturation with the health system may be naturally limited. New immigrants tend to prioritize their needs differently from the more established immigrants and assign higher priorities to the needs that are necessary for social adaptation and economic survival and health needs usually rank low (Asian American Health & Forum, 1990). Many times, the links among religious, cultural, and traditional medical practices are inseparable, especially among recent immigrants from traditional and rural societies (Penn et al., 1995).

One potential confounding aspect of psychosocial assessment is that Asian American clients may express psychiatric distress somatically (Sue & Sue, 1990). Assessment of quality of life with this population may be difficult if the patient is culturally predisposed to be reluctant to talk about psychological constructs. The medical aspects of good seizure control may be more acceptable to the patient in doctor–patient discussions. It would be up to the clinician to determine if somatic concerns are manifestations of stress associated with the physical aspects of seizures or stress associated with the psychosocial adjustment to epilepsy, and to determine treatment accordingly.

Hispanic Americans

Hispanic Americans are a rapidly growing population. Unfortunately, health statistics on this group of Americans have been lacking on a national level (Flack et al., 1995). As with the Asian American population, there is a great diversity of ethnicity within the Hispanic American community. Mexican Americans are the largest Hispanic group, followed by Puerto Ricans, Cubans, and Central and South Americans.

There is evidence that the health status of Hispanics of all groups declines among immigrants with increased stay in the United States. Infant mortality, low birthweight, adolescent pregnancy, use of cigarettes and alcohol, illicit drug use, and depression increase with acculturation (Flack et al., 1995). The abandonment of culturally tied health-related beliefs and the loss of culturally tied resources and social support networks seem to place Hispanic Americans at greater health risk (Flack et al., 1995).

The Hispanic American patient, as with many other ethnic groups, comes from a culture where collectivistic thinking and expression is the norm (Hays, 1997). Therefore data gathering for seizure diagnosis, treatment, and followup is enhanced if the individual is viewed in the context of their family (extended as well as immediate) and community. Indeed, an individual interview and neuropsychological testing techniques may be uncomfortable for the patient and adjustments may need to be made.

Native Americans/American Indians

American Indians are the only ethnic group of individuals in the United States with which the federal government has had a special obligation to provide health services. This is probably where the ability to group American Indians on health status ceases because the diversity extends to over 500 distinct tribal groups scattered over thousands of miles (Flack et al., 1995). The public health service achieved success in the past decades in controlling infectious disease in this population, but was ill-prepared for coping with pressing demands for long-term care for the elderly, management of problems in youth, and prevention and treatment of alcohol and drug abuse (Flack et al., 1995). DeBruyn (1990) suggests that the Indian Health Service has provided inadequate care to American Indian children with epilepsy.

Among Tewa Indians there is a reluctance to discuss traditional beliefs and healing practices with clinicians (DeBruyn, 1990). A traditional Navajo belief is that individuals with epilepsy have transgressed moral norms (such as sibling incest) and they are sanctioned by illness that causes seizures. This, in turn, causes parents to withdraw from the child with epilepsy and subsequent adjustment problems are common (Levy, 1987). Traditional Navajo healers attribute negative social attributes to persons suffering generalized seizures, therefore acculturated Navajos who are trained as mental health workers are healers of choice (Levy, 1979). Navajos with epilepsy do have higher rates of death, criminal activity, and alcoholism (which is especially problematic in seizure disorders; Hauser, 1990) than Navajos with psychiatric diagnoses (Neutra et al., 1977). On the other hand, Pueblo Indians try to treat their epileptic children as normally as possible (Levy, 1987). Much more research is needed with different American Indian tribes regarding perceptions about epilepsy because of the diversity of what constitutes quality of life within this ethnic group.

Summary and Conclusion

Neuropsychology is indebted to the epilepsies for our current knowledge of brain behavior relationships and neuropsychology has contributed greatly to the diagnosis, treatment, and evaluation of individuals with epilepsy. Much of the world's population of individuals with epilepsy do not have access to treatment and are victim to the medical and social sequelae of their untreated seizure disorders.

In the United States, appropriate diagnosis, treatment, and followup of epilepsy is dependent on the individual's ability to gain access to the health care system. Those of lower socioeconomic status tend to seek treatment later on in the development of the seizure disorder, and tend to seek treatment from emergency medical facilities that are not designed to coordinate the multidimensional and long-term aspects of epilepsy treatment.

The diagnosis of epilepsy is dependent on a productive relationship between the diagnosing clinicians and the patient. This relationship must be a vehicle for culturally competent communication that translates not only the medical aspects of good seizure control, but also the quality of life of the patient. The concept of quality of life is culture bound and must be treated as such.

The neuropsychological assessment research literature is just starting to examine cultural validity of neuropsychological test instruments that not only measure brain–behavior functioning but also quality of life as well. Eventually, the assessment of quality of life will also have to be tied to measures of acculturation for individuals of ethnic groups that are not representative of white American culture. In addition, the assessment and treatment of women, children, elderly, and ethnic groups differ from traditional treatment. Each group has specific diagnostic and quality-of-life issues that affect treatment outcome.

It would be preferable that the future direction of epilepsy research in the United States continue with sound and culturally competent prevention policies based on appropriate incidence and prevalence studies. In addition, the specialization of knowledge about how different groups react to and engage with antiepileptic medications, quality-of-life issues, treatment compliance, assessment instruments, and access to health care must be researched. Perhaps highly developed countries such as the United States can lead the way in culturally competent research, education, and funding so that the world's 30 million individuals with untreated epilepsy can come out of the shadows, and perhaps the direction of 4,000 years of ignorance, superstition, and stigma can be changed.

References

Alper, K., Devinsky, O., Perrine, K., Vazquez, B., & Luciano, D. (1993). Nonepileptic seizures and childhood sexual and physical abuse. *Neurology, 43,* 1950–1953.

American Academy of Neurology (1999). *New guidelines offer recommendations for women with epilepsy.* St. Paul, MN: Author.

Asian American Health Forum. (1990). *Asian and Pacific Islander American population statistics* (Monograph Series 1). San Francisco: Author.

Baumann, R. J., Wison, J. F., & Wiese, H. J. (1995). Kentuckians's attitudes toward children with epilepsy. *Epilepsia, 36,* 1003–1008.

Bennett, T. L., & Maile, R. Ho. (1997). The neuropsychology of pediatric epilepsy and antiepileptic drugs. In C. R. Reynolds & E. Fletcher-Janzen (Eds.), *Handbook of clinical child neuropsychology* (2nd ed.; pp. 517–538). New York: Plenum.

Bharucha, N. E., & Shorvon, S. D. (1997). Epidemiology in developing countries. In J. Engel & T. A. Pedley (Eds.), *Epilepsy: A comprehensive textbook* (pp. 105–118). Philadelphia: Lippincott-Raven.

Black, K. C., & Hynd, G. W. (1995). Epilepsy in the school aged child: Cognitive-Behavioral characteristics and effects on academic performance. *School Psychology Quarterly, 10,* 345–358.

Boivin, M. J., Chounramany, C., Giordani, B., Xaisida, S., Choulamountry, L., Pholsena, P., Crist, C. L., & Olness, K. (1996). Validating a cognitive ability testing protocol with Lao children for community development applications. *American Psychologist, 10,* 588–599.

Bourgeois, B. F. D. (1998). Antiepileptic drugs, learning, and behavior in childhood epilepsy. *Epilepsia, 39,* 913–921.

Carrazana, E., De Toledo, J., Tatum, W., Rivas-Vasquez, R., Rey, G., & Wheeler, S. (1999). Epilepsy and religious experiences: Voodoo possession. *Epilepsia, 40,* 239–241.

Centers for Disease Control and Prevention. (1993). Use of race and ethnicity in public health surveillance summary of the CDC/ATSDR workshop. *MMWR Weekly* (No. RR-10).

Centers for Disease Control and Prevention. (1994). *Health United States.* Washington, DC: Author.

Centers for Disease Control and Prevention. (1995). Current trends prevalence of self-reported epilepsy—United States, 1986–1990. *MMWR Weekly, 43,* 810–811.

Chaplin, J. E., & Malmgren, K. (1999). Cross-cultural adaptation and use of the Epilepsy Psychosocial Effects Scale: Comparison between the psychosocial effects of chronic epilepsy in Sweden and the United Kingdom. *Epilepsia, 40,* 951–954.

Chen, J., & Gardner, H. (1997). Alternative assessment from a multiple intelligences theoretical perspective. In D. P. Flanagan, J. L. Genshaft, & P. L. Harrison (Eds.), *Contemporary Intellectual Assessment* (pp. 105–121). New York: Guilford.

Cooper, W. O., Federspiel, C. F., Griffin, M. R., & Hickson, G. B. (1997). New use of anticonvulsant medication among children enrolled in the Tennessee Medicaid Program. *Archives of Pediatric Adolescent Medicine, 151,* 1242–1246.

Cramer, J. A., Perrine, K., Devinsky, O., Bryant-Comstock, L., Meador, K., & Hermann, B. (1998). Development and cross-cultural translations of a 31-item Quality of Life in Epilepsy Inventory. *Epilepsia, 39,* 2148–2159.

DeBruyn, L. M. (1990). Tewa children who have epilepsy: A health care dilemma. *American Indian and Alaska Native Mental Health Research, 4*(2), 25–42.

Devinsky, O., Vicrey, B. G., Cramer, J., Perrine, K., Hermann, B., Meador, K., & Hays, R. D. (1995). Development of the Quality of Life in Epilepsy Inventory. *Epilepsia, 36,* 1089–1104.

Dhanak, M. (1996). Racial differences in leukocyte counts. *American Journal of Psychiatry, 153,* 586–587.

Dodrill, C. B. (1978). A neuropsychological battery for epilepsy. *Epilepsia, 19,* 611–623.

Dodrill, C. B. (1992). Neuropsychological aspects of epilepsy. *Psychiatric Clinics of North America, 15,* 383–394.

Dodrill, C. B., & Batzel, L. W. (1994). The Washington Psychosocial Seizure Inventory and quality of life in epilepsy. In M. R. Trimble & W. E. Dodson (Eds.), *Epilepsy and quality of life* (pp. 109–122). New York: Raven.

Dodrill, C. B., Batzel, L. W., Queisser, H. R., & Temkin, N. R. (1980). An objective method for the assessment of psychological and social difficulties among epileptics. *Epilepsia, 21,* 123–135.

Dodrill, C., & Matthews, C. G. (1992). The role of neuropsychology in the assessment and treatment of persons with epilepsy. *American Psychologist, 47,* 1139–1142.

Ellis, B. B., & Kimmel, H. D. (1992). Identification of unique cultural response patterns by means of item response theory. *Journal of Applied Psychology, 77,* 177–184.

Epilepsy Foundation of America (1999a). *Epilepsy: A report to the nation.* Landover, MD: Author.

Epilepsy Foundation of America (1999b). *Epilepsy facts and figures.* Landover, MD: Author.

Epilepsy Foundation of America (1999c). *Women and epilepsy initiative.* Landover, MD; Author.

Epilepsy Ontario (1999). *Women and epilepsy.* Ontario, Canada: Author.

Everitt, A. D., & Sander, J. W. (1998). Incidence of epilepsy is now higher in elderly people than children. *British Medical Journal, 3,* 780.

Fisher, R. S. (1994). *Imitators of epilepsy.* New York: Demos.

Flack, J. M., Amaro, H., Jenkins, W., Kunitz, S., Levy, J., Mixon, M., & Yu, E. (1995). Epidemiology of minority health. *Health Psychology, 14,* 592–600.

Greenfield, P. M. (1997). You can't take it with you: Why ability assessment doesn't cross cultures. *American Psychologist, 52,* 115–124.

Griebel, M. L., Roscoe, A., Dykman, R. A., & Williams, J. (1997). *Demographic factors related to treatment compliance in pediatric patients with new onset seizures.* Poster Session at American Epilepsy Society Annual Meeting, December 7–10, San Francisco, CA.

Hauser, W. A. (1990). Epidemiology of alcohol use and epilepsy: The magnitude of the problem. In R. J. Porter & R. Mattson (Eds.), *Alcohol and seizures: Basic mechanisms and clinical concepts* (pp. 12–21). Philadelphia: F. A. Davis.

Hauser, W. A. (1994). Seizures and epilepsy in the elderly. In A. Martin & J. Knoefel (Eds.), *Clinical neurology of aging* (2nd ed., pp. 595–610). New York: Oxford.

Hauser, W. A. (1997). Incidence and prevalence. In J. Engel & T. A. Pedley (Eds.), *Epilepsy: A comprehensive textbook* (pp. 47–57). Philadelphia: Lippincott-Raven.

Hauser, W. A., & Hesdorffer, D. C. (1990). *Epilepsy: Frequency, causes and consequences.* New York: Demos.

Hauser, W. A., Morris, M. L., Heston, L. L., & Anderson, V. E. (1986). Seizures and myoclonus in patients with Alzheimer's disease. *Neurology, 36,* 1226–1230.

Hays, P. (1997). Culturally responsive assessment with diverse older clients. *Professional Psychology: Research and Practice, 27*(2), 188–193.

Hermann, B. P., Whitman, S., & Anton, M. (1992). A multietiological model of psychological and social dysfunction in epilepsy. In T. L. Bennett (Ed.), *The neuropsychology of epilepsy* (pp. 39–57). New York: Plenum.

Hempal, A. M., Risse, G. L., Frost, M. D., & Ritter, F. (1994). The utility of neuropsychological testing for identifying lateralization of the epileptogenic region in children. *Epilepsia, 35*(Suppl. 84), 80.

Hubert, T. J. (1992). Classroom performance and adaptive skills in children with Epilepsy. *Journal of School Psychology, 30,* 331–342.

International Epilepsy Commission (1989). Classification of epilepsy syndromes. *Epilepsia, 30,* 389–399.

Jones, B. P., Duncan, C. C., Mirsky, A. F., Post, R. M., & Theodore, W. H. (1998). Neuropsychological profiles in bipolar affective disorder and complex partial seizure disorder. *American Psychologist, 8,* 55–64.

Kale, R. (1997). Bringing epilepsy out of the shadows. *British Medical Journal, 3*(15), 2–3.

Klein, P., & Herzog, A. G. (1997). Endocrine aspects of partial seizures. In S. C. Schachter & D. L. Schomer (Eds.), *The comprehensive evaluation and treatment of epilepsy* (pp. 207–232). Boston: Academic Press.

Krumholz, A., Grufferman, S., Orr, S. T., & Stern, B. J. (1989). Seizures and seizure care in an emergency department. *Epilepsia, 30,* 175–181.

Lesser, R. P. (1996). Psychogenic seizures. *Neurology, 46,* 1499–1507.

Levy, J. E. (1987). Psychological and social problems of epileptic children in four southwestern Indian tribes. *Journal of Community Psychology, 15,* 307–315.

Levy, J. E., Neutra, R., & Parker, D. (1979). Life careers of Navajo epileptics and convulsive hysterics. *Social Science and Medicine, 13B*(1), 53–66.

Lin, K.-M., Anderson, D., & Poland, R. E. (1995). Ethnicity and psychopharmacology: Bridging the gap. *Psychiatric Clinics of North America, 18,* 635–647.

Manly, J. J., Jacobs, D. M., Sano, M., Bell, K., Merchant, C. A., Small, S. A., & Stern, Y. (1998). Cognitive test performance among nondemented elderly African Americans and whites. *Neurology, 50,* 1238–1245.

McKenzie, K. (1996). Describing race, ethnicity, and culture in medical research. *British Medical Journal, 312,* 1054.

McLin, W. M. (1992). Introduction to issues in psychology and epilepsy. *American Psychologist, 47*, 1124–1125.

Medina, M. T., Rosas, E., Rubio-Donnadieu, F., & Sotelo, J. (1990). Neurocysticercosis as the main cause of late-onset epilepsy in Mexico. *Archives of Internal Medicine, 150*, 325–327.

Minh-Thu, T., & Rausch, R., (1996). *Stress and employment status among multiple ethnic groups of individuals with epilepsy.* Poster Session at American Epilepsy Society Annual Meeting, December 7–10, San Francisco, CA.

Mitchell, W. G., Scheier, L. M., & Baker, S. A. (1994). Psychosocial, behavioral and medical outcomes in children with epilepsy: A developmental risk factor model using longitudinal data. *Pediatrics, 94*, 471–477.

Murphy, J. V., & Dehkharghani, F. (1994). Diagnosis of childhood seizure disorders. *Epilepsia, 35*(Suppl. 2), S7–S17.

Murphy, C. C., Trevathan, E., & Yeargin-Allsopp, M. (1995). Prevalence of epilepsy and epileptic seizures in 10-year-old children: Results from the Metropolitan Atlanta Developmental Disabilities Study. *Epilepsia, 36*, 866–872.

National Institute of Neurological Disorders and Stroke (1999). *Epilepsy.* Bethesda, MD: National Institutes of Health Office of Communications and Public Liaison.

Neutra, R., Levy, J. E., & Parker D. (1977). Cultural expectations versus reality in Navajo seizure patterns and sick roles. *Culture, Medicine and Psychiatry, 1*, 255–275.

Novelly, R. A. (1992). The debt of neuropsychology to the epilepsies. *American Psychologist, 47*, 1126–1129.

Oquendo, M. A. (1995). Differential diagnosis of ataque de nervios. *American Journal of Orthopsychiatry, 65*(1), 60–65.

Pedley, T. A. (1995). Epilepsy and education. *Epilepsia, 36*(Suppl. 8), S18–S22.

Penn, N. E., Kar, S., Kramer, J., Skinner, J., & Zambrana, R. E. (1995). Ethnic minorities, health care systems, and behavior. *Health Psychology, 14*, 641–646.

Sander, J. W., & O'Donoghue, M. F. (1997). Epilepsy: Getting the diagnosis right. *British Medical Journal, 312*, 158.

Serge, P. L. J. C. (1996). *Epilepsy in a large urban public hospital in the Midwest.* Poster Session at American Epilepsy Society Annual Meeting, December 7–10, San Francisco, CA.

Shafer, P. O. (1998). Counseling women with epilepsy. *Epilepsia, 39*(Suppl. 8), S38–S44.

Shamansky, S. L., & Glaser, G. H. (1979). Socioeconomic characteristics of childhood seizure disorders in the New Haven area: An epidemiologic study. *Epilepsia, 20*, 457–474.

Simpson, G., Bloom, B., Cohen, R. A., & Parsons, E. (1993). *Access to health care Part 1: Children.* Vital and Health Statistics Data from the National Health Interview Survey No. 191. Hyattsville, MD: U.S. Department of Health and Human Services.

Smith, P. E. M. (1998). The teenager with epilepsy. *British Medical Journal, 317*, 960–961.

Snyder, P. J., & McConnell, H. W. (1997). Neuropsychological aspects of epilepsy in the elderly. In P. D. Nussbaum (Ed.), *Handbook of neuropsychology of aging* (pp. 271–279). New York: Plenum.

Stauss, E., Hunter, M., & Wada, J. (1995). Risk factors for cognitive impairment in epilepsy. *Neuropsychology, 9*, 457–463.

Stein, R. A., & Strickland, T. L. (1998). A review of the neuropsychological effects of commonly used prescription medicine. *Archives of Clinical Neurology, 13*, 259–284.

Strickland, T. L., Ranganath, V., Lin, K.-M., & Poland, R. E. (1991). Psychopharmacological considerations in the treatment of black American populations. *Psychopharmacology Bulletin, 27*, 441–448.

Sue, D. W., & Sue, D. (1990). *Counseling the culturally different* (2nd ed). New York: Wiley. (1981, 1st ed.)

Tohen, M. (1996). Blood dyscrasias with carbamazepine and valproate: A pharmacoepidemiological study of 2, 228 patients at risk: Reply. *American Journal of Psychiatry, 153*, 587.

Trostle, J. A., Hauser, W. A., Sharbrough, F. W. (1989). Psychologic and social adjustment to epilepsy in Rochester, Minnesota. *Neurology, 39*, 633–637.

Tucker, R. (1998). Seizure disorders presenting with psychiatric symptomatology. *Psychiatric Clinics of North America, 21*, 625–635.

Watanabe, M., Iwahashi, K., Kugoh, T., & Suwaki, H. (1998). The relationship between phenytoin pharmacokinetics and the CYP2C19 genotype in Japanese epileptic patients. *Clinical Neuropharmacology, 21*, 122–126.

Williams, J., Roscoe, D., Griebel, M. L., Lange, B., & Bates, S. (1996). *AED effects on cognition and behavior in children.* Poster Session at American Epilepsy Society Annual Meeting, December 7–10, San Francisco, CA.

World Health Organization (1995). *Epilepsy demographics.* Geneva, Switzerland: Author.

World Health Organization (1997a). *Epilepsy: Historical overview* (Fact Sheet N 168). Geneva, Switzerland: Author.

World Health Organization (1997b). *Epilepsy: Aetiology, epidemiology and prognosis* (Fact Sheet N 165). Geneva, Switzerland: Author.

World Health Organization (1997c). *Bringing epilepsy out of the shadows* (Press Release WHO/48). Geneva, Switzerland: Author.

World Health Organization (1997d). *Epilepsy: social consequences and economic aspects* (Fact Sheet N166). Geneva, Switzerland: Author.

13

Considerations of Culture for Understanding the Neuropsychological Sequelae of Medical Disorders

RALPH E. TARTER

It is generally recognized that there is substantial variation in the population with respect to level and style of cognitive functioning. One obvious example illustrating the wide range of individual differences is in the area of intelligence where IQ scores in the population vary between 20–160 for 99% of the population. Considering the whole population, there is thus approximately an eightfold variation with respect to intellectual capacity.

Virtually all biobehavioral processes are characterized by interindividual variability. Not surprisingly, therefore, cognitive processes directly reflecting the integrity of brain functioning are, like other psychological processes, highly variable in the general population.

Among particular segments of the population, cognitive functioning does not, however, necessarily map to the whole population. For example, there is convincing evidence that females, left-handed people, and children of alcoholics demonstrate, on average, skewed scores on certain cognitive processes (Filskov & Catanese, 1986; Giancola, Martin, Tarter, Moss, & Pelham, 1996). The extent to which cultural factors are associated with variation in neurocognitive functioning has not been systematically investigated. In consideration of the lacuna of empirical literature, this discussion broadly outlines a research strategy for investigating the cultural factors that underlie variation in cognitive functioning among subpopulations having medical disorders.

Complicating this task is the dilemma that numerous subpopulations have been presumed to exist based on superficial biological, behavioral, or social characteristics. Classifying the general population into categories or subgroups based on unfounded criteria (e.g., physical appearance) has lead to a search for differences where, in fact, the typology is based on criteria that are not meaningful or discriminative, and thereby lack validity. For example, classification of the population into races is ill-founded from a biological perspective inasmuch as the types

RALPH E. TARTER • University of Pittsburgh School of Pharmacy, Pittsburgh, Pennsylvania 15261.

Handbook of Cross-Cultural Neuropsychology, edited by Fletcher-Janzen, Strickland, and Reynolds. Kluwer Academic/Plenum Publishers, New York, 2000.

are based on superficial physical attributes. With respect to culture—the organizing values, symbols and traditions of a subpopulation—is there any reason to believe that there are distinctive biological differences that would be expressed in brain organization and cognitive functioning? This question remains to be addressed. However, should it prove possible to meaningfully categorize the population into valid subgroups, the grouping parameters are useful only to the extent that they afford a more generalized understanding of cognitive processes than afforded by an analysis at the individual level.

With respect to cognitive capacities, there is strong evidence pointing to variation in the distribution of capacities among various subpopulations. In the field of neuropsychology, this has been most frequently documented with respect to differences in cognitive functioning among left-handed compared to right-handed people. Male and female subpopulations have also been studied and shown in many studies to differ in cognitive functioning. Clearly, not all subpopulations are discriminable from the total population from which they are derived. For example, although not as yet empirically demonstrated, it is extremely unlikely that subpopulations classified according to hair color are discriminable on cognitive processes. Thus, at the descriptive level, a major task is to identify the distinguishing characteristics defining the subpopulations of interest. Next, it needs to be demonstrated that these characteristics are associated with variation in cognitive capacities. These tasks have not, to date, been undertaken with respect to delineating variation in cognitive functioning according to cultural parameters.

Determining the presence and origins of group variation requires at the outset an understanding of the causes of individual variation. The following discussion examines the basis of human individuality with respect to cognitive functioning as well as all other biobehavioral processes.

Origins of Individual Differences

The factors underlying individual variation are easy to conceptualize but extraordinarily difficult to analyze empirically. As shown in Figure 1, all phenotypes (defined as the measured characteristics of an individual) are determined jointly by genetic and environmental factors.

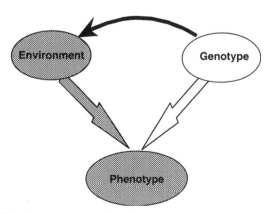

FIGURE 1. Gene–environment interactions determining cognitive phenotypes.

With respect to cognitive processes, there is no dispute that they are the product of both genetic and environmental factors (Plomin, Fulker, Corley, & DeFries, 1997) although there is currently very little understanding of the interaction between specific genes and particular environmental conditions that underlie specific capacities. Part of this difficulty stems from the fact that the cognitive architecture in relation to neuroanatomical functional organization has yet to be specified. Moreover, because the cognitive architecture has not yet been fully explicated, the universe of phenotypes (characteristics) that differentiate particular subpopulations (e.g., cultures) currently remains unknown. This lacuna notwithstanding, across the spectrum of cognitive processes, of which a subset of capacities are commonly the focus of a neuropsychological evaluation, it is commonly recognized that genetic and environmental factors jointly determine cognitive functioning.

At the subpopulation level of analysis, differences between groups are due to the differential interplay among genetic and environmental factors. For some groups the genetic anomaly is present and specifiable (e.g., Turner's syndrome, Kleinfelter syndrome), however, the fact that there is variation of cognitive capacities *within* any particular group underscores the integral influence of the environment on cognitive functioning. In situations where the environment is marked by extreme deprivation (e.g., sensory stimulation, nutrition), the genetic potential is not realized. In this circumstance the average level of cognitive functioning of the group is reduced. Notably, the Head Start program is based on the premise that enriching the environment of disadvantaged youth potentiates genetic potential that would otherwise be thwarted.

Cognitive processes, because they are complex, are the product of the interaction among manifold genetic and environmental factors. Neuropsychological test scores reflecting brain functioning need to be understood in the context of the genetic factors coding for distinct capacities interacting with the environment to affect brain development and integrity. However, complicating the research agenda at both the individual and subpopulation levels of analysis is the heterogeneity of causal factors defining a particular phenotype. Disaggregating the relative contribution of genetic and environmental factors on continuous variables or traits (IQ, face recognition, motor speed, etc.) is extraordinarily difficult because of the interplay of many genes and manifold environments. However, in order to delineate the basis of individual as well as group differences, both facets have to be considered. Combining individuals into a group (subpopulation) for any medical disorder without accounting for the sources of genetic and environmental variation obscures elucidating the basis of brain–behavior relationships within and between cultural groups. For example, diabetes, hypertension, and cancer are the products of genetic and environmental influence. Combining individuals into a single group based on this overt characteristic without taking into consideration the relative contribution of genetic and environmental causal mechanisms works against clarifying the association between medical disease and cognition. In effect, even though individuals may have the same phenotype (e.g., asthma), the factors determining the phenotypes can be very different. This principle is applicable to understanding all the causal mechanisms underlying medical disorder and associated cognitive sequelae for all putative subpopulations categorized according to cultural or ethnic characteristics.

Cognitive Traits

Each phenotype represents an underlying trait. By definition, everyone in the population has every trait; differences between individuals and groups are confined to phenotypic expression. For example, everyone has the trait of motor speed, face recognition, working memory, and so forth. Differences between individuals and groups are evident with respect to capacity and efficiency. In neuropsychological assessment the test score is generally accepted to reflect the person's phenotype for the trait. Because cognitive traits are determined by many genes interacting with numerous environments, the distribution of phenotypes in the population would be expected to be normal according to the central limits theorem. However, it should be emphasized that the various cognitive traits comprising the overall architecture are determined by a wide range of unique, as well as shared and overlapping, genetic and environmental factors. For instance, genes coding for memory are not likely to be confined to the same exact genes coding for other neuropsychological processes. Similarly, the environmental determinants vary; for example, the social contexts contributing to language skills are, in all probability, not entirely different from environmental contexts that foster motor skills.

Cognitive processes are continuous traits characterized by a normal distribution. Using IQ for illustration purposes, it is commonly understood that it is a complex trait consisting of a number of constituent traits. For example, Full Scale IQ on the Wechsler Adult Intelligence Scale is based on the aggregation of eleven tests, each of which measures one or more cognitive traits. Based on level of functioning, the whole population can be partitioned into subpopulations (e.g., average, superior, etc.) according to their IQ score; these categories, although somewhat arbitrary, are used for clinical diagnosis.

Numerous investigations have demonstrated that IQ is the product of both genetic and environmental factors. Much attention has also been devoted to determining whether the profile of subtest scores comprising the overall IQ differs among subgroups in the population. For example, substantial neuropsychological research has inquired into the extent that gender and lesion location contribute to population variation in scores. Where a subpopulation does not map to the general population, it is necessary to disaggregate the contribution of genetic and environmental influences determining the skewed distribution in the subpopulation.

Understanding the mechanisms underlying differences in cognitive functioning among various ethnic, demographic, and cultural groupings requires at the outset specification of the similarities and differences on the cognitive traits of interest. In other words, it needs to be established, at the descriptive level, that a difference between subpopulations or between a subpopulation and the general population indeed exists.

At first glance, this task would appear to be straightforward. A major obstacle in this effort, however, is that the neurocognitive tests employed may not be free of cultural bias. In effect, what appears overtly as a real group difference is due to method variance. Hence, one research agenda for investigating culture influences on cognition is to devise and standardize assessment instruments that are psychometrically valid across subpopulations. Once the psychometric properties of a test of cognitive functioning are shown to be comparable across different ethnic groups, investigations into the differential impact of exogenous and endogenous factors on differences in capacity can be initiated. However, two additional points are also noteworthy: First, all members within a putative ethnic group may not share the characteristics assumed to define a distinctive cultural entity. For example, the Hispanic population in the United States varies dramatically according to country of origin. Individuals from Peru, Mexico, Puerto Rico, and the Canary Islands, although all sharing roots in Spanish language, culture, and traditions, and living currently in the same adopted country, are quite different. A more robust example perhaps is the well-known fact that Tay-Sachs disease is overrepresented in Ashkenazic but not Sephardic Jews. The point is that even within a particular culture, there is substantial variation with respect to liability for medical disorder. Generalizations about specific cultural groups may, therefore, be potentially misleading in view of the vast heterogeneity of its constituent membership. Second, the signs and symptoms as well as overall prevalence of medical disease are, in part, manifest according to the person's cultural identification. It is well established, for example, that psychiatric and psychosomatic diseases are not equally distributed across all cultural groups. In effect, the type of disorder as well as its natural history may be moderated by the person's habits and traditions acquired within a particular culture. This important topic is discussed below.

The Influence of Culture on Medical Disorders

Identification

Participation with other individuals in behaviors that unite the person to a group is referred to as *cultural identification*. Cultural identification has the potential to augment or reduce the risk for medical illness. A high-fat diet, for example, that is common in eastern European culture, predisposes to cardiovascular disease which, in turn, can induce neuropsychological impairment. Identification with a culture can also be protective; for example, the prohibition against smoking among Mormons reduces the risk for pulmonary disease and ultimately hypoxia-induced neuropsychological deficits.

Attachment

It has long been known that emotional and social support afforded by connection to a group having shared values and beliefs promotes health. Under this circumstance, reducing the risk of disease via social support has the effect of indirectly lowering the risk for neuropsychological impairment. This is especially salient for medical disorders that are stress-induced, or where stress is a moderating factor on the pathophysiology.

Knowledge

Implementing the customs of a culture requires knowledge of its norms and rituals. Diseases that ensue are determined in part by knowledge of risks associated with a particular culturally accepted behavior. A dramatic example is kuru, a degenerative neurological disease caused by consumption of virus-infected human brains of dead tribal members as part of ritual practice. Numerous disease enhancing behaviors (e.g., diet, alcohol consumption) comprise routine aspects of cultural expression. Cultures, over many centuries of experience, codify and sanction correct and incorrect behavior. Washing hands before meals might be a religious ritual but clearly it is also a health promoting activity.

In summary, culture can increase or decrease the risk for disease and ultimately neurocognitive impairment. Each of the three facets of culture noted above can have either risk enhancing or risk attenuating impacts. Importantly, the three facets of culture are not independent, hence the manner in which culture mediates or moderates the association between medical illness and neuropsychological deficit is highly variable and complex.

Distribution of Diseases in Subpopulations

Various subpopulations, interacting with cultural influences, are differentially susceptible to a wide array of diseases for many different reasons. For example, demography linked to culture is important. To illustrate one etiological pathway from myriad possibilities, low-income inner-city dwelling families are more exposed to lead particles and atmospheric neurotoxic chemicals which impair cognitive functioning. As a result of socioeconomic disadvantage, African Americans are more likely to live in the inner city compared to most other subpopulations. Other diseases having a primarily genetic contribution are more prevalent in certain ethnic groups. For example, sickle cell disease has the highest prevalence rate among African Americans; this disorder is associated with severe neuropsychological deficits.

For most medical disorders producing cognitive deficits, the genetic contribution is polygenic and the environmental contribution is chronic. For example, hypertension has been shown to be associated with reduced performance on neuropsychological tests (Bird, Blizard, & Mann, 1990). It is well-established that the prevalence of hypertension is higher among African Americans. In attempting to delineate the mechanisms responsible for the neuropsychological deficits, it is necessary to determine the relative genetic and environmental contribution underlying the medical disorder which, in turn, produces the cognitive deficit. Moreover, on average, African Americans experience more severe and persisting social stress compared to European Americans. The extent to which stress potentiates genetic liability resulting in a higher prevalence of disease that ultimately affects cognitive capacity remains to be determined. The point is that whereas a particular group may manifest a higher prevalence of medical disorder and cognitive deficit than other subpopulations, it cannot be concluded to reflect simply innate individual differences. Rather, the cognitive profile must be understood as the endpoint of interacting genetic and environmental factors predisposing to the medical disorder which, within cultural and other contextual factors, culminates in cognitive impairment. The genetic propensity among individuals comprising a particular culture may be the product of multiple generations of intrapopulation mating. The multifaceted environmental contributions include both physical and social contextual factors impacting on the person from the moment of conception and operating through the lifespan.

In summary, it is well-established that the prevalence of disease is not equally distributed in the general population. Subpopulations vary in the degree of risk for a variety of medical disorders. For the reasons noted above, different subpopulations vary with respect to types of diseases, and accordingly, the prevalence of neuropsychological deficits. As yet, epidemiological investigations of neuropsychological functioning have not been conducted. The central task in elucidating the mechanisms underlying group differences is to explicate the genetic–environment interactions that underlie the particular disease which, in turn, are responsible for the cognitive deficit. The following discussion articulates a conceptual framework that extends beyond merely descriptively contrasting population subgroups on neurocognitive tests but rather emphasizes the underlying causal mechanisms originating in genetic–environment interactions.

Heuristic Model for Cross-Cultural Neuropsychological Research

Figure 2 depicts the conceptual framework for delineating the impact of culture on neuropsychological functioning. As can be seen, ethnic or cultural factors can operate through multiple pathways. Genetic factors operate at two levels, by contributing to variation in normal cognitive functioning (G_1) and by contributing to variation in risk for medical disease (G_2). The cultural environment (E_c) in conjunction with G_1 and G_2 produces cognitive phenotypes, measured as capacity and efficiency across the overall cognitive architecture. The endophenotypes characterize the level of cognitive functioning conjointly determined by premorbid

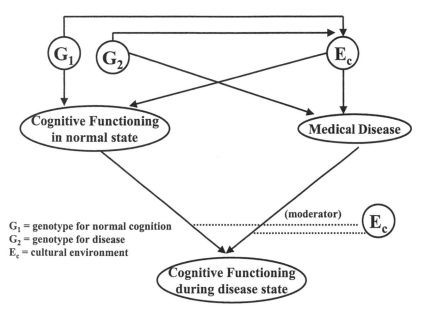

FIGURE 2. Path model illustrating the role of culture on cognitive functioning in medical disease.

cognitive status and disease determined cognitive sequelae. Cultural environment, for the reasons previously discussed, moderates the association between normal and disease related cognitive functioning to determine the course, severity, and profile of deficit.

Enriched environments foster superior cognitive capacity. In contrast, disadvantaged environments attenuate genetic potential that is ultimately manifest as cognitive deficit. Many studies have shown that severe environmental deprivation (e.g., inadequate nutrition, limited sensory experience, and low frequency of social interaction) predisposes to permanent and severe negative consequences on cognitive development. In studies of animals and humans, suboptimal environment interactions is a salient factor contributing to neurodevelopmental deficiency. For example, deprivation of vision during neuromaturation has a permanent effect by reducing perceptual capacity even if vision is subsequently restored. Lack of exposure to the sound "r" during childhood mitigates learning to enunciate this sound in everyday speech as adults. While it is generally recognized that the physical environment is integral to acquisition of cognitive capacities, little is known about the impact of cultural interactions and influences. It is reasonable to conclude that attachment to a culture provides enriching environmental interactions which in turn potentiates cognitive development. However, direct research on this topic is lacking.

Numerous investigations have, however, demonstrated an association between socioeconomic status and cognitive ability. This factor is relevant to this discussion because particular cultural groups comprise an overrepresentation of immigrants who are commonly poor and thus exposed to more limited environmental opportunities. Other cultures may prefer lifestyles in small or isolated communities, thereby limiting environmental exposure necessary for optimal cognitive development. In effect, culture and socioeconomic status are not independent. The extent to which culture, independent of socioeconomic status, is associated with specific cognitive capacities has not been studied with respect to medical diseases and their neuropsychological sequelae.

Contextualism

Patterns of behavior are formalized into sanctioned customs and rituals by the various ethnic and cultural groups. These so-called folkways and mores comprise the distinctive features of a culture. Certain customs foster disease (e.g., a high-fat diet). Other health risk behaviors (e.g., smoking) are negatively sanctioned by certain cultures. Hence, cultural expectations and compliance with cultural norms influence behavior so as to potentially augment as well as attenuate the likelihood of disease. For example, alcohol consumption is prohibited to Muslims and Mormons. Consequently, alcoholic cirrhosis is practically absent in these groups and accordingly the prevalence of alcohol-related neurological pathology (dementia, Wernicke–Korsakoff syndrome) and hepatic encephalopathy is extremely low.

Interactions with the cultural environment occur in two ways which predispose to or protect the person from diseases that have neuropsychological sequelae. First, the environment impinges on the person; that is, it exerts a *contagion* influence. In effect, other people in the particular cultural group affect the person in a fashion that increases or decreases the risk for disease. Ambivalence about alcohol consumption may produce frequent opportunities to drink thereby placing the person at increased risk for alcohol-related diseases. Alternatively, the culture can provide a supportive environment by buffering the effects of stress, thereby diminishing the risk for stress-induced medical disease and associated cognitive sequelae.

The second mode of interaction with the environment pertains to *selection*. That is, based on phenotypic characteristics the person seeks out particular social contexts, some of which may foster disease. Multiple sexual partners involving unprotected sex, exposure to tobacco smoke directly or secondhand, and a diet containing high levels of fat and salt, are examples of environmental selection that predisposes to infectious and systemic disease. Culture provides explicit sanctions (e.g., Mormons do not smoke) and prohibits certain modes of conduct (e.g., premarital sex). The extent to which a particular culture defines the behavioral norms and regulates the person's behavior is a major factor on the type and frequency of environments that are selected which increase the risk of medical disease. The individual's adherence to cultural norms thus exerts a major influence on the risk of developing medical disease and associated neuropsychological sequelae.

Summary

This chapter described an interactionist framework for understanding the origins of neuropsychological deficit concomitant to medical disease. Whereas neuropsychologists have traditionally emphasized, indeed confined their interest to, the measurement of the individual, it is evident from this discussion that it is essential to understand the person in the context of interactions with the environment. Culture has a regulatory influence on the person by providing the norms determining the quality of the person's interactions with the environment. These interactions contribute to the risk for a variety of different diseases related to behavior. However, all disease to more or less a degree involves genetic–environment interaction. Understanding the differential prevalence of disease in different cultural groups requires, therefore, disaggregating genetic–environmental interactions. In this framework, culture is a macrosystem influence which, combined with other environmental systems (e.g., family, neighborhood, workplace, peers, and so forth) influences the risk for many diseases and ultimately cognitive impairment.

References

Bird, A., Blizard, R., & Mann, A. (1990). Treating hypertension in the older person: An evaluation of the association of blood pressure level and its reduction with cognitive performance. *Journal of Hypertension, 8,* 147–152.

Filskov, S., & Catanese, R. (1986). Effects of sex and handedness on neuropsychological testing. In S. Filskor and T. Boll (Eds.), *Handbook of clinical neuropsychology* (pp. 198–212). New York: Wiley.

Giancola, P., Martin, C., Tarter, R., Moss, H ., & Pelham, W. (1996). Executive cognitive functioning and aggressive behavior in preadolescent boys at high risk for substance abuse/dependence. *Journal of Studies on Alcohol, 57,* 352–359.

Plomin, R., Fulker, D., Corley, R., & DeFries, J. (1997). Nature, nurture, and cognitive development from 1 to 16 years: A parent-offspring adoption study. *Psychological Science, 8,* 442–447.

14

HIV-1 Infection Spectrum Disease

Neuropsychological Manifestations and Cross-Cultural Considerations in Adulthood, Adolescence, and Childhood

ANTOLIN M. LLORENTE, CHRISTINE M. LOPRESTI,

CHRISTINE R. GUZZARD, PAUL SATZ,

AND GWENDOLYN EVANS

Neuropsychological manifestations associated with human immunodeficiency virus (HIV-1) infection and relevant cultural factors warrant special consideration in a handbook of this nature. This unique merit stems partially from the increasing incidence and cumulative prevalence of this infectious disease affecting ethnic-minority populations in the United States and abroad (Centers for Disease Control and Prevention, 1996; Mann, Tarantola, & Netter, 1992; World Health Organization, 1996), and partially from the deleterious effects of HIV upon the central nervous system (CNS) of adults (Grant et al., 1987; McArthur, 1994; Navia, Jordan, & Price, 1986; Snider et al., 1983) and children (Belman, 1990; Epstein et al., 1986; Falloon, Eddy, Wiener, & Pizzo, 1989; Pizzo & Wilfert, 1994), and their neuropsychological and neurobehavioral sequelae (Bayés, 1995; Brouwers, Belman, & Epstein, 1991, 1994; Brouwers, Moss, Wolters, Eddy, & Pizzo, 1989; Chase et al., in press; Llorente, LoPresti, Levy, & Fernandez, 2000; Llorente, LoPresti, & Satz, 1997; Llorente et al., 1998; Miller et al., 1990; Navia et al., 1986; Tross et al., 1988; van Gorp, Miller, Satz, & Visscher, 1989).

This chapter initially surveys pediatric and adult HIV-1 diagnostic classification. Subsequently, a review of U.S. and worldwide epidemiological data is presented, which depicts the pandemic scope of this disease, particularly as it applies to ethnic-minority populations. A review of clinicopathological, neuropsychological, and behavioral manifestations of HIV and AIDS is followed by specific considerations relevant to ethnic-minority populations. Select

ANTOLIN M. LLORENTE • Baylor College of Medicine, Houston, Texas 77030.   **CHRISTINE M. LOPRESTI** • UCLA School of Medicine, Los Angeles, California 90095.   **CHRISTINE R. GUZZARD** • University of Southern California, Los Angeles, California 90089.   **PAUL SATZ** • UCLA School of Medicine, Los Angeles, California 90095; and Charles R. Drew University of Medicine and Science, Los Angeles, California 90059.   **GWENDOLYN EVANS** • Walden House, Inc., San Francisco, California 94103.

Handbook of Cross-Cultural Neuropsychology, edited by Fletcher-Janzen, Strickland, and Reynolds. Kluwer Academic / Plenum Publishers, New York, 2000.

issues related to the treatment of HIV-associated neurobehavioral and neuropsychological problems in these populations are then briefly addressed.

Diagnostic Nosology

In 1994, the Centers for Disease Control and Prevention (CDC) updated the pediatric classification criteria for the spectrum of HIV diseases (CDC, 1994). Diagnosis of HIV in children less than 13 years of age is based on infection, immunologic, and clinical status. The three infection-related diagnostic groups are "HIV infected (I), perinatally exposed (E), and seroreverter (SR)." Children are diagnosed as HIV infected under the following conditions: A child who is younger than 18 months is diagnosed as infected if he or she is born to an HIV+ mother and (a) has had positive laboratory results on two HIV detection tests, or (b) has an AIDS-defining illness based on the 1987 CDC surveillance case definition. A child 18 months or older is diagnosed as infected if either born to an HIV+ mother or infected through any route of transmission (see, deMartino, 1994 and Friedland & Klein, 1987) and has repeatedly tested HIV+ by antibody tests. A perinatally exposed child is one who is (a) under 18 months of age and is HIV-seropositive by antibody tests, or (b) is born to an HIV+ mother but has unknown antibody status. A seroreverter is a child born to an HIV+ mother but who is antibody-negative, has no laboratory evidence of viral infection, and has not had an AIDS-defining illness.

Children who are infected or perinatally exposed based on the criteria described above are further classified according to both immunologic and clinical status. Immunologic categories are established on both age and level of immunosuppression and are based on CD4+ counts and percent of total lymphocytes (Table 1). Categorically, they range from "no evidence of suppression to severe suppression." Clinical categories are based on the presence and severity of symptomatology and range from asymptomatic to severe signs and symptoms (CDC, 1994).

With regard to adolescents and adults, two immunologic classification systems describing the progressive stages of HIV infection are currently in use, namely the Walter Reed (WR) (Redfield, Wright, & Tramont, 1986) and the Centers for Disease Control and Prevention (1993) classifications, the latter being the most commonly used in the U.S. These nosologic systems use CD4+ lymphocyte counts (e.g., CDC, 1993: $\geq 500/\mu L$, $200–499/\mu L$, $< 200/\mu L$) and three clinical levels of symptomatology (Category A [asymptomatic], Category B [minor opportunistic infections and symptoms], and Category C [AIDS-defining conditions])

TABLE 1. CDC Immunologic Classification System for Human Immunodeficiency Virus Infection in Infancy and Childhood

	Age-specific CD4+ T-lymphocyte count categories					
	< 12 months		1–5 years		6–12 years	
Immunologic category	T-cells/μL	%	T-cells/μL	%	T-cells/μL	%
No evidence of suppression	≥1500	≥25	≥1000	≥25	≥500	≥25
Evidence of moderate suppression	750–1499	15–24	500–999	15–24	200–499	15–24
Severe suppression	<750	<15	<500	<15	<200	<15

Source: Adapted from Centers for Disease Control and Prevention, 1994.

TABLE 2. CDC Immunologic Classification System for Human Immunodeficiency Virus Infection in Adulthood and Adolescence

Immunologic category	CD4+ T-lymphocyte count categories		
	≥ 500 T-cells/μL	200–499 T-cells/μL	< 200 T-cells/μL[a]
Asymptomatic (A), acute HIV	A1	A2	A3
Symptomatic (B), not (A) or (C) status	B1	B2	B3
AIDS-defining conditions (C)	C1	C2	C3

Source: Adapted from Centers for Disease Control and Prevention, 1993.
[a]Indicates AIDS-defining CD4+ count.

(Table 2) as the basis for categorization. Classification and definition of HIV-related neurological manifestations are based on the American Academy of Neurology nomenclature and vary from the earliest level of cognitive impairment now termed HIV-1-Associated Minor Cognitive/Motor Disorder to HIV-1-Associated Dementia (American Academy of Neurology Task Force, 1991).

The neurocognitive profiles of ethnic-minority children, adolescents, and adults infected with HIV are quite heterogeneous. This heterogeneity may be a consequence of viral characteristics (e.g., viral load present, viral strain) and/or environmental, medical, and host-related factors (drug use, level of education, onset of symptomatic disease, socioeconomic status (SES) and its impact on cognitive profiles after infection), transmission mode (vertical vs. horizontal transmission in children), quality of treatment, and so forth (Brouwers, Moss, Wolters, & Schmitt, 1994; Fama, Pace, Tiempiero, & Bornstein, 1992; see also Satz et al., 1993). Although it is not being advocated that HIV infection, per se, has differential expression in minority groups relative to mainstream populations (this is an issue open to empirical investigation; see Samson et al., 1996 for differential CCR5 chemokine response to HIV infection in Caucasian relative to black populations in Africa), several factors, including those noted above, may have significant modulating impact in disease expression in these groups (e.g., timing of disease detection and onset of treatment).

HIV and Its Impact on Ethnic-Minority Populations: U.S. and Worldwide Epidemiology Summary

The population of HIV infected children and adults has spiraled dramatically in the United States since the first cases were reported to the CDC. As of June 1996, 7,296 children under the age of 13 had been diagnosed with AIDS, accounting for 1.3% of the total number of reported AIDS cases in the U.S., including territories outside the U.S. mainland. Adults/adolescents (540,806) accounted for the remainder of cases reported. In the 24- to 44-year-old age group, AIDS is now the leading cause of death in men and the third leading cause of death in women (CDC, 1996). Infant and childhood mortality resulting from AIDS has also experienced a dramatic increase worldwide (Mann et al., 1992; Novello, Wise, Willoughby, & Pizzo, 1989). This rise in the number of cases and deaths, whether the result of better surveillance techniques or the rapid spread of the disease, has led to enormous social and economic consequences (Mann et al., 1992). With regard to morbidity and mortality as a result of HIV in the U.S., Kranczer (1995) notes that HIV infection has contributed to the first known reduction in average life expectancy in this country.

Five states have accounted for over half of the pediatric and adult/adolescent AIDS cases reported in the U.S.: New York, California, Florida, Texas and New Jersey. New York has reported the largest percentage of both children (25%) and adults/adolescents (19%) with AIDS in the country (CDC, 1996). Through June 1996, African Americans (31%) and Hispanics (17%) accounted for almost half of the 462,152 male adult/adolescent AIDS cases, despite the fact that these populations comprise only 13% and 10%, respectively, of the overall U.S. population (CDC, 1996)! Most of the remaining cases were Caucasian males (51%). Sex with other males and injecting-drug use were the risk factors associated with 89% of AIDS cases in adult and adolescent males. The pattern of exposure to HIV, however, varied within racial/ethnic groups. Roughly equal proportions of African American and Hispanic males were infected through sex with males as were infected through injecting-drug use, while the vast majority (81% to 94%) of males in all other groups were infected through sex with other males (CDC, 1996).

Females account for 15% of all adult/adolescent AIDS cases in the U.S. As with males, selective minority groups are disproportionally affected, with African American and Hispanic women accounting for 55% and 20%, respectively, and Caucasian women 24%, of reported AIDS cases (CDC, 1996). The fastest growing mode of HIV transmission in adult/adolescent females across all racial/ethnic groups is heterosexual contact, with most of these women becoming infected via sexual activity with men who inject drugs. From July 1995 through June 1996, 40% of females were exposed to HIV through sex with males, while 36% were infected through their own intravenous drug use. Cumulative statistics indicate that Hispanic females accounted for the greatest proportion (45%) of women infected through heterosexual contact, compared with African American (35%) and Caucasian (38%) women (CDC, 1996).

In the U.S., 90% of children with AIDS were vertically infected. Forty-four percent of their mothers acquired HIV through injecting-drug use or sex with an injecting-drug user (CDC, 1996). This rise in vertically infected cases probably reflects the increasing number of infected women and the relative decreases in other methods of transmission, including infection from blood and blood products (Andiman & Modlin, 1991). For this reason, vertical transmission can be expected to account for virtually all cases of pediatric HIV infection in the future. Because most children are exposed to HIV through their mothers, the disproportionate impact on selective minority groups observed in women is also reflected in the distribution of children with AIDS. Through June 1996, 81% of pediatric AIDS cases were accounted for by African American and Hispanic children, 58% and 23%, respectively, while Caucasian children comprised 18% of the cases. Among both pediatric and adult/adolescent cases, nearly 1% of cases were accounted for by Asian/Pacific Islanders and American Indian/Alaskan Natives (CDC, 1996).

Although domestic epidemiological data are informative, these figures misrepresent the magnitude of the HIV epidemic in ethnic-minority populations in terms of worldwide prevalence. Since the late 1970s to early 1980s, approximately 25.5 million adults and more than 2.4 million children are estimated to have been infected with HIV. It is estimated that approximately 21 million adults and 800,000 children are currently living with HIV/AIDS, with sub-Saharan Africa accounting for more than half of the cases, followed in descending order of prevalence by South and Southeast Asia, Latin America and the Caribbean, North America, Western Europe, North Africa and the Middle East, East Asia and the Pacific, Eastern Europe and Central Asia, and Australia (Table 3) (WHO, 1996). These data clearly demonstrate that areas highly populated with individuals from ethnic-minority backgrounds, and in many cases

TABLE 3. Worldwide Epidemiolgical Data (Adults and Children)—HIV Seroprevalence Estimate in Total Number of Cases

Region	Estimated number of cases
Sub-Saharan Africa	14,000,000
South and southeast Asia	4,800,000
Latin America and the Caribbean	1,600,000
North America	780,000
Western Europe	470,000
North Africa and the Middle East	200,000
East Asia and the Pacific	35,000
Eastern Europe and Central Asia	30,000
Australia	13,000

Source: Adapted from the World Health Organization, 1996.

from countries with elevated ethnic populations with limited financial and medical resources, have been substantially affected by this disease. Similarly, the United Nations Council on AIDS has reported that the devastating effects of HIV infection on select sub-Saharan nations (e.g., Zimbabwe) will decimate as much as a third of their population.

In the survey of the clinicopathological manifestations of HIV infection that follows, an attempt has been made to encompass a substantive portion of HIV investigations that incorporated ethnic minorities. However, it should be noted that several of the studies reported below may not have included these populations as part of their investigations. It also should be noted that certain variables capable of moderating medical factors (e.g., differential chemokine response) could very well limit the applicability of these investigations as they relate to ethnic minorities (even general disease progression differs across ethnic groups probably as a result of access to insurance and medical treatment, quality of medical care [see Tuckson, 1994], and/or cultural stigma associated with this infectious disease).

Clinicopathological Findings Associated with CNS HIV-1 Infection

Ample evidence (Brouwers et al., 1994; Gottlieb et al., 1981; Grant et al., 1987; Ho et al., 1985; Koenig et al., 1986; Navia et al., 1986; Navia, Cho, Petito, & Price, 1986; Pang et al., 1990; Resnick, Berger, Shapshak, & Tourtellete, 1988; Snider et al., 1983) from multiple lines of research (cognitive assessment, neuroimaging, neuropathology, etc.) suggests that the human immunodeficiency virus invades the CNS of adults and children. The invasion occurs shortly after initial systemic infection, eventually causing dramatic behavioral, cognitive, and neuropathological disturbances in a large number of infected individuals (Belman, 1990; Belman et al., 1984; McArthur, 1994).

Neurological Findings

HIV-related neurological manifestations experienced by children vary substantially. Some children exhibit mild alterations in cognition and motor skills. More severe expressions of the disease are manifested through childhood encephalopathy capable of causing substantial deviations from normal development (Sharer et al., 1986; Ultmann et al., 1987). Belman et al. (1988) and Belman (1990) described two forms of encephalopathy, namely progressive and static HIV-related encephalopathy. *Progressive encephalopathy* is subcategorized into two different types (*Sub-Acute* and *Plateau*) to describe the distinct rates of disease progression observed in infants and children. *Sub-acute progressive encephalopathy*, most commonly seen in infants and young children (Belman et al., 1988), is the most crippling developmental neurological expression of HIV infection. It is marked by a gradual and progressive decline across most domains of neurological functioning. Its greatest impact is observed in overall cognition, expressive functions including motor and language skills, and adaptive functioning in preschool-age children, or loss of already attained developmental milestones in infants and younger children with lack of further development usually leading to death (Epstein et al., 1985). Subacute encephalopathy causes serious CNS debilitation including profound cerebral atrophy and microcephaly (acquired as a result of lack of continued CNS development) (Epstein et al., 1985, 1986; see also DeCarli et al., 1991). In contrast, *plateau encephalopathy* is often observed in infants and young children who fail to acquire new developmental milestones, or acquire them very slowly. Unlike youngsters experiencing progressive subacute encephalopathy, children suffering from plateau course encephalopathy typically do not display losses from previously acquired levels of functioning (Belman et al., 1989). Belman (1990) reported that these children suffer from motor deficits as well as declines in overall cognitive functioning.

Static encephalopathy is characterized by continued acquisition of skills at rates below expected levels of normal development but commensurate with their level of functioning. Furthermore, the delays observed during static encephalopathy remain relatively stable over time from initial levels of functioning (Belman et al., 1985; Brouwers, Moss et al., 1994; Epstein et al., 1986; Epstein, Sharer, & Goudsmit, 1988). The gradual decline or lack of gains in development observed during progressive encephalopathy is not seen in children with static encephalopathy. The American Academy of Neurology recently combined the various categorizations of HIV-related encephalopathy under one category termed HIV-associated encephalopathy of childhood (American Academy of Neurology AIDS Task Force, 1991). Some researchers (Brouwers, Belman, & Epstein, 1994) argue that the singular categorization fails to account for the different neurological presentations associated with the various types of encephalopathy, contending that the classification proposed by Belman et al. (1988) better characterizes the various courses of disease progression observed during each of the three types of childhood encephalopathy. Regardless of the existing categorization of HIV-related encephalopathy, recent research has attempted to examine early neurodevelopmental indicators of encephalopathy in infancy and early childhood with promising success, including HIV-related changes in head circumference and Babinski response (see Blasini et al., 1998).

Although the actual frequency of these disorders is not high relative to adults, other neurological diseases associated with an HIV-induced immunodeficient state have also been observed in children (Belman, 1990), including opportunistic infections and other CNS complications (e.g., neoplasia), typically observed in children who have developed encephalopathy (Belman, 1990). For example, neoplasms have been documented in the literature, primary CNS lymphoma being the most common (Belman, 1990; Epstein et al., 1988). Neoplasia have been observed in children between ages 6 months and 10 years, but occur chiefly after the first birthday (Epstein et al., 1988). Their most prominent locations are in the basal ganglia and areas surrounding the third ventricle (Belman, 1990). Secondary CNS lymphomas also have been noted (Dickson et al., 1989), as well as cerebrovascular complications, including infarctions (Belman, 1990; Frank, Lim & Kahn, 1989) and strokes (Park et al.,

1988). Although there is consensus regarding the infrequency of CNS opportunistic infections in children (Epstein et al., 1988), they have been nonetheless reported in the neurological literature (Belman et al., 1988; Dickson et al., 1989). Of these, bacterial meningitis, *Candida* meningitis, and acquired cytomegalovirus (CMV) have been the most common. In contrast, HIV-related CNS toxoplasmosis, commonly observed in adults (McArthur, 1994), has rarely been reported in children (Belman, 1990; Nicholas, 1994).

In adulthood, the spectrum of neurological problems varies from a lack of neurological symptoms in most HIV-positive asymptomatic patients (McArthur et al., 1989) to HIV-related dementia in late-stage disease (McArthur, 1994; Navia et al., 1986). In some cases, primary neurological symptoms, including neuropathies, have been observed in the absence of consti-tutional symptoms in asymptomatic patients (McArthur, 1994). Acute aseptic meningitis also has been reported as a primary neurological problem in a number of patients (Cooper et al., 1985). Although motoric and myelopathic disturbances have been found to commonly occur as a result of HIV-1 infection, the most compromising primary neurological sequela associated with this infectious disease is HIV-1-related dementia secondary to HIV encephalopathy (Navia et al., 1986) with a clinical presentation marked by cognitive slowing, depression, and memory loss (Navia et al., 1986; Navia, Cho, et al., 1986) similar to symptoms ascribed to the subcortical dementias described by Cummings and Benson (1983; cf. Filley, 1994). Within an HIV-1-related dementing state, several clinical stages of impairment have been postulated from mild to end-stage (Price and Brew, 1988).

Secondary CNS neuropathology, including opportunistic infections (cytomegalovirus [CMV], progressive multifocal Leukoencephalopathy [PML], toxoplasmosis, cryptococcal meningitis, etc.), malignancies (Kaposi's sarcoma), and neoplasms (lymphoma) have been commonly reported in adults with AIDS. Of these potential complications, cerebral toxoplas-mosis caused by *Toxoplasma gondii* and cerebral cryptococcal meningitis (caused by *Crypto-coccus neoformans*) are the most prevalent nonviral forms of CNS infections observed (Bredesen, Levy, & Rosenblum, 1988; Levy & Fernandez, 1997), whereas PML (Fong & Toma, 1995; Miller et al., 1982) and acquired CMV (Bredesen et al., 1988) are the most common secondary coexisting viral infections. Non-Hodgkin's lymphoma is the primary CNS neoplastic manifestation associated with AIDS (Bredesen et al., 1988). Cerebrovascular problems may result from viral or bacterial vasculitis (Brightbill et al., 1995) or from cerebral infarcts secondary to nonbacterial thrombotic endocarditis (Bredesen et al., 1988). These complications may occur at any time due to immune compromise but they are usually asso-ciated with late-stage HIV disease and/or significant immunosuppression (CD4+ counts < 200 per cubic millimeter). They may initially present as a focal or diffuse process. In addition, they may at first present as a cognitive or affective disturbance (Levy & Fernandez, 1997).

Findings from Neuroimaging Studies

Several investigators have found abnormalities in the brains of HIV-infected children (Tardieu, 1991) using various neuroradiological procedures. Belman et al. (1985) noted cere-bral atrophy of varying degrees, marked by cortical atrophy with dilation of the ventricular system and calcification of the basal ganglia and frontal white matter in an 8-month-old with AIDS, using computed tomography (CT). These abnormalities were again observed longi-tudinally at 18 and 21 months. CT studies conducted by Belman et al. (1988) also found cortical atrophy and white matter abnormalities (basal ganglia [bilaterally] and frontal calcification) in children with AIDS or AIDS-related complex (ARC). In addition, sixteen of seventeen participants who were longitudinally evaluated in the study showed progressive levels of atrophy. These results were substantiated by DeCarli and his colleagues (1993). They found bilateral symmetrical calcification of the basal ganglia and frontal white matter calcification on CT in 100 children with symptomatic HIV infection. Furthermore, a recent study reported a significant relationship between white-matter abnormalities on CT and neuropsychological functioning. With children matched on level of cortical atrophy, Brouwers et al. (1995) found greater cognitive dysfunction in the group with white-matter abnormalities relative to the children with no cerebral calcification. Studies using magnetic resonance imaging (MRI) also have revealed CNS abnormalities associated with pediatric-HIV infection. Belman et al. (1986) detected decreased and increased signal intensities on T1- and T2-weighted images, respectively, as a result of bilateral white-matter atrophy in the basal ganglia and cerebral atrophy in a 10-year-old male. Similar results using T2-weighted imaging were evidenced by other investigators (see Epstein et al., 1986). A study examining cerebral metabolism through the use of positron emission tomography (PET) has supported the findings obtained with the structural neuroradiological techniques described above. Pizzo et al. (1988), while conducting a study assessing the effects of AZT pharmacotherapy, reported diffuse cortical, focal right-frontal, and right-superior-temporal hypometabolism prior to treatment in an 11-year-old male with HIV-1 infection.

Structural (qualitative and quantitative) and functional neuroimaging procedures have revealed abnormalities most likely associated with HIV-spectrum disease in adults (Dooneief et al., 1992; Flowers et al., 1990; Sacktor et al., 1995). In fact, as early as 1983, Whelan et al. (1983) reported remarkable cerebral manifestations associated with AIDS using computed tomography. In another study employing CT, Post et al. (1988) reported cortical atrophy and ventricular enlargement in 95% and 61%, respectively, of a sample of 21 patients with HIV encephalitis. Levin et al. (1990) reported structural (CT) abnormalities marked by small focal lesions (< 1 cm) in 25% of their symptomatic HIV-positive group (CDC II–IV). In addition, these investigators observed the presence of brain atrophy, particularly in their CDC IV group relative to the other diagnostic groups. Equally important, a significant relation was found between atrophy as measured by the CT and psychomotor retardation assessed using neuropsychological procedures (reaction time, RT). More recently, Post, Berger, and Quencer (1991) used qualitative MRI methods and found abnormalities in 13% of the asymptomatic participants and 46% of the symptomatic subjects in a sample of 119 HIV-positive patients. In particular, this study revealed white-matter lesions present in the neurologically-symptomatic group that were larger and more numerous relative to those found in the asymptomatic group. It is interesting to note that several factors, including drug use and a history of head injury, were not correlated with the abnormalities found in these patients, but a correlation was found between decreased CD4+ count and cortical atrophy. A quantitative (morphometric) MRI study (Jernigan et al., 1993) revealed the presence of brain-volume loss associated with HIV infection in the HIV-positive symptomatic group but not in the asymptomatic group employed in their investigation. This study also revealed that a large amount of the volume loss in the symptomatic seropositive group was the result of white-matter loss despite the fact that the subjects were free of clinical (neurological) signs. Cerebral gray-matter losses were also reported in this investigation.

Finally, similar to the results obtained by Belman et al. (1986) with children, Aylward et al. (1993) reported the presence of atrophy in basal ganglia structures in adults with HIV dementia using quantitative MRI procedures. With regard to functional imaging, Rottenberg et al. (1987) used resting state PET (flurodeoxyglucose, FDG) to study glucose metabolism in a group of 12 patients diagnosed with AIDS dementia complex and a group of 18 HIV-negative controls. The results of that study revealed evidence for increased thalamic and basal ganglia metabolic activity in patients with mild HIV-related encephalopathy relative to controls. In contrast, the remaining patients with more advanced dementia exhibited both decreased cortical and subcortical metabolism when compared to controls. Similarly, van Gorp and his colleagues (1992) investigated resting-state cerebral glucose metabolism through PET with 17 AIDS patients diagnosed with and without dementia using Sidtis and Price's (1990) AIDS Dementia Rating Scale and a group of 14 uninfected individuals. Only thalamic and basal ganglia metabolism differed significantly between the AIDS group and controls, the former exhibiting hypermetabolism as had been the case in Rottenberg and colleagues' (1987) study. Perfusion defects have also been found in HIV-positive, relative to HIV-negative adults using single-photon emission computed tomography (SPECT) (Krammer & Sanger, 1990; LaFrance et al., 1988). Altogether, neuroimaging studies with adults and children have revealed that both CT and MRI are capable of detecting atrophy and ring-enhancing lesions as well as certain aspects of white-matter compromise. Whereas MRI has been proven to be superior in detecting focal signal intensities in gray and white matter areas using T2-weighted procedures (Dooneief et al., 1992), it has not been found useful in detecting structural correlates of asymptomatic infection (Post et al., 1991). PET, SPECT, and magnetic resonance spectroscopy (MRS) have been able to capture regional functional abnormalities reflecting metabolism, brain perfusion, and biochemical function, respectively.

Electroencephalographic Correlates

Given the abnormalities observed in the CNS using other functional diagnostic procedures (e.g., imaging), remarkable findings from electroencephalographic (EEG) studies with HIV-positive adults and children are not surprising. Abnormalities on this functional modality are most commonly present during the late stages of the disease.

In a study conducted by Belman et al. (1985) with six children with AIDS, five of the six displayed EEG abnormalities consistent with the imaging results. Three of the five showed mild diffuse slowing, and the other two displayed moderate diffuse slowing. Four of the six also displayed abnormalities in brainstem evoked potential (BAEP) marked by abnormal rate function ($n = 1$) and prolongation ($n = 3$) of the I–V interwave latency. Other pediatric studies have found similar abnormalities (Ultmann et al., 1985).

EEG abnormalities in adults have also been reported in the literature (Darko et al., 1995; Gazbuda, Levy, & Chiappa, 1988; Leuchter, Newton, van Gorp, & Miller, 1989). As early as 1986, Navia, Cho et al. (1986) noted the presence of diffuse slowing in the late stages of HIV-related dementia. Leuchter and his colleagues studied a group of 28 individuals with AIDS and 56 HIV-negative controls using quantitative EEG coherence. Subjects with AIDS exhibited significantly higher EEG coherence in the 6–10-Hz band relative to the seronegative controls. Although EEG investigations have demonstrated increased abnormalities in the EEG traces of individuals with significant impairments (e.g., AIDS), Nuwer et al. (1992) noted the absence of increased abnormalities in asymptomatic HIV-positive subjects during their large prospective investigation. In a similar vein, McArthur (1987) noted that in less advanced stages of dementia the EEG traces can be normal in up to 50% of that population of patients. Most recently, Darko et al. (1995) demonstrated sleep disturbances associated with HIV infection (using sleep paradigms in adults) (see also Wiegand et al., 1991).

Neuropathological Findings

Measurable neuropathology has been observed in microscopic and gross specimens of the brain and spinal cord. As early as 1988, several investigators reported abnormalities in the brains of children diagnosed with HIV. Sharer, Cho, and Epstein (1985) conducted autopsies on 11 children infected with HIV. The results of these autopsies revealed diminished gross brain weight for their ages, inflammatory cell infiltrates, multinucleated cells and multinucleated giant cells, cerebrovascular calcification, vascular and perivascular calcification, and white-matter changes. In addition, inflammatory and vascular lesions were most pronounced in the basal ganglia and pons (Sharer et al., 1985). Similar results have been obtained by subsequent investigators (Belman et al., 1988; Epstein et al., 1988). The investigation by Epstein and his colleagues (1988) revealed diminished brain weight for age under gross examination in the children who had died of AIDS-related progressive encephalopathy. Microscopic examination indicated the presence of inflammatory cell infiltrates, multinucleated giant cells, white-matter changes, and vascular calcification supporting earlier reports by Sharer et al. (1985). On autopsy, Sharer et al. (1990) found 9 spinal cords with inflammatory cell infiltrates and 6 spinal cords with multinucleated cells, as part of a study with 18 children (16 spinal cords were autopsied) who died as a result of HIV-1 infection. They also identified myelin pallor in the corticospinal tracts in nearly half of the cases, consistent with previous studies (e.g., Dickson et al., 1989). Several studies have identified viral particles or HIV-related antigen in the multinucleated cells and other cells (Epstein et al., 1985; Koenig et al., 1986). As discussed earlier, it appears that the neuropathological effects of HIV infection on the developing brain are so devastating that they often can be detected under gross examination.

Price and his colleagues (Brew, Sidtis, Petito, & Price, 1988; Navia, Cho, et al., 1986) initially noted substantial atrophy marked by ventricular enlargement, involvement of the white-matter and subcortical structures, as well as vacuolar myelopathy of the spinal cord in adults with AIDS. Vinters, Tomiyasu, and Anders (1989) found neuropathological abnormalities in 70% to 90% of the brains of adult subjects with AIDS. Among their various findings, diffuse pallor of the white matter was the most common abnormality found. The subcortical gray-matter structures most frequently reported as showing involvement include the basal ganglia, thalamus, and the temporal–limbic centers. In contrast to the data supporting the presence of subcortical gray-matter and white-matter abnormalities, Wiley et al. (1991) and other researchers (see Everall, Luther, & Lantos, 1991, 1993) have documented the presence of neuronal loss in cortical areas as well. Using quantitative histological analysis, this group of investigators (Masliah et al., 1992) noted losses of neocortical dendritric areas of up to 40% and a correlation of these losses with levels of HIV gp41 immunoreactivity (Masliah et al., 1992). More recent studies conducting extensive reviews of autopsy data of individuals diagnosed with AIDS continue to support these findings (Masliah, Ge, Achim, & Wiley, 1995).

Neuropathological differences that may be associated with developmental factors emerge when comparing adults and children . Although similar findings have been observed in both groups, white-matter pallor is difficult to identify in children relative to adults, and periventricular infiltrates and multinucleated giant cells are common in both (McArthur, 1994).

Findings from Other CNS Correlates

Other abnormalities thought to be the result of HIV-1 infection have been identified in various CNS biological markers. Cerebrospinal fluid (CSF) has been one such index targeted (Brew et al., 1992; Brouwers et al., 1993; Carrieri, Indaco, Maiorino, & Buscaino, 1992; Epstein et al., 1987; McArthur et al., 1992).

Brouwers et al. (1993) found a high correlation between CSF levels of quinolinic acid (QUIN) and degree of encephalopathy in 40 children with HIV infection relative to 16 controls. In addition, this study revealed decreasing levels of overall mental abilities (Bayley Scales [MDI], McCarthy Scales [GCI] and WISC-R [FSIQ]) to be associated with increasing levels of QUIN. Similarly, in a study assessing levels of serum tumor necrosis factor alpha (TNFα), Mintz (1989) found elevated levels of this marker related to progressive encephalopathy in children with AIDS. Tardieu, Blanche, Duliege, Rouzioux, and Griscelli (1989), using antigen-capture assays specific to HIV-1-p24, also found detectable levels of this marker in the CSF of children. In the same year, Hutto et al. (1989) reported abnormalities in the CSF of children infected with HIV.

Investigations examining CSF composition (Heyes et al., 1991) also have detected elevated levels of QUIN in HIV-infected adults. In fact, Martin, Heyes, et al. (1992) reported significant correlations between elevated CSF excitotoxic quinolinic acid and decreased motor performance. Resnick et al. (1985) and Resnick et al. (1988) were able to isolate HIV in the cerebrospinal fluid of infected adult subjects. More important, CSF β-2 microglobulin absolute levels and CSF/serum ratios have exhibited some specificity in discriminating between HIV-1-Associated Dementia and multiple sclerosis or other CNS disorders (Carrieri et al., 1992).

Neurobehavioral, Neurodevelopmental, and Neuropsychologic Findings in HIV-1 Disease

Neurodevelopmental, neurobehavioral, and neuropsychological sequelae as a result of HIV infection have been frequently reported in the developmental and adult literature (Brouwers, Belman, & Epstein, 1994; Brouwers et al., 1994; Chase et al., in-press; Cohen et al., 1991; Diamond et al., 1987; Fernandez, 1988; Fowler, 1994; Grant & Martin, 1994; Levin, Berger, Didona, & Duncan, 1992; Levy & Fernandez, 1997; Llorente et al., 1998, 2000; McArthur et al., 1989; Miller et al., 1990; Navia, Jordan, & Price, 1986; Perdices & Cooper, 1989; van Gorp et al., 1989, 1993). Therefore, the remainder of this chapter reviews neuropsychological and neurobehavioral correlates associated with this infectious disease, with findings from studies which included ethnic-minority populations. Although an attempt will be made to integrate the clinicopathological findings presented above with the neuropsychological literature, thus describing the brain–behavior relationships associated with this disease, the reader is cautioned regarding the generalization of these findings due to the scarcity of studies addressing the impact of HIV on cognitive and neuropsychologic functions in these ethnic groups. In addition, recent studies have indicated that cultural factors may modulate neuropsychological performance in groups of ethnic minority persons with HIV-1 disease.

Overall Intellectual Functioning

Several studies have found impairments in overall levels of cognitive abilities as a result of HIV infection in children and adults. A lowering in overall intellectual functioning within the borderline and mild mental retardation range has been reported by several researchers in children (Boivin et al., 1995; Brouwers et al., 1991; see Fowler, 1994, for review) and lowering of intellectual abilities in children is most often associated with encephalopathy (Manly et al., 1998). In adults, van Gorp et al. (1989) reported data noting lower WAIS-R Full Scale and Verbal IQ scores in a group of symptomatic HIV-positive subjects in the U.S., some of which were ethnic minorities (e.g., Hispanics) albeit fully fluent in English, relative to a group of HIV-negative participants. Similar findings were reported by Rubinow, Berttini, Brouwers, and Lane (1988) for the WAIS-R Full Scale IQ score. In general, however, no differences in measures of global intellectual functioning have been found between asymptomatic HIV-positive subjects and HIV-negative controls (McAllister et al., 1992; Stern et al., 1991) including studies which examined ethnic minorities (e.g., see McArthur et al., 1989 and Miller et al., 1990 for an investigation [MACS] evaluating the natural history of HIV infection in men where approximately 9% of their cohort were persons from ethnic-minority backgrounds).

In summary, it appears that HIV infection may be capable of causing impairments in the overall cognitive abilities of some children and adults regardless of ethnicity. The degree of intellectual impact in select patients is consistent with the magnitude of neuropathology sometimes observed in this disease process, including HIV-related cerebral atrophy and acquired microcephaly in the case of some infants and children, and opportunistic diseases in the case of adults. These debilitating CNS insults are quite capable of accounting for the global dampening in intellectual functioning observed in some of these patients, particularly during the late symptomatic stage of the disease process (Heaton et al., 1995).

Attention and Concentration

A study by Brouwers et al. (1989) investigating attentional processes in children with HIV infection examined the WISC-R Freedom from Distractibility factor (Kaufman, 1975). The results from this investigation revealed that HIV-positive children experienced "relative weaknesses" on this factor. However, Brouwers, Moss, et al. (1994) cautioned that these deficits could very well have been the result of other factors not related to HIV involvement per se, such as potential confounds (e.g., the high base rates of attention difficulties in children for this age group in the general population). Furthermore, although behavioral assessment has revealed that these children may indeed suffer from attentional deficits (Hittelman et al., 1991), the children studied in these investigations were quite young. In another investigation using cluster analytic procedures, one group of symptomatic HIV-infected children revealed a cluster that could be identified as a result of attention deficits (Brouwers et al., 1992). Although further studies need to be conducted with children infected with the human immunodeficiency virus to determine whether the attention deficits observed during neuropsychological testing are the result of the disease process versus other etiologies (diseases in general; see Tarter, Edwards, & van Thiel, 1988), given the fragile nature of these processes (Lezak, 1978), the probability is high that these mechanisms may be indeed compromised by this infectious disease. In addition, from a brain–behavior perspective, during severe expressions of the disease in children, white-matter involvement has been identified as a neuropathological hallmark of HIV, especially pontine calcification (Sharer et al., 1985). Therefore, it is possible that HIV affects ascending pathways from the reticular activating system or other deep-matter substrates involved in attentional functions, and is responsible for the deficits observed in this domain.

Disturbances in attention and concentration represent a hallmark manifestation of this disease in adults (Butters et al., 1990; Heaton et al., 1995; Levy & Fernandez, 1997; Miller et al., 1990; Navia et al., 1986b; Stern et al., 1991), particularly as they relate to attentional mechanisms such as complex divided and sustained attention as measured by the Paced Auditory Serial Addition Test (PASAT) during late disease stages (Grant et al., 1987; van Gorp et al., 1989). Some investigators, however, have reported deficits in complex attentional skills even during the asymptomatic stage of HIV disease, though usually identifying subtle differences on variables such as reaction time, which may have little clinical and adaptational significance (see Stern et al., 1990). In contrast to deficits found on procedures assessing complex attentional processes, results from neuropsychological tests of simple attention (e.g.,

WAIS-R, Digit Span) have not revealed impairment in either asymptomatic or symptomatic adults (Miller et al., 1990; van Gorp et al., 1989). Similar results have been noted in studies which included a significant number of ethnic minorities. For example, deficits in simple attention span were not observed in the controlled investigation that utilized "ethnicity" (Hispanics) as a research variable by Levin and her colleagues (Levin et al., 1992). Although a quasi-experimental study (Klusman, Moulton, Hornbostel, Picano, & Beattier, 1991) examining attentional processes in HIV-positive asymptomatic military personnel (including ethnic minorities as part of their "Black" and "Mixed Ethnic" groups) found significant differences on the WAIS-R Digit Span subtest, particularly Digits Backward, between white and black participants, favoring the former group, no differences were observed between the white and mixed-ethnic groups. In summary, simple attentional processes may be spared in both asymptomatic and symptomatic groups, with deficits in complex attentional mechanisms, such as divided and sustained attention, most commonly observed in late-stage HIV disease. As was the case with children, alterations in attention and concentration should be interpreted with care in adult populations since neuropsychiatric disturbances (e.g., anxiety and depression) commonly observed during HIV infection (Fernandez, 1989) could account for a portion of the attentional deficits attributed to primary concentration/attention mechanisms (van Gorp et al., 1993).

Learning and Memory

Infection with HIV may cause direct memory deficits in children (Bellman et al., 1988; Diamond, 1989; Levenson, Mellins, Zawadzki, Kairam, & Stein, 1992). Boivin et al. (1995) reported impairments in verbal and visual memory in a group of African (Zairian) children 2 years old and older. Specifically, HIV-positive participants, relative to controls and HIV-negative children born to infected mothers, obtained significantly lower levels of performance on the K-ABC Immediate Recall and Spatial Memory subtests (these measures assess, among other functions, emerging immediate verbal and visual recall, respectively). Significant differences were also observed on another measure of visual immediate recall (K-ABC, Hand Movements). In summary, although it is difficult to define what constitutes memory in very young children, or to what extent the difficulties observed in recall in these populations are driven by attentional deficits, relative to memory impairments proper, it appears that HIV infection may be capable of causing disturbances in attentional as well as memory mechanisms (verbal and visual) in childhood.

Although conflicting results have been reported in the literature regarding the extent of verbal and visual memory difficulties in adults (van Gorp et al., 1993), different aspects of these abilities have been observed to undergo compromise during HIV infection. Janssen et al. (1989) reported that a group of symptomatic HIV-seropositive subjects performed worse than seronegative controls on the Wechsler Memory Scale's passages recall (Logical Prose subtest). Miller et al. (1990) found symptomatic seropositive subjects to perform worse on the Rey Auditory Verbal Learning Test relative to seronegative controls (see Harris, Cullum, and Puente [1995] with regard to the effects of bilingualism on verbal learning tasks). Although somewhat against expectations due to their asymptomatic state, Wilkie et al. (1990) found a group of infected participants to perform significantly lower relative to controls on a task assessing delayed recall of passages, whereas Levin et al. (1992) found Hispanic infected participants to perform lower than noninfected, non-Hispanic subjects on a list learning task (California Verbal Learning Test, Trial 5).

With regard to visual memory, several investigations have noted impairments in performance in groups of HIV-symptomatic subjects relative to seronegative controls on various measures assessing this domain. For example, van Gorp et al. (1989) and Ollo and Pass (1988) reported significantly lower recall on the Wechsler Memory Scales (WMS-R), Visual Reproduction subtest, and on the delayed recall portion of the Rey–Osterrieth Complex Figure on the part of symptomatic HIV-seropositive subjects relative to seronegative controls. Despite the unfortunate fact that their study did not use a control group (quasi-experimental), Klusman et al. (1991) found lower performance on the WMS-R, Visual Reproduction Subtest (Immediate recall), in their "Black" and "Mixed Ethnic" asymptomatic group relative to their group of Caucasian asymptomatic participants (see Ardila, Rosselli, & Rosas [1989] for a discussion on the effects of illiteracy on visual–spatial and memory skills in general). Pending further research, the aforementioned findings combined (children and adults) buttress a hypothesis suggesting that memory compromises may be a manifestation of HIV infection (Ryan, Paolo, & Skrade, 1992).

Language and Auditory Processing

Declines and deficits in language, specifically expressive language difficulties, and auditory processing delays associated with HIV infection have been reported in the developmental literature (Bellman et al., 1985; Wolters, Brouwers, Moss, & Pizzo, 1994). Language-related deficits in infancy and childhood are to a certain extent modulated by the mode of viral transmission in conjunction with the degree of disease progression and age of the child. A vertically infected infant who suffers from progressive encephalopathy will display delays in acquiring and developing language, whereas an older child who becomes infected with HIV horizontally may eventually develop regression or complete loss of speech, slurred speech (probably confounded with oral–motor difficulties), as well as regression in other language skills from previous levels of functioning.

Although deficits in both receptive and expressive language have been reported in the pediatric literature (see Epstein et al., 1986), the majority of insult occurs in the expressive domain with relatively spared receptive skills (Brouwers, Moss, et al., 1994). Data-based evidence for this observation was also reported by Wolters and associates (Wolters et al., 1994). They demonstrated, as part of a study of adaptive functioning using the Vineland Adaptive Behavior Scales, that expressive skills suffered greater insult relative to receptive abilities.

In contrast to findings in the pediatric literature, language functions have largely been found to be spared in adulthood using a variety of tasks such as confrontation naming (Boston Naming Test), word-list generation (controlled oral–word fluency test), and vocabulary tests (WAIS-R), even when comparing symptomatic HIV-positive subjects to seronegative controls (Miller et al., 1990; Stern, Sano, Williams, & Gorman, 1989; Tross et al., 1988; van Gorp et al., 1989). Two investigations, however, yielded results indicating language impairments. Differences in the WAIS-R Vocabulary subtest were found between asymptomatic HIV-positive subjects and controls (Heaton el al., 1995) and between symptomatic seropositive subjects and controls (Heaton et al., 1995; Saykin et al., 1988), as well as between symptomatic seropositive subjects relative to controls on a word-list generation test. Levin and her colleagues (1992) also found language differences not only as a result of serostatus (asymptomatic seropositive subjects performed poorer on these measures relative to seronegative controls) but secondary to "ethnicity" (Hispanics scored lower than non-Hispanics) on the Boston Naming Test, Controlled Oral–Word Fluency Test (Food), and WAIS-R Vocabulary subtest.

Motor, Psychomotor, Speeded Functions, and Executive Skills

Given the striking and profound involvement observed with neuroradiological and neuropathological techniques in the basal ganglia complex of children with HIV infection and AIDS, specifically calcific vasculopathy and inflammatory CNS diseases, it is not surprising to detect motor deficits in these children during developmental and neuropsychological evaluation. As a result, gross- and fine-motor delays are prominent in symptomatic immunosuppressed infants and older children and are often some of the most frequent aspects of functioning to fall prey to the disease process (Chase et al., in press; Fowler, 1994; Hittelman et al., 1990, 1991; Ultmann, 1985). Specifically, infants display muscle tone abnormalities as well as delays across all other aspects of this domain. Even seemingly unaffected asymptomatic HIV-positive infants less than 2 years of age have been observed to suffer from motor delays (Boivin et al., 1995). Older children, including preschoolers and school-age children, also display abnormalities in this domain, initially marked by disturbances in gait and balance (Brouwers, Belman, et al., 1994). However, according to Fowler (1994), in contrast to infants and toddlers, older children and adolescents tend to suffer only from mild neurologic impairments, including motor dysfunction (e.g., fine-motor tremor) until the latter stages of the disease process. In more severe cases, the ability to ambulate is lost due to pronounced gross-motor deficits in the lower extremities, most likely associated with neuropathological processes affecting the basal ganglia complex. Brouwers, Moss, et al. (1994) reported, as might be expected, that more serious deficits in this domain may be observed, including spastic quadriparesis and pyramidal tract signs, with greater levels of CNS involvement such as progressive encephalopathy (see Belman et al., 1988).

In summary, pronounced delays in motor functioning are evidenced in symptomatic immunocompromised infants and older children, including motor tone abnormalities and other motor delays, with greater arrest in development correlated with increasing levels of disease involvement, particularly progressive encephalopathy. Even seemingly unaffected HIV-positive asymptomatic infants may display mild delays in this domain. Although rare, due to the low incidence of these diseases in children, abrupt onset of motor difficulties, different from those described above, are sometimes seen in those with acquired opportunistic diseases (e.g., lymphoma) as a result of their immunocompromised condition.

Navia, Jordan, and colleagues (1986) considered motor difficulties to be one of the hallmark symptoms of the AIDS Dementia Complex, and gross-motor impairment is commonly found in late-stages of HIV dementia. Results on neuropsychological indices of fine-motor skills, however, have been mixed. Motor speed (finger tapping) and fine-motor coordination as measured by the Grooved Pegboard Test (Kløve, 1963) failed to show impairments in groups of symptomatic HIV-positive research participants in studies conducted by Claypoole et al. (1990), Franzblau et al. (1991), and Stern et al. (1989). In contrast, relative to controls, symptomatic HIV-seropositive subjects displayed slower performance on the Grooved Pegboard Test in investigations conducted by Miller et al. (1990) and Tross et al. (1988). Klusman et al. (1991) also found motor and psychomotor differences (finger tapping asymmetry) favoring "White" relative to "Black" and "Ethnically-Mixed" asymptomatic participants. Therefore, it is evident that at least a subsample of HIV-infected individuals display fine-motor impairments, particularly during the advanced stages of the disease, and in some cases during early mildly symptomatic stages (CDC Group A, Heaton et al., 1995; Levy & Fernandez, 1997), and that these difficulties do indeed represent one of the cardinal abnormalities observed in HIV infection in adulthood (Navia, Jordan, et al., 1986; Martin et al., 1994; Selnes & Miller, 1994; Butters et al., 1990).

Combined with these motor difficulties, pronounced slowing of information processing (Hart, Wade, Klinger, & Levenson, 1990; Llorente et al., 1998; Martin et al., 1992), even after controlling for the effects of peripheral neuropathy and other putative confounds (e.g., mood) (Llorente et al., 1998), slowed psychomotor speed (Perdices & Cooper, 1989; Selnes & Miller, 1994), and impaired cognitive flexibility (e.g., Llorente et al., 1998; Martin et al., 1992) have also been considered chief signs of symptomatic HIV-1 disease in adulthood. Martin and colleagues (Martin et al., 1992) and Llorente et al. (1998), using procedures known to assess information processing mechanisms, such as a Stroop Color-Word Test and complex sequential reaction time tasks, have shown slowing of these mechanisms subsequent to symptomatic HIV infection (see Figure 1).

Although the findings have been more equivocal (see Stern et al., 1989), other executive skills in adults have been shown in some investigations to be impaired in seropositive subjects relative to controls on tasks including the Wisconsin Card Sorting Test and the Trailmaking Test B (Claypoole et al., 1990; Grant et al., 1987; Klusman et al., 1991). However, a recent investigation using a Stroop Interference Task, Trailmaking Test B, and complex reaction time tasks, measures requiring frontal system skills including inhibitory processes, found no differences between asymptomatic HIV-positive (ASYMHIV+)and HIV-negative participants after controlling for age, education, depressive symptomatology, peripheral neuropathy, and other potential confounds (Llorente et al., 1998). In contrast, significant differences were found between HIV+ symptomatic participants relative to both normal controls and HIV+ asymptomatic participants on this measure (see Llorente et al., 1998).

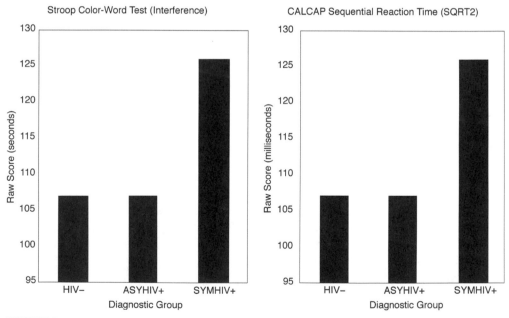

FIGURE 1. Mean sequential reaction time (CALCAP, SQRT2) and Stroop Color-Word Test (interference) scores across diagnostic groups depicting the selective information process slowing evidenced during the symptomatic stage of infection (SYMHIV+). Also note the similarities in information processing scores in the HIV-negative (HIV−) and asymptomatic HIV-positive groups (ASYMHIV+). In this study, 10%, 17%, and 14%, respectively, of the HIV−, ASYMHIV+, and SYMHIV+ participants were ethnic-minority individuals. (Adapted from Llorente et al., 1998; reprinted with permission.)

From a correlative viewpoint, the deficits observed in neuropsychological performance subserved by frontal skills in adulthood are consistent with neuropathological findings. For example, Everall et al. (1991) reported neuronal loss in the frontal cortex of symptomatic and more impaired (dementing) individuals infected with HIV. Nevertheless, care should be exercised in grouping together findings from different procedures assessing frontal systems as if they were homogenous since each of the neuropsychological instruments used may be measuring different aspects of frontal skills. Finally, caution must be exercised not to readily generalize these findings to minority groups as only a small number of minorities have been used in these investigations.

Adaptive, Behavioral, and Neuropsychiatric Manifestations

Other areas of psychological functioning have been shown to undergo dramatic alterations associated with adult and pediatric HIV infection and/or its treatment (Bayés, 1995; Brouwers, Belman, et al., 1994; Fernandez, 1988; Fernandez et al., 1988; Perry, 1990). These disturbances may be capable of further impacting neuropsychological performance. For example, indirect effects (Brouwers, Moss, et al., 1994) associated with environmental factors and stressors, coupled with host variables (e.g., psychological resources, educational level, coping strategies), synergistically operating with the disease process (e.g., undergoing multiple medical procedures and hospitalizations as part of radiation treatment for an opportunistic disease; see Tarter et al., 1988) may impact upon the child's overall level of functioning. These behavioral and adaptive factors play a major role in the way that HIV symptoms exhibit themselves from patient to patient and must be taken into consideration when evaluating them, performing research with these populations, or providing rehabilitative interventions. Similarly, a large portion of ethnic-minority children infected with HIV, whether in the U.S. or abroad, come from low SES and underserved backgrounds (Tuckson, 1994) for which there is sometimes little normative data or for which inferences made on the data available would be invalid for the purposes at hand or the population under investigation. For these reasons, caution must be exercised when interpreting neuropsychological findings, in light of these potential confounds, since children with HIV infection tend to display augmented behavioral disturbances (Ultmann et al., 1985).

Mood and anxiety disorders have been assessed in adult individuals with HIV infection and appear to be the most common of all neuropsychiatric disorders to affect this population. Fernandez (1988), Fernandez et al. (1988), and Levy and Fernandez (1997) have reported elevations on measures assessing these domains. Miller et al. (1990) reported elevations on the CES-D in their group of symptomatic patients relative to controls (MACS) of which approximately 9% of the sample were of ethnic-minority origin. Van Gorp and his colleagues (1990) also reported elevations on the Beck Depression Inventory and on Scale 2 of the MMPI-168 in a group of clinically-referred symptomatic seropositive individuals relative to controls. Although equivocal findings were reported by several investigators in the literature (Janssen et al., 1989; van Gorp et al., 1989), a recent report by Heaton and his colleagues (1995) noted significant elevations on the Hamilton Anxiety and Depression Scales and the BDI in their HIV-positive group relative to controls. Nevertheless, it should be noted that several studies failed to find a significant relationship of mood dysfunction to cognitive compromise (e.g., van Gorp et al., 1989).

Finally, extreme caution should be exercised not to attribute neurological (e.g., frontal-systems dysfunction) signs and symptoms sometimes associated with increased immunosuppression (e.g., disinhibition, poor planning, difficulties shifting set/perseverations) to a primary psychiatric disorder (e.g., personality disorders). This is an important differential-diagnosis since the former is capable of mimicking symptoms of the latter, and to complicate matters, they often occur concurrently in people with HIV-1 infection. This caution is particularly important when assessing African American and Latina women (see LoPresti, Llorente, Guzzard, & Brumm, 1998, in which 58% of the sample were ethnic-minority women).

Special Considerations for Research and Clinical Evaluations with HIV+ Ethnic-Minority Populations

Although other chapters in this volume will articulate in a more comprehensive manner some of the specific topics covered in this section, they are now briefly addressed as they are closely associated with HIV infection and ethnic-minority populations. General cross-cultural issues unique to the assessment of neurobehavioral disorders in these groups, and as expounded by other investigators (Ardila, Rosselli, & Puente, 1994; Pontón & Ardila, 1999), should be strongly considered.

With regard to the evaluation process, an assessment posture should be adopted addressing *level of acculturation* (Marín & Marín, 1991; Stern et al., 1992), problems posed by *linguistic* issues including bilingualism (Harris et al., 1995; Laosa, 1984; Marín & Marín, 1991), *SES* (Pérez-Arce, 1994), *level of formal education* (Ardilla et al., 1989; see Satz et al., 1993 for low level of education as a risk factor for cognitive abnormalities in HIV-1), *examiner characteristics*, as well as factors capable of modulating these variables (see Llorente, Pontón, Taussig, & Satz, [1999] for a discussion of the impact of American immigration patterns upon the process of normative data acquisition and inference for Hispanics).

When conducting assessments with ethnic-minority toddlers and preschool children from families whose primary language is not English, problems with rapport may occur when the evaluation is conducted through an interpreter (see Likely, 1987 for this topic in general) or when the clinician is unfamiliar with sociocultural issues relevant to the population. A nonstandardized administration is often conducted, translating items into the child's language (e.g., Spanish), which then further limits the inferences that can be made from test results. Even when administering tests and procedures in English, the level of acculturation is one factor which influences the degree to which valid and reliable interpretations can be made. For example, children from primarily Spanish-speaking families often demonstrate increased familiarity with the English language after enrolling in school. Improvements noted on subsequent evaluations, rather than indicating beneficial response to treatment, may simply reflect greater understanding and expression of the English language; for children who have not attended preschool settings, improvements upon retest may reflect greater comfort level with elements of the evaluation, such as sitting at a child's table and attending in a sustained manner to activities presented by the examiner. The lack of neuropsychological measures developed and standardized on ethnic-minority children and adults and the dearth of appropriate normative data are also major obstacles which greatly limit the validity of inferences that can be made from test results. In sum, level of acculturation, education, language, and other cross-cultural issues in neuropsychological assessment can have indirect consequences on the examinations of the HIV-positive minority individual.

The setting in which neuropsychological services are provided is critical as well (see van Gorp et al., 1995). For example, research providing neuropsychological consultation in community mental health centers has revealed that staff in those centers tend to attribute HIV-related cognitive symptomatology to psychiatric and personality variables rather than to HIV-related CNS impediments (LoPresti et al., 1998). This is an important issue since a large portion of the patient populations in these clinics is comprised of African American and Latina women and adolescents.

Although a detailed exposition is beyond the scope of this chapter, the issue of drug use in HIV infection should be given special attention, as a large number of men, women, and adolescents from ethnic-minority backgrounds are exposed to the virus through intravenous drug use. In particular, a disproportionate number of African American and Hispanic males, relative to all other ethnic or racial groups, became infected through intravenous drug use (IVDU) (CDC, 1996). While some researchers have suggested that the effect of HIV on the immune system serves to worsen the neurocognitive impairment associated with drug use (McKegney et al., 1990; Silberstein et al., 1987), other investigators (Royal et al., 1991; Selnes et al., 1992) have argued that the presence of HIV infection in drug users is incapable of accounting for the majority of neuropsychological deficits observed and does not increase the sequelae associated with drug use. Further research will have to elucidate the complex reactions between HIV infection and drug use on the brain.

HIV-related neuropsychological sequelae in women also deserves special attention, particularly in ethnic-minority women. Consistent with early reports (see Mann et al., 1992), present trends in the epidemiology of HIV infection continue to indicate that women, more than any other group infected with HIV, represent the leading cohort of newly reported infected cases (CDC, 1996). More akin to this chapter, of the entire population of women infected with HIV, women of color, particularly African American and Latinas, comprise 75% of the HIV+ female cohort (CDC, 1996; see also Dicks, 1994). Yet, women with HIV infection have received little attention (Long & Leger, 1995; Wofsy, 1987) and have not been included in studies in sufficient numbers to permit gender comparisons (Fox, Ethier, Cerreta, & Ickovics, 1995). Although recent efforts have increased the participation of women in research and clinical trials, as late as 1992 women had not been included in many of the trials used to develop antiretroviral medications (Wofsy, 1987). This is unfortunate since HIV disease expression in women may be different from that observed in men (Schuman & Sobel, 1993). Indeed, neurocognitive findings from studies reporting gender-specific results suggest that women's cognitive profiles may be different as well (Dorfman, Handelsman, Williams, Kincaid, & Hauser, 1995; Stern et al., 1995). Few studies are available, however, that have addressed neurobehavioral functioning specifically in infected women.

In a study group primarily comprised of African American and Caucasian women, Stern and colleagues (1998) found no differences between HIV+ asymptomatic and seronegative women in attention, information-processing speed, executive functioning, fine-motor dexterity/ speed, visuoconstructive skills, learning and memory, and apathy, fatigue, and mood. It is noteworthy, however, that a high percentage of women in both groups demonstrated impairment on a number of cognitive and mood-related measures, although there was no significant difference in the number of seropositive or seronegative women who scored in the impaired range. In contrast to findings in select groups of asymptomatic HIV-positive men (White et al., 1995), asymptomatic women did not demonstrate subtle impairment on measures assessing speeded information processing/reaction time. Symptomatic women, however, demonstrated greater cognitive impairment than groups of infected gay men and infected IVDUs, even when controlling for age, level of education, and other comorbid factors (Dorfman et al., 1995). A well-designed longitudinal neuropsychological study with ethnic-minority women is under-way and it will soon yield informative data (see Durvasala & Miller, 1997). Additional neurocognitive studies that have included women but have not reported specific gender-related findings will not be described here.

Two studies by Brown and Rundell (1990, 1993) reported psychiatric diagnoses in primarily African American and Caucasian females in the U.S. Air Force. As a group, the military women studied share fewer characteristics with HIV+ women described in epidemiologic studies, in that they are middle-class, relatively better educated, and employed. Brown and Rundell (1990) found that none of the asymptomatic women met criteria for a major mood disorder, but half received diagnoses that included personality disorders, hypoactive sexual desire disorder, and organic mental disorder which was described as mild cognitive changes consistent with an early dementing process. A later report by these authors (Brown & Rundell, 1993) found that women were more likely to receive a psychiatric diagnosis at reevaluation (76%) than at the time of study entry (41%), with the increase accounted for primarily by additional women being diagnosed with hypoactive sexual desire at the followup point (from 14% to 44%). Overall, a low level of mood-related symptoms and alcohol/substance disorders was reported.

More impairment has been found in studies of HIV-positive women in hospital-based clinics and community clinics. These women represent primarily ethnic/racial minority groups (with African American women comprising the largest percentage) and have less education and lower SES than women who participated in the studies described above. Significant levels of depression were found in HIV-positive women who underwent clinical diagnostic interview (James, Rubin, & Willis, 1991; McDaniel, Cohen-Cole, Farber, Summerville, & Fowlie, 1995; Taylor, Amodei, & Mangos, 1996) or completed self-report questionnaires (Coons, Spence, Harwell, Walsh, & Spriepe, 1995; Kaplan, Marks, & Mertens, 1997; LoPresti et al., 1998; Moore et al., 1995; Orr, Celentano, Santelli, & Burwell, 1994). In these studies, 20% to 50% of women were found to have a significant level of depressive symptomatology. Anxiety has also been reported in HIV-positive women (Kaplan, Marks, & Mertens, 1997). In the only study describing gender-related differences in mood and substance abuse, roughly equivalent numbers of men and women had a depressive disorder (47% and 40%, respectively), but men received a broader range of psychiatric diagnoses and reported abusing a broader range of substances (McDaniels et al., 1995).

Factors such as current or prior substance abuse and a history of psychiatric condition have not been consistently assessed by investigators, but substantial disturbances were noted in several studies. Active substance abuse was present in one-third of pregnant ethnic-minority women who had just learned of their HIV status (James, Rubin, & Willis, 1991), in one-third of women who were newly referred to a large, outpatient infectious-disease clinic (McDaniel et al., 1995), and in nearly one-half of women referred to an AIDS clinic by community practitioners (Taylor, Amodei, & Mangos, 1996). In contrast, women who had established ties to community-based centers that provide substantial supportive services to individuals and families living with HIV/AIDS reported a much lower level of active substance use, with only 15% of women indicating sporadic drug use (LoPresti et al., 1998). A large percentage of women also have reported histories positive for both substance abuse and mood disturbances (LoPresti et al., 1998; McDaniels et al., 1995).

Relative to women without substance abuse histories, HIV-positive women who reported a history of IVDU had more psychiatric disorders (Clark & Bessinger, 1997), psychological distress (Franke, Jager, Thomann, & Beyer, 1992; Mellers, Marchand-Gonod, King, Laupa, & Smith, 1994), and mood or personality disorders (James et al., 1991). In a sample of male and female IVDUs comprised of both HIV+ and seronegative individuals, Lipsitz and colleagues (1994) found roughly equivalent numbers of HIV+ compared with seronegative women who were depressed (26% vs. 30%), while depression was significantly more prevalent in infected men relative to uninfected men (33% vs. 16%).

In summary, studies of neurobehavioral functioning in women are only beginning to emerge. Early evidence of gender-related differences (Dorfman et al., 1995; Lipsitz et al., 1994; McDaniels et al., 1995; Stern et al., 1998) highlights the need to devote more attention to women, particularly women of color, since they comprise the majority of HIV-infected females. It is of particular importance to note that a large percentage of women reported histories of substance abuse and psychological distress, with multiple chronic psychosocial stressors in their lives that predated their HIV diagnoses. Women with previous or current drug/alcohol abuse also reported the highest levels of current depressive symptoms. This type of behavioral presentation is quite common in women who present at social service agencies with a need for assistance with comprehensive management of medical and social services. In our study of women referred from community agencies for evaluation due to concerns from staff that women were experiencing HIV-related neurobehavioral changes (LoPresti et al., 1998), we found striking discrepancies between staffs' perceptions of women's cognitive functioning and actual findings from neuropsychological evaluations. In discussions with agency staff, it became clear that problems with adaptive functioning that would have been attributed to substance use, unfamiliarity with bureaucratic systems, and overtaxed coping strategies *in the absence of an HIV diagnosis* were almost routinely being interpreted by staff as resulting from HIV-related dementia when such a neurocognitive dysfunction was not present.

Several researchers (Bornstein, 1994; Brouwers et al., 1994; Butters et al., 1990; Selnes & Miller, 1994) have addressed critical issues associated with the neuropsychologic assessment of HIV infection throughout the lifespan that also apply to research and clinical assessment with ethnic-minority populations. Butters and his colleagues (1990) alluded to the need to assess a broad set of functions typically affected by prototypical subcortical dementias (e.g., Supranuclear Palsy) as described by Cummings and Benson (1983). To this end, they recommend procedures that would assess attention, executive skills (abstraction), language, memory (verbal and visual), motor abilities, psychomotor speed and speed of processing, and visuospatial/visuoperceptive skills. Bornstein (1994) discussed the importance of variables such as adequate sample size, the need for repeated assessment, and issues associated with impairment and exclusion criteria. Selnes and Miller (1994) also addressed important methodological concerns, including the need for comprehensive assessment while simultaneously minding issues associated with fatigue in individuals with HIV, the need for longitudinal assessment, the assessment of a wide range of neuropsychological domains, and the robustness of neuropsychological tests to serial repetition. Given that cognitive slowing is one of the principal symptoms of HIV-related cognitive impairment, speed of processing also should be a focus of assessment (see Llorente et al., 1998).

Methodological issues relevant to longitudinal assessment of HIV infected infants and children must also be considered. Brouwers et al. (1991) discussed the importance of using a comprehensive test battery with interim monitoring using a smaller number of tests to ensure that treatment effects and/or disease progression are monitored while at the same time minimizing practice effects. Brouwers et al. (1991) also highlighted the need to interpret serial assessments within the context of normal developmental growth, possible AIDS-related deterioration, and sociocultural factors. In addition, they provided suggestions for modifying testing procedures to accommodate chronically ill children who are functioning below age level (commonly seen in children with progressive encephalopathy) or have other handicapping conditions.

Although a detailed coverage of the treatment of HIV-related neurobehavioral and neuropsychological sequelae is beyond the scope of this chapter, interventions with the HIV-infected ethnic-minority patient should be multidisciplinary in scope. A multifactorial treatment approach should address medical and cognitive aspects with the aid of state of the art

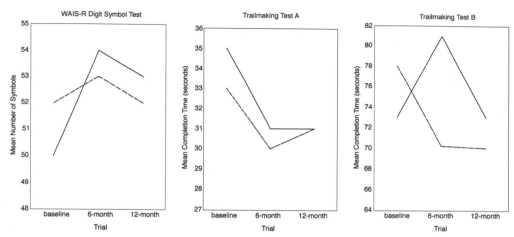

FIGURE 2. Longitudinal (baseline-12 month) neuropsychological data from a randomized, double-blind, placebo-controlled trial of zidovudine (AZT). Note the lack of sustained neuropsychological improvements (increased or no change in completion time on Trailmaking Test A & B and reduction or no change in the number of symbols copied on WAIS-R, Digit Symbol) as a result of protracted high-dose (1500 mg) AZT administration to mildly symptomatic HIV-positive individuals (——) and control participants (– – –). (Adapted from Llorente et al., 1994; reprinted with permission.)

antiretroviral medication regimens including zidovudine (AZT) and other antiretrovirals (e.g., ddI), protease inhibitors, or combinations thereof under the care of a physician knowledgeable in the treatment of infectious diseases including HIV-1 infection (Hamilton et al., 1992; Mappou, Lane, Wagner, Malone, & Skillman, 1996; Sidtis et al. 1993; Wolters et al., 1990, 1991, 1994). Medication regimens should be monitored regularly to assess their efficacy and outcome in a formal objective fashion with the aid of specialized neuropsychological examinations, carefully addressing the benefits of antiretrovirals and similar treatments on cognitive functions, bearing in mind the limitations associated with these treatments (e.g., the transient nature of cognitive improvement subsequent to antiviral treatments in some patients) (see Llorente, Stern, & van Gorp, 1994, and Figure 2). In addition to pharmacological treatment, the HIV-infected ethnic-minority patient, and particularly the immunocompromised and constitutional symptomatic patient, should receive therapy addressing pragmatic aspects of daily living and social functioning (Buckingham & van Gorp, 1988; Harris, 1992; Wiener & Septimus, 1994), as well as cognitive rehabilitation (Levy & Fernandez, 1997). Support groups may also be of aid to some patients and should be given due weight (see Grant, 1988).

Longstanding psychosocial difficulties in women must also be considered, with comprehensive treatment potentially including referrals to medical specialists, drug/alcohol-treatment programs, mental-health providers, support groups, social workers who may provide assistance with housing and finances, and legal aid (Morokoff, Mays, & Coons, 1997). In addition, for women with children, treatment may require focus on issues around parenting and school consultation.

Conclusions

The study of the neuropsychological sequelae of HIV-1 infection and cultural factors associated with this disease in adults, adolescents, and children warrants unique consideration.

This unique merit is derived from the documented effects of HIV on the CNS in conjunction with the epidemic nature of this disease worldwide, and in particular, with its staggering impact on individuals from ethnic-minority backgrounds in the U.S and abroad. Clinicopathological correlates and neuropsychological sequelae indicate the proclivity of the virus to enter and infect the brain early in the disease process, exhibiting subtle if any manifestation during the asymptomatic stage but more dramatic sequelae subsequent to the development of constitutional symptomatology or a significant immunocompromised state. At its most pernicious expression, neurological and neuropsychological findings suggest that HIV is capable of producing significant impairments throughout the lifespan marked by encephalopathy in infants and children, while mimicking normal aging or subcortical dementias in adults predominantly by infringing on speeded psychomotor and information processing functions. Although tempting, caution must be exercised in subsuming groups of individuals falling within the same categorical labels on the basis of their serological status (i.e., asymptomatic, symptomatic) as homogeneous, particularly with regard to their cognitive and neuropsychological status.

Recent research has indicated that specific biological responses (e.g., chemokine response) may be responsible for differential disease expression in ethnic groups, and may have implications for neuropsychology as well. Cultural variables are also relevant in the assessment of the HIV-positive ethnic-minority patient, and while such issues may not have direct impact on neurobehavioral examinations, a modulating effect can be expected at the very least. Using an analogy, level of acculturation, language, and other cross-cultural issues in neuropsychological assessment may be thought of as modulating factors in the same way that a severely handicapping condition affects the assessment of those people (e.g., deaf individuals). As the degree of the handicapping condition (e.g., deafness) increases in an individual, it increasingly modulates the fashion in which the assessment of such an individual is conducted (e.g., not administering the verbal scales of an intelligence test). In the same fashion, although not a handicapping condition in the traditional sense, ethnicity, level of acculturation and language, for example, modulate the fashion in which an evaluation should be conducted with ethnic-minority individuals. As the level of acculturation and language of the person undergoing assessment increasingly differ from that of the examiner and/or the mainstream population, the greater the alterations and changes that must be made to the evaluation of the ethnic-minority person, including the selection of assessment procedures, normative data, and related factors as they affect the outcome of such an examination in individuals with HIV infection.

Despite the moderate strides in understanding the neurocognitive effects of HIV infection since the initial reports of AIDS in the early 1980s, further research is necessary, particularly with ethnic-minority populations, in an attempt to elucidate in greater detail the complex manifestations and brain–behavior relationships of this infectious disease. In particular, research focusing on certain aspects of disease response and its differential impact on the cognitive and neuropsychologic abilities of individuals of various ethnic and racial backgrounds deserves closer attention.

ACKNOWLEDGMENTS.   Portions of this chapter were supported in part by a grant from the UCLA CIRID–Fogarty AIDS International Foundation to Antolin M. Llorente and a National Institutes of Health, National Institute of Allergy and Infectious Diseases, grant to Texas Children's Hospital, Section of Allergy and Immunology.

The authors wish to express their sincere thanks to Eric N. Miller, Ph.D., Department of Psychiatry and Biobehavioral Sciences, University of California, Los Angeles, for his suggestions on an earlier draft of this manuscript.

References

American Academy of Neurology AIDS Task Force. (1991). Nomenclature and research case definition for neurologic manifestations of human immunodeficiency virus-type 1 infection. *Annals of Neurology, 41,* 778–785.

Andiman, W. A., & Modlin, J. F. (1991). Vertical transmission. In P. A. Pizzo & K. M. Wilfert (Eds.), *Pediatric AIDS: The challenge of HIV infection in infant, children, and adolescents* (pp. 140–155). Baltimore, MD: Williams & Wilkins.

Ardilla, A., Rosselli, U. M., & Puente, A. E. (1994). *Neuropsychological evaluation of the Spanish speaker.* New York: Plenum.

Ardilla, A., Rosselli, M., & Rosas, P. (1989). Neuropsychological assessment of illiterates: Visuospatial and memory abilities. *Brain and Cognition, 11,* 147–166.

Aylward, E. H., Henderer, J. D., McArthur, J. C., Brettschneider, P. D., Barta, P. E., & Pearlson, G. D. (1993). Reduced basal ganglia atrophy in HIV-1 associated dementia complex: Results from quantitative neuroimaging. *Neurology, 43,* 2099–2104.

Bayés, R. (1995). *Sida.* Barcelona: Martínez Roca.

Belman, A. L. (1990). AIDS and pediatric neurology. *Neurology Clinics, 8,* 571–603.

Belman, A. L., Diamond, G., Dickson, D., Horoupian, D., Liena, J., Lantos, G., & Rubinstein, A. (1988). Pediatric acquired immunodeficiency syndrome. *American Journal of Diseases of Children, 142,* 29–35.

Belman, A., Diamond, G., Park, Y., Nozyce, M., Douglas, C., Cabot, T., Bernstein, L., & Rubinstein, A. (1989). Perinatal HIV infection: A prospective longitudinal study of the initial CNS signs. *Neurology, 39*(Suppl. 1), 278–279. (Abstract).

Belman, A. L., Lantos, G., Horoupian, D., Novick, B. E., Ultmann, M. H., Dickson, D. W., & Rubinstein, A. (1986). AIDS: Calcification of the basal ganglia in infants and children. *Neurology, 36,* 1192–1199.

Belman, A. L., Novick, B., Ultmann, M. H., Spiro, A. J., Rubinstein, A., Horoupian, D. S., & Cohen, H. (1984). Neurologic complications in children with AIDS. *Annals of Neurology, 16,* 414. (Abstract).

Belman, A. L., Ultmann, M. H., Horoupian, D., Novick, B., Spiro, A. J., Rubinstein, A., Kurtzbert, D., & Cone-Wesson, B. (1985). Neurological complications in infants and children with acquired immune deficiency syndrome. *Annals of Neurology, 18,* 560–566.

Blasini, I., Velez-Boras, J., Hittelman, J., Ware, J., Smith, R., Chase, C., Llorente, A., Moye, J., & Fowler, M. (1998, June). *Early neurodevelopmental indicators of encephalopathy in vertically HIV-infected children.* Paper presented at the Annual Neuroscience in HIV Infection Conference, Chicago, IL.

Boivin, M. J., Green, S. D. R., Davies, A. G., Giordani, B., Mokili, J. K. L., & Cutting, W. A. M. (1995). A preliminary evaluation of the cognitive and motor effects of pediatric HIV infection in Zairian children. *Health Psychology, 14,* 13–21.

Bornstein, R. A. (1994). Methodological and conceptual issues in the study of cognitive change in HIV infection. In I. Grant & A. Martin (Eds.), *Neuropsychology of HIV infection* (pp. 146–160). New York: Oxford University Press.

Bredesen, D. E., Levy, R. M., & Rosenblum, M. L. (1988). The neurology of human immunodeficiency virus infection. *Quarterly Journal of Medicine, 68,* 665–677.

Brew, B. J., Bhalla, R. B., Paul, M., Sidtis, J. J., Keilp, J. J., Sadler, A. E., Gallardo, H., McArthur, C., Schwartz, M., & Price, P. W. (1992). Cerebrospinal fluid β2 microglobulin in patients infected with AIDS dementia complex: An expanded series including response to zidovudine treatment. *AIDS, 6,* 461–465.

Brew, B. J., Sidtis, J. J., Petito, C. K., & Price, R. W. (1988). The neurologic complications of AIDS and human immunodeficiency virus infection. In F. Plum (Ed.), *Advances in contemporary neurology* (pp. 1–49). Philadelphia: F. A. Davis.

Brightbill, T. C., Ihmeidan, I. H., Post, M. J. D., Berger, J. K., & Katz, D. A. (1995). Neurosyphilis in HIV-positive and HIV-negative patients. Neuroimaging findings. *American Journal of Neuroradiology, 16,* 703–711.

Brouwers, P., Belman, A. L., & Epstein, L. G. (1991). Central nervous system involvement: Manifestations and evaluation. In P. A. Pizzo & K. M. Wilfert (Eds.), *Pediatric AIDS: The challenge of HIV infection in infants, children, and adolescents* (pp. 318–335). Baltimore, MD: Williams & Wilkins.

Brouwers, P., Belman, A. L., & Epstein, L. (1994). Central nervous system involvement: Manifestations, evaluation, and pathogenesis. In P. A. Pizzo & K. M. Wilfert (Eds.), *Pediatric AIDS: The challenge of HIV infection in infants, children, and adolescents* (2nd ed., pp. 433–455). Baltimore, MD: Williams & Wilkins.

Brouwers, P., DeCarli, C., Civitello, L., Moss, H., Wolters, P., & Pizzo, P. (1995). Correlation between computed tomographic brain scan abnormalities and neuropsychological function in children with symptomatic human immunodeficiency virus disease. *Archives of Neurology, 52,* 39–44.

Brouwers, P., Heyes, M., Moss, H., Wolters, P., Poplack, D., Markey, S., & Pizzo, P. (1993). Quinolinic acid in the cerebrospinal fluid of children with symptomatic HIV-disease: Relationships to clinical status and therapeutic response. *Journal of Infectious Diseases, 168,* 1380–1386.

Brouwers, P., Moss, H., Wolters, P., Eddy, J., & Pizzo, P. (1989). Neuropsychological profile of children with symptomatic HIV infection prior to antiretroviral therapy. *Proceedings from the V International Conference on AIDS, 1,* 316 (Abstract).

Brouwers, P., Moss, H., Wolters, P., el-Amin, D., Tassone, E., & Pizzo, P. (1992). Neurobehavioral typology of school-age children with symptomatic HIV disease. *Journal of Clinical and Experimental Neuropsychology, 14,* 113 (Abstract).

Brouwers, P., Moss, H., Wolters, P., & Schmitt, F. A. (1994). Developmental deficits and behavioral change in pediatric AIDS. In I. Grant & A. Martin (Eds.), *Neuropsychology of HIV infection* (pp. 310–338). New York: Oxford University Press.

Brown, G. R., & Rundell, J. R. (1990). Prospective study of psychiatric morbidity in HIV-seropositive women without AIDS. *General Hospital Psychiatry, 12,* 30–35.

Brown, G. R., & Rundell, J. R. (1993). A prospective study of psychiatric aspects of early HIV disease in women. *General Hospital Psychiatry, 15,* 139–147.

Buckingham, S., & van Gorp, W. (1988). AIDS-dementia complex: Implications for practice. *Social Casework: The Journal of Contemporary Social Work, 69,* 371–375.

Butters, N., Grant, I., Haxby, J., Fudd, L. L., Martin, A., McClelland, J., Pegvegnant, W., Schachter, D., & Stover, E. (1990). Assessment of AIDS-related cognitive changes: Recommendations of the NIMH workshop on neuropsychological assessment approaches. *Journal of Clinical and Experimental Neuropsychology, 12,* 963–978.

Carrieri, P. B., Indaco, A., Maiorino, A., & Buscaino, G. A. (1992). Cerebrospinal fluid beta-2-microglobulin in multiple sclerosis and AIDS dementia complex. *Neurological Research, 14,* 282–283.

Centers for Disease Control and Prevention (1993). *HIV/AIDS Surveillance Report, 5,* 1–19.

Centers for Disease Control and Prevention. (1994). Revised classification system for human immunodeficiency virus (HIV) infection in children less than 13 years of age. *Morbidity and Mortality Weekly, 43,* 1–10.

Centers for Disease Control and Prevention. (1996). *HIV/AIDS Surveillance Report, 8*(1), 1–33.

Chase, C., Ware, J., Hittelman, J., Blasini, I., Smith, R., Llorente, A., Anisfeld, E., Diaz, C., Fowler, M. G., Moye, J., & Almy, S. (in press). Early cognitive and motor development among infants born to women infected by human immunodeficiency virus. *Pediatrics.*

Clark, R.A., & Bessinger, R. (1997). Clinical manifestations and predictors of survival in older women infected with HIV. *Journal of Acquired Immune Deficiency Syndromes and Human Retrovirology, 15,* 341–345.

Claypoole, K., Townes, B., Collier, A., Combs, R., Longstreth, W., Cohen, W., Marra, C., Gerlack, H., Maravilla, K., Bahls, F., White, D., Murphy, V., Maxwell, C., & Handheld, H. (1990, February). *Neuropsychological aspects of early HIV infection.* Presented at the eighteenth annual International Neuropsychological Society Conference, Orlando, FL.

Cohen, S., Mundy, T., Karrassik, B., Lieb, L., Ludwig, D., & Ward, J. (1991). Neuropsychological functioning in human immunodeficiency virus type 1 seropositive children infected through neonatal blood transfusion. *Pediatrics, 88,* 58–68.

Coons, H. L., Spence, M. R., Harwell, T. S., Walch, S. E., & Spriepe, M. I. (February, 1995). *Psychosocial adjustment of women with HIV/AIDS.* Presented at the HIV Infection in Women: Setting a New Agenda conference, Washington, D.C.

Cooper, D. A., Gold, J., Mclean, P., Donovan, B., Finlayson, R., Barnes, T. G., Michelmore, H. M., Brooke, M., & Penny, R. (1985). Acute AIDS retrovirus infection: Definition of a clinical illness associated with seroconversion. *Lancet, 1,* 537–540.

Cummings, J. L., & Benson, D. F. (1983). *Dementia: A clinical approach.* Boston: Butterworth's.

Darko, D. F., Miller, J. C., Gallen, C., White, J., Koziol, J., Brown, S. J., Hayduk, R., Atkinson, J. H., & Ascmus, J. (1995). Sleep encephalogram delta-frequency amplitude, night plasma levels of tumor necrosis factor α, and human immunodeficiency virus infection. *Proceedings of the National Academy of Science of the USA, 92,* 12080–12084.

DeCarli, C., Civitello, L. A., Brouwers, P., & Pizzo, P. A. (1993). The prevalence of computed axial tomographic abnormalities of the cerebrum in 100 consecutive children symptomatic with the HIV. *Annals of Neurology, 34,* 198–205.

DeCarli, C., Fugate, L., Falloon, J., Eddy, J., Katz, D. A., Friedland, R. P., Rapoport, S. I., Brouwers, P., & Pizzo, P. A. (1991). Brain growth and cognitive improvement in children with human immune deficiency virus-induced encephalopathy after six months of continuous infusion with azidothymidine therapy. *Journal of Acquired Immune Deficiency Syndromes, 4,* 585–592.

de Martino, M. (1994). Human Immunodeficiency Virus type 1 infection and breast milk. *Acta Paediatrica Supplement, 400,* 51–58.

Diamond, G. W. (1989). Developmental problems in children with HIV infection. *Mental Retardation, 27,* 213–217.

Diamond, G. W., Kaufman, J., Belman, A. L., Cohen, L., Cohen, H. J., & Rubinstein, A. (1987). Characterization of cognitive functioning in a subgroup of children with congenital HIV infection. *Archives of Clinical Neuropsychology, 2,* 245–256.

Dicks, B. A. (1994). African American women and AIDS: A public health/social work challenge. *Social Work in Healthcare, 19,* 123–143.

Dickson, D. W., Belman, A. L., Park, Y. D., Wiley, C., Horoupian, D. S., Llena, J., Kure, K., Lyman, W. D., Morecki, R., & Mitsudo, S. (1989). Central nervous system pathology in pediatric AIDS: An autopsy study. *Acta Pathologica Microbiologica et Immunologica Scandinavica (Suppl), 8,* 40–57.

Dooneief, G., Bello, J., Todak, G., Mun, J. K., Marder, K., Malouf, R., Gorman, J., Hilal, S., Stern, Y., & Mayeux, R. (1992). A prospective controlled study of magnetic resonance imaging of the brain in gay men and parental drug users with human immunodeficiency virus infection. *Archives of Neurology, 49,* 38–43.

Dorfman, D., Handelsman, L., Williams, D., Kincaid, J., & Hauser, A. (1995). HIV-infected women show neuropsychological impairment earlier than men. *Proceedings from the HIV Infected Women's Conference,* P125.

Durvasala, R. S., & Miller, E. (1997). Neuropsychological performance and HIV serostatus in women. *Proceedings from the National Conference on Women and HIV,* p. 115. (Abstract #114.4).

Epstein, L. G., Goudsmit, J., Paul, D. S., Morrison, S. H., Connor, E. M., Oleske, J. M., & Holland, B. (1987). Expression of human immunodeficiency virus in cerebrospinal fluid of children with progressive encephalopathy. *Annals of Neurology, 21,* 397–401.

Epstein, L. G., Sharer, L. R., Joshi, V. V., Fogas, M. M., Koenigsberger, M. R., & Oleske, J. M. (1985). Progressive encephalopathy in children with acquired immune deficiency syndrome. *Annals of Neurology, 17,* 488–496.

Epstein, L. G., Sharer, L. R., Oleske, J. M., Connor, E. M., Goudsmit, J., Bagdon, L., Robert-Guroff, M., & Koenigsberger, M. R. (1986). Neurologic manifestations of human immunodeficiency virus infection in children. *Pediatrics, 78,* 678–687.

Epstein, L. G., Sharer, L. R., & Goudsmit, J. (1988). Neurological and neuropathological features of human immunodeficiency virus infection in children. *Annals of Neurology, 23*(Suppl.), S19–S23.

Everall, I., Luthert, P. J., & Lantos, P. L. (1991). Neuronal loss in the frontal cortex in HIV infection. *Lancet, 337,* 1119–1121.

Everall, I., Luthert, P. J., Lantos, P. L. (1993). A review of neuronal damage in human immunodeficiency virus infection: Its assessment, possible mechanism and relationship to dementia. *Journal of Neuropathology and Experimental Neurology, 52,* 561–566.

Falloon, J., Eddy., J., Wiener, L., & Pizzo, P. A. (1989). Human immunodeficiency virus infection in children. *Journal of Pediatrics, 114,* 1–30.

Fama, R., Pace, P. L., Tiempiero, A. M., & Bornstein, R. A. (1992). Effects of alcohol and drug use on neuropsychological performance in HIV asymptomatic individuals. *Journal of Clinical and Experimental Neuropsychology, 14,* 79.

Fernandez, F. (1988). Psychiatric complications in HIV-related illnesses. *American Psychiatric Association AIDS primer.* Washington, DC: American Psychiatric Association Press.

Fernandez, F. (1989). Anxiety and the neuropsychiatry of AIDS. *Journal of Clinical Psychiatry, 50*(Suppl.), 9–14.

Fernandez, F., Adams, F., Levy, J. K., Holmes, V. F., Neidhart, M., & Mansell, P. W. (1988). Cognitive impairment due to AIDS-related complex and its response to psychostimulants. *Psychosomatics, 29,* 38–46.

Fernandez, F., Levy, J. K., & Pirozzolo, F. J. (1989). *Neuropsychological and immunological abnormalities in advanced HIV infection.* Fifth International Conference on AIDS. Montreal, Canada.

Filley, C. M. (1994). Neurobehavioral aspects of cerebral white matter disorders. In B. S. Fogel, R. S. Schiffer, & S. M. Rao (Eds.), *Neuropsychiatry: A comprehensive textbook.* Baltimore, MD: Williams & Wilkins.

Flowers, C. H., Mafee, M. F., Crowell, R., Raofi, B., Arnold, P., Dobben, G., & Wycliffe, N. (1990). Encephalopathy in AIDS patients: Evaluation with MR imaging. *American Journal of Neuroradiology, 11,* 1235–1245.

Fong, I. W., & Toma, E. (1995). The natural history of progressive multifocal leukoencephalopathy in patients with AIDS. *Clinical Infectious Diseases, 20,* 1305–1310.

Fowler, M. G. (1994). Pediatric HIV infection: Neurologic and neuropsychological findings. *Acta Paediatrica Supplement, 400,* 59–62.

Fox, K. A., Ethier, K. A., Cerreta, C., & Ickovics, J. R. (1995). *Women and HIV/AIDS: Representation in neurological and neuropsychological research.* Presented at the HIV Infection in Women: Setting a New Agenda conference, Washington, DC.

Frank, K. Y., Lim, W., & Kahn, E. (1989). Multiple ischemic infarcts in children with AIDS, varicella zoster infection and cerebral vasculitis. *Pediatric Neurology, 5,* 64–67.

Franke, G. H., Jager, H., Thomann, B., & Beyer, B. (1992). Assessment and evaluation of psychological distress in HIV-infected women. *Psychology and Health, 6,* 297–312.

Franzblau, A., Letz, R., Hershman, D., Mason, P., Wallace, J. I., & Bekesi, G. (1991). Quantitative neurologic and neurobehavioral testing of persons infected with human immunodeficiency virus type 1. *Archives of Neurology, 48,* 263–268.

Friedland, G., & Klein, R. (1987). Transmission of the human immunodeficiency virus. *New England Journal of Medicine, 317*, 1125–1135.

Gazbuda, D. H., Levy, S. R., & Chiappa, K. H. (1988). Electroencephalography in AIDS and AIDS-related complex. *Clinical Electroencephalography, 19*, 1–6.

Gottlieb, M., Schroff, R., Schanker, H., Weisman, J., Fan, P., Wolf, R., & Saxon, A. (1981). *Pneumocystis carinii* pneumonia and mucosal candidiasis in previously healthy homosexual men: Evidence of a newly acquired cellular immunodeficiency. *New England Journal of Medicine, 305*, 1425–1430.

Grant, D. (1988). Support groups for youth with the AIDS virus. *International Journal of Group Psychotherapy, 38*, 237–250.

Grant, I., Atkinson, J. H., Hesselink, J. R., Kennedy, C. J., Richman, D. D., Spector, S. A., & McCutchan, J. A. (1987). Evidence for early central nervous system involvement in the acquired immunodeficiency syndrome (AIDS) and other human immunodeficiency virus (HIV) infections. *Annals of Internal Medicine, 107*, 828–836.

Grant, I., & Martin, A. (1994). Introduction: Neurocognitive disorders associated with HIV-1 infection. In I. Grant & A. Martin (Eds.), *Neuropsychology of HIV infection* (pp. 3–19). New York: Oxford University Press.

Hamilton, J.D., Hartigan, P. M., Simberkoff, M. S., Day, P. L., Diamond, G. R., Dickinson, G. M., Drusano, G. L., Egovin, M. J., George, W. L., Gordin, F. M., Hawkes, C. A., Jensen, P. C., Kilmas, N. G., Labriola, A. M., Lahort, C. J., O'Brien, W. A., Oster, C. N., Weinhold, K. J., Wray, N. P., Zolla-Pazner, S. B., & the Veterans Affairs Cooperative Study Group on AIDS Treatment. (1992). A controlled trial of early versus late treatment with Zidovudine in symptomatic human immunodeficiency virus infection. *New England Journal of Medicine, 326*, 437–443.

Harris, J. G., Cullum, C. M., & Puente, A. E. (1995). Effects of bilingualism on verbal learning and memory in Hispanic adults. *Journal of the International Neuropsychological Society, 1*, 10–16.

Harris, M. H. (1992). Habilitative and rehabilitative needs of children with HIV infection. In A. C. Crocker, H. J. Cohen, & T. A. Kastner (Eds.), *HIV infection and developmental disabilities: A resource for service providers* (pp. 85–94). Baltimore, MD: Brookes.

Hart, R. P., Wade, J. B., Klinger, R. L., & Levenson, J. L. (1990). Slowed information processing as an early cognitive change associated with AIDS and ARC. *Journal of Clinical and Experimental Neuropsychology, 12*, 72.

Heaton, R. K., Grant, I., Butters, N., White, D. A., Kirson, D., Atkinson, J. H., McCutchman, J. A., Taylor, M. J., Kelly, M. D., Ellis, R. J., Wolfson, T., Velin, R., Marcotte, T. D., Hesselink, T. L., Venigan, J., Chandlier, J., Wallace, M., Abramson, I., & the HNRC Group. (1995). The HNRC 500-neuropsychology of HIV infection at different disease stages. *Journal of the International Neuropsychological Society, 1*, 231–251.

Heyes, M. P., Brew, B. J., Martin, A., Price, R. W., Salazar, A. M., & Sidtis, J. J. (1991). Quinolinic acid in cerebrospinal fluid and serum in HIV-1 infection: Relationship to clinical neurological status. *Annals of Neurology, 29*, 202–209.

Hittelman, J., Willoughby, A., Mendez, H., Nelson, N., Gong, J., Holman, S., Muez, L., Goedert, J., & Landesman, S. (1990). Neurodevelopmental outcome of perinatally-acquired HIV infection on the first 15 months of life. *Proceedings from the VI International Conference on AIDS, 3*, 130. (Abstract).

Hittelman, J., Willoughby, A., Mendez, H., Nelson, N., Gong, J., Mendez, H., Holman, S., Muez, L., Goedert., J., & Landesman, S. (1991). Neurodevelopmental outcome of perinatally-acquired HIV infection on the first 24 months of life. *Proceedings from the VI International Conference on AIDS, 1*, 65. (Abstract).

Ho, D. D., Rota, T. R., Schooley, R. T., Kaplan, J. C., Allan, J. D., Groopman, J. E., Resnick, L., Felsenstein, D., Andrews, C. A., & Hirsch, M. S. (1985). Isolation of HTLV-III from cerebrospinal fluid and neural tissues of patients with neurologic syndromes related to the acquired immunodeficiency syndrome. *New England Journal of Medicine, 313*, 1493–1497.

Hutto, C., Scott, G., Parks, E., & Frschl, M. (1989, June 1–5). Cerebrospinal fluid (CSF) studies in adults and pediatric HIV infections. *Proceedings from the Third International Conference on AIDS*. Washington, DC.

James, M.E., Rubin, C.P., & Willis, S.E. (1991). Drug abuse and psychiatric findings in HIV-seropositive pregnant patients. *General Hospital Psychiatry, 13*, 4–8.

Janssen, R., Saykin, J., Cannon, L., Campbell, J., Pinsky, P. F., Hessol, N., O'Malley, P. M., Lifson, A. R., Doll, L. S., Rutherford, G. N., & Kaplan, J. (1989). Neurologic and neuropsychologic manifestations of human immunodeficiency virus (HIV-1) infection: Association with AIDS-related complex but not asymptomatic HIV-1 infection. *Annals of Neurology, 26*, 592–600.

Jernigan, T. T. L., Archibald, S., Hesselink, J. R., Atkinson, J. H., Velin, R. A., McCutchan, J. A., Chandler, J., & Grant, I. (1993). Magnetic resonance imaging morphometric analysis of cerebral volume loss in human immunodeficiency virus. The HNRC group. *Archives of Neurology, 50*, 250–255.

Kaplan, M. S., Marks, G., & Mertens, S. B. (1997). Distress and coping among women with HIV infection: Preliminary findings from a multiethnic sample. *American Journal of Orthopsychiatry, 67*(1), 80–91.

Kaufman, A. S. (1975). Factor analysis of the WISC-R at 11 age levels between 6½ and 16½ years. *Journal of Consulting and Clinical Psychology, 43*, 135–147.

Kløve, H. (1963). Clinical neuropsychology. In F. M. Foster (Ed.), *The Medical Clinics of North America*. New York: W.B. Saunders.

Klusman, L. E., Moulton, J. K., Hornbostel, L. K., Picano, J. J., & Beattie, M. T. (1991). Neuropsychological abnormalities in asymptomatic HIV seropositive military personnel. *Journal of Neuropsychiatry, 3*, 422–428.

Koenig, S., Gendelman, H. E., Orenstein, J., Dal Canto, M. C., Pezeshkpour, G. H., Yungbluth, M., Janotta, F., Aksamit, A., Martin, M. A., & Fauci, A. S. (1986). Detection of AIDS virus in macrophages in brain tissue from AIDS patients with encephalopathy. *Science, 233*, 1089–1093.

Kramer, E. L., & Sanger, J. J. (1990). Brain imaging in acquired immunodeficiency syndrome dementia complex. *Seminars in Nuclear Medicine, 20*, 353–363.

Kranczer, S. (1995). U.S. longevity unchanged. *Statistical Bulletin, 76*, 12–20.

LaFrance, N., Pearlson, G., Shaerf, F., McArthur, J., Polk, B., Links, J., Bascom, M., Knowles, M., & Galen, S. (1988). I-123 IMP-SPECT in HIV-related dementia. *Advances in Functional Neuroimaging, Fall*, 9–15.

Laosa, L. M. (1984). Ethnic, socioeconomic and home language influences upon early performance on measures of abilities. *Journal of Educational Psychology, 76*, 1178–1198.

Leuchter, A., Newton, T., van Gorp, W., & Miller, E. (1989, May). *Early detection of HIV effects on brain function.* Paper presented at the 142nd Annual Meeting of the American Psychiatric Association, San Francisco, CA.

Levenson, R. L., Jr., Mellins, C. A., Zawadzki, R., Kairam, R., & Stein, Z. (1992). Cognitive assessment of human immunodeficiency virus-exposed children. *American Journal of Diseases in Children, 146*, 1479–1483.

Levin, B. E., Berger, J. R., Didona, T., & Duncan, R. (1992). Cognitive function in asymptomatic HIV-1 infection: The effects of age, education, ethnicity, and depression. *Neuropsychology, 6*, 303–313.

Levin, H. S., Williams, D. H., Borucki, M. J., Hillman, G. R., Williams, M. B., Guinto, F. C., Amparo, E. G., Crow, W. N., & Pollard, R. B. (1990). Magnetic resonance imaging and neuropsychological findings in human immunodeficiency virus infection. *Journal of Acquired Immune Deficiency Syndrome, 3*, 757–762.

Levy, J. K., & Fernandez, F. (1997). Human immunodeficiency virus infection of the central nervous system: Implications for neuropsychiatry. In S. C. Yudofsky & R. E. Hales (Eds.), *Textbook of neuropsychiatry* (3rd. ed., pp. 663–692). Washington, DC: American Psychiatric Press.

Lezak, M. D. (1978). Subtle sequelae of brain damage: Perplexity, distractibility, and fatigue. *American Journal of Physical Medicine, 57*, 9–15.

Likely, J. J. (1987). Forensic psychological evaluations through an interpreter: Legal and ethical issues. *American Journal of Forensic Psychology, 5*, 29–43.

Lipsitz, J. D., Gorman, J. M., Sorrell, S., Goetz, R., el Sadr, W., Bradbury, M., Remien, R. H., Rabkin, J. G., & Williams, J. B. (1994). Psychopathology in male and female intravenous drug users with and without HIV infection. *American Journal of Psychiatry, 151*(11), 1662–1668.

Llorente, A. M., LoPresti, C. E., Levy, J. K., & Fernandez, F. (2000). Neurobehavioral and neuropsychological manifestations of HIV infection: Assessment considerations with Hispanic populations. In M. O. Ponton & J. Leon-Carrion (Eds.), *Neuropsychology and the Hispanic patient* (pp. 322–337). Hillsdale, NJ: Erlbaum.

Llorente, A. M., LoPresti, C. E., & Satz, P. (1997). Neuropsychological and neurobehavioral sequelae associated with pediatric HIV infection. In C. R. Reynolds & E. Fletcher-Janzen (Eds.), *Handbook of clinical child neuropsychology* (2nd ed., pp. 634–650). New York: Plenum.

Llorente, A. M., Miller, E. N., D'Elia, L. F., Selnes, O. A., Wesch, J., Becker, J. T., & Satz, P. (1998). Slowed information processing in HIV-1 disease. *Journal of Clinical and Experimental Neuropsychology, 20*, 60–72.

Llorente, A. M., Pontón, M. O., Taussig, I. M., & Satz, P. (1999). Patterns of American immigration and their influence on the acquisition of neuropsychological norms for Hispanic groups. *Archives of Clinical Neuropsychology, 14*, 603–614.

Llorente, A. M., Stern, M. J., & van Gorp, W. G. (1994, April). *Long-term effect of AZT on neuropsychological performance.* Poster presented at the NIH (Office on AIDS) sponsored Pathogenesis of HIV Infection of the Brain: Impact on Function and Behavior conference, Chantilly, VA.

Long, I. L., & Leger, J. A. (1995, February). *Women's access to government-sponsored AIDS/HIV Clinical Trials.* Presented at the HIV Infection in Women: Setting a New Agenda conference, Washington, DC.

LoPresti, C. M., Llorente, A. M., Guzzard, C. R., & Brumm, V. L. (1998, August). *Neuropsychological functioning in HIV+ women: Consultation with community-based organizations.* Poster presented at the 106th Annual Meeting of the American Psychological Association, Chicago, IL.

Manly, J. J., Miller, S. W., Heaton, R. K., Byrd, D., Reilly, J., Velasquez, R. J., Saccuzzo, D. P., & Grant, I. (1998). The effect of African American acculturation on neuropsychological test performance in normal and HIV-positive individuals. *Journal of the International Neuropsychological Society, 4*, 291–302.

Mann, J. M., Tarantola, D. M., & Netter, T. W. (1992). *AIDS in the world.* Cambridge, MA: Harvard University Press.

Mapou, R. L., Law, W. A., Wagner, K., Malone, J. L., & Skillman, D. R. (1996). Neuropsychological effects of Interferon Alfa-n3 treatment in asymptomatic human immunodeficiency virus-1-infected individuals. *Journal of Neuropsychiatry and Clinical Neurosciences, 8*, 74–81.

Marín, G., & Marín, B. V. (1991). *Research with Hispanic populations.* Newbury Park, CA: Sage.

Martin, A. (1994). HIV, cognition, and the basal ganglia. In I. Grant & A. Martin (Eds.), *Neuropsychology of HIV infection* (pp. 234–269). New York: Oxford University Press.

Martin, A., Heyes, M. P., Salazar, A. M., Kampen, M. S., Williams, J., Law, W. A., Coats, M. E., & Markey, S. P. (1992). Progressive slowing of reaction time and increasing cerebrospinal fluid concentrations of quinolinic acid in HIV-infected individuals. *Journal of Neuropsychiatry and Clinical Neuroscience, 4,* 270–279.

Martin, E. M., Robertson, L. C., Edelstein, H. E., Jagust, W. J., Sorenson, D. J., SanGiovanni, D., & Chirurgi, V. A. (1992). Performance of patients with early HIV-1 infection on the Stroop Task. *Journal of Clinical and Experimental Neuropsychology, 14,* 857–868.

Masliah, E., Achim, C. L., Ge, N., DeTerresa, R., Terry, R. D., & Wiley, C. A. (1992). Spectrum of human immunodeficiency virus associated neocortical damage. *Annals of Neurology, 32,* 321–329.

Masliah, E., Ge, N., Achim, C. L., & Wiley, C. A. (1995). Differential vulnerability of calbindin-immunoreactive neurons in HIV encephalitis. *Journal of Neuropathology and Experimental Neurology, 54,* 350–357.

McAllister, R. H., Herns, M. V., Harrison, M. J. G., Newman, S. P., Connolly, S., Fowler, C. J., Fell, M., Durrance, P., Manji, H., & Kendall, B. E. (1992). Neurologic and neuropsychologic performance in HIV seropositive men without symptoms. *Journal of Neurology, Neurosurgery and Psychiatry, 55,* 143–148.

McArthur, J. C. (1987). Neurologic manifestations of AIDS. *Medicine (Baltimore), 66,* 407–437.

McArthur, J. C. (1994). Neurological and neuropathological manifestations of HIV infection. In I. Grant & A. Martin (Eds.), *Neuropsychology of HIV infection* (pp. 56–107). New York: Oxford University Press.

McArthur, J. C., Cohen, B. A., Selnes, O. A., Kumar, A. J., Cooper, K., McArthur, J. H., Soucy, G., Cornblath, D. R., Chmiel, J. S., & Wang, M. C. (1989). Low prevalence of neurological and neuropsychological abnormalities in otherwise healthy HIV-1-infected individuals: Results from the Multicenter AIDS Cohort Study. *Annals of Neurology, 26,* 601–611.

McArthur, J. C., Nance-Sproon, T. E., Griffin, D. E., Hoover, D., Selnes, O. A., Miller, E. N., Margolick, J. B., Cohen, B. A., Furzadagan, H., & Saah, A. (1992). The diagnostic utility of elevation in cerebral spinal fluid β2-microglobulin in HIV-1 dementia. *Neurology, 42,* 1707–1712.

McDaniel, J. S., Cohen-Cole, S. A., Farber, E. W., Summerville, M. B., & Fowlie, E. (1995). An assessment of rates of psychiatric morbidity and functioning in HIV disease. *General Hospital Psychiatry, 17,* 346–352.

McKegney, F. P., O'Dowd, M. A., Feiner, C., Selwyn, P., Drucker, E., & Friedland, G. H. (1990). A prospective comparison of neuropsychologic function in HIV-seropositive and seronegative methadone-maintained patients. *AIDS, 4,* 565–569.

Mellers, J. D. C., Marchand-Gonod, N., King, M., Laupa, V., & Smith, J. R. (1994). Mental health of women with HIV infection: A study in Paris and London. *European Psychiatry, 9,* 241–248.

Miller, E. N., Selnes, O. A., McArthur, J. C., Satz, P., Becker, J. T., Cohen, B. A. Sheridan, K., Machado, A. M., van Gorp, W. G., & Visscher, B. (1990). Neuropsychological performance in HIV-1 infected homosexual men: The Multicenter AIDS Cohort Study (MACS). *Neurology, 40,* 197–203.

Miller, J. K., Barrett, R. E., Britton, C. B., Tapper, M. L., Bahr, G. S., Bruno, P. J., Marquardt, M. D., Hays, A. P., McMurty, J. G., III, Weissman, J. P., & Bruno, M. S. (1982). Progressive multifocal leukoencephalopathy in a male homosexual with T-cell immune deficiency. *New England Journal of Medicine, 307,* 1436–1438.

Mintz, M. (1989). Elevated serum levels of tumor necrosis factor associated with progressive encephalopathy in children with acquired immunodeficiency syndrome. *American Journal of Diseases of Children, 143,* 771–774.

Moore, J., Solomon, L., Schoenbaum, E., Boland, B., Zeiler, S., & Smith, D. (1995, February). *Factors associated with stress and distress among HIV-infected and uninfected women.* Presented at the HIV Infection in Women: Setting a New Agenda conference, Washington, DC.

Morokoff, P. J., Mays, V. M., & Coons, H. L. (1997). HIV infection and AIDS. In S. J. Gallant, G. Puryear-Keita, & R. Royak-Schaler (Eds.), *Health care for women* (pp. 273–293). Washington, DC: American Psychological Association.

Navia, B., Cho, E. S., Petito, C. K., & Price, R. W. (1986a). The AIDS dementia complex: II. Neuropathology. *Annals of Neurology, 19,* 525–535.

Navia, B., Jordan, B., & Price, R. (1986b). The AIDS dementia complex: I. Clinical features. *Annals of Neurology, 19,* 517–524.

Nicholas, S. W. (1994). The opportunistic and bacterial infections associated with pediatric human immunodeficiency virus disease. *Acta Paediatrica Supplement, 400,* 46–50.

Novello, A. C., Wise, P. H., Willoughby, A., & Pizzo, P. A. (1989). Final report of the United States Department of Health and Human Services Secretary's Work Group on pediatric human immunodeficiency virus infection disease: Content and implications. *Pediatrics, 84,* 547–555.

Nuwer, M. R., Miller, E. N., Visscher, B. R., Niedermeyer, E., Packwood, J. W., Carlson, L. G., Satz, P., Jankel, W., & McArthur, J. C. (1992). Asymptomatic HIV infection does not cause EEG abnormalities: Results from the Multicenter AIDS Cohort study (MACS). *Neurology, 42,* 1214–1219.

Ollo, C., & Pass, H. (1988, February). *Neuropsychological performance in HIV disease. Effect of depression and chronic CNS infection*. Paper presented at the 16th annual meeting of the International Neuropsychological Society, New Orleans, LA.

Orr, S. T., Celentano, D. D., Santelli, J., & Burwell, L. (1994). Depressive symptoms and risk factors for HIV acquisition among black women attending urban health centers in Baltimore. *Education and Prevention, 6,* 230–236.

Pang, S., Koyanagi, Y., Miles, S., Wiley, C., Vinters, H., & Chen, I. (1990). High levels of unintegrated HIV-1 DNA in brain tissue of AIDS dementia patients. *Nature, 343,* 85–89.

Park, Y., Belman, A., Dickson, D., Llena, J., Josephina, F., Lantos, G., Diamond, G., Bernstein, L., & Rubinstein, A. (1988). Stroke in pediatric AIDS. *Annals of Neurology, 24,* 279 (Abstract).

Perdices, M., & Cooper, D. (1989). Simple and choice reaction time in patients with human immunodeficiency virus infection. *Annals of Neurology, 25,* 460–467.

Pérez-Arce, P. (1994). The role of culture and SES on cognition. *The Clinical Neuropsychologist, 8,* 350.

Perry, S. W. (1990). Organic mental disorders caused by HIV: Update on early diagnosis and treatment. *American Journal of Psychiatry, 147,* 696–710.

Pizzo, P., Eddy, J., Falloon, J., Balis, F., Murphy, R., Moss, H., Wolters, P., Brouwers, P., Jarosinski, P., Rubin, M., Broder, S., Yarchoan, R., Brunetti, A., Maha, M., Nusinoff Lehrman, S., & Poplack, D. (1988). Effect of continuous intravenous infusion of zidovudine (AZT) in children with symptomatic HIV infection. *New England Journal of Medicine, 319,* 889–896.

Pizzo, P. A., & Wilfert, C. M. (Eds.). (1994). *Pediatric AIDS: The challenge of HIV infection in infants, children, and adolescents* (2nd ed.). Baltimore, MD: Williams & Wilkins.

Pontón, M. O., & Ardila, A. (1999). The future of Hispanic neuropsychology in the U.S. *Archives of Neuropsychology, 14,* 565–580.

Post, M. J. D., Berger, J. R., & Quencer, R. M. (1991). Asymptomatic and neurologically symptomatic HIV-seropositive individuals: Prospective evaluation with cranial MR imaging. *Radiology, 178,* 131–139.

Post, M., Tate, L., Quencer, R., Hensley, G., Berger, J., Sheremata, W., & Maul, G. (1988). CT, MR, and pathology in HIV encephalitis and meningitis. *American Journal of Radiology, 151,* 373–380.

Price, R. W., & Brew, B. J. (1988). The AIDS dementia complex. *Journal of Infectious Diseases, 158,* 1079–1083.

Prober, C., & Gershon, A. (1991). Medical management of newborns and infants born to seropositive mothers. In P. A. Pizzo & C. M. Wilfert (Eds.), *Pediatric AIDS: The challenge of HIV infection in infants, children, and adolescents* (pp. 516–530). Baltimore, MD: Williams & Wilkins.

Redfield, R. R. , Wright, D. C., & Tramont, E. C. (1986). The Walter Reed staging classification of HTLV-III/LAV infection. *New England Journal of Medicine, 314,* 131–132.

Resnick, L., Berger, J. R., Shapshak, P., & Tourtellete, W. W. (1988). Early penetration of blood-brain barrier by HIV. *Neurology, 38,* 9–14.

Resnick, L., diMarzio-Veronese, F., Schüpback, J., Tourtellete, W. W. , Ho, D., Müller, F., Sharpshak, P., Vogt, M., Groopman, J. E., & Markham, P. D. (1985). Intra-blood-brain-barrier synthesis of HTLV-III specific IgG in patients with neurological symptoms associated with AIDS or ARC. *New England Journal of Medicine, 313,* 1498–1504.

Rottenberg, D., Moeller, J., Sidtis, J., Navia, B., Dhawan, V., Ginos, Z., & Price, R. (1987). The metabolic pathology of the AIDS dementia complex. *Annals of Neurology, 22,* 700–706.

Royal, W., III, Updike, M., Selnes, O. A., Proctor, T. V., Nance-Sproson, L., Salomon, L., Vlahov, D., Cornblath, D. R., & McArthur, J. C. (1991). HIV-1 infection and nervous system abnormalities among a cohort of intravenous drug users. *Neurology, 41,* 1905–1910.

Rubinow, D., Berettini, C., Brouwers, P., & Lane, H. (1988). Neuropsychiatric consequences of AIDS. *Annals of Neurology, 23*(Suppl.), S24–S26.

Ryan, J. J., Paolo, A. M., & Skrade, M. (1992). Rey Auditory Verbal Learning Test performance of a federal corrections sample with acquired immunodeficiency syndrome. *International Journal of Neuroscience, 64,* 177–181.

Sacktor, N., van Heertum, R. L., Dooneief, G., Gorman, J., Khandji, A., Marder, K., Novr, R., Todak, G., Stern, Y., & Mayer, R. (1995). A comparison of cerebral SPECT abnormalities in HIV-positive homosexual men with and without cognitive impairment. *Archives of Neurology, 52,* 1170–1173.

Samson, M., Libert, F., Doranz, B. J., Rocker, J., Liesnard, C., Farber, C. M., Saragasti, S., Lapoumeroulie, C., Cognaux, J., Forceille, C., Muyldermans, G., Verhofstede, C., Burtonboy, G., Georges, M., Imai, T., Rana, S., Yi, Y., Smyth, R. J., Collman, R. G., Doms, R. W., Vassart, T. G., & Parmantier, M. (1996). Resistance to HIV-1 infection in caucasian individuals bearing mutant alleles of the CCR-5 chemokine receptor gene. *Nature, 382,* 722–725.

Satz, P., Morganstern, H., Miller, E. N., D'Elia, L. F., van Gorp, W., & Visscher, B. (1993). Low education as a possible risk factor for cognitive abnormalities in HIV-1: Findings from the Multicenter AIDS Cohort Study (MACS). *Journal of Acquired Immune Deficiency Syndrome, 6,* 503–511.

Saykin, A., Janssen, R., Sphren, G., Kaplan, J., Spira, T., & Weller, P. (1988). Neuropsychological dysfunction in HIV-infection: Characterization in a lymphadenopathy cohort. *International Journal of Clinical Neuropsychology*, *10*, 81–95.

Schuman, P., & Sobel, J. D. (1993). Women and AIDS. *The Australian and New Zeland Journal of Obstetrics and Gynecology*, *33*, 341–350.

Selnes, O. A., McArthur, J. C., Royal, W., III, Updike, M. L., Nance-Sproson, T., Concha, M., Gordon, B., Solomon, L., & Vlahov, D. (1992). HIV-1 infection and intravenous drug use: Longitudinal neuropsychological evaluation of asymptomatic subjects. *Neurology*, *42*, 1924–1930.

Selnes, O. A., Jacobson, L., Machado, A. M., Becker, J. T., Wesch, J., Miller, E. N., Visscher, B., & McArthur, J. C. (1991). Normative data for a brief neuropsychological screening battery. Multicenter AIDS Cohort Study. *Perceptual and Motor Skills*, *73*, 539–550.

Selnes, O. A., & Miller, E. N. (1994). Development of a screening battery for HIV-related cognitive impairment: The MACS experience. In I. Grant & A. Martin (Eds.), *Neuropsychology of HIV infection* (pp. 176–187). New York: Oxford University Press.

Sharer, L., Cho, E. S., & Epstein, L. G. (1985). Multinucleated giant cells and HTLV-III in AIDS encephalopathy. *Human Pathology*, *16*, 760.

Sharer., L. R., Dowling, P., Micheals, J., Cook, S., Menonna, J., Blumberg, B., & Epstein, L. (1990). Spinal cord disease in children with HIV-1 infection: A combined biological and neuropathological study. *Neuropathology of Applied Neurobiology*, *16*, 317–331.

Sharer, L. R., Epstein, L. G., Cho, E., Joshi, V. V., Meyenhofer, M. F., Rankin, L. F., & Petito, C. K. (1986). Pathologic features of AIDS encephalopathy in children: Evidence for LAV/HTLV-III infection of brain. *Human Pathology*, *17*, 271–284.

Sidtis, J. J., Gastonis, C., Price, R. W., Singer, E. J., Collier, A. C., Richman, D. D., Hirsch, M. S., Schaert, F. W., Fischl, M. A., Kieburtz, K., Simpson, D., Koch, M. A., Feinberg, J., Dafni, V., & The AIDS Clinical Trial Group. (1993). Zidovudine treatment of the AIDS dementia complex: Results of a placebo-controlled trial. AIDS Clinical Trials Group. *Annals of Neurology*, *33*, 343–349.

Sidtis, J. J., & Price, R. W. (1990). Early HIV-1 infection and the AIDS dementia complex. *Neurology*, *40*, 323–326.

Silberstein, C. H., McKegney, F. P., O'Dowd, M. A., Selwin, P. A., Schoenbaon, E., Drucker, E., Feiner, C., Cox, C. P., & Friedland, C. (1987). A prospective longitudinal study of neuropsychological and psychosocial factors in asymptomatic individuals at risk of HTLV-III/LAV infection in a methadone program: Preliminary findings. *International Journal of Neuroscience*, *32*, 669–676.

Snider, W., Simpson, D., Nielsen, S., Gold, J., Metroka, C., & Posner, J. (1983). Neurological complications of acquired immune deficiency syndrome: Analysis of 50 patients. *Annals of Neurology*, *14*, 403–418.

Stern, R. A., Arruda, J. E., Somerville, J. A., Cohen, R. A., Boland, R. J., Stein, M. D., & Martin, E. M. (1998). Neurobehavioral functioning in asymptomatic HIV-1 infected women. *Journal of the International Neuropsychological Society*, *4*, 172–178.

Stern, R. A., Singer, N. G., Silva, S. G., Rogers, J. H., Perkins, D. O., Hall, C. D., van der Hart, C. M., & Evans, D. L. (1992). Neurobehavioral functioning in a nonconfounded group of asymptomatic HIV-seropositive homosexual men. *American Journal of Psychiatry*, *149*, 1099–1102.

Stern, Y., Marder, K., Bell, K., Chen, J., Dooneief, G., Goldstein, S., Mindry, D., Richards, M., Sano, M., Williams, J., Gorman, J., Ehrhardt, A., & Mayeux, R. (1991). Mulitdisciplinary baseline assessment of homosexual men with and without human immunodeficiency virus infection. III: Neurologic and neuropsychological findings. *Archives of General Psychiatry*, *48*, 131–138.

Stern, Y., Sano, M., Morder, K., Mindrey, D., Goldstein, S., Richards, M., & Gorman, J. (1990). Subtle neuropsychological changes in HIV+ gay men. *Journal of Clinical and Experimental Neuropsychology*, *12*, 48.

Stern, Y., Sano, M., Williams, J., & Gorman, J. (1989). Neuropsychological consequences of HIV infection. *Journal of Clinical and Experimental Neuropsychology*, *11*, 78.

Tardieu, M. (1991, June). Brain imaging in pediatric HIV infection. In A. Belman & A. M. Laverda (Chairs), *Pediatric HIV-1 infection: Neurological and neuropsychological aspects*. Symposium conducted at the meeting of the Neuroscience of HIV Infection: Basic and Clinical Frontiers, Padova, Italy.

Tardieu, M., Blanche, S., Duliege, A., Rouzioux, C., & Griscelli, C. (1989). Neurologic involvement and prognostic factors after materno-fetal infection. *Proceedings of the V International Conference on AIDS*, *1*, 194 (Abstract).

Tarter, R. E., Edwards, K. L., & van Thiel, D. H. (1988). Perspective and rationale for neuropsychological assessment of medical disease. In R. E. Tarter, D. H. van Thiel, & K. L. Edwards (Eds.), *Medical neuropsychology: The impact of disease on behavior* (pp. 1–10). New York: Plenum.

Taylor, E. R., Amodei, N., & Mangos, R. (1996). The presence of psychiatric disorders in HIV-infected women. *Journal of Counseling and Development*, *74*, 345–351.

Tross, S., Price, R., Navia, B., Thaler, H., Gold, J., & Sidtis, J. (1988). Neuropsychological characterization of the AIDS dementia complex: A preliminary report. *AIDS, 2,* 81–88.

Tuckson, R. (1994). Health care perceptions and needs of America's poor. In P. A. Pizzo & K. M. Wilfert (Eds.), *Pediatric AIDS: The challenge of HIV infection in infants, children, and adolescents* (2nd ed., pp. 963–973). Baltimore, MD: Williams & Wilkins.

Ultmann, M. H., Belman, A. L., Ruff., H. A., Novick, B. E., Cone-Wesson, B., Cohen, J. J., & Rubinstein, A. (1985). Developmental abnormalities in infants and children with acquired immune deficiency syndrome (AIDS) and AIDS-related complex. *Developmental Medicine and Child Neurology, 27,* 563–571.

Ultmann, M. H., Diamond, G. W., Ruff, H. A., Belman, A. L., Novick, B. E., Rubinstein, A., & Cohen, H. J. (1987). Developmental abnormalities in children with acquired immunodeficiency syndrome (AIDS): A follow up study. *International Journal of Neuroscience, 32,* 661–667.

van Gorp, W., Hinkin, C., Freeman, D., Satz, P., Weisman, J., Rothman, P., Scarsella, A., & Buckingham, S. (1990). *Depressed vs. non-depressed mood and its effect on neuropsychological test performance among HIV-1 seropositive individuals.* Paper presented at the conference on neurological and neuropsychological complications on HIV infection: A satellite conference to the VI international AIDS conference, Monterey, CA.

van Gorp, W., Hinkin, C. H., Moore, L. H., Miller, E. N., Marcotte, T. D., Satz, P., & Weisman, J. (1995). Subject ascertainment bias and neuropsychological performance in HIV disease. *Neuropsychology, 9,* 206–211.

van Gorp, W. G., Hinkin, C., Satz, P., Miller, E., & D'Elia, L. F. (1993). Neuropsychological Findings in HIV infection, encephalopathy, and dementia. In R. W. Parks, R. F. Zec, & R. S. Wilson (Eds.), *Neuropsychology of Alzheimer's disease and other dementias* (pp. 153–185). New York: Oxford University Press.

van Gorp, W., Mandelkern, M., Gee, M., Hinkin, C., Stern, C., Paz, D., Dixon, W., Evans, G., Flynn, F., Frederick, C., Ropchan, J., & Bland, W. (1992). Cerebral metabolic dysfunction in AIDS: Findings in an AIDS sample with and without dementia. *Journal of Neuropsychiatry and Clinical Neurosciences, 4,* 280–287.

van Gorp, W. G., Miller, E. N., Satz, P., & Visscher, B. (1989). Neuropsychological performance in HIV-1 immuno-compromised patients: A preliminary report. *Journal of Clinical and Experimental Neuropsychology, 11,* 763–773.

Vinters, H. V., Tomiyasu, U., & Anders, K. H. (1989). Neuropathological complications of infection with the human immunodeficiency virus (HIV). *Progress in AIDS Pathology, 1,* 101–130.

Whelan, M. A., Kricheff, M., Handler, M., Ho, V., Crystal, K., Gopinathan, G., & Laubenstein, L. (1983). Acquired immunodeficiency syndrome: Cerebral computed tomographic manifestations. *Radiology, 149,* 477–484.

White, D. A., Heaton, R. K., Monsch, N. D., & the HNRC Group. (1995). Neuropsychological studies of asymptomatic immunodeficiency virus-type-1 infected individuals. *Journal of the International Neuropsychological Society, 1,* 304–315.

Wiegand, M., Möller, A. A., Schreiber, W., Krieg, J. C., & Holsboer, F. (1991). Alterations of nocturnal sleep in patients with HIV infection. *Acta Neurologica Scandinavica, 83,* 141–142.

Wiener, L., & Septimus, A. (1994). Psychosocial support for child and family. In P. A. Pizzo & K. M. Wilfert (Eds.), *Pediatric AIDS: The challenge of HIV infection in infants, children, and adolescents* (2nd ed., pp. 809–829). Baltimore, MD: Williams & Wilkins.

Wiley, C. A., Masliah, E., Morey, M., Lemere, C., DeTerasa, R., Grafe, M., Hanson, L., & Terry, R. (1991). Neocortical damage during HIV infection. *Annals of Neurology, 29,* 651–657.

Wilkie, F. L., Eisdorfer, C., Morgan, R., Loewenstein, D. A., & Szapocznik, J. (1990). Cognition in early human immunodeficiency virus infection. *Archives of Neurology, 43,* 433–440.

Wofsy, C. (1987). Intravenous drug use and women's medical issues. *Report of the Surgeon General's Workshop on Children with HIV infection and their families* (pp. 32–34). Washington, DC: U.S. Department of Health and Human Services, Public Health Service.

Wolters, P., Brouwers, P., Moss, H., el-Amin, D., Eddy, J., Butler, K., Husson, R., & Pizzo, P. (1990). The effect of 2'3' dideoxyinosine (ddI) on the cognitive functioning of infants and children with symptomatic HIV infection. *Proceedings of the VI International Conference on AIDS, 3,* 130 (Abstract).

Wolters, P., Brouwers, P., Moss, H., el-Amin, D., Gress, J., Butler, L., & Pizzo, P. (1991). The effect of dideoxyinosine on the cognitive functioning of children with HIV infection after 6 and 12 months of treatment. *Proceedings from the VII International Conference on AIDS, 2,* 194 (Abstract).

Wolters, P., Brouwers, P., Moss, H., & Pizzo, P. (1994). Adaptive behavior of children with symptomatic HIV infection before and after Zidovudine therapy. *Journal of Pediatric Psychology, 19,* 47–61.

World Health Organization. (1996). *Weekly Epidemiological Record, 71,* 205–212.

IV

Cross-Cultural Applications
of Neuropsychological Assessment
Instruments

15

Methods for Detecting and Evaluating Cultural Bias in Neuropsychological Tests*

CECIL R. REYNOLDS

Since the early 1900s, near the time of Binet's first offering, intelligence tests have been scrutinized for cultural biases in a variety of forms. Indeed, the issues of bias (or its potential) in psychological testing have been a source of recurring, characteristically intense, social controversy throughout the history of mental measurement (e.g., see Reynolds & Brown, 1984, for a review of early to mid-1900s controversies). Discussions of cultural bias in tests, especially aptitude and ability measures such as are common to neuropsychological examinations, frequently are accompanied by strongly emotion-laden polemics decrying the use of mental tests with members of ethnic minorities. Courts, legislatures, and the media have all become involved in the questions surrounding potential cultural bias in testing (e.g., see Brown, Reynolds, & Whitaker, in press; Elliott, 1987; Spitz, 1986).

The issue of cultural bias has been prompted by the well documented findings (now seen consistently in over 100 years of research) that members of different ethnic groups have different levels and patterns of performance on a host of cognitive tests and most prominently on IQ measures (e.g., Elliott, 1987; Gutkin & Reynolds, 1981; Reynolds, Chastain, Kaufman, & McLean, 1987). The reason or reasons for these differences are crucial to the interpretation of performance by minority-ethnic groups. The differences may be due to genetic influences, environmental influences, or various combinations of genetics and environment (including transactional and reciprocal models of development), or they may be due to cultural bias in tests. If due to cultural bias versus other explanations, then scores must be corrected or new tests devised for ethnic minorities since the differences in performance are artifacts of the tests and not truly representative of skill, ability, or knowledge of the examinee. This leads directly to what has become known as the cultural test bias hypothesis (CTBH) (Brown, Reynolds, &

*This chapter is based substantively on a number of prior works of the author, most notably Reynolds (1982a), Reynolds and Kaiser (1992), Reynolds (1999), and Reynolds, Lowe, and Saenz (1999).

CECIL R. REYNOLDS • Texas A&M University, College Station, Texas 77843-4225; and Bastrop Mental Health Associates, Bastrop, Texas 78602.

Handbook of Cross-Cultural Neuropsychology, edited by Fletcher-Janzen, Strickland, and Reynolds. Kluwer Academic/Plenum Publishers, New York, 2000.

Whitaker, in press; Reynolds, 1982a, 1982b; Reynolds & Brown, 1984). The CTBH at its essence argues that differences in mean levels of performance across ethnic groups or gender are due to artifacts of the test or the measurement process and do not reflect real differences among these groups.

Although mean differences in level of performance are well documented on a variety of neuropsychological tests (e.g., see Grey-Little & Kaplan, 1998, and Reynolds 1997), neuropsychology has been relatively immune from attack on this issue. It was not uncommon in texts in the field into the 1990s for the issue of ethnic differences on neuropsychological test performance to be ignored altogether. It was not until the mid-1990s that research into ethnic differences on neuropsychological tests began in earnest, but it still lags other areas (Ardila, Rosselli, & Puente, 1994; Mayfield & Reynolds, 1997; Reynolds, 1997). Thus far, neuropsychological tests have fared well in test bias investigations (Reynolds, 1997) but much, much more remains to be done.

What Is Bias?

The term "bias" carries many different connotations for the lay public and for professionals in a number of disciplines. To the legal mind, bias denotes illegal discriminatory practices, while to the lay mind it may conjure notions of prejudicial attitudes. Much of the rancor in psychology and education regarding proper definitions of test bias is due to the divergent uses of this term in general (Reynolds & Brown, 1984), but especially by professionals in the same and related academic fields. Contrary to certain other opinions that more common or lay usages of the term bias should be employed when using the word in definitions or discussions of bias in educational and psychological tests, bias as used in the present chapter is defined in its widely recognized, distinct statistical sense. Bias denotes constant or systematic error, as opposed to chance or random error, in the estimation of some value; for purposes here, this constant or systematic error is alleged to be due to group membership or some other nominal variable, and occurs in the estimation of a score on a psychological or educational test or performance criterion. This definition is consistent with the position of the CTBH.

Other uses of the term bias in research on the differential or cross-group validity of tests are unacceptable from a scientific perspective for two reasons: (1) the imprecise nature of other uses of bias makes empirical investigation and rational inquiry exceedingly difficult, and (2) other uses of the term invoke specific moral value systems that are the subject of intense, polemic, emotional debate without a mechanism for rational or scientific resolution. The present chapter will proceed by presenting empirically assessable definitions of test bias and discussing the appropriate methodology for researching bias under the proffered definition.

Mean score differences in performance on tests do not define bias. A popular lay view has been that differences in mean levels of scoring on cognitive, achievement, or personality tests among groups constitute bias in tests; however, such differences alone clearly are not evidence of bias. A number of writers in the professional literature have also taken this position (Adebimpe, Gigandet, & Harris, 1979; Alley & Foster, 1978; Chinn, 1979; Guilford Press, 1997; Hilliard, 1979; G. D. Jackson, 1975; Mercer, 1976; Padilla, 1988; Williams, 1974; Wright & Isenstein, 1977). Those who support this definition of test bias correctly state that there is no valid a priori scientific reason to believe that intellectual or other cognitive performance levels should differ across race. It is the inference that tests that demonstrate such differences are inherently biased because there can, in reality, be no differences that is fallacious. Just as there are no a priori bases for deciding that differences exist, there is no a priori basis for deciding that differences do not exist. From the standpoint of the objective methods of science, a priori or premature acceptance of either hypothesis (differences exist vs. differences do not exist) is untenable. As stated by Thorndike (1971), "The presence (or absence) of differences in mean score between groups, or of differences in variability, tells us nothing directly about fairness" (p. 64). Some adherents of the "mean score differences as bias" viewpoint also require that the distribution of test scores in each population or subgroup be identical before one can assume that the test is fair: "Regardless of the purpose of a test or its validity for that purpose, a test should result in distributions that are statistically equivalent across the groups tested in order for it to be considered nondiscriminatory for those groups" (Alley & Foster, 1978, p. 2). Portraying a test as biased regardless of its purpose or validity is psychometrically naive. Mean score differences and unequivalent distributions have been the most uniformly rejected of all criteria examined by sophisticated psychometricians in investigating the problems of bias in assessment (see especially Reynolds, 1999a and 1982b).

What Are the Possible Sources of Bias?

Black, Hispanic, and other minority psychologists have raised many legitimate objections to the use of educational and psychological tests with minorities. Unfortunately, these objections are frequently stated as facts on rational rather than empirical grounds (Ardila, Rosselli, & Puente, 1994; Chambers, Barron, & Sprecher, 1980; Dana, 1996; Helms, 1993; Hilliard, 1979). The most frequently stated problems fall into one of the following categories:

Inappropriate Content.   African Americans and other minorities have not been exposed to the material in the test questions or other stimulus materials. The tests are geared primarily toward the majority class' homes, vocabulary, and values. Different value systems among cultures may produce cognitively equivalent answers, which are scored as incorrect because of prejudicial value judgements, not differences in ability (Bond, 1987; Butler-Omololu, Doster, & Lahey, 1984).

Inappropriate Standardization Samples.   Ethnic minorities are underrepresented in standardization samples used in the collection of normative reference data. Proportionate sampling with stratification by ethnicity is the herald for standardization samples for tests and is done to enhance the accuracy of parameter estimations for scaling purposes. Thus, although represented proportionately, ethnic minorities may appear in test standardization samples in small absolute numbers, and this may bias item selection (e.g., Harrington, 1975, 1976) and also fails to have any impact of significance from these ethnic groups on the tests themselves (Greenlaw & Jensen, 1996). In earlier years, it was not unusual for standardization samples to be all white (e.g., the 1937 Binet and 1949 WISC), disallowing any minority impact.

Examiners' and Language Bias.   Most psychologists in the United States are European in origin and speak only standard English, and they may intimidate people from other cultural groups. They are also unable to communicate accurately with minority children—to the point of being intimidating and insensitive to ethnic pronunciation of words on the tests. Lower test scores for minorities, then, may reflect only this intimidation and difficulty in the communication process, not lower ability (Clarizio, 1982; Emerling, 1990; Isern, 1986).

Inequitable Social Consequences.   As a result of bias in educational and psychological tests, minority group members, already at a disadvantage in the educational and vocational markets because of past discrimination and being thought unable to learn, are disproportionately relegated to dead-end educational tracks. Labeling effects also fall under this category (Chipman, Marshall, & Scott, 1991; Payne & Payne, 1991).

Measurement of Different Constructs.   Related to the issue of inappropriate content, this position asserts that tests measure different attributes when used with children from other than the majority culture, the culture on which the tests are largely based, and thus are not valid measures of minority skill, intelligence, or personality.

Differential Predictive Validity.   Although tests may accurately predict a variety of outcomes for members of the majority culture, they do not predict successfully any relevant behavior for minority-group members. Furthermore, there are objections to the use of the standard criteria against which tests are validated with minority cultural groups. For example, scholastic or academic attainment levels in white, middle-class schools are themselves considered by a variety of African American psychologists to be biased as criteria (see discussions in Reynolds, 1982a, 1982b).

Qualitatively Distinct Minority and Majority Aptitude and Personality.   Championed by Helms (1992), but not a new argument at all (e.g., Lonner, 1985), this position leads to the conclusion that ethnic minorities and the majority culture are so different as to require different conceptualizations of ability and of personality. Helms, for example, argues the potential existence of a "White g" factor that is separate from "African g" (p. 1090), which would necessitate separate tests for these groups.

Contrary to the situation of the late 1960s and 1970s, when the current controversies resurfaced after some decades of simmering, research has examined these areas of potential bias, especially in intelligence assessment and achievement testing. Extensive reviews of this literature are available, particularly with regard to measures of aptitude and cognitive skill (see especially Frisby & Braden, in press; Reynolds, 1982b, 1999a; Reynolds, Lowe, & Saenz, 1999); far less data are available on the CTBH and personality and behavioral measures; and even less data are available for neuropsychological tests. The overall findings of research directly addressing the CTBH are that well constructed, properly standardized tests of aptitude or cognitive skill are not biased against native-born American ethnic minorities (Brown, Reynolds, & Whitaker, in press; Frisby & Braden, in press; Reynolds, 1999a, in press; Reynolds, Lowe, & Saenz, 1999). The remainder of this chapter will focus on methods for investigating the CTBH, not on outcome literature or specific investigations of bias on neuropsychological tests. There is little actual research on what most consider exclusively neuropsychological tests (e.g., the Halstead–Reitan Neuropsychological Test Batteries, Luria–Nebraska Neuropsychological Battery) and the CTBH.

Methods for Investigating Cultural Bias in Neuropsychological Tests

The seven objections to testing with ethnic minorities noted above and the CTBH all resolve to issues of validity. Classically, validity has been discussed in its tripartite conceptualization of content, construct, and criterion-related (also encompassing predictive) validity components. This artificial division of validity has been for convenience and it is at times misleading. Validity is referenced to a test often as well, typically as a means of shorthand. Validity actually is a characteristic of the interpretation or meaning assigned to performance on a test (the latter typically represented as a test score). The CTBH may then be seen as proposing that the traditional interpretation of test scores for a majority group in a population cannot be generalized to minority groups for the reasons noted above. If there exists systematic error in the estimation of test scores, which are believed to represent some latent aspect of brain function, as a function of some nominal characteristic such as ethnicity or gender, then it follows that a common interpretation of test performance across such groups would be in error. Such errors logically would lead to overdiagnosis of central nervous system (CNS) psycho-pathology among minorities on some occasions and underdiagnosis on others.

A significant battery of methods has evolved to detect bias in mental tests and many of these methods are now applied by publishers during the development of new tests. Any bias detected in score estimation can then be eliminated, but cross-validation of the end product and careful examination of older tests, devised prior to the advent of research on bias in tests, are necessary. Methods for examination of individual test items for bias are presented first, under the general rubric of examining the test's content, followed by methods for examining tests as a whole to see if bias exists in the scores obtained (construct validity and criterion-related validity).

Bias in Content Validity

Bias in the item content of tests is one of the favorite topics of those who decry the use of standardized tests with minorities (e.g., Hilliard, 1979; Jackson, 1975; Williams, 1974; Wright & Isenstein, 1977). The earliest work in cultural test bias centered on content. Typically, critics review the items of a test and single out specific items as being biased because: (1) the items ask for information that an ethnic minority or a disadvantaged person has not had equal opportunity to learn, (2) the scoring of the item is improper since the test's author has arbitrarily decided on the only correct answer, and ethnic minorities are inappropriately penalized for giving answers that would be correct in their own culture but not that of the author, and/or (3) the working of the questions is unfamiliar, and an ethnic minority who may "know" the correct answer may not be able to respond because he or she does not understand the question. Each of these and related criticisms, when accurate, have the same basic empirical result: The item becomes relatively more difficult for ethnic minority group members than for the majority population; for example, an ethnic minority and a member of the majority culture with the same standing on the construct in question will respond differently to such biased items. Cronbach (1990) refers to such properties as irrelevant difficulties. (Test developers are always working to remove irrelevant difficulties on all fronts because they lower item reliability.) This leads directly to a definition of content bias for aptitude tests that allows empirical assessment of the phenomenon:

> An item or subscale of a test is considered to be biased in content when it is demonstrated to be relatively more difficult for members of one group than for members of another when the general ability level of the groups being compared is held constant and no reasonable theoretical rationale exists to explain group differences on the item (or subscale) in question.

With regard to achievement tests, the issue of content bias is considerably more complex. Exposure to instruction, the general ability level of the group, and the accuracy and specificity of the sampling of the domain of items are important variables in determining whether the content is biased (see Schmidt, 1983). Research into item (or content) bias with achievement tests has typically, and perhaps mistakenly, relied on methodology appropriate for determining item bias in aptitude tests. Nevertheless, research that examines both types of instruments for content bias has yielded quite comparable results. Items on personality tests may be perceived differently across cultures as well, or appropriate responses may vary dramatically and quite properly deserve different interpretations cross-culturally. If so, the items will behave differently across groups for individuals with the same relative standing. This, too, is detectable through analyses of item response data across groups.

One method of locating "suspicious" test items requires item difficulties to be determined separately for each group under consideration. If any individual item or series of items appears to be exceptionally difficult relative to other items on the tests for the members of any group, the item is considered potentially biased and removed from the test. Analyses of variance (ANOVA) and several closely related procedures, in which the group-by-item interaction term is of interest (Angoff & Ford, 1973; Cardall & Coffman, 1964) were once thought to be more exacting and were widely used to identify biased items; until the late 1980s ANOVA was the most popular empirical approach (Camilli & Shepard, 1987).

ANOVA Methods

The definition of content bias just presented actually requires that the relative differences in item difficulty between groups be the same for every item on the test. Thus, in the ANOVA procedures, the group-by-item interaction should not yield a significant result. Whenever the differences in items are not uniform (a significant group-by-item interaction does exist), one may contend that these are biased items. Earlier in this area of research it was hoped that the empirical analysis of tests at the item level would result in the identification of a category of items having similar content as biased and that such items could then be avoided in future test development (Flaugher, 1978). Very little similarity among items determined to be biased has been found. No one has been able to identify those characteristics of an item that cause it to be biased. It does seem that poorly written, sloppy, and ambiguous items tend to be identified as biased with greater frequency than those items typically encountered in a well-constructed, standardized instrument. The variable at issue, then, may be the item reliability. Item reliabilities are typically not large, and poorly written or ambiguous test items easily can have problems with low reliability; low item reliabilities have long been known to increase the probability of the occurrence of bias (Linn & Werts, 1971). Informal inventories and locally derived tests are much more likely to be biased than professionally written standardized tests.

The ANOVA methodology is appealing conceptually but has some significant problems, even though it was the dominant methodological approach to the issue of item bias through the 1980s. Camilli and Shepard (1987) have provided convincing examples, although using contrived data, that ANOVA methods often miss biased items, in both directions, and identify some items as biased that are not. An algebraic demonstration of the reasons for this is provided in Camilli and Shepard (1994), who conclude that ANOVA should no longer be used. However, common content of biased items has not been revealed by any statistical method, so the failure to determine classes or even a class of content that creates bias is not an artifact of ANOVA methods.

IRT Methods

Based on their thorough and compelling analyses of methods for detecting biased items, Camilli and Shepard (1994) recommend methods derived from item response theory to detect what has come to be known as differential item functioning (DIF). The DIF statistics work by identifying all items in a test that function differently from the standards for different groups. Ideally, once these items are identified, a logical analysis is conducted to determine why they are relatively more difficult for one or more groups. Based on the analysis, subsets of DIF items are identified as biased and are eliminated from the test. Therefore, DIF indexes are merely raw or uninterpretable indexes that detect multidimensionality of an item set in a test or subtest. Significant DIFs do not necessarily mean that particular items are biased. Biased items are determined according to the interpretation of the items within a coherent and substantive framework about their relevance to the construct being measured. In other words, if items tap traits irrelevant to the intended construct, as determined through careful judgement and additional empirical investigation, these items are considered to be biased. For example, if baseball is the topic of a reading passage on the reading comprehension section of a comprehensive examination of aphasia, and items relating to baseball on the reading comprehension section produce significant DIFs when comparing males and females, further analysis would need to be conducted to determine if these items were measuring reading comprehension or tapping some other trait, such as prior knowledge about baseball, which might introduce irrelevant difficulties for females. Through careful deliberations and further empirical study, if it is found that these items are tapping the examinees' prior knowledge about baseball instead of reading comprehension, these items would be labeled as biased and would be removed from the test.

Item response theory (IRT) is primarily concerned with the probability of occurrence of a particular response to a test item as a function of the examinee's relative position on the latent trait. The IRT's principal conceptual unit, the item characteristic curve (ICC), represents this relationship. The ICC is determined by three parameters: a, b, and c. The a parameter represents the discrimination power of an item (i.e., how well an item distinguishes examinees who score high or low on the latent trait). Discrimination corresponds to the slope of the ICC. The b parameter represents the difficulty of an item and is measured in the same scale units as the latent trait. The b parameter is located along the latent trait scale at the point where the probability of a correct response is equal to $(1 + c)/2$. The c parameter, the guessing parameter, represents the probability of examinees who score low on the latent trait answering a test item correctly. The c parameter is the lower asymptote of the ICC. These three parameters determine the shape of the ICC. Diagrammatic representation of one group's ICC for one item is depicted in Figure 1.

Different IRT models are derived from estimates of these three different parameters. The three-parameter (3P) model is made up of the three parameter estimates and is the most commonly used and recommended IRT model, especially with multiple-choice items because of the complexity of the data (Camilli & Shepard, 1994). Multiple-choice tests are a common occurrence in neuropsychological testing. A few prominent examples include the Wisconsin Card Sorting Test, Speech Sounds Perception Test, and the Seashore Rhythm Test. However, open-ended questions, such as the Weschler Scales Information and Comprehension items, also are affected by guessing, and guessing parameters are especially crucial to assess in the Boston process approach to these tests. A two-parameter (2P) model and one-parameter (1P), also known as the Rasch model, also exist. Camilli and Shepard (1994) and Hambleton, Swaminathan, and Rogers (1991) describe these models more extensively. The selection of an appropriate IRT model is critical, as failure to use an adequate model will lead to inaccurate estimates of item parameters and decrease the utility of IRT techniques. Computer programs are available for estimating item and latent parameters, such as LOGIST and BILOG, using joint maximum likelihood (JML) or marginal maximum likelihood (MML) techniques, respectively.

In applying IRT to DIF, the ICCs of the two different groups (group A and group B) are compared on the same item. Conceptually, the ICCs for the two groups are plotted on the same

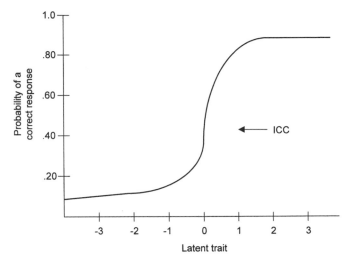

FIGURE 1. Example of an ICC or item characteristic curve.

scale, and the area between the two ICCs is measured to determine the degree of DIF. The area between the two ICCs, for group A and group B, DIF, is depicted in Figure 2. The DIF procedure requires not only equating item and latent parameter estimates for the two different groups but also selecting appropriate IRT measures and tests for DIF. If the DIF index is significant, further analysis of this item and all the other items with significant DIFs are needed to determine if they are biased.

To plot the two ICCs on the same scale, the parameters or estimates of the item and latent parameters must be equated or scaled in the same metric. There are two techniques for equating the item parameter estimates; the anchor-test method and separate-sample method. The latter requires running the IRT analyses separately for each group and then transforming the parameter estimates so they can be placed on a common scale. This method involves explicit equating. A more implicit equating approach, recommended by Camilli and Shepard (1994), is the anchor-test method, which requires that estimated parameters for both groups be simultaneously equated during a single computer estimation run by using MML. During the computer run, all items except the item of interest, known as the anchor item, are constrained. This procedure is repeated for each item on the test so that biased items will not spoil the estimation of the examinee's latent trait.

To determine the degree of DIF, an IRT method for measuring the size of the area or differential performance of the two groups on a test is needed. The IRT measures of DIF include simple area indexes, b parameter difference indexes, pseudo-IRT indexes, and probability difference indexes. In the probability difference indexes, the area between the ICCs is weighted. The probability difference statistics, signed probability difference controlling for the latent trait (SPD-O) and unsigned probability difference controlling for the latent trait (UPD-O), are calculated for uncrossed or crossed ICCs, respectively, to determine the degree of DIF. According to Camilli and Shepard (1994), probability difference indexes have more stability and power and are the preferred methods for determining the degree of DIF because they have outperformed the other measures of DIF in accurate, replicable detection of DIF.

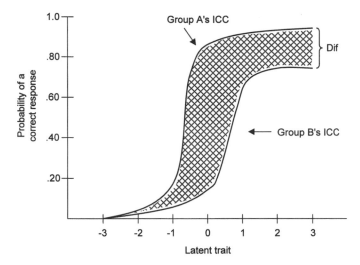

FIGURE 2. ICCs for 2 groups on a common item showing DIF across groups.

Once the degree of DIFs is measured, an IRT statistical test is used to determine if DIF is statistically significantly different from the null hypothesis. The IRT statistical tests include the test of b differences, item drift method, Lord's chi-square, bootstrap, and jackknife methods, and model comparison measures. Descriptions of these IRT statistical tests are found in Camilli and Shepard (1994), which remains an excellent source for item bias detection methods.

Model comparison procedures are the recommended approaches to test for significance of DIF, according to numerous researchers and psychometricians (Camilli & Shepard, 1994; Judd & McClelland, 1989; Thissen, Steinberg, & Wainer, 1993). In this approach, the relative fit of the compact model and augmented model are compared. The compact model is a model in which all of the estimated parameters of an item, a, b, and c, for all of the groups are identical, yielding a single ICC for all groups. In contrast, the augmented model allows one, two, or all three of the estimated parameters to vary, yielding different ICCs for the different groups. To determine which model provides a better fit of the data, an inferential test statistic based on a natural log transformation of a likelihood ratio that is approximately distributed as a chi-square is calculated. If the inferential test statistic is significant, significant DIF exists for that one item. This procedure is repeated for all items on a test. Once this procedure is completed, those items with significant DIFs undergo further empirical study and deliberation to determine if they are biased. If the items are biased, they should be removed from the test. If the analyses are postpublication, a sufficient degree of DIF should cast considerable doubt on use of the scale altogether.

The IRT methods provide the most sensitive tests for DIF when the models accurately describe the data. These are the preferred approaches in research to obtain generalizable results, however, these methods are computer-intensive and require large samples for testing the model fit. As a result, contingency table (CT) approaches, using nonparametric methods, are often used to detect DIF in applied settings during test development when sample size, resources, time, and programming experience are limited.

In comparison to the IRT methods, CT approaches correspond closely to the visual inspection of the area between the ICC curves (Camilli & Shepard, 1994). In addition, these approaches use observed scores rather than measures of latent traits in statistical analyses (Ackerman, 1991). Contingency table methods for testing DIF include summed chi-square, Mantel–Haenszel chi-square, and logistic regression. Camilli and Shepard provide a detailed description of these CT methods of testing for DIF. Both CT and IRT methods have their advantages, however, the decision whether to use one or the other often boils down to sample size.

As a relevant example of the CT approach, the Mantel–Haenszel technique was used to examine possible racial, ethnic, and gender bias on the Guide to the Assessment of Test Session Behavior (GATSB). Only 10 out of 80 items were found to have significant DIFs, and the 10 significant DIF items barely exceeded the chance rate. This result lends support to the notion that the GATSB shows no signs of item bias across gender and ethnicity (Nandakumar, Glutting, & Oakland, 1993). More importantly, these authors provide a good explanation of the application of the method, making it more readily accessible.

The IRT models, such as those to detect DIF, are conceptually similar to other models, such as ANOVA. The IRT models to detect DIF are primarily superior to previous methods because they are less sample-dependent, and they allow one to estimate multiple-item statistics more precisely than a technique like ANOVA, which has special problems when main effects are present along with interaction effects. Using the item characteristics curves, DIF more accurately and readily detects when the probability of a particular response changes as a function of some nominal variable (e.g., ethnicity or gender) for individuals with the same relative standing on the latent trait being assessed.

Partial Correlation

A partial correlation procedure developed independently by Stricker (1982) and Reynolds, Willson, and Chatman (1984) has been used to study systematically DIF in a variety of aptitude and cognitive tests. Computationally much simpler than IRT or ICC models, the partial correlation method is widely accessible through SPSS, SAS, BMD, STATA, and virtually any other statistical software package including an ordinary least squares regression component.

In the partial correlation procedure, the partial correlation between item score and the nominal variable of interest (e.g., gender) is calculated, partialling the correlation between total test score (subtest of a larger battery or the total score on a unidimensional test) and the nominal variable. This procedure effectively holds total score constant across groups and reveals whether an item is more or less difficult for members of one nominal group versus another when the members being compared possess a common level of skill or ability on the latent trait in question. If the partial r value differs significantly from zero, then the item can be seen to possess irrelevant difficulties for some group(s) (i.e., difficulties unrelated to the skill or ability being tested). The partial r may be squared to provide an immediate and viable estimate of an effect size as well. The partial correlation method is the simplest of the methods available and the most powerful, but will also tend to overidentify potentially as biased items that are not confirmed by IRT. When using the partial correlation methods, controls for experiment-wise error rates must be employed and effect sizes should be viewed in making final decisions about bias in an item. An additional example of the application of the partial r procedure to problems in neuropsychology is given in Willson, Nolan, Reynolds, and Kamphaus (1989).

P-Decrements

Jensen (1976) has pursued another approach to the identification of biased items. According to Jensen, if a test contains items that are disproportionately more difficult for one group of examinees than another, the correlations of P-decrements between adjacent items will be low for the two groups. (P-decrement is the difference in the difficulty index, P, from one item of a test to the next item. Typically, ability test items are arranged in ascending order of difficulty.) Jensen (1974, 1976) also contends that if a test contains biased items, the correlation between the rank order of item difficulties for one race with another will also be low. Clear examples of the use of this approach may be found in Jensen (1974, 1976, 1977). In these studies, Jensen calculated cross-racial correlations of item difficulties for large samples of black and white children on five major intelligence tests: Peabody Picture Vocabulary Test (PPVT), Raven's Progressive Matrices (the Raven), Revised Stanford–Binet Intelligence Scale Form L-M, WISC-R, and Wonderlic Personnel Test. Cross-racial correlations of P-decrements were reported for several of the scales. He found little evidence to support any consistent content bias in any of the scales. A correlation between P-decrements of .90 or higher indicates a general lack of content bias in the instruments as a whole.

This method has proved popular with some test publishers who want to look at the items on a test as a group, despite the fact that this approach may be overly sensitive. Using the Detroit Tests of Learning Aptitude (DTLA-3), Hammill (1991) reported correlations of P-decrements exceeding .90 for all subtests, with most exceeding .95. Similar results have been reported for other aptitude measures. On the 14 subtests of the Test of Memory and Learning (TOMAL), Reynolds and Bigler (1994) report correlations across P-decrements by gender and ethnicity that all exceed .90, with most again above .95.

The method of correlated P-decrements is very sensitive to changes in relative positions of items across nominal groups, but is a poor choice for the identification of specific items contributing to any potential bias in test content. Although one can inspect the rank-ordering of the items across groups and certainly pick out items with large differences in P-decrements, determining bias for an individual item is too subjective using these procedures. Nevertheless, the technique is useful in evaluating the success of a test developer in removing biased items. The method of correlated P-decrements is used best near the end of the test development process to assess the item bank as a whole, testing the relative success of the individual item identification procedures and to determine whether the items, taken as a whole, display significant variation in relative difficulty across groups.

Multiple Choice Items and Distractor Attractiveness

With multiple-choice tests, another level of complexity is added to the examination of content bias. With a multiple-choice question, three or four distractors are typically given, in addition to the correct response. Distractors may be examined for their attractiveness (the relative frequency with which they are chosen) across groups. When distractors are found to be disproportionately attractive for members of any particular group, the item may be defined as biased. When items are constructed to have an equal distribution of responses to each distractor for the total test population, chi-square can be used to examine the distribution of choices for each distractor for each group (Burrill, 1975).

As an example, Jensen (1976) investigated the distribution of wrong responses for two multiple-choice intelligence tests, the PPVT and the Raven. These two tests were individually administered to 600 Anglo-American and 400 African American children between the ages of 6 and 12. The analysis of incorrect responses for the PPVT indicated that the errors were distributed in a nonrandom fashion over a large number of items. However, no cultural bias in response patterns occurred because the disproportionate choice of distractors followed the same pattern for African Americans and European Americans. On the Raven, African Americans made different types of errors than European Americans, but only on a small number of items. To try to understand the outcome in more detail, Jensen followed up these items and compared the African American response pattern to the response pattern of European American children at a variety of age levels. For every item showing differences in response patterns, the African American response patterns could be duplicated by the response patterns of European Americans approximately two years younger than the African Americans. Follow up and evaluation to determine the reasons for DIF is always useful.

Veale and Foreman (1983) have advocated inspecting multiple-choice tests for bias in distractor or "foil" response distribution as a means of refining tests *before* they are finalized for the marketplace. They note that there are many instances in which unbiased external criteria (such as achievement or ability) or culturally valid tests are not readily accessible for detecting bias in the measure under study. They add that inspection of incorrect responses to distractor items can often lead to greater insight into cultural bias in any given question than would inspection of the percentage of correct responses across groups. Veale and Foreman provide the statistical analyses for their "overpull probability model," along with the procedures for measuring cultural variation and diagramming the source of bias in any given item.

Expert Approaches

A common practice in recent times has been a return to the expert judgment of professionals and members of minority groups in the item selection for new psychological and educational tests. This approach was used in development of the K-ABC, the revision of the Wechsler Preschool and Primary Scale of Intelligence (WPPSI-R), the PPVT-R, and a number of other contemporary tests. The practice typically asks for an "armchair" inspection of individual items as a means of locating and expurgating biased components in the measure under development. The federal judge in *PASE vs. Hannon* (Reschley, 2000) applied this method himself, reviewing items from the WISC and the Binet, dismissing most expert testimony, and determining which items were biased based upon his own reading of the items (see Elliott, 1987). In a televised interview in 1997, a Texas Education Agency statewide testing director defended the agency's competency tests as possessing no biased items because members of minority groups read the items in advance and tell the agency which are biased (Brown, Reynolds, & Whitaker, in press). Since, as previously noted, no detectable pattern or common characteristics of individual items statistically shown to be biased has been observed (given reasonable care in the item-writing stage), it seems reasonable to question this approach.

The bulk of scientific data since the pioneering work of McGurk (1951) has not supported the position that anyone can—upon surface inspection—detect the degree to which any given item will function differentially across groups. Several researchers since McGurk's time have identified items as being disproportionately more difficult for minority group members than for members of the majority culture and have subsequently compared their results with a panel of expert judges. The data have provided some interesting results.

Although examples of the failure of judges to identify biased items now abound (Camilli & Shepard, 1994; Reynolds, 1982b) and show that judges are right about an item almost as often as they are wrong, two studies demonstrate this failure most clearly. After identifying the eight least and most racially discriminating items on the Wonderlic Personnel Test, Jensen

(1976) asked panels of five black psychologists and five white psychologists to sort the eight most and eight least discriminating items when only these 16 items were presented to them. The judges sorted the items at a level no better than chance. Sandoval and Mille (1979) conducted a more extensive analysis, using items from the WISC-R. These researchers had 38 black, 22 Mexican American, and 40 white university students from Spanish, history, and education classes identify items from the WISC-R that would be more difficult for a minority child than a white child and items that would be equally difficult for each group. A total of 45 WISC-R items were presented to each judge, including the 15 most difficult items for blacks as compared to whites, the 15 most difficult items for Mexican Americans as compared to whites, and the 15 items with the most nearly identical difficulty indexes for minority and white children. The judges were asked to read each question and determine whether they thought the item was (1) easier for minority than for white children, (2) easier for white than for minority children, or (3) of equal difficulty for white and minority children. Sandoval and Mille's results indicated that the judges were not able to differentiate accurately between items that were more difficult for minorities and items that were of equal difficulty across groups; minority and nonminority judges did not differ in their ability to identify biased items accurately, nor did they differ with regard to the type of incorrect identification they tended to make. Sandoval and Mille concluded: "(1) judges are not able to detect items which are more difficult for a minority child than an Anglo child, and (2) the ethnic background of the judge makes no difference in accuracy of item selection for minority children" (p. 6). In each of these studies, the most extreme items were used, which should have given the judges an advantage.

Anecdotal evidence is also available to refute the assumption that armchair analyses of test bias in item content are accurate. By far the most widely cited example of a biased intelligence test item is item 6 of the WISC-R Comprehension subtest: "What is the thing to do if a boy (girl) much smaller than yourself starts to fight with you?" This item is generally considered to be biased against African American children in particular because of the scoring criteria. According to the item's critics, the most logical response for an African American child is to "fight back," yet this is a zero-point response. The correct (two-point) response is to walk away and avoid fighting with the child—a response that critics claim invites disaster in black culture, where children are taught to fight back and would not know the so-called correct white response. Black responses to this item have been investigated empirically in several studies, with the same basic results: the item is relatively easier for black children than for white children. When all items on the WISC-R are ranked separately according to difficulty level for blacks and whites, this item is the forty-second least difficult item (where one represents the easiest item) for black children and the forty-seventh least difficult item for white children (Jensen, 1976). Miele (1979) in a large N study of bias, reached a similar conclusion, stating that this item "is relatively easier for Blacks than it is for Whites" (p. 163). The results of these empirical studies with large samples of black and white children in the United States are unequivocal: when matched for overall general intellectual skill, more black than white children will answer this item correctly—the very item most singled out as a blatant example of the inherent bias of intelligence tests against blacks (see also Reynolds & Brown, 1984).

Even without empirical support for its accuracy, a number of prestigious writers support the "face validity" approach of using a panel of minority judges to identify "biased" test items (Anastasi, 1982; Cronbach, 1990; Kaufman, 1979; Sandoval & Mille, 1979). Those who support the continued use of this technique see it as a method of gaining greater rapport with the public. As pointed out by Sandoval and Mille, "Public opinion, whether it is supported by empirical findings or based on emotion, can serve as an obstacle to the use of a measurement instrument" (p. 7). The elimination of items that are offensive or otherwise objectionable to any substantive segment of the population for whom the test is intended seems an appropriate action that may aid in the public's acceptance of new and better psychological assessment tools. However, the subjective judgment approach should not be allowed to supplant the use of more sophisticated analyses in the determination of biased items. The subjective approach should serve as a supplemental procedure, and items identified through this method (provided that some interrater agreement can be obtained, an aspect of the subjective methods yet to be demonstrated) can be eliminated when a psychometrically equivalent (or better) item can be obtained as a replacement and the intent of the item is kept intact (e.g., with a criterion-referenced measure, the new item must be designed to measure the same objective).

Summary

Statistical estimates of DIF, although central to the question of item bias, do not, as Camilli and Shepard (1994) so aptly instruct us, provide immediate evidence of bias. A test statistic indicating a statistically significant level of DIF is no more than reason to suspect an item to be biased. A variety of contributions may be at work including multidimensionality, unreliability of the method itself (all DIF statistics have their own Type I and Type II error rates), errors of parameter estimation, and violation of any assumptions about the data that are necessary to the analysis. There will always be some degree of subjective judgment in determining whether an item with a significant DIF statistic is biased or not. The search for bias is a search for irrelevant, but systematic, difficulties at the item level. Camilli and Shepard (1994, Chapter 6) provide an extended discussion of various levels of analysis to apply in estimation of bias or irrelevant difficulty in an item designed to measure a particular cognitive attribute. (This discussion is highly recommended for those who pursue item bias research in neuropsychological testing.) For statistical methods, IRT/ICC 3P models and the partial correlation procedures are recommended. The expert approaches to item bias are not recommended and may be worse than no analysis at all if substituted for other, reliable procedures with the caveat that minority experts should review items for culturally objectionable content (which it turns out, does not tend to create irrelevant difficulties but which should nevertheless be removed as offensive).

Methods for Investigating Bias in Construct Validity

The construct validity of a test refers to the extent to which the test in question may be interpreted to measure a given construct or trait (e.g., constructional praxis, intelligence, executive function, attention, memory, etc.). Construct validity is easily the most complex but most central of all conceptualizations of test validity and requires greater inference and argument by reason than do other traditionally conceived categories of validity. The defining of bias in construct validity then requires a general, but operational, statement that can be researched from a variety of viewpoints with a broad range of methodology. The following definition has been proffered by Reynolds (1982a):

> Bias exists in regard to construct validity when a test is shown to measure different hypothetical traits (psychological constructs) for one group than another or to measure the same trait but with differing degrees of accuracy. (p. 194)

The question of bias in construct validity is of substantial concern, not only to practitioners in neuropsychology, but to the researcher and theoretician alike. Indeed, if bias in construct validity across groups for males and females, or blacks and whites, upper- and lower-SES (socioeconomic status) groups, or other popular nominal groupings of individuals for research purposes occurs with any consistency, then much of the research of differential psychology of the present century must be discarded as confounded and major theories abandoned as primarily artifactual (Reynolds, 1980a; Reynolds & Brown, 1984). This would present a difficult situation at best since the psychology of individual differences is the basic science underlying much of applied psychology, including clinical neuropsychology.

As befitting the complexity of a concept such as construct validity, many methods have been employed to examine existing psychological tests for potential bias in construct validity.

Factor Analysis Methods

One of the more popular and necessary empirical approaches to investigating construct validity is factor analysis (Anastasi, 1982; Cronbach, 1990). Factor analysis, as a procedure, identifies clusters of test items or clusters of subtests of psychological or educational tests that correlate highly with one another and less so or not at all with other subtests or items. Factor analysis then allows one to determine patterns of relationships of performance within and between groups of individuals. For example, if several subtests of an intelligence scale load highly on (are members of) the same factor, then if a group of individuals scores at a high level on one of these subtests, the group would be expected to score highly on other subtests that load highly on that factor. Psychologists attempt to determine through a review of the test content and correlates of performance on the factor in question what psychological trait(s) underlie performance, or, in a more hypothesis-testing approach, they will make predictions concerning the pattern of factor loadings. Hilliard (1979), one of the more vocal critics of IQ tests on the basis of cultural bias, has pointed out one of the potential areas of bias dealing with the comparison of the factor-analytic results of test studies across race.

"If the IQ test is a valid and reliable test of 'innate' ability or abilities, then the factors which emerge on a given test should be the same from one population to another, since 'intelligence' is asserted to be a set of *mental* processes. Therefore, while the configuration of scores of a particular group on the factor profile should be expected to differ, logic would dictate that the factors themselves would remain the same" (Hilliard, 1979, p. 53). Given that neuropsychological tests attempt to assess brain function, perhaps an even stronger statement would be appropriate for many tests used by neuropsychologists.

While not agreeing that identical factor analyses of an instrument speak to the innateness of the abilities being measured, *consistent factor analytic results across populations do provide strong evidence that whatever is being measured by the instrument is being measured in the same manner and is in fact the same construct within each group*. If factor analytic results (i.e., the relationships of the variables comprising the test) are constant across groups, then one may have greater confidence that the individuals in each group perceive and interpret the test materials in a similar manner. The information derived from comparative factor analysis across populations then is directly relevant to the use of neuropsychological tests in diagnostic and other decision-making functions. In order to make consistent interpretations of test score data, neuropsychologists must be certain that the test(s) measures the same variable across populations.

Comparative factor analysis is not without its own set of methodological and statistical problems. Camilli and Shepard (1994) downplay this approach as having many of the same problems of ANOVA and related regression approaches. Factor analysis is kindred to these approaches and is steeped in ordinary least squares (OLS) methods. In reviewing the criticisms of Camilli and Shepard (1994) of factor analytic approaches, they seem to apply best to using the method to identify biased items, but the method may also overestimate the presence of bias. When bias is not detected, the evidence is then even stronger. However, the search for potential bias and biasing factors requires multiple methods and factor analysis is useful in identifying latent structures that may correspond to real *abilities* or skills we seek to measure. Factor analysis also helps us address the problem of differences in dimensionality across groups.

It is common in neuropsychological research on various tests to contrast groups of individuals with central nervous system (CNS) compromise, be it traumatic injury, stroke, or disease, with groups having no known CNS problems. Differences in test scores are then interpreted along specific dimensions of cognitive function. In individual differences research, groups are often compared across ethnicity or gender on various psychological tests. In order for such comparisons to make psychological sense, one must demonstrate (although more commonly researchers simply assume) that the tests have a common latent structure and are measuring the same construct in the subgroups being compared. In the absence of such a demonstration there are too many competing interpretations. For purposes here, one competing interpretation would be that the groups do not differ on the construct in question, despite differences in mean level of performance on a common test, because the test is measuring something different in the two groups. For example, a group of patients with highly focal prefrontal lesions and a group of focal occipital lesion patients may show comparable levels of impairment, relative to a matched normal control sample, on the Trailmaking Test, Part A. However, for those groups, an interpretation of attentional deficits in the two TBI groups may or may not be appropriate. Deficits on Trailmaking may be representing attentional deficits in a prefrontal group and visual search problems in the occipital group. Separate, comparative factor analyses of the proper group of tests, including Trailmaking, for each of those three groups would help answer the question of what interpretation is most appropriate. The same may well be true between genders and among various ethnic groups, and without studies of the comparability of the latent structure of test batteries across groups, questions remain. Some work has been done in this regard. For example, in evaluating ethnic differences in mean levels of performance on 14 memory tests, Mayfield and Reynolds (1997) first presented a comparative factor analysis of the tests by gender and ethnicity.

In assessing the outcome of factor analysis across groups, there are two fundamental approaches. One approach addresses the question of the similarity of the outcome of the analyses, that is, how closely do the latent structures of the test battery correspond across groups. The second approach asks whether there is a statistically significant difference in the results of the analyses for the two groups. In the context of test interpretation, the former question is of inherently greater interest, especially given the sample sizes needed for stable factor analysis results. In such large *N* studies, inconsequential differences (i.e., minimal or even trivial effect sizes) may be statistically significant.

Assessing Differences

Chi-Square Goodness-of-Fit

The most sophisticated approach to the latter questions has been the work of Jöreskog (1969, 1971; Jöreskog & Sorbom, 1989; McGaw & Jöreskog, 1971) in simultaneous factor analysis in several populations. Jöreskog employs the chi-square test for goodness-of-fit across the factor analytic results for several groups to determine whether there is a "fit" or the results differ significantly across groups. A full treatment of Jöreskog's techniques is certainly beyond the scope and intent of the present chapter. The computational procedure is quite complex and the comparison of factors very sensitive. As yet, little research has been reported in the bias literature using Jöreskog's method. One could apply confirmatory factor analysis (CFA) in this situation, taking the solution of either of the two groups as the target solution and assess the fit of the other group's solution using a test of the statistical significance of the difference. If the effect size is small (and effect size estimation is quite subjective in CFA), there are substantive difficulties in determining the proper interpretation of the results. Assessing similarity is preferred, but there are other approaches to evaluating differences in factor analytic results.

A related but computationally simpler method for determining the significance of the difference between individual factors for two groups, also employing a chi-square technique, has been presented by Jensen (1980) and has ben employed by Miele (1979) and Reynolds and Streur (1982). Once corresponding factors have been located, all factor loadings are converted to Fisher z scores. The z scores for corresponding factors are paired by variable and subtracted. The differences in factor loadings, now expressed as differences between z scores, are squared, summed, and the mean of the squared differences derived. The mean difference must then be divided by the standard error of measurement of the difference between factor loadings, calculated to be the quantity

$$\frac{1}{N_1 - 3} + \frac{1}{N_2 - 3} \tag{1}$$

where N_1 is the number of subjects in group one and N_2 represents the number of subjects in group two. This division of the mean of the squared differences by the standard error of the difference will be distributed as chi-square with one degree of freedom. Special cases of this test are described in Jensen (1980, Chapter 9), though the above general form is applicable in most cases.

Comparing Correlation Matrices

Factor analysis is typically, though not always, based on a correlation matrix for a set of variables. For this reason, it may be desirable to test for the significance of the difference between correlation matrices. As Jensen (1980) points out, however, there is no direct test for equivalence of two correlation matrices across samples from different populations, though such a test may be approximated by a form of the above test. To test for the significance of the difference between correlation matrices, correlations in each matrix are transformed to Fisher zs. Corresponding pairs of correlations in each matrix, now expressed as z scores, are then contrasted, the difference squared, and the mean of the squared differences derived. This value then becomes the numerator for the procedure described above. The denominator remains the same (Eq. 1). The test statistic thus derived will approximately be distributed as chi-square with one degree of freedom. Since this test is only approximate, Jensen (1980) properly warns that interpretation of differences should precede cautiously unless $p \leq .01$. More exact, yet computationally complex, procedures are available for comparing correlation matrices across groups (Timm, 1975). Most statistical programs (e.g., SAS, SPSS, BMD) will also compare covariance matrices, but with the extreme power of these tests with large N samples trivial differences that are statistically significant are common.

Significant Differences between Factor Loadings: Conclusion

Methods for determining the significance of the difference in the size and pattern of variable loadings on corresponding factors between samples, while appropriate in certain circumstances, suffer from two major related drawbacks when addressing the more practical problems of test interpretation. With the very large samples necessary for stability of factor analysis results, small, practically negligible differences between factors can easily produce "significant" results. When interpreting test scores across groups, the degree of similarity of factors takes on greater importance for the practitioner; tests for statistically significant differences cannot sufficiently answer questions of similarity. Although psychology and research in most social sciences tend to emphasize differences, similarities may occur in greater frequency and magnitude and deserve close scrutiny and attention. Thus, in answering most practical questions of test bias, it is more informative to evaluate the degree of similarity of factor structures across groups in evaluating whether test score interpretation may be undertaken without regard for the nominal variable in questions.

Determining Degree of Similarity between Factors

A number of methods for determining factorial similarity across groups exist. These methods differ primarily along two lines: whether they allow estimates of shared variance between factors, and the various assumptions underlying their use. With large samples, these various indices of factorial similarity typically produce quite consistent findings (Reynolds & Harding, 1983). In small sample studies, multiple methods of evaluation are necessary to guard against the overinterpretation of what may simply be sampling error.

Katzenmeyer and Stenner (1977) have described a technique for determining the similarity of factors across groups that is biased essentially on *factor score comparisons*. A factor score is a composite score derived by summing an individual's weighted scores on each variable that appears on a factor. Weights are derived from the factor analysis procedure and are directly related to the factor loadings of the variables. Katzenmeyer and Stenner propose that factor scores be derived on a factor analysis of the combined groups of interest. Then, the scores of each group are factor-analyzed separately and factor scores again determined. The Pearson product–moment coefficient of correlation between the factor scores based on the total group analysis and the factor scores of the single group analysis is then used as an estimate of the factorial similarity of the test battery across groups. The method is actually somewhat more complex as described by Katzenmeyer and Stenner (1977) and has not been widely employed in the test bias literature, yet it is a practical technique with many utilitarian implications, especially when factor scores are likely to be employed. This method should receive more attention in future work on bias in tests.

The *Pearson correlation* can also be used to examine directly the comparability of factor loadings on a single factor for two groups. The correlation coefficient between pairs of factor loadings for corresponding factors has been used in some previous work, however, in the comparison of factor loadings, assumptions of normality or linearity are likely to be violated. Transforming the factor loadings to Fischer zs prior to computing r helps to correct some of these flaws but is not completely satisfactory. Other technical problems in the use of the Pearson r for determining factorial similarity are detailed by Cattell (1978). Other, more appropriate indices of factorial similarity exist and are no more difficult to determine than the Pearson r in most cases. The use of the Pearson r between factor loadings (or transformations of factor loadings) as a measure of factorial similarity is thus *not* recommended.

One popular index of factorial similarity, which is similar to the Pearson r, based on the relationship between pairs of factor loadings for corresponding factors is the *coefficient of congruence* (r_c). When determining the degree of similarity of two factors, an r_c value of .90 or higher is typically, though arbitrarily, taken to indicate equivalency of the factors in question or factorial invariance across groups (Cattell, 1978; Harman, 1976; Mulaik, 1972). The coefficient of congruence is given by the following equation:

$$r_c = \frac{\sum_{1}^{N} a_1 \cdot a_2}{\sqrt{\sum_{1}^{N} a_1^2 \sum_{1}^{N} a_2^2}} \tag{2}$$

where a_1 represents the factor loading of a variable for one sample and a_2 represents the factor loading of the same variable for the second sample. Although significance tables are provided for r_c (Cattell, 1978), significance levels can only be approximated for r_c since its distribution will vary as a function of the number of factors in the analysis, the number of variables each factor has in common for each group, and certain other factors. Significance levels are of little importance in the interpretation of r_c in detecting test bias when initial samples for factoring are sufficiently large; the actual magnitude of r_c is of primary concern.

Some concerns have been expressed regarding the use of r_c to compare factors extracted from a correlation matrix with the variances for each variable not constant across groups. Differences in covariance matrices can result that can alter the distribution of r_c. Some disquietude has also been expressed regarding the comparison of orthogonal factors (Mulaik, 1972). Most of the problems in the calculation and interpretation of r_c act to attenuate its value, so overinterpretation should not be a problem in such cases.

Covariance matrices can be compared as noted earlier. If the covariance matrices differ, then the factor analysis should be conducted based on the covariance matrices for each group and r_c, calculated on the basis of factor loadings derived from this procedure. With large samples, however, the effects on r_c are minimal at best (Gutkin & Reynolds, 1981; Reynolds & Harding, 1983). This procedure is sometimes difficult to interpret and is not common in the test bias literature. Another procedure to consider, if using r_c when equivalence of covariance matrices is in doubt, is to supplement the interpretation of r_c with a nonparametric measure of factorial similarity (e.g., Reynolds & Paget, 1981).

Cattell (1978; Cattell & Baggaley, 1960) has described a useful nonparametric index for factor comparison known as the *salient variable similarity index* (s). The calculation of s is straightforward with one exception. In the determination of s, one first proceeds by classifying each variable by its factor loading as being salient or nonsalient and as being positive or negative, depending on the sign of the variable's loading. After reviewing several other options, Cattell (1978) recommends a cutoff value of $\pm$ .10 to indicate a variable with a salient loading. While this is likely the best choice for analyses of items (or with subscales, in the case of personality scales), this value is probably too liberal when examining subscales of cognitive batteries with high subtest reliabilities and a large general factor, especially given the sensitive nature of questions of potential bias. In the latter case, investigators should consider adopting more conservative values between .15 and .25 for positive salience and $-.15$ to $-.25$ for negative salience. Once the cutoff value has been determined, variable classification should be undertaken and Table 1 completed.

Once Table 1 has been completed, s is given by the following equation (from Cattell, 1978, p. 260);

TABLE 1. Tabulation Table for Use in Calculating
the Salient Variable Similarity Index(es) in Studies of Test Bias

	Factor for group two		
Factor for group one	Positive salient variable	Hyperplane variable (variable with a nonsalient loading)	Negative salient variable
Positive salient variable	$f_{11}{}^{a}$	f_{12}	f_{13}
Hyperplane variable (variable with a nonsalient loading)	f_{21}	f_{22}	f_{23}
Negative salient variable	f_{31}	f_{32}	f_{33}

Source: Adapted, with permission, from R. B. Cattell (1978, p. 257).
[a]Joint frequency, for example, the number of variable with positive salient loadings on the factor in both groups. The variables in the analysis must be the same when examining the test's bias.

$$s = \frac{f_{11} + f_{33} - f_{13} - f_{31}}{f_{11} + f_{33} + f_{13} + f_{31} + \frac{1}{2}(f_{12} + f_{21} + f_{23} + f_{32})} \qquad (3)$$

The various f values in the above formula correspond to the frequency of variables in the cells of Table 1 for the designated f. The value of s can range from -1.00 to $+1.00$, with either extreme traditionally taken to indicate perfect agreement between factors since any factor may be reflected 180°, thereby changing the signs of all variables. When examining for test bias, however, a significant negative s must be considered strong evidence of bias, although with very large negative values the appropriate corrective measures become obvious. Additionally, such an occurrence is extremely unlikely with well-developed cognitive scales when the variables are common across groups and factors are rotated to orthogonal solutions; if a negative s occurs under these conditions, the investigator would be wise to recheck the data to be sure they were all coded correctly and there were no errors in the mathematical calculations.

The nature of s, as opposed to indices more similar to the Pearson r, requires a significance test of its deviation from zero (when its value $\neq \pm 1.00$). There is no established cutoff value such as with r_c which is accepted as indicating total similarity of factors. Tables for evaluating the significance of an obtained value for s are found in Cattell (1978). When s is significantly different from zero, one may be confident that the two factors in question are indeed constant across groups, especially if r_c also has reached a value of .90 or higher.

Many other methods of determining the similarity of factors exist, and a complete review of these techniques cannot be undertaken here. Configurative matching methods (e.g., Kaiser, Hunka, & Bianchini, 1971) or the use of Cattell's (Cattell, 1978; Cattell, Coulter, & Tsujioka, 1966) coefficient of pattern similarity (r_c) are but two prominent examples. The methods reviewed above, however, will be adequate for the vast majority of cases, especially if analyses can be based on covariance matrices, and are certainly the most common procedures in the test bias literature.

Factor Extraction and Interpreting Indices of Similarity

Before moving to the next aspect of evaluating construct bias for a test, at least two more issues should be addressed: (1) interpreting indices of factorial similarity (e.g., r_c) in small N studies, and (2) determining the number of factors to rotate in studies of bias. With small sample studies (e.g., the subject:variable ratio is less than 10:1 or the N for each group is less than 200), the standard error of the correlation of a variable with a factor can be quite substantial. Thus, when indices of similarity fall below established cutoff or significance levels, a test for significance of the difference between factor loadings of the two factors that takes this error into account is a necessary supplement prior to concluding that the factors are dissimilar. An r_c value of .80 is typically taken to indicate a lack of factorial similarity or invariance (.90 denotes invariance and values of .81–.89 are marginal and require additional evidence from other studies of construct validity for an adequate interpretation), yet in small sample studies, or studies where the Ns are disproportionate across groups, such a finding easily could be attributable to sampling error. Clearly, a method for determining the reliability of such a finding with small Ns is a necessary adjunct to the analysis.

Determining the number of factors to extract and rotate is a much debated issue. The most popular methods seem to be the "eigenvalue one" criterion, the scree test, and the "whatever solution most appeals to the investigator's theoretical bent" technique. Regardless of which method is chosen, neither nonjudicious use of rigid cutoffs nor totally subjective methods should be allowed to infiltrate the investigation of test bias. One obvious example of inappropriate conclusions that can be drawn from the use of rigid techniques when analyses are totally separate for each group is the following: An investigator conducts a factor analysis of a popular intelligence scale separately for a group of 6½-year-olds and a group of 9½-year-olds. Wanting to avoid accusations of subjective influence in the analysis, the investigator adopts a criterion of extracting only factors with eigenvalues of 1.00 or higher. For the younger group, the eigenvalues of the first four factors are 3.12, 2.01, 1.01, and .89. For the older group they are 3.24, 1.96, 0.99, and .87. Since the younger group has three factors with eigenvalues above 1.00 and the older group has only two, the investigator concludes that the factor structure of the test is quite different for the younger and older children since not even the same number of factors result. Obviously, the difference of .02 in eigenvalues of the third factors can hardly support such a conclusion, yet how can the investigator support comparing the third factor without accusations of biasing the outcome of the study? The use of purely subjective review of factor loadings to determine the proper number of factors boggles the imagination with possibilities for such difficult circumstances. Two methods of avoiding such problems can immediately be applied.

Once having decided on a method for determining the proper number of factors, the investigator can analyze the scores of the major group. The same factor solution can then be applied to the minor group and the two solutions compared, as discussed above. Another, apparently superior, method is available, however. Once having decided on the method for determining the proper number of factors, the investigator can collapse the major and minor groups and derive a factor solution on the combined groups. The factor solution should then be determined separately for each group in the analysis and the resulting solutions compared across groups. The latter method is desirable for a number of reasons, the most notable being the greater sample size available to increase the stability of the solution. The use of this method will also remove the ambiguity of situations such as that described above.

Comparing Internal Consistency Estimates

The previously offered definition of bias in construct validity requires equivalency in the "accuracy" of measurements across groups for nonbiased assessment. Essentially, this means that any error due to domain sampling in the choice of items for the test must be constant across groups. The proper test of this condition is the comparison of internal consistency reliability estimates (r_{xx}) or alternate form correlations (r_{ab}) across groups. Different statistical procedures are necessary for the comparison of r_{xx} across groups and the comparison of r_{ab} across groups. Internal consistency reliability estimates are such coefficients as Cronbach's alpha, Kuder–Richardson 20 (KR_{20}), KR_{21}, odd–even correlations with length corrections, or estimates derived through analysis of variance. Typically, the preferred estimate of r_{xx} is Cronbach's coefficient alpha or KR_{20}, a special case of alpha. Alpha has a variety of advantages; for example, alpha can be shown to be the mean of all possible split-half correlations for a test and is also representative of the predicted correlation between true alternate forms of a test. Feldt (1969) has provided a technique that can be used to determine the *significance of the difference between alpha or KR_{20} reliabilities on a single test for two groups*. Feldt originally devised this method as a test of the hypothesis that alpha or KR_{20} is the same for two tests. The assumptions underlying the test, however, are even more closely met by the use of a single psychological test and two independent samples (Feldt, personal communication, 1980). The test statistic is given by the ratio of $1 - $ alpha for the first group over $1 - $ alpha for the second group as shown in Eq. 4:

$$F = \frac{1 - \text{alpha}_1}{1 - \text{alpha}_2} \tag{4}$$

Where alpha_1 is the reliability coefficient of some test x as determined for group 1 and alpha_2 is the same reliability coefficient as calculated based on the responses of the second group. Kuder–Richardson 20 reliabilities may be used in Eq. 4 as well. The test statistic will be distributed as F with $N_1 - 1$ degrees of freedom in the numerator and $N_2 - 1$ degrees of freedom in the denominator. The quantity $1 - r_{xx}$ represents an error variance term, and the larger variance is always placed over the smaller variance term. The complete development of this technique is described in Feldt (1969). Whenever Eq. 4 reveals a statistically significant discrepancy in reliability estimates, the test in question must be considered biased since errors due to domain sampling are different across groups creating disparities in the ability of the test to measure the trait in question for all groups. True score estimates will vary with a common obtained score for two or more groups.

Comparisons of Correlations between Alternate Forms

Comparisons of correlations between alternate forms of a test across groups may be needed in cases where alpha or KR_{20} is inappropriate or for some reason they are not available. Alternate form reliability estimates assume that the items on the two scales have been randomly sampled from the same domain of items and that a less-than-perfect relationship between the two measures represents errors of domain sampling. The Pearson correlation between the two sets of scores is then taken as the "alternate form reliability coefficient" of the test. With two samples, alternate form correlations are calculated separately for each group, producing two independent correlations. Since the standard error of the difference between independent correlations is non normal and difficult to estimate precisely, to test for the significance of the difference between correlations for two groups, the correlations must first be transformed to Fisher zs. The standard error of the difference between Fisher zs is normally distributed and is relatively easy to calculate. Equation 5 can be used to produce a Z statistic that is then referred to a table of the normal curve. The numerator of the equation is the difference between the correlations, expressed as Fisher z scores. The denominator is the standard error of the difference between Fisher z scores.

$$Z_c = \frac{z_1 - z_2}{\sqrt{\dfrac{1}{N_1 - 3} + \dfrac{1}{N_2 - 3}}} \tag{5}$$

where:

z_1 = correlation for group 1 expressed as a Fisher z,
z_2 = correlation for group 2 expressed as a Fisher z,
N_1 = sampling size for group 1, and
N_2 = sampling size for group 2.

When a significant difference between alternate form reliability estimates for two groups occurs, several other factors must be considered prior to concluding that bias exists. The tests under consideration must be shown to be in reality alternate forms for at least one of the two groups. Before two tests can be considered alternate forms, they must in fact be sampling items from the same domain. Other methodological problems that apply generally to the investigation of alternate form reliability also will apply.

Comparison of Test–Retest Correlations

Comparison of test–retest correlations across groups may also be of interest and can be conducted using Eq. 5 as well. Whether a test–retest correlation is an appropriate measure of a test's reliability, however, should carefully be evaluated. Unless the trait the test is measuring is assumed to be completely static, test–retest correlations speak more directly to the stability of the trait under consideration than to the accuracy of the measuring device (Reynolds, 1999b). Certainly there are few psychological traits that would be considered totally unchanging, yet only under this circumstance can differences in test–retest correlations for two groups be considered as evidence for bias in domain sampling for the two groups.

Other Methods of Examining for Construct Bias

A variety of other logically derived methods may be determined when examining for bias in construct validity. Indeed, the richness and complexity of construct validation demands ingenuity in research and evaluation of the meaning of psychological test scores (Cronbach, 1990). These techniques will generally not have the broader applicability of the above techniques.

Correlations of Age with Raw Scores

A potentially valuable yet seldom-employed technique for investigating the construct validity of aptitude of intelligence tests is the evaluation of the relationship between raw scores and age. Scores on tests of mental ability during childhood are believed to increase with age in almost all theories of early cognitive development. The original Binet Intelligence Scale relied quite heavily on the relationship between chronological age and the various tasks Binet created to measure intelligence. The location of an item on Binet's scale was determined by the percentage of children passing the item at several age levels. For many neuropsychological tests, performance may decline at older-adult ages. If a test is measuring some construct of mental ability in a uniform manner across groups with which the test is used (as it must to be free of bias according to the above definition), the correlation of raw scores with chronological age should be constant across groups. The test of this condition is to calculate the correlation of age with raw scores separately for each group under consideration, and then test for the significance of the difference between the two correlations. The method of transforming correlations to Fisher z scores and dividing by the standard error of the difference between z scores should be applied as described above.

Care must be taken, however, with the interpretation of such analyses. If mean differences in total scores are present, the researcher must be certain that the test has enough floor and ceiling at all ages. A nonsignificant difference also does not "prove" the test is nonbiased; it only adds to other evidence. As with most tests of bias, we cannot prove the null hypothesis, only retain it for further evaluation. Contrary to what will be presented later with regard to a test's predictive validity, differences in slopes of the regression between age and raw-score performance indicate only differences in the rate of cognitive development across groups and are unrelated to bias. Jensen (1980) has a number of interesting observations to offer on the interpretation of the relationship between raw scores on ability tests and age when used to evaluate cultural bias. The reader considering the use of this method would do well to review his comments (Jensen, 1980, Chapter 9).

Kinship Correlations and Differences

Jensen (1980) has proposed that "the construct validity of a test in any two population groups is reinforced if the test scores show the same kinship correlations (or absolute differences) in both groups" (p. 427). The evaluation of this test of bias is relatively complex and involves the much debated calculation of heritability estimates across groups. While this method of evaluating test bias is of little utility to the practitioner, it is a valid technique for investigating the construct validity of tests that are purported to be measures of g.

Multitrait–Multimethod Validation

One of the most convincing techniques for establishing the construct validity of performance-interpretations on a psychological test is through the use of a multitrait–multimethod validation matrix (Campbell & Fiske, 1959). This technique evaluates both the convergent and divergent validity of a test with multiple methods of assessment; that is, predictions regarding what will correlate with the test score are evaluated along with predictions regarding what the test *will not* correlate with (an equally important facet of validity), using multiple methods of assessment so that the observed relationships are not artifacts of a common assessment method.

A square matrix can be produced which is amenable to evaluation through factor analysis. When evaluating for bias, it is best to put the test reliabilities in the diagonal of the matrix. It would be necessary to establish a multitrait–multimethod matrix for a test separately for each group under consideration. Each matrix could then be factor-analyzed and the results of the factor analysis compared using techniques described above. In the evaluation for bias, all methods or tests in the matrix, other than the specific test being evaluated, must be nonbiased, a potential drawback to the use of this technique. When correctly carried out, however, this procedure has the greatest potential for the ultimate resolution of the question of bias.

Comparative Item Selection

Reynolds (1998) has proposed an additional method of evaluating the comparability of tests across groups. In Reynolds' approach to determining construct validity across groups, items are selected using either traditional true score theory or IRT models separately from the initial item pool for each group under consideration. For example, suppose 100 items are standardized for a test of inductive reasoning, an aspect of executive function. The researcher determines that 50 items (of this 100) provide adequate measurement of the construct. To assess comparability across groups, the 50 best items (i.e., items with the best item statistics) are selected separately based on the responses of each group (e.g., African Americans, Anglo/

European Americans, Hispanics, etc.). The overlaps in items selected, represented as a proportion of items chosen using the pooled standardization or item selection sample, provides a measure of the appropriateness of the pooled item test across groups. Overlap in items between each group and the pooled group should approximate 90%. However, the less reliable the items are for all groups, the less likely this will happen. Poor item reliabilities will reflect a poor test generally that should not be used with any group. This method requires large Ns for stable results. A complete explanation and example application appears in Reynolds (1998).

Obviously, many techniques for evaluating construct validity can be derived. Research on construct validity is limited only by the investigator's ingenuity and imagination. Any method that can be derived for investigating construct validity can be applied ultimately to the question of bias. (One very common procedure of appraising construct validity, correlation of a test score with an external criterion, will be discussed in the next section on predictive bias.) The search for other methods of investigation should continue. Many procedures may prove unique to the instrument in question, but should nevertheless be employed.

Methods for Investigating Bias in Predictive and Criterion-Related Validity

Evaluating bias in predictive validity of neuropsychological tests is less related to the evaluation of group mental test score differences than to the evaluation of individual test scores in a more absolute sense. This is especially true for cognitive and related diagnostic tests where the primary purpose of administration is the prediction of some specific future outcome or behavior, or other criteria such as membership in a diagnostic class. Internal analyses of bias (such as in content and construct validity) are less confounded than analyses of bias in predictive validity, however, due to the potential problems of bias in the criterion measure. Predictive validity is also strongly influenced by the reliability of criterion measures, which frequently is poor. The degree of relationship between a predictor and a criterion is restricted as a function of the square root of the product of the reliabilities of the two variables, that is, the maximum r.

Arriving at a consensual definition of bias in predictive validity has seemingly been a difficult task, as has already been discussed. Yet, from the standpoint of the practical applications of neuropsychological tests to decisionmaking, predictive validity is the most crucial form of validity in relation to test bias, and the debate in professional journals concerning bias in predictive validity has centered around models of selection rather than errors of prediction. There is very limited discussion of bias in diagnosis as a function of bias in tests outside of the school psychology literature. If one remains concerned with constant or systematic errors of prediction, however, only one definition is logically or statistically permissible. Since the present section is concerned with statistical bias, and not the social or political justification of any one particular selection model, the Cleary, Humphreys, Kendrick, and Wesman (1975) definition, with only slight restatement, provides a clear, direct statement of test bias with regard to predictive validity:

> A test is considered biased with respect to predictive validity when the inference drawn from the test score is not made with the smallest feasible random error or if there is constant error in an inference or prediction as a function of membership in a particular group.

Evaluating Bias in Prediction

The evaluation of bias in prediction under the Cleary et al. (1975) definition (the regression definition) is quite straightforward. With simple regressions, predictions take the form of $\hat{Y}_i = aX_i + b$, where a is the regression coefficient and b is some constant. When this equation is graphed (forming a regression line), a represents the slope of the regression line and b the Y intercept. Since our definition of bias in predictive validity requires errors in prediction to be independent of group membership, the regression line formed for any pair of variables must be the same for each group for whom a prediction is to be made. Whenever the slope or the intercept differs significantly across groups, there is bias in prediction if one attempts to use a regression equation based on the combined groups. When the regression equations for two (or more) groups are equivalent, prediction is the same for all groups. This condition is referred to as homogeneity of regression across groups (or simultaneous regression or nonbiased prediction). This is illustrated in Figure 3. In this case, the single regression equation is appropriate with all groups, any errors in prediction being random with respect to group membership (i.e., residuals are uncorrected with group membership). When homogeneity of regression does not occur, separate regression equations must be used for each group for nonbiased prediction to occur.

In actual clinical neuropsychological practice, regression equations are seldom actually generated for the prediction of future performance. Clinicians essentially establish mental prediction equations that are assumed to be equivalent across race, sex, and other factors. While these mental equations cannot readily be tested across groups, the actual form of criterion prediction can be compared across groups in several ways. Errors in prediction must be independent of group membership. If regression equations are equal, this condition is met. To test the hypothesis of simultaneous regression, both slopes and intercepts must be compared. In the evaluation of slope and intercept values, two basic techniques have been most often employed in the research literature. Gulliksen and Wilks (1950) first described methods (that remain current and are available is most omnibus statistical packages such as SPSS or SAS) for separately testing regression coefficients and intercepts for significant differences across groups. Using separate, independent tests for these two values considerably increases the probability of a decision error and unnecessarily complicates the decision-making process. Potthoff (1966) has described a useful technique allowing one simultaneously to test the equivalence of regression coefficients and intercepts across K independent groups with a single F ratio. If a significant F results, the researcher may then test the slopes and intercepts

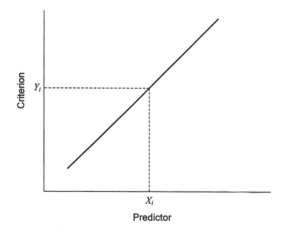

FIGURE 3. An illustration of equal slopes and equal intercepts when $y = ax_i + b$ is the same for two groups. The regression line represents the graph of the equation for group a, group b, and for the combined groups.

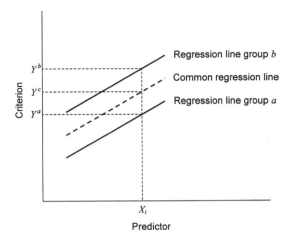

FIGURE 4. When slopes are equal (*a*) but intercept values (*b*) differ across groups, regression lines are parallel and yield constant errors in prediction of *y* across all values of *x*; and always in the same direction.

separately if he or she desires information concerning which value differs. When homogeneity of regression does not occur, three basic conditions can result: (1) intercept constants differ, (2) regression coefficients (slopes) differ, or (3) slopes and intercepts differ. These conditions are depicted in Figures 4–6.

Significantly Different Intercepts

The regression coefficient is related to the correlation (which, when scores are expressed in the metric of the unit normal distribution, is the regression coefficient) between the two

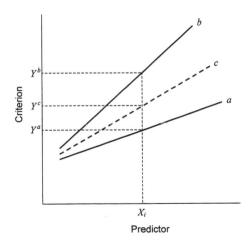

FIGURE 5. When slopes are unequal but intercept values are constant across groups, one group's criterion score will always be underestimated but the degree of underestimation will change as a function of x_i.

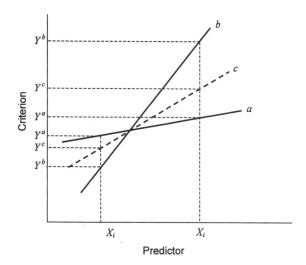

FIGURE 6. When slopes and intercept values are both unequal, the direction of bias in prediction of the criterion and the size of the error in prediction of y both vary as a function of x_i.

variables and is one measure of the strength of the relationship between two variables. When intercepts differ and regression coefficients do not, a situation such as that in Figure 4 results. Relative accuracy of prediction is the same for the two groups (a and b), yet the use of a regression equation derived by combining the two groups results in bias that works against the group with the higher mean-criterion score. Since the slope of the regression line is the same for all groups, the degree of error in prediction remains constant and does not fluctuate as a function of an individual's score on the independent variable. That is, regardless of group member b's score on the predictor, the degree of underprediction in performance on the criterion is the same. As illustrated in Figure 4, the use of the common regression equation results in the prediction of a criterion score of Y^b for a score of X_i. This score (Y^b) overestimates how well members of group a will perform and underestimates the criterion performance of members of group b.

Significantly Different Slopes

Figure 5, nonparallel regression lines, illustrates the case where intercepts are constant across groups but the slope of the line is different for each group. Here, too, the group with the higher mean-criterion score is typically underpredicted when a common regression equation is applied. The amount of bias in prediction that results from using the common regression line is not constant in this case, but rather varies as a function of the distance of the score from the mean.

Significantly Different Slopes and Intercepts

Figure 6 represents a more difficult, complex case of bias, showing the result of significant differences in slopes and intercepts. Not only does the amount of bias in prediction accruing from use of a common equation vary in this instance, the actual direction of bias can reverse depending upon the location of the individual's score in the distribution of the independent variable. Only in the case of Figure 6 do members of the group with the lower mean-criterion score run the risk of having their performance on the criterion variable underpredicted by the application of a common regression equation.

Testing for Cross-Group Differences in Regression

As noted above, Potthoff (1966) has provided the most efficient method for determining whether the regression equation relating any two variables is constant across groups. Slopes and intercepts are first simultaneously evaluated and then, if a significant difference is revealed, separate tests of these factors may be undertaken if this information is desired. Potthoff's F-test for homogeneity of regression can be determined through SAS as a component of its general linear model (GLM) programs and also through SPSS. Some modification of model specifications that can be confusing to those not conversant with SPSS or with SAS are required in these programs. Potthoff's original formulas are available in several sources, however, and are easily programmed in SAS or SPSS as well (e.g., see Potthoff, 1966; Reynolds, 1982a). Pedhazur and Schmelkin (1991) also present several models (see especially Chapters 3 and 21) for evaluating regression equations and differential prediction that follow the above recommendations.

The Case of More than One Independent Variable

Potthoff (1966) has provided extensions of the above procedures to account for the situation of more than a single test being used to predict the criterion. The procedure is derived directly from the above technique and will readily be reduced by the statistician. Others who wish to use this approach when more than one test is employed should consult Potthoff (1966).

Potthoff's (1966) extension has some slight difficulties in the estimation of exact probability levels that increase the probability of a Type I error being made by the investigator. Another method that may prove easier and more exact has been used by Reynolds (1980c) and involves a direct examination of residual or error terms for each individual by group membership. In this procedure, a multiple regression equation for the prediction of performance on the criterion variable is determined using all independent variables with a single collapsed-group of subjects. Using this equation based on the total sample, the investigator predicts criterion scores and calculates a residual score $(\hat{Y}_i - Y_i)$ for each individual. Standardized residual scores are then examined by ANOVA with group membership as a main effect to determine if there are any mean differences in errors of prediction as a function of group membership. If there is no constant or systematic error in the prediction of the criterion variable for members of a particular group, the ANOVA will yield nonsignificant results and the mean residual for each group will approach zero. With multiple independent variables, the ANOVA approach has certain advantages, allowing for the examination of interactions and the direct evaluation of variances of each cell. Virtually any ANOVA design can be used with the standardized residuals, and effect sizes are readily determined (e.g., Pedhazur & Schmelkin, 1991). The direct examination of residuals is also more readily interpretable to nonstatistical audiences.

The Case of More than One Dependent Variable

As Potthoff (1966) has noted, when more than one dependent or criterion variable is being predicted, the test in question may be a nonbiased predictor of one variable but a biased predictor of another variable. Separate tests of bias can be conducted with regard to each dependent variable and alpha levels can be adjusted for the multiple comparison to control Type I error rates. This procedure is probably adequate when only two or three dependent measures are involved. A more exact, appropriate procedure would be a multivariate test for bias simultaneously across all dependent measures. Potthoff (1966, Section 7) presents the necessary formulas and matrices for carrying out the multivariate test for bias. A multivariate analog of the procedure described in the preceding section of this chapter could also be used. With multiple independent and multiple dependent variables, comparisons of canonical analysis outcomes may prove useful as well.

Path Analysis as a Modeling Method for Criterion-Related Bias

Another model that can be useful in detecting bias in prediction under the conditions of simple or multiple independent or dependent variables is derived from structural equation modeling and is generally referred to as path analysis (Pedhazur & Schmelkin, 1991). Path analysis allows the determination of direct and indirect effects of multiple variables on one or more dependent variables. In one sense it is comparable conceptually to the partial-correlation procedure introduced earlier for detecting DIF. Path analysis can calculate the associations among several variables in a manner specified by the model of the investigator and then look for associations with residual terms that would indicate bias (if there were associations between a nominal variable such as ethnicity or gender and a residual variable), since true residual terms are randomly distributed across nominal groupings.

Keith and Reynolds (1990) have suggested the use of path analysis as an alternative model for assessing bias in predictive validity. In such a path model, ability would be proposed to predict achievement, and group membership would be assessed as a moderating variable. Diagrammatic representations of biased and unbiased models are shown in Figures 7–9.

Figure 7 shows a path model of nonbias in which scores on an intelligence test serve as the predictor variable and the scores on the achievement test serve as the criterion. Group membership is the dichotomous bias variable coded 0 for all individuals who are members of one group (e.g., the minority group or females). The true-ability variable is the latent trait or factor. In the nonbiased model, group membership affects intelligence-test scores and achievement-test scores only through true ability, the latent trait. In contrast, Figure 8 shows a path-model of bias in which group membership affects not only true ability but also intelligence-test scores independent of true ability. In other words, the path that connects group membership to intelligence-test scores (i.e., the relationship between group membership and intelligence-test scores) deviates from 0. To the extent that the path deviates from 0, the

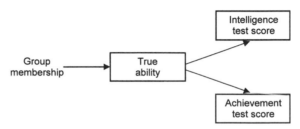

FIGURE 7. Path-model illustrating no bias as a function of group membership.

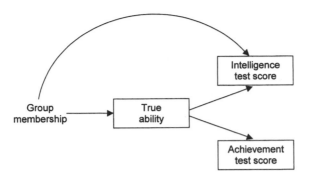

FIGURE 8. A path-model illustrating bias in which group membership affects measured IQ independent of true ability.

intelligence test is considered biased and errors of measurement are associated with group membership (Keith & Reynolds, 1990).

The path-model of bias depicted in Figure 8 is probably not an accurate or a realistic diagrammatic representation, as the direct effect of group membership on true achievement has not been included. That is, group membership affects achievement test scores directly through true achievement, a latent trait variable, or indirectly through true ability. Bias occurs when group membership affects intelligence-test scores independent of true achievement. In other words, the path directly connecting group membership to achievement-test scores deviates from 0. The extent to which these paths deviate from 0 provides evidence that the intelligence test and/or achievement test is biased and the errors of measurement are related to

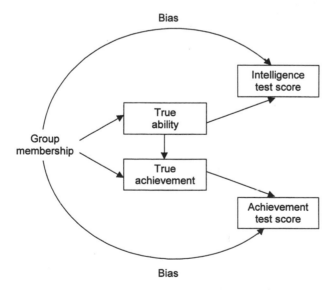

FIGURE 9. A more comprehensive path model of bias in which group membership affects measured IQ directly and achievement test performance, biasing both variables.

group membership. Figure 9 illustrates this more complete path-model of bias (Keith & Reynolds, 1990).

An example of a path-model of bias that affects achievement-test scores occurs when one group of high-school students completes more academic coursework than another group of high-school students. The coursework variable would affect achievement test scores directly. The direct path between group membership and achievement-test scores would deviate from 0, and evidence of bias would be present (Keith & Reynolds, 1990).

As noted, bias in prediction exists when group membership affects measured ability *independent* of true ability and/or when group membership affects measured achievement *independent* of true achievement; that is, errors of measurement in testing of ability and/or achievement would be correlated with group membership.

Testing for Equivalence of Validity Coefficients

The correlation between a test score and a criterion variable, whether measured concurrently or at a future time, is typically referred to as a validity coefficient (r_{xy}) and is a direct measure of the strength and magnitude of the relationship between two variables. Another method for detecting bias in predictive validity is the comparison of validity coefficients across groups. The procedure described in an earlier section of this chapter for comparing alternate-form reliabilities may also be used to test the hypothesis that (r_{xy}) is the same for two groups.

Some researchers, in evaluating validity coefficients across groups, have compared each correlation to zero and, if one correlation deviates significantly from zero and the other does not, have concluded that bias exists. As Humphreys (1973) has explained so eloquently, this is not the correct comparison. To determine whether two correlations are different, they must be compared directly with one another and not separately against hypothetical population values of zero. The many defects in the latter approach are explained amply in Humphreys (1973) and will not be reiterated further here. Other factors must be considered in comparing the correlations directly with one another, however, such as whether to make corrections for unreliability, restriction of range, and other study-specific elements, prior to making the actual comparisons. The particular question involved and whether theory or practice is being assessed will influence the outcome of these deliberations. If corrections for unreliability are appropriate, and they would be in most studies of bias in evaluation of the CTBH (but would not if one did not intend to generalize outside of the sample under investigation), the validity coefficients for each group are corrected by dividing each by the square root of the product of the reliability coefficients of each measure calculated for the group represented by each respective validity coefficient.

Comparing Standard Errors of Estimate

Since the correlation between two variables such as a test and a criterion is almost always less than perfect (± 1.00), there is invariably some error involved in the prediction of the criterion variable. This error has been referred to above as the *residual term*. The standard deviation of the residuals within a sample is known as the *standard error of estimate* (SE_{est}) and should also be equal. The SE_{est} is directly related to the size of the correlation between two variables (in conjunction with the standard deviation of the dependent variable), and if the correlations are identical, SE_{est} should also be equal. The SE_{est} can, however, be compared across groups in several ways; the SE_{est} must be equivalent across groups prior to concluding that there is no bias. One method of comparing SE_{est} across groups has already been discussed, which is to compare cell variances for the residuals in the ANOVA procedure. Unfortunately, this will not always be convenient. The SE_{est} for a set of predicted scores is given by Eq. 6 below,

$$SE_{est} = SD_y \sqrt{(1 - r_{xy}^2) \frac{(N - 1)}{(N - 2)}} \qquad (6)$$

where SD_y represents the standard deviation of the scores of Y, r_{xy}^2 represents the squared validity coefficient, and N represents the sample size on which r_{xy} is based. The test for the difference between independent SE_{est} derived from two samples is simply the F ratio formed by the variance errors of estimate, or

$$F = \frac{SE_{est1}^2}{SE_{est2}^2}$$

where SE_{est1}^2 represents the square of SE_{est} for group 1 and SE_{est2}^2 represents the square of SE_{est} for group 2. The test statistic is referred to the F distribution with $N_1 - 2$ and $N_2 - 2$ degrees of freedom. This is essentially the F test for homogeneity of variance that would be used to test variances from the ANOVA referred to above. With multiple groups, some variation such as Hartley's F_{max} may be used (also see Pedhazur & Schmelkin, 1991).

Diagnostic Utility

Especially in the case of diagnostic testing (e.g., classification of patients into diagnostic groups such as depressed, Alzheimer's disease, Korsakoff's, etc.), companions of the sensitivity and specificity of a neuropsychological test or battery across groups would be useful. A test that leads a clinician to diagnose dementia may be biased if it leads to diagnosis more often than justified for one ethnic group or gender than another (or to the failure to diagnose, which may be more harmful to the individual patient). Since various ethnic groups and genders perform differently on some neuropsychological tests, that is, have different means (e.g., see Mitrushina, Boone, & D'Elia, 1999) and experience different prevalence rates of many forms of psychopathology (e.g., see DSM IV [American Psychiatric Association, 1994]), this form of bias may go unnoticed without direct examination.

The best methods for examining bias in determination of diagnostic category are to: (1) compare rates of sensitivity and specificity across ethnic groups and gender for known diagnostic groups and (2) to compare logistic regression models predicting group membership across ethnic groups and gender. The second approach (the logistic regression model) is a direct extension of the prediction problem posited earlier and can be answered via an extension of Potthoff's (1966) well-known model. The first question, regarding sensitivity and specificity, is even more easily addressed.

Sensitivity and specificity are simple proportions as statistics (e.g., see Reynolds, 1997). Sensitivity refers to the proportion of correct detections of a disorder when it is present, that is, the probability that the disorder will be diagnosed when a patient has the disorder. It is calculated to be the ratio of true-positive findings to the sum of true-positive and false-negative findings in a diagnostic group. This proportion can be calculated separately for the nominal groups of concern (male, female; white, Hispanic, black) and compared by any of several z-tests for the significance of the difference between two proportions. One version, requiring about 5 minutes with most handheld calculators, may be found in Bruning and Kintz (1968,

Section 5.2). If the proportions differ in any meaningful way, a test may lack sensitivity in one or more groups or lead to systematic under- or overdiagnosis in some groups versus others.

Specificity refers to the ability to differentiate among conditions, or, in essence, to detect the absence of a disorder. Specificity is also a proportion and is the ratio of true-negative classifications to the sum of true-negative decisions and false-positive diagnoses. As a proportion, this value can be contrasted across nominal groups, as noted above. A significant finding would indicate the presence of systematic error in the probability of obtaining the correct diagnosis. Overall diagnostic accuracy (true-positives plus true-negatives divided by the number of subjects in the total of groups) can be assessed in the same manner.

Concluding Comments

Neuropsychology, of the clinical specialties in psychology (clinical, counseling, school, clinical health, and clinical neuropsychology), has paid the least attention to empirical evaluation of the CTBH. As American culture becomes increasingly diverse, it becomes increasingly imperative for us to do so. More so than other clinical disciplines, neuropsychologists are more likely to apply actuarial methods (and for good reason, e.g., see Grove & Meehl, 1998). Actuarial methods paradoxically are the most directly testable of models to assess the CTBH. Tests showing mean differences in levels of performance by ethnicity or gender are common in our field (Mitrushina, Boone, & D'Elia, 1999) and we must apply the research methods reviewed in this chapter to understand how these differences are best interpreted and whether they bias our ability to diagnose patients accurately, design proper rehabilitation programs, or make proper predictions of future performance and recovery.

References

Adebimpe, V. R., Gigandet, J., & Harris, E. (1979). MMPI diagnosis of black psychiatric patients. *American Journal of Psychiatry, 136*, 85–87.

Ackerman, T. A. (1991). A didactic explanation of item bias, item impact, and item validity from a multidimensional perspective. *Journal of Educational Measurement, 29*(1), 67–91.

Alley, G., & Foster, C. (1978). Nondiscriminatory testing of minority and exceptional children. *Focus on Exceptional Children, 9*, 1–14.

American Psychiatric Association. (1994). *Diagnostic and statistical manual of mental disorders*, 4th ed: DSM-IV. Washington, DC: Author.

Anastasi, A. (1982). *Psychological testing* (5th ed.). New York: Macmillan.

Angoff, W. H., & Ford, S. R. (1973). Item–race interaction on a test of scholastic aptitude. *Journal of Educational Measurement, 10*, 95–106.

Ardila, A., Rosselli, M., & Puente, A. E. (1994). *Neuropsychological evaluation of the Spanish speaker*. New York: Plenum.

Bond, L. (1987). The golden rule settlement: A minority perspective. *Educational Measurement: Issues and Practice, 6*(2), 23–25.

Brown, R. T., Reynolds, C. R., & Whitaker, J. S. (in press). Bias in mental testing since "Bias in Mental Testing." *School Psychology Quarterly.*

Bruning, J., & Kintz, B. (1968). *Computational handbook of statistics*. Glenview, IL: Scott, Foresman.

Burrill, L. E. (1975). *Statistical evidence of potential bias in items and tests assessing current educational status.* Paper presented at the annual meeting of the Southeastern Conference on Measurement in Education, New Orleans, LA.

Butler-Omololu, C., Doster, J., & Lahey, B. (1984). Some implications for intelligence test construction and administration with children of different racial groups. *Journal of Black Psychology, 10*(2), 63–75.

Camilli, G., & Shepard, L. A. (1987). The inadequacy of ANOVA for detecting test bias. *Journal of Educational Statistics, 12*, 87–99.

Camilli, G., & Shepard, L. A. (1994). *Methods for identifying biased test items*. Thousand Oaks, CA: Sage.

Campbell, D. F., & Fiske, D. W. (1959). Convergent and discriminant validation by the multitrait-multimethod matrix. *Psychological Bulletin, 56*, 85–105.

Cardall, C., & Coffman, W. E. (1964). *A method of comparing the performance of different groups on the items in a test (RB- 64-61)*. Princeton, NJ: Educational Testing Service.

Cattell, R. B. (1978). *The scientific use of factor analysis in behavioral and life sciences*. New York: Plenum.

Cattell, R. B., & Baggaley, A. R. (1960). The salient variable similarity index for factor matching. *British Journal of Statistical Psychology, 13*, 33–46.

Cattell, R. B., Coulter, M. A., & Tsujioka, B. (1966). The taxonomic recognition of types and functional emergents. In R. B. Cattell (Ed.), *Handbook of multivariate experimental psychology* (pp. 288–329). Chicago: Rand McNally.

Chambers, J. S., Barron, F., & Sprecher, J. W. (1980). Identifying gifted Mexican-American students. *Gifted Child Quarterly, 24*, 123–128.

Chinn, P. C. (1979). The exceptional minority child: Issues and some answers. *Exceptional Children, 46*, 532–536.

Chipman, S., Marshall, S., & Scott, P. (1991). Content effect on word-problem performance: A possible source of test bias? *American Educational Research Journal, 28*, 897–915.

Clarizio, H. (1982). Intellectual assessment of Hispanic children. *Psychology in the Schools, 19*(1), 61–71.

Cleary, T. A., Humphreys, L. G., Kendrick, S. A., & Wesman, A. (1975). Educational uses of tests with disadvantaged students. *American Psychologist, 30*, 15–41.

Cronbach, L. J. (1990). *Essentials of psychological testing* (5th ed.). New York: Harper & Row.

Dana, R. H. (1996). Culturally competent assessment practices in the United States. *Journal of Personality Assessment, 66*, 472–487.

Elliott, R. (1987). *Litigating intelligence*. Dover, MA: Auburn House.

Emerling, F. (1990). An investigation of test bias in nonverbal cognitive measures for two ethnic groups. *Journal of Psychoeducational Assessment, 8*(1), 34–41.

Feldt, L. S. (1969). A test of the hypothesis that Cronbach's alpha or Kuder–Richardson coefficient twenty is the same for two tests. *Psychometrika, 34*, 363–373.

Flaugher, R. L. (1978). The many definitions of test bias. *American Psychologist, 33*, 671–679.

Frisby, C., & Braden, J. (Eds.). (in press). Bias in mental testing. A special, topical issue of *School Psychology Quarterly*.

Gray-Little, B., & Kaplan, D. A. (1998). Interpretation of psychological tests in clinical and forensic evaluations. In J. Sandoval et al. (Eds.), *Test interpretation and diversity* (pp. 141–178). Washington, DC: American Psychological Association.

Greenlaw, R., & Jensen, S. (1996). Race norming and the Civil Rights Act of 1991. *Public Personnel Management, 25*(1), 13–24.

Grove, W., & Meehl, P. A. (1998). Comparative efficiency of informal (subjective, impressionistic) and formal (mechanical, algorithmic) prediction procedures: The clinical-statistical controversy. *Psychology, Public Policy, and Law, 2*, 293–323.

Guilford Press. (1997). Culturally sensitive assessment: Paying attention to cultural orientation. *Child Assessment News, 6*, 8–12.

Gulliksen, H., & Wilks, S. S. (1950). Regression tests for several samples. *Psychometrika, 15*, 91–114.

Gutkin, T. B., & Reynolds, C. R. (1981). Factorial similarity of the WISC-R for white and black children from the standardization sample. *Journal of Educational Psychology, 73*, 227–231.

Hambleton, R. K., Swaminathan, H., & Rogers, H. J. (1991). *Fundamentals of item response theory*. Newbury Park, CA: Sage.

Hammill, D. (1991). *Detroit tests of learning aptitude* (3rd ed.). Austin, TX: PRO-ED.

Harman, H. (1976). *Modern factor analysis* (2nd ed.). Chicago: University of Chicago Press.

Harrington, G. M. (1975). Intelligence tests may favor the majority groups in a population. *Nature, 25*(8), 708–709.

Harrington, G. M. (1976, September). *Minority test bias as a psychometric artifact: The experimental evidence*. Paper presented at the annual meeting of the American Psychological Association, Washington, DC.

Helms, J. E. (1992). Why is there no study of cultural equivalence in standardized cognitive ability testing? *American Psychologist, 47*, 1083–1101.

Hilliard, A. G. (1979). Standardization and cultural bias as impediments to the scientific study and validation of "intelligence." *Journal of Research and Development in Education, 12*, 47–58.

Humphreys, L. G. (1973). Statistical definitions of test validity for minority groups. *Journal of Applied Psychology, 58*, 1–4.

Isern, M. (1986). An investigation of bias in tests of writing ability for bilingual Hispanic college students. Doctoral dissertation, University of Miami. *Dissertation Abstracts International, 47*, 2135A.

Jackson, G. D. (1975). Another view from the Association of Black Psychologists. *American Psychologist, 30*, 88–93.

Jensen, A. R. (1974). How biased are cultural loaded tests? *Genetic Psychology Monographs, 90*, 185–224.

Jensen, A. R. (1976). Test bias and construct validity. *Phi Delta Kappan, 58*, 340–346.

Jensen, A. R. (1977). An examination of culture bias in the Wonderlic Personnel test. *Intelligence, 1*, 51–64.

Jensen, A. R. (1980). *Bias in mental testing*. New York: Free Press.

Jöreskog, K. G. (1969). A general approach to confirmatory maximum likelihood factor analysis. *Psychometrika, 34*, 183–202.

Jöreskog, K. G. (1971). Simultaneous factor analysis in several populations. *Psychometrika, 36*, 409–426.

Jörsekog, K. G., & Sorbom, D. (1989). *LISREL 7: A guide to the program and applications*. Mooresville, IN: Scientific Software.

Judd, C. M., & McClelland, G. H. (1989). *Data analysis: A model comparison approach*. San Diego, CA: Harcourt Brace Jovanovich.

Kaiser, H., Hunka, S., & Bianchini, J. (1971). Relating factors between studies based upon different individuals. *Multivariate Behavioral Research, 6*, 409–422.

Katzenmeyer, W. G., & Stenner, A. J. (1977). Estimation of the invariance of factor structures across race and sex with implications for hypothesis testing. *Educational and Psychological Measurement, 37*, 111–119.

Kaufman, A. S. (1979). *Intelligent testing with the WISC-R*. New York: Wiley-Interscience.

Keith, T. Z., & Reynolds, C. R. (1990). Measurement and design issues in child assessment research. In C. R. Reynolds & R. W. Kamphaus (Eds.), *Handbook of psychological and educational assessment of children* (pp. 29–61). New York: Guilford.

Linn, R. L., & Werts, C. E. (1971). Considerations for studies of test bias. *Journal of Educational Measurement, 8*, 1–4.

Lonner, W. J. (1985). Issues in testing and assessment in cross-cultural counseling. *The Counseling Psychologist, 13*, 599–614.

Mayfield, J. W., & Reynolds, C. R. (1997). Black-white differences in memory test performance among children and adolescents. *Archives of Clinical Neuropsychology, 12*, 111–122.

McGaw, B., & Jöreskog, K. G. (1971). Factorial invariance of ability measures in groups differing in intelligence and socioeconomic status. *British Journal of Mathematical and Statistical Psychology, 24*, 154–168.

McGurk, F. V. J. (1951). *Comparison of the performance of Negro and white high school seniors on cultural and noncultural psychological test questions*. Washington, DC: Catholic University of America Press.

Mercer, J. R. (1976, August). *Cultural diversity, mental retardation, and assessment: The case for nonlabeling*. Paper presented to the Fourth International Congress of the International Association for the Scientific Study of Mental Retardation, Washington, DC.

Miele, F. (1979). Cultural bias in the WISC. *Intelligence, 3*, 149–164.

Mitrushina, M. N., Boone, K. B., & D'Elia, L. F. (1999). *Handbook of normative data for neuropsychological assessment*. Oxford: Oxford University Press.

Mulaik, S. A. (1972). *The foundation of factor analysis*. New York: McGraw-Hill.

Nandakumar, R., Glutting, J. J., & Oakland, T. (1993). Mantel–Haenszel methodology for detecting item bias: An introduction and example using the guide to the assessment of test session behavior. *Journal of Psychoeducational Assessment, 11*(2), 108–119.

Padilla, A. M. (1988). Early psychological assessment of Mexican American children. *Journal of the History of the Behavioral Sciences, 24*, 113–115.

Payne, B., & Payne, D. (1991). The ability of teachers to identify academically at-risk elementary students. *Journal of Research in Childhood Education, 5*(2), 116–126.

Pedhazur, E. J., & Schmelkin, L. P. (1991). *Measurement, design, and analysis*. Hillsdale, NJ: Erlbaum.

Potthoff, R. F. (1966). *Statistical aspects of the problem of biases in psychological tests* (Institute of Statistics Mimeo Series No. 479). Chapel Hill: Department of Statistics, University of North Carolina.

Reschley, D. (2000). PASE v. Hannon. In C. R. Reynolds & E. Fletcher-Janzen (Eds.), *Encyclopedia of special education* (2nd ed., pp. 1325–1326). New York: Wiley.

Reynolds, C. R. (1980a). In support of "Bias in Mental Testing" and scientific inquiry. *Behavioral and Brain Sciences, 3*, 352.

Reynolds, C. R. (1980b). Differential construct validity of intelligence as popularly measured: Correlations of age with raw scores on the WISC-R for blacks, whites, males, and females. *Intelligence, 4*, 371–379.

Reynolds, C. R. (1980c). An examination for bias in a preschool battery across race and sex. *Journal of Educational Measurement, 17*, 137–146.

Reynolds, C. R. (1982a). Construct and predictive bias. In R. A. Berk (Ed.), *Handbook of methods for detecting test bias* (pp. 199–227). Baltimore, MD: Johns Hopkins University Press.

Reynolds, C. R. (1982b). The problem of bias in psychological assessment. In C. R. Reynolds & T. B. Gutkin (Eds.), *The handbook of school psychology* (pp. 178–208). New York: Wiley.

Reynolds, C. R. (1997). Measurement and statistical problems in neuropsychological assessment of children. In C. R. Reynolds & E. Fletcher-Janzen (Eds.), *Handbook of child clinical neuropsychology* (pp. 180–203). New York: Plenum.

Reynolds, C. R. (1998). Need we measure anxiety differently for males and females. *Journal of Personality Assessment, 70,* 212–221.

Reynolds, C. R. (1999a). Cultural bias in testing of intelligence and personality. In A. Bellack, M. Hersen (Series Eds.), & C. Celar (Vol. Ed.), *Comprehensive clinical psychology: Vol. 10: Sociocultural and individual differences* (pp. 53–92). New York: Pergamon.

Reynolds, C. R. (1999b). Fundamentals of measurement and assessment in psychology. In A. Bellack, M. Hersen (Series Eds.), & C. R. Reynolds (Vol. Ed.), *Comprehensive clinical psychology: Vol. 4: Assessment* (pp. 33–56). New York: Pergamon.

Reynolds, C. R. (in press). Why do we ignore research on bias in mental testing? *Psychology, Public Policy, and Law.*

Reynolds, C. R., & Bigler, E. D. (1994). *Test of memory and learning.* Austin, TX: PRO-ED.

Reynolds, C. R., & Brown, R. T. (1984). Bias in mental testing: An introduction to the issues. In C. R. Reynolds & R. T. Brown (Eds.), *Perspectives on bias in mental testing* (pp. 1–39). New York: Plenum.

Reynolds, C. R., Chastain, R., Kaufman, A. S., & McLean, J. (1987). Demographic influences on adult intelligence at ages 16 to 74 years. *Journal of School Psychology, 25,* 323–342.

Reynolds, C. R., & Harding, R. E. (1983). Outcome in two large sample studies of factorial similarity under six methods of comparison. *Educational and Psychological Measurement, 43,* 723–728.

Reynolds, C. R., & Kaiser, S. (1992). Test bias in psychological assessment. In T. B. Gutkin & C. R. Reynolds (Eds.), *The handbook of school psychology* (2nd ed., pp. 487–525). New York: Wiley.

Reynolds, C. R., Lowe, P. A., & Saenz, A. (1999). The problem of bias in psychological assessment. In T. B. Gutkin & C. R. Reynolds (Eds.), *The handbook of school psychology* (3rd ed., pp. 549–595). New York: Wiley.

Reynolds, C. R., & Paget, K. D. (1981). Factor structure of the revised Children's Manifest Anxiety Scale for blacks, whites, males, and females with a national normative sample. *Journal of Consulting and Clinical Psychology, 49,* 352–359.

Reynolds, C. R., & Streur, J. (1982). Comparative structure of the WISC-R for emotionally disturbed and normal children. *The Southern Psychologist, 1,* 27–35.

Reynolds, C. R., Willson, V. L., & Chatman, S. P. (1984). Item bias on the 1981 revision of the Peabody Picture Vocabulary Test using a new method of detecting bias. *Journal of Psychoeducational Assessment, 2,* 219–221.

Sandoval, J., & Miller, M. (1979). *Accuracy judgements of WISC-R item difficulty for minority groups.* Paper presented to the annual meeting of the American Psychological Association.

Schmidt, W. H. (1983). Content biases in achievement tests. *Journal of Educational Measurement, 20,* 165–178.

Spitz, H. (1986). *The raising of intelligence.* Hillsdale, NJ: Erlbaum.

Stricker, L. J. (1982). Identifying test items that perform differentially in population subgroups: A partial correlation index. *Applied Psychological Measurement, 6,* 261–273.

Thissen, D., Steinberg, L., & Wainer, H. (1993). Detection of differential item functioning using the parameters of item response models. In P. W. Holland & H. Wainer (Eds.), *Differential item functioning: Theory and practice* (pp. 67–113). Hillsdale, NJ: Erlbaum.

Thorndike, R. L. (1971). Concepts of culture-fairness. *Journal of Educational Measurement, 8,* 63–70.

Thorndike, R. M. (1978). *Correlational procedures for research.* New York: Gardner.

Timm, N. H. (1975). *Multivariate analysis with applications in education and psychology.* Monterey, CA: Brooks/Cole.

Veale, J. R., & Foreman, D. F. (1983). Assessing cultural bias using foil response data: Cultural variation. *Journal of Educational Measurement, 20,* 249–258.

Williams, R. L. (1974). From dehumanization to black intellectual genocide: A rejoinder. In G. J. Williams & S. Gordon (Eds.), *Clinical child psychology: Current practices and future perspectives.* New York: Behavioral.

Willson, V. L., Nolan, R. F., Reynolds, C. R., & Kamphaus, R. W. (1989). Race and gender effects on item functioning on the Kaufman Assessment Battery for Children. *Journal of School Psychology, 27,* 289–296.

Wright, B. J., & Isenstein, V. R. (1977, reprinted 1978). *Psychological tests and minorities* [DHEW Pub. No. (ADM) 78-482]. Rockville, MD: National Institute of Mental Health, Department of Health, Education and Welfare.

16

Cross-Cultural Applications of the Halstead–Reitan Batteries

JOVIER D. EVANS, S. WALDEN MILLER,
DESIREE A. BYRD, AND ROBERT K. HEATON

Introduction

The Halstead–Reitan battery (HRB) has been extensively used in clinical neuropsychology and numerous research studies have demonstrated its validity for neurodiagnostic and other applications (Reitan & Wolfson, 1993). The HRB typically includes the Wechsler Adult Intelligence Scale (WAIS) or one of its revisions (WAIS-R or WAIS-III), as well as several other measures: the Lateral Dominance Examination, a measure to determine left versus right preference for the hand, foot, and eye; the Reitan–Indiana Aphasia Screening Test, a modification of the Halstead–Wepman Aphasia Screening test to monitor various aspects of language function such as naming, repetition, and comprehension; the Finger Tapping Test, a test of motor speed with the upper extremities; the Hand Dynamometer test of grip strength; the Sensory-Perceptual Examination, a series of subtests to measure tactile, visual, and auditory function; the Tactile Form Recognition Test; the Seashore Rhythm Test and Speech Sounds Perception Test, measures of auditory attention and the ability to discriminate among auditory stimuli; the Trailmaking Test—Parts A and B, which measure sustained attention, perceptual–motor speed, and flexibility of thinking; the Tactual Performance Test, a measure of perceptual–motor problem solving, learning, and incidental memory; the Category Test, a complex test of abstraction and problem solving; and a version of the Minnesota Multiphasic Personality Inventory (MMPI) (Reitan & Wolfson, 1993). Often the HRB is supplemented by various tests of learning and memory such as the Wechsler Memory Scale (WMS) or one of its versions (WMS-R or WMS-III). A somewhat modified version of the HRB also has been developed and validated for use with older children (ages 9 to 14), and there is a much more extensively modified Reitan–Indiana Neuropsychological Test Battery for young children (ages 5 to 8; Reitan & Wolfson, 1993).

JOVIER D. EVANS • Department of Psychology, Indiana University-Purdue University, Indianapolis, Indiana 46202.   S. WALDEN MILLER, AND ROBERT K. HEATON • Department of Psychiatry, University of California, San Diego, California 92616-2292.   DESIREE A. BYRD • San Diego State University/University of California, San Diego, California 92616-2292.

Handbook of Cross-Cultural Neuropsychology, edited by Fletcher-Janzen, Strickland, and Reynolds. Kluwer Academic/Plenum Publishers, New York, 2000.

A review of the literature noted that the HRB has been validated at least 39 times for the detection of brain damage (Russell, 1995). Reitan and Wolfson (1993) state that the utility of this approach has been proven in "thousands" of clinical settings all over the world. Nevertheless, few investigations have examined the cross-cultural uses of this battery.

Vega and Parsons (1967) argued that many tests in the HRB would have trouble with cross-validation among different geographic regions and socioeconomic classes in the U.S., due to the lack of appropriate normative data. A meta-analysis of normative studies of the HRB up to the mid-1980s (Steinmeyer, 1986) determined that the greatest amount of empirical data were derived on primarily middle-aged, well-educated (presumably Caucasian) individuals and that normative data were needed across the lifespan and for various education levels. Heaton, Grant, and Matthews (1991) addressed this need by developing normative standards with demographic corrections based on age, education, and gender. While this research has established and has begun to correct for the influence of the aforementioned demographic variables on neuropsychological test performance, none of these studies examined these issues in nonwhite samples.

Race, Ethnicity, Culture, and Socioeconomic Status in Cognitive Ability Testing

This relative lack of diversity in normative samples is true with most neuropsychological tests used within the United States. A review of the literature provides few studies of HRB performance across culture or within different ethnic-minority groups in this country. However, a more fundamental concern is the confounded and unclear notions of race, ethnicity, culture, and socioeconomic status (SES). Researchers have argued that, if these variables have been considered at all, unclear definitions have been employed in research studies of cognitive ability tests and the idea of examining them independently or in combination has been woefully lacking (Helms, 1995, 1997). For example, most studies attempt to control for these variables by characterizing groups based on race, but not examining relevant cultural and socioeconomic factors that may account for differences in performance on most cognitive assessments. According to some researchers (Betancourt & Lopez, 1995; Lin, Poland, & Nakasaki, 1993) race has been used to denote groups that are biologically (and presumably genetically) determined, whereas culture represents attributes that are learned and passed down from generation to generation (e.g., work and recreational activities, celebration of religious holidays). Characteristics that are racially determined (such as skin color) are theoretically inherited and immutable, whereas traditions and customs shape culturally determined traits. However, the use of the term *race* has come under sharp criticism because it may convey a misleading sense of biological distinctiveness among different groups that might not even exist in any meaningful form. Jones (1991) argued that the concept of race is fraught with problems. Specifically, there are more within-group differences in the characteristics used to define the "three races" than between-group differences. These researchers go on to state that the use of racial characteristics to define groups, which are purely phenotypic expressions, to explain the differences in psychological phenomena fails to recognize the social and cultural influences which are likely to shape the psychological factors being examined.

Ethnicity, however, connotes groups of individuals who typically share a common ancestry and culture as well as a sense of identity (Bettancourt & Lopez, 1995; McGoldrick, Pearce, & Giordano, 1982). Ethnicity often is used interchangeably with both race and culture. Bettancourt and Lopez (1995) suggest that ethnicity refers to the ethnic quality or affiliation of a group, which is normally defined in terms of culture. This affiliation is also bidirectional in the sense that cultural background can determine ethnic identity and ethnic affiliation can also determine culture, through specific means such as ethnic identification, perceived discrimination, and bilingualism, for example. In summary, race, ethnicity, and culture are all linked and future studies of cross-cultural assessment approaches need to develop adequate modes of operationalizing these constructs to deal with a multicultural and multiethnic environment.

Socioeconomic status is another influence affecting the measurement of cognitive ability that should be considered more in studies examining ethnic differences in neuropsychological performance (Grubb & Ollendick, 1986). SES connotes the degree of educational, vocational, and financial attainment, all of which are likely to be associated with differences in cognitive development. For example, SES directly affects the quality of educational opportunities, the financial resources necessary for adequate access to healthcare, good nutritional standards, and exposure to important cultural institutions (e.g., museums, music). People of a lower SES may not have had these opportunities and may have trouble passing these opportunities on to successive generations. Grubb and Ollendick (1986) found that when examining African American and Caucasian performance on the WAIS-R, the Peabody Picture Vocabulary Test (PPVT), the Booklet Category Test, and the Memory Drum Recall and Recognition Test (a measure of auditory learning and memory), Caucasians scored significantly higher on the WAIS-R Full Scale IQ, Verbal IQ, and PPVT than African Americans, and that African Americans scored higher than whites on the Memory Drum Recall Test. Controlling for SES (social exposure, home dwelling conditions, fathers' occupational level, parental attitude toward education, and parental supervision) eliminated the differences seen in performance on the WAIS-R scores. This study provides a compelling example of the influence of SES on the cognitive performances of both African American and Caucasian subjects.

Most people considered to have achieved "middle-class" SES would be expected to do better on standardized cognitive assessment than otherwise similar people of a lower SES background since the predominant normative standards used are Western European, presumably middle or higher class. Controlling for the effects of SES, however, may not be sufficient to eliminate cultural or even biological (e.g., nutrition) differences seen in neuropsychological assessments.

Etic versus Emic Approaches to Psychological Assessment

Given the issues of culture and environment and their impact on psychological assessment, several methodological issues become important to consider. For example, what is the best way to characterize the constructs of "intelligence" or "abstract problem solving" in different cultures? Furthermore, how does one develop instruments, which are intrinsically culture dependent (usually Western), to be applicable and useful across cultures. These issues regarding culture and the search for universalism in cognitive constructs have introduced additional difficulties in the construction and development of psychological instruments. Okazaki and Sue (1995) review several methodological problems inherent in research with ethnic minorities. One major issue is the appropriate selection and method of scientific study. This debate has led to the "etic–emic" controversy in psychological assessment. An emic approach to assessment views the construct under study from within the culture one is examining. This involves identifying a hypothesized construct within a particular culture and determining its meaning, operations, and consequences from within that culture. This is in contrast to an etic perspective, which seeks to identify "universals" from outside the culture under study (Berry, 1995; Dana, 1993).

Dana (1993) notes that American psychologists generally adopt an etic perspective, but only in the sense that they assume universals among human beings by using assessment procedures from one culture and applying those procedures to other cultures. The predominant comparison group is generally Anglo middle-class American subjects. By applying this standard to non-Anglo populations, Dana notes "cultural differences can be treated as statistical differences that describe a departure from normality" (page 21).

This etic–emic distinction, in addition to other problems in assessment of different cultures, is one of the more difficult barriers to adequate neuropsychological assessment facing the field. It is clear that culture does play a role in neuropsychological performance and that no test can be considered culture-free (Anastasi, 1988; Manly, 1996). Other researchers have noted various problems with bias and cultural equivalence in assessment instruments (Helms, 1995; van de Vijver, 1994). For example, van de Vijver (1997) notes that if instruments are differentially appropriate across groups, this represents bias in the test. He identifies three types of bias in assessment: construct bias, method bias, and item bias. Construct bias can be demonstrated when behaviors associated with a construct are not identical across cultural groups. The second type, method bias represents measurement problems at the test level, such as mastery of the testing language or familiarity with the test stimuli. Many tests assume a mastery of the language of the test, even when this language mastery is not equivalent across groups. In addition, previous exposure to psychological tests or similar tasks has a considerable effect on performance. Finally, item bias refers to differential item functioning across groups. This is taken to mean that groups with the same level of ability do not have an equal probability of getting the same answer on a test. Most tests use local idioms and expressions to aid in ease of administration of the test; however, these idioms may be incomprehensible in translation (van de Vijver, 1994, 1997). For example, the expression, "One swallow doesn't make a summer," from the Comprehension subtest of the WAIS-R, may be meaningless to someone from sub-Saharan Africa.

In summary, problems inherent in cross-cultural research may have a profound impact on tests of cognitive ability when applied to different cultures. These dilemmas may emerge at the test development, normative, and validation stages due to one or all of the aforementioned problems. Issues of construct validity across cultures, problems with appropriate behavioral and cognitive operational definitions, and inherent sources of bias that have not been adequately controlled for need to be examined in future research of cognitive abilities across cultures.

The following review will present studies of components of the HRB applied to various cultures outside of the U.S., followed by cross-cultural applications within the U.S. among different ethnic groups, and then by recent studies which have attempted to examine the moderating influences of culture on neuropsychological test performance.

Cross-Cultural Applications of the Wechsler Scales

The Wechsler intelligence scales are an important component of (or adjunct to) the HRB. Reitan and Wolfson (1993) note that measures of intelligence serve as indications of basic aptitude and achievement typically learned in school. Furthermore, the specific WAIS (or WAIS-R, or WAIS-III) subtests provide information concerning the relationship of these aptitudes and abilities to other "biological" forms of intelligence, such as abstract reasoning and problem solving which are assessed more extensively by the HRB. The concept of intelligence and how we define and measure the construct has been the topic of extensive debate in the literature for many years (Herrnstein & Murray, 1994; Yee, Fairchild, Wiezmann,

& Wyatt, 1993). Traditionally, the WAIS summary measures have been considered indices of global intelligence or "*g*." Horn and Cattell (1967) have proposed that fluid (novel problem-solving with little impetus on learning experiences) and crystallized (cognitive functioning which is dependent to some extent on a person's formal educational experiences) intelligence are major components of *g*. A revision of this theory has been expanded to include nine broad dimensions of cognitive ability, which include: 1) fluid reasoning, 2) acculturation knowledge, 3) short-term apprehension–retention, 4) visual processing, 5) auditory processing, 6) processing speed, 7) correct decision speed, 8) quantitative knowledge, and 9) fluency of retrieval from long-term storage (see Horn & Noll, 1997 for a more detailed discussion). Other researchers have argued that intelligence is a multidimensional construct and that the Wechsler scales may only tap part of the overall concept of "intelligent behavior" (Chen & Gardner, 1997). Chen and Gardner (1997) have proposed the theory of Multiple Intelligences (MI) which go beyond traditional measures of fluid versus crystallized domains to include other aspects of cognitive performance, such as spatial abilities, musical ability, and athletic prowess. Sternberg (1997) proposes a triarchic theory of intelligence, which integrates three subtheories to explain the various manifestations of intelligent thought. In his view, the components of intelligence are in all cultures and are thus universal. The representation of these universal components, however, is mediated by 1) the internal world of the individual; 2) the unique experience of the individual in his or her world, and 3) the external world or environment of the individual. This debate has expanded research into intelligence to examine factors related to the individual in his or her cultural context.

The Wechsler scales have been used extensively in northern America, northern European countries and Japan (Flynn, 1987; Hattori & Lynn, 1997; Kaufman, 1990; Warner, Ernst, Townes, Peel, & Preston, 1987). Attempts have also been made to adapt these scales for use in Nigeria (Omotoso, 1996). The debate continues, however, with regard to the cultural appropriateness of these measures in other countries. In China, for example, some researchers have begun to question if the assessment of intelligence using "Western" tests of mental abilities accurately measures the same attributes of intelligence in Chinese people and that alternative methods of assessment may be more appropriate (Chan, 1991).

Much of the work done with cross-cultural applications of the Wechsler scales has examined ethnic differences on the WAIS-R within the U.S. population (Kaufman, 1990). Nevertheless, the standardization sample of the WAIS-R contains very few ethnic-minority subjects other than African Americans. Thus, it is still the case that relatively little is known about different ethnic-minority groups' (in the U.S.) performances on the WAIS-R.

People of Hispanic descent are the fastest growing ethnic-minority population in the U.S. However, few studies have examined the cognitive performance of this large, heterogeneous population on standard neuropsychological assessment. This may be due to the fact that Hispanics in the U.S. vary widely in terms of socioeconomic status, cultural background, educational attainment, and even racial background. For example, Mexican Americans may be culturally distinct from Cuban Americans in terms of religious practices, communication styles, and level of acculturation into the predominant American society (Perez-Arce & Puente, 1996). In terms of intellectual assessment, evidence from the standardization sample of the WAIS-R suggests that the whites outscore English-speaking Hispanics by 6–7 IQ points (Kaufman, 1990).

The most widely used test with Spanish-speaking Hispanic Americans is the Spanish translation of the WAIS, the Escala de Inteligencia Wechsler para Adultos (EIWA) (Wechsler, 1968). The EIWA was standardized on a sample of 1,127 Puerto Ricans from predominantly rural and poor economic backgrounds to provide a Spanish translation equivalent of the WAIS.

Most of the subtest items were altered to achieve both linguistic and cultural similarity between the EIWA and the WAIS. Two subtests were unaltered (Digit Span and Object Assembly). Resulting studies of the factor structure of the EIWA found a two-factor solution supporting both the Verbal and Performance factors similar to that found in the WAIS (Gomez, Piedmont, & Fleming, 1992). Unfortunately, there are several problems with using this instrument. The marked differences in the conversion from raw scores to scaled scores between the EIWA and the WAIS result in an overestimation of IQ (compared to U.S. norms) in samples of Hispanic subjects by as much as 20 points (Lopez & Romero, 1988). Melendez (1994) states that the EIWA may represent a major ethical problem if used in clinical assessment with Hispanic populations. He suggests that it should be avoided in clinical assessments of Hispanics living in the U.S. and, if used at all, it should be interpreted with extreme caution.

Reynolds, Chastain, Kaufman, and McLean (1987) examined the influence of the stratification variables of gender, race, educational level, occupational group, and urban versus rural residence on WAIS-R performance. Results indicated significant influences of gender, education, occupational level (unskilled workers versus professional and technical), and racial differences between African Americans and whites. In this study, 1,664 whites and 192 African Americans in the WAIS-R standardization sample were compared on the composite IQ scores. Whites outscored African Americans by almost 13.5 points on Verbal IQ, 14 points on Performance IQ, and 14.5 points on Full Scale IQ, all roughly equivalent to one standard deviation on the WAIS-R. Furthermore, these differences were fairly consistent across age and gender distributions of the standardization sample. It should be noted, however, that the differences in IQ varied across educational levels. The smallest discrepancies were noted in people with fewer than 8 years of education (7 IQ points) and only reached the one standard deviation discrepancy for highly educated groups (greater than 13 years of education). However, these conclusions are tentative at best due to the small sample-cell size of African Americans in this group ($n = 20$). The racial differences also varied according to occupational level. Groups of persons within middle-class occupations had a 10–12 point difference in IQ, while working-class groups had a slightly lower 9–11 point difference, with whites outscoring African Americans in both groups. Within each group, however, differences also were evident across class distinctions, with the middle-class groups performing better than the working-class subjects (Reynolds et al., 1987). It should be noted that the relatively small sample size of the African Americans in this study limits other comparisons with regard to regional differences (urban versus rural) and more extensive normative data with African American samples is needed. Another analysis of the WAIS-R subtests also found significant racial differences, with whites outscoring African Americans on all 11 subtests (Kaufman, McLean, & Reynolds, 1988). Significant racial differences in IQ performance remain even after controlling for age and education (Heaton, Ryan, Grant, & Matthews, 1996).

Vincent (1991) found that while the one standard deviation discrepancy between blacks and whites was seen in adults' WAIS-R performances, children in studies published after 1980 had differences on the WISC-R that were half as large as those seen in adults. Vincent concludes that these IQ differences are a barometer of educational and economic opportunity. Thus, the young children in the normative studies conducted after 1980 may be benefiting from the improvements in educational opportunities afforded them. With the recent development and standardization of the WAIS-III, this hypothesis can now be examined in a new sample of both young and old African Americans.

Another line of research in this area is to validate the Wechsler scales by conducting factor analytic studies among different ethnic/racial groups to determine construct validity across groups. Factor analytic studies of the WAIS-R standardization sample have provided confirmation of three basic constructs underlying the WAIS-R: Verbal Comprehension (Verbal), Perceptual Organization (Performance), and Freedom from Distractibility (Kaufman, McLean, & Reynolds, 1991). Theorists propose that the construct validity of the WAIS scales in different ethnic/racial groups would be established if similar factor structures were found in these samples. As mentioned previously, the EIWA displayed a similar factor structure to the WAIS (Gomez et al, 1992), yet the EIWA is seriously limited in its utility with Hispanics in the U.S. Other studies have found a similar factor structure in African American children and adults with both the WAIS-R and WISC-R (Kaufman et al., 1991; Kush & Watkins, 1997), although this has not been examined in Native Americans (Dana, 1995). Factorial similarity across ethnic groups is a necessary but not sufficient condition to prove that a test is not biased. For a standardized test to be considered fair and appropriate for use across groups, the following conditions must be met: 1) the regression lines of the distributions of scores (on the same test, with criterion measures[1]) must be parallel across groups, and 2) the correlation between the criteria and the test scores must be similar across groups (Cleary, Humphrey, Kendricks, & Wesman, 1975, as cited in Dent, 1996).

The HRB across Cultures

The HRB has been used in other, predominately northern European countries. An early cross-cultural validation of this assessment battery was conducted in Norway (Klove, 1974). Klove and his colleagues administered the HRB to groups of Norwegian control and brain-damaged subjects and compared them to groups of control and brain-damaged subjects from Wisconsin in the U.S. Results of this analysis found high rates of discrimination among brain-damaged and control subjects in both samples of patients. The authors speculated that factors such as different language and different cultural background have little influence on the discriminative power of these tests. A review of the literature uncovered a study which found limited evidence for HRB application in Czechoslovakia (Preiss & Hynek, 1991) with a mixed sample (psychiatric outpatients, epileptic patients, and "disability" patients) of clinical patients, however, no information regarding its results with neurologically normal subjects was discussed. Further review of the PsychInfo database revealed a few other studies attempting to cross-validate the HRB in Czechoslovakian children (Preiss, 1994), Chinese children (Xie & Gong, 1993), and Chinese adults (Gong, 1986).

In the Chinese adult study (Gong, 1986), the authors modified the HRB battery for use with 885 normal male and female subjects (age range 16– 45+) and 350 subjects with brain lesions. Normative data were collected on the subtests, and cutoff scores and a "damage quotient" were computed. The diagnostic validity of this revised battery was examined in terms of sensitivity, specificity, and the ability to detect left versus right hemispheric lesions. Findings support the use of the HRB to detect neurological impairment with this population in terms of both overall sensitivity (brain damaged vs. normal) and hemispheric localization. The later study of children examined the following aspects of the HRB modified for Chinese culture: dominant hemisphere function, aphasia, grip strength, tactual performance, musical rhythm, finger tapping, line-linking capability, speech sounds perception, and the different senses (Xie & Gong, 1993). This study examined 914 normal school age children (9–14 years old), and 111 children with brain dysfunction. Reliability and validity were examined, and

---

[1]Criterion measures are defined as measures that could be used to determine the accuracy of a decision.

means, standard deviations, and standard T-scores were reported. Again, the results suggest that the HRB is useful in documenting neurological impairment in Chinese children. What is unknown in these two studies is what the actual modifications consisted of and what demographic factors, if any, may have been controlled for in developing the standard T-scores in the child study.

In summary, a limited number of cross-cultural validation studies of the HRB have been attempted in European and Asian cultures to determine the utility of this neuropsychological assessment approach in countries other than the U.S. These studies have provided evidence of the usefulness of the HRB battery to detect neurological dysfunction in these differing cultural contexts. However, we have very little direct knowledge regarding the modifications and revisions to these instruments and if these modifications may have, in fact, altered the basic structure of the cognitive processes being assessed. Cognitive abilities, at least as measured by neuropsychological tests, are culturally as well as biologically influenced abilities, and performance on these tests is under the influence and control of several moderating factors such as language, educational level, and overall cultural environment (Ardila, 1995).

More investigators have attempted to cross-validate specific tests of the HRB in different cultures. In one study by Cuevas and Osterich, (1990), NATO pilots, pilot instructors, and their spouses were administered the booklet version of the Category Test (DeFilippis, McCampbell, & Rogers, 1979). The volunteers were men and women from Denmark ($n = 19$), the Netherlands ($n = 23$), the United States ($n = 26$), Germany ($n = 22$), Italy ($n = 19$), and Norway ($n = 22$). Results indicated that European women made significantly more errors on the booklet version of the Category test as compared to American women and both European and American men, suggesting gender-related differences across cultures for this test (Cuevas & Osterich, 1990).[2]

Another study examined the performance of Zairian children on the Tactual Performance Test (TPT) in comparison to a sample of American and Canadian children (Boivin, Giordani, & Bornefeld, 1995). The TPT was chosen because it was presumed to be a more fundamental assessment of the integrity of brain–behavior development and function. The hypothesis was that the TPT would be a more culturally fair assessment instrument due to its reliance on manual dexterity and coordination, covert visualization, spatial-cognitive mapping, flexibility in problem solving, and the ability to share information across cerebral hemispheres (Boll, 1981) without the *necessary* use of language or other culturally determined abilities. One hundred ninety-five rural, right-handed Zairian children (aged 5–12) were administered the TPT as part of a larger assessment battery. Their performance was compared to a sample of American schoolchildren from Michigan, and to the published TPT norms for children aged 5–12 which were collected in Ontario, Canada (Spreen & Strauss, 1991). There were no significant differences between the Canadian and the American children's performance on the TPT. However, both the Canadian and American samples had faster performance times than the Zairian children in terms of time per correctly placed block on all three trials (dominant, nondominant, and both hands), and they showed improvement between the first (dominant) and second (dominant) trials while the Zairian children did not. In addition, the Zairian children scored significantly lower on the TPT memory measures as compared to both the Canadian-based normative sample and the American children. It could well be that the stimulus material (blocks with geometric shapes) was much less familiar to the Zairian children than their North American peers. Sensitivity to brain damage was not assessed. These results suggest that there may be cultural influences at work in the TPT that may limit its utility when comparing groups of children from other cultures, particularly in nonindustrialized

---

[2]No gender differences were found in a U.S. sample as documented in Heaton et al., (1991).

settings. The authors note that this test may be useful within some specific cultures, provided there are appropriate normative standards to compare performance.

In Spain, Leon-Carrion (1989) sought to establish norms for the Trailmaking Test. The Trailmaking Test was administered to 268 healthy children between the ages of 10 and 15, and their performance was compared to published normative data (Reitan, 1971). Significant differences were found in mean performance levels between the two samples, suggesting that this test of perceptual–motor speed and information processing may not be free of cultural influences. Specifically, the Spanish children took longer to complete both Trails A and Trails B compared to the American children. The author did suggest that the original normative sample was small ($n = 98$) and that no information regarding the socioeconomic and cultural makeup of the American sample was provided to determine if the two samples were comparable on these variables. Furthermore, the author suggested that the processes underlying successful performance on Trails may be conditioned by culturally specific educational, environmental, or both types of influences.

Taken together, these studies have highlighted the need for normative data to be collected on neuropsychological measures across cultures, and that information regarding the moderating influences of such factors as environment, socioeconomic status, and level of education be included as areas of empirical study. In addition, more (e.g., factor analytic) work should be done to verify the construct validity of different test measures in different cultures. In addition, the sensitivity of measures to brain damage needs to be established within each population with which these tests may be used. The next section will focus on the work being done in the U.S. with regard to cross cultural assessment.

The HRB and Ethnic Minorities in the U.S.

Relatively few attempts have been made to examine ethnic differences in performance on neuropsychological tests in the U.S. (Adams, Boake, & Crain, 1982; Bernard, 1989; Boyar & Tsushima, 1975). These studies have noted that failure to consider subject characteristics (i.e., race, SES) in neuropsychological assessment may lead to diagnostic errors due to the bias of the normative data being used. Adams et al. (1982) found that, using published norms, 39% of their nonwhite (Mexican and African American) and 27% of their white controls were misclassified as brain damaged on the Bender-Gestalt Test due to factors such as age, education, and race. Another study noted a high level of misclassification (22%) of African American controls with the standard normative data on the Visual Naming Subtest of the Multilingual Aphasia Examination (Roberts & Hamsher, 1984). Another study of the HRB found differences between white, Hispanic and African American male college students on selected tests of the battery (Bernard, 1989). In this study, traditional cutoffs resulted in 11% (Category Test) to 71% (Finger Tapping) of these normal subjects being misclassified as impaired. When the Impairment Index (a summary measure of performance on seven subtests of the HRB) was calculated, however, the original cutoffs did not result in a high prevalence (15%) of misclassification among these normal subjects. Nevertheless, significant racial differences were noted on the Category test, the Seashore Rhythm test, and Finger Tapping. Black males scored lower on the Category test, and higher on the Seashore Rhythm test, as compared to both white and Hispanic males. Hispanic males were significantly better in their Finger Tapping performances compared to both black and white males. These differences were offset, however, by the fact that all scores of the relatively young and well-educated subjects were still within the "normal" range on both the Category and Rhythm tests.

Racial differences have been found in other neuropsychological domains, such as confrontation naming (Lichtenberg, Ross, & Christensen, 1994; Ross, Lichtenberg, & Christensen, 1995), and abstraction and memory (Inouye, Albert, Mohs, Sun, & Berkman, 1993). Most of these studies have documented significant differences in level of performance between ethnic minorities and Caucasians on these neuropsychological domains. In response to the lack of ethnic-minority representation in most normative samples, and the resulting misclassification of the groups into diagnostic categories, normative studies have been completed with African American and Caucasian elderly-community samples of both patients and controls using the CERAD neuropsychological battery (Unverzagt et al., 1996; Welsh et al., 1995).

Another study sought to cross-validate the HRB with the heterogeneous population found in Hawaii (Boyar & Tsushima, 1975). In this study, 120 subjects (all patients seen in a private medical setting) were evaluated with the HRB, a neurological examination, EEG, and skull x-rays. They were divided into three groups: a "normal" group of subjects who presented with symptoms consistent with a neurological disorder but were found to be without neurological pathology; a "neurological" group of subjects who had documented brain impairment on the basis of neurological exam; and a "neurosurgical" group with documented brain impairment on the basis of exam and definitive pathological findings based on surgery, brain scans, or autopsy. The ethnic makeup of the study was typical of the population of Hawaii, with patients of European, Chinese, Japanese, Korean, Filipino, Hawaiian, "other" Polynesian, and multiracial backgrounds. It was found that 83% of the neurological patients and 100% of the neurosurgical patients were impaired on the HRB tests, yet over 37% of the "normal" group of patients were classified as impaired using the existing norms. This high degree of false-positive diagnoses of neurological impairment across ethnic groups emphasizes the need for comprehensive normative data among nonwhite samples. In addition, the high degree of ethnic heterogeneity within this sample points out other problems in this area of work. For example, is it correct to collectively group Japanese, Chinese, Korean, and Polynesian subjects as simply nonwhite or ethnic-minority subjects?

In summary, this work clearly highlights the need for adequate normative data across ethnic and cultural groups to improve diagnostic accuracy in cognitive assessment. Research with minority participation is woefully lacking and too often members of minority groups are labeled as "impaired" in their cognitive performance when, in reality, there is a dearth of appropriate normative data with which to make accurate diagnostic judgments. Furthermore, the construct validity of most of these cognitive measures has not been thoroughly examined across different ethnic/racial groups within the U.S. More neuropsychological research is needed to examine the basic issues of reliability and validity of these neuropsychological instruments among different ethnic groups in the U.S. In possible cases where cross-cultural validity cannot be established there may be a need for the development of new culturally "appropriate" instruments to be used in a multicultural society.

The HRB and Acculturation

Another approach to the issue of cross-cultural assessment has been to examine the effects of acculturation on neuropsychological test performance among different ethnic minorities in the U.S. Acculturation refers to the culture change that results from continuous, firsthand contact between two distinct cultural groups (Redfield, Linton, & Herskovits, 1936, as cited in Berry, 1994). Through this change, immigrants or people of the nondominant culture begin to adopt the cultural behaviors, mores, and attitudes of the dominant culture

(Manly, 1996). Arnold, Montgomery, Castaneda, and Longoria (1994) examined the influence of level of acculturation on the test performance of 150 Mexican, Mexican American and Anglo college students on selected tests of the HRB. These three groups were categorized on a continuum of acculturation into the dominant American culture, ranging from total Mexican acculturation to biculturalism to Anglo acculturation using the Acculturation Rating Scale for Mexican Americans (ARSMA) (Cuellar, Harris, & Jasso, 1980). The ARSMA is a 20-item scale with four derived factors: 1) language familiarity, usage, and preference, 2) ethnic identity and generation, 3) reading, writing, and cultural exposure, and 4) ethnic interaction. Five tests from the HRB were administered to all subjects: the Category Test, the Tactual Performance Test, the Finger Tapping Test, the Seashore Rhythm Test, and the Trailmaking Test. Results indicated a significant effect of acculturation on performance of the Tactual Performance Test (Dominant, Nondominant, and Total times), the Seashore Rhythm Test, and the Category Test. Anglos had fewer errors on the Category Test and scored higher (better) on the three TPT measures. Mexican Americans, however, scored higher than either the Mexican or Anglo groups on the Seashore Rhythm test. Measures not affected by acculturation included Finger Tapping, Trailmaking, and Memory and Location scores of the Tactual Performance Test. Findings from this study support the use of acculturation measures as moderating influences of neuropsychological test performance in future normative studies with Hispanics. The study also demonstrates that the effects of culture are not uniform across all measures used in neuropsychological assessment, and that these differences remain after controlling for other demographic influences (such as age and education) on test performance.

Recently, work has been undertaken to examine the influence of acculturation on African American test performance (Manly, 1996; Manly et al., 1998). The purpose of the study was to determine: 1) if acculturation would be related to performance on formal neuropsychological tests among a group of normal African Americans, and 2) if this acculturation measure would moderate any differences in neuropsychological test performance in medically ill patients at risk for disease-related cognitive impairment. The African American Acculturation Scale (AAAS) (Landrine & Klonoff, 1995, 1996) was used to assess the level of acculturation in a sample of 170 normal African American adults who were subjects in the African American Neuropsychological Test Normative Project (AANP) undertaken by the second author (S.M.), and a matched sample of white and African American HIV-infected individuals who were part of a larger study examining neurocognitive effects of HIV infection. The AAAS has been found to examine key dimensions of the African American cultural experience, including traditional childhood experiences, religious beliefs and practices, preferences for African American music, media, and people, and preparation and consumption of traditional foods. The AAAS measures acculturation on a continuum (range 33–231) with low scores representing individuals who are acculturated to the American mainstream (high acculturation) and high scores representing traditional African American values (low acculturation). Individuals with middle-level scores are considered to be bicultural and hold beliefs, values, and practices from both cultures. All subjects were administered an expanded HRB assessment battery (Heaton et al., 1991; Reitan & Wolfson, 1993), which included the HRB and other tests of language skills, information processing, learning, and memory.

Acculturation was related to both demographic influences (education and gender), as well as performance on the neuropsychological evaluation. Specifically, individuals with fewer years of education were also more traditionally African American in their beliefs. Furthermore, women reported significantly more traditional religious beliefs and food practices than men did. In terms of neuropsychological performance, acculturation variables accounted for a significant amount of variance in performance on the Category Test, Trails A and B time,

Boston Naming Test, WAIS-R Information, Block Design, and Digit Symbol subtests, Grooved Pegboard (dominant hand), and learning components of the Story and Figure Memory Tests. Furthermore, after controlling for age, education, and sex, acculturation still accounted for a significant degree of variance in performance on the Boston Naming Test and the WAIS-R Information subtest, suggesting that these two tests are highly culturally loaded to a Western/European framework.

In the second study, acculturation (AAAS summary score) was used as a covariate in the analyses of neuropsychological performance between the two matched groups of HIV-infected individuals (African American and Caucasian). When the AAAS measure was used as a covariate, the previously detected differences on Category Test performance, Trails B time, Figure Learning, and WAIS-R Vocabulary and Block Design subtests became nonsignificant. The only significant difference that remained was in performance on the Story Memory Test. Taken together, these results suggest intraethnic differences in neuropsychological performance are moderated to some extent by acculturation. On many neuropsychological tests, persons who are more highly acculturated to the normative standards tend to perform better than people who are more traditional in their cultural beliefs and practices do. Furthermore, by accounting for this cultural variable, significant differences in clinical manifestations of illness between ethnic groups are likely to be more clearly detected, increasing diagnostic accuracy.

Another aspect of the Manly et al. (1998) study examined the rate of "impairment" of the normal African Americans in this study based on the Heaton et al. (1991) norms which correct for age, education, and gender. It should be stressed, again, that the Heaton et al. norms are based on a mostly Caucasian sample of individuals. Results indicated that a large proportion of these healthy, normal individuals scored more than one standard deviation below the normative mean (T-score less than 40), suggesting impairment on many of the tests in the expanded HRB. For example, 10 out of the 16 test measures had rates of impairment over 30%. Given the wide variability in the false-positive rates of impairment, it would seem that the appropriate normative standard to gauge African American performance would be that of an African American sample (Campbell et al., 1996; Heaton et al., 1996; Manly et al., 1998). In fact, this was the main purpose of the AANP Project, which will provide such norms in forthcoming publications.

Future Directions

While this review has not been exhaustive, it does highlight several key areas of research that need to be conducted in the future to ensure the utility of clinical neuropsychology in a multicultural society. First, at a minimum, more normative studies need to be conducted with other ethnic groups that have been traditionally neglected in psychological research. In addition, these groups need to be examined not only in terms of racial composition, but other cultural factors such as educational level, SES, language and cultural backgrounds to determine what, if any, moderating influences these factors may have on cognitive performance. Perez-Arce and Puente (1996) argue that more studies need to specifically examine the influence of non-European cultural variables and non–Anglo-Saxon languages on performance on current neuropsychological assessment batteries. Other researchers have argued that it is unethical to conduct neuropsychological assessments with persons who speak another language due to obvious threats to test standardization and construct validity (Artiola i Fortuny & Mullaney, 1998).

Helms (1997) suggests that tests themselves may be culturally biased and may not be measuring the same constructs across cultural groups. In other words, many ability tests fail to demonstrate cultural (i.e., racial, ethnic, cultural, or socioeconomic conditions of socialization) equivalence. She goes on to propose that the following types of cultural equivalence be considered when developing cognitive ability tests: 1) *functional equivalence*, or the extent to which the test scores have the same meaning in different cultural groups and measure the underlying psychological construct with equal accuracy within these groups; 2) *conceptual equivalence*, or whether the groups are equally familiar or unfamiliar with the content of test items and therefore assign the same meaning to them; 3) *linguistic equivalence*, or the extent to which the language used in the tests has equivalent meaning across cultural groups; 4) *psychometric equivalence*, or the extent to which tests measure the same thing at the same level across groups; 5) *testing condition equivalence*, or that the idea of testing and the testing procedures are equally familiar and acceptable across groups; 6) *contextual equivalence*, or evidence that the cognitive ability being assessed is comparable across environments; and 7) *sampling equivalence*, which refers to the samples of subjects representing different racial or ethnic groups being comparable at each level of test construction, that is, test development, validation, and interpretation (Helms, 1995; Helms, 1997). Whether or not it is necessary to develop entirely new tests for use across cultures or, in some cases, to carefully translate or develop new, ethnicity-specific norms are important questions for future research.

As noted earlier in this chapter, some neuropsychologists are beginning to examine the effects of acculturation on neuropsychological performance (Arnold et al., 1994; Manly et al., 1998). This is a good beginning. Acculturation measures may not, however, fully encompass all the important aspects underlying cultural/ethnic differences in test performance. Helms (1997) contends that most acculturation measures do not conceive of acculturation as a cognitive process and only use it to measure the extent to which various ethnic minorities are traditionally acculturated. She argues that a more beneficial approach would be to consider the degree to which ethnic minorities have been acculturated into the dominant (Western) culture of the cognitive ability tests. Cognitive abilities may be determined, at least partly, by the ecological demands for that ability (Manly, 1996). Therefore, traditional neuropsychological tests may be evaluating skills which have some implicit value for mainstream Western culture, but which may have less value (or even no value) for ethnic minorities or different cultural groups. Furthermore, controlling for some of these cultural factors may not control for other factors influencing ethnicity differences in cognitive performance. For example, controlling for level of acculturation may still not eliminate differences due to SES and other environmental influences (e.g., nutritional deprivation or quality of educational experiences) on cognitive development.

Another focus has been on minimizing cultural bias. One recent study of the World Health Organization (WHO) sought to develop culturally fair neuropsychological assessments to detect the clinical manifestations of HIV-infection (Maj et al., 1993). This study developed the WHO/UCLA Auditory Verbal Learning Test and Color Trails 1 and 2 to be used in Zaire, the U.S., Germany, Kenya, and Brazil. The two tests were found to be sensitive to HIV-associated cognitive impairment and to be culturally fair across both developed and developing countries.

A major challenge in the study of the effects of culture on neuropsychological test performance is the identification and reliable measurement of the proper variables. Only recently has neuropsychology begun to recognize the importance of demographic/environmental variables and their effects on test performance. While it is clear that large discrepancies exist between the scores of Caucasians and most ethnic minorities on tests of cognitive functioning, the reasons for this difference remain unclear. The answer to this important question does not lie in identifying test bias, construct validity, invalid normative samples, or acculturation alone. It is more likely that all of the aforementioned factors, as well as some yet unidentified factors, interact together to produce such discrepant findings between cultural groups. The challenge to neuropsychologists is to realize the complexity of these issues and dedicate scientific resources toward working for a solution. Until this issue is properly addressed, ethnic minorities risk being underserved by the field of neuropsychology.

As neuropsychology enters the next century, it is incumbent upon us to deal with the issues of a multicultural society and develop instruments and procedures that will not unduly penalize persons from other than traditional Western backgrounds. We must develop techniques and methods of assessment that will be able to document and describe brain–behavior relationships across racial, ethnic and, cultural boundaries.

ACKNOWLEDGMENTS.   This work was supported in part by NIMH grants #5 P30 MH49671, #5 R37 MH43693, #5-P30 MH49671-01S1, #1 R03 MH51200, and 5 R01 MH49550-04. The authors gratefully acknowledge the assistance of Jennifer J. Manly, Ph.D., for her help with the collection of relevant literature.

References

Adams, R. L., Boake, C., & Crain, C. (1982). Bias in a neuropsychological test classification related to education, age, and ethnicity. *Journal of Consulting and Clinical Psychology*, *50*, 143–145.

Anastasi, A. (1988). *Psychological testing*. New York: Macmillan.

Ardila, A. (1995). Directions of research in cross-cultural neuropsychology. *Journal of Clinical and Experimental Neuropsychology*, *17*, 143–150.

Arnold, B.R., Montgomery, G.T., Castaneda, I., Longoria, R. (1994). Acculturation and performance of Hispanics on selected Halstead–Reitan neuropsychological tests. *Assessment*, *1*, 239–248.

Artiola i Fortony, L., & Mullaney, H. A. (1998). Assessing patients whose language you do not know: Can the absurd be ethical? *The Clinical Neuropsychologist*, *12*, 113–126.

Bernard, L. C. (1989). Halstead-Reitan neuropsychological test performance of black, Hispanic, and white young adult males from poor academic backgrounds. *Archives of Clinical Neuropsychology*, *4*, 267–274.

Berry, J. W. (1994). Acculturation and psychological adaptation: An overview. In A. M. Bouvy, F. van de Vijver, P. Boski, & P. Schmitz (Eds.), *Journeys into cross-cultural psychology* (pp. 129–141). Berwyn, PA: Swets & Zeitlinger.

Berry, J. W. (1995). Psychology of acculturation. In N. R. Goldberger & J. B. Veroff (Eds.), *The culture and psychology reader* (pp. 457–488). New York: New York University Press.

Betancourt H. & Lopez, S. R. (1995), The study of culture, ethnicity, and race in American psychology. In N. R. Goldberger & J. B. Veroff (Eds.), *The culture and psychology reader* (pp. 87–107). New York: New York University Press.

Boivin, M. J., Giordani, B., & Bornefeld, B., (1995). Use of the Tactual Performance Test for cognitive ability testing with African children. *Neuropsychology*, *9*, 409–417.

Boll, T. J. (1981). The Halstead–Reitan neuropsychology battery. In S. B. Filskov & T. J. Boll (Eds.), *Handbook of clinical neuropsychology* (pp. 577–607). New York: Wiley.

Boyar, J. I., & Tsushima, W. T., (1975). Cross-validation of the Halstead–Reitan neuropsychological battery: Application in Hawaii. *Hawaii Medical Journal*, *34*(3), 94–96.

Campbell, A., Rorie K., Dennis G., Wood D., Combs S., Hearn L., Davis H., Brown A., & Weir R. (1996) Neuropsychological assessment of African Americans: Conceptual and methodological considerations. In R. L. Jones (Ed.), *Handbook of tests and measurements for black populations* (Vol. 2; pp. 75–84). Hampton, VA: Cobb & Henry.

Chan, J. (1991). Are the western-type mental tests measuring Chinese mental faculties? *Bulletin of the Hong Kong Psychological Society*, Jan–Jul (26–27), 59–70. Abstract from: Melvyl File: PsychINFO.

Chen, J., & Gardner, H. (1997). Alternative assessment from a multiple intelligences theoretical perspective. In D. P.

Flanagan, J. L. Genshaft, & P. L. Harrison (Eds.), *Contemporary intellectual assessment* (pp. 105–121). New York: Guilford.

Cuellar, I., Harris, L.C., & Jasso, R. (1980). An acculturation scale for Mexican American normal and clinical population. *Hispanic Journal of Behavioral Science, 2*, 199–217.

Cuevas, J. L., & Osterich, H. (1990). Cross-cultural evaluation of the booklet version of the Category test. *International Journal of Clinical Neuropsychology, 12*(3–4), 187–190.

Dana, R. H. (1993). *Multicultural assessment perspectives for professional psychology.* Boston: Allyn & Bacon.

Dana, R. H. (1995). Impact of the use of standard psychological assessment on the diagnosis and treatment of ethnic minorities. In J. F. Aponte, R. Young Rivers, & J. Wohl (Eds.), *Psychological interventions and cultural diversity* (pp. 57–73). Boston: Allyn & Bacon.

DeFilippis, N. A., McCampbell, E., & Rogers, P. (1979). The development of a booklet form of the Category Test: Normative and validity data. *Journal of Clinical Neuropsychology, 1*, 339–342.

Dent, H.E. (1996). Non-biased assessment or realistic assessment? In R.L. Jones (Ed.), *Handbook of tests and measurements for black populations* (Vol. 1; pp. 103–122). Hampton, VA: Cobb & Henry.

Flynn, J. R. (1987). Massive IQ gains in 14 nations: What IQ tests really measure. *Psychological Bulletin, 101*, 171–191.

Gong, Y. (1986). The Chinese revision of Halstead–Reitan neuropsychological test battery for adults. *Acta Psychologica Sinica, 18*, 433–442. Abstract from Melvyl File: PsychINFO.

Gomez, F. C., Jr., Piedmont, R. L., & Fleming, M. Z. (1992). Factor analysis of the Spanish version of the WAIS: the Escala de Inteligencia Wechsler para Adultos (EIWA). *Psychological Assessment, 4*, 317–321.

Grubb, H. J., & Ollendick, T. H. (1986). Cultural-distance perspective: An exploratory analysis of its effect on learning and intelligence. *International Journal of Intercultural Relations, 10*, 399–414.

Hattori, K., & Lynn, R. (1997). Male–female differences on the Japanese WAIS-R. *Personality and Individual Differences, 23*, 531–533.

Heaton, R. K., Grant, I., & Matthews, C. G. (1991). *Comprehensive norms for an expanded Halstead–Reitan Battery: Demographic corrections, research findings, and clinical applications.* Odessa, FL: Psychological Assessment Resources.

Heaton, R. K., Ryan, L., Grant, I., & Matthews, C. G. (1996). Demographic influences on neuropsychological test performance. In I. Grant & K. M. Adams (Eds.), *Neuropsychological assessment of neuropsychiatric disorders* (2nd ed.; pp. 141–163). New York: Oxford University Press.

Helms, J. E. (1995). Why is there no study of cultural equivalence in standardized cognitive ability testing. In N. R. Goldberger & J. B. Veroff (Eds.), *The culture and psychology reader* (pp. 674–719). New York: New York University Press.

Helms, J. E. (1997). The triple quandary of race, culture, and social class in standardized cognitive ability testing. In D. P. Flanagan, J. L. Genshaft, & P. L. Harrison (Eds.), *Contemporary intellectual assessment* (pp. 517–532). New York: Guilford.

Herrnstein, R. J., & Murray, C. (1994). *The bell curve: Intelligence and class structure in American life.* New York: Free Press.

Horn, J. L., & Cattell, R. B. (1967). Age differences in fluid and crystallized intelligence. *Acta Psychologica, 26*, 107–129.

Horn, J. L., & Noll, J. (1997). Human cognitive capabilities: Gf-Gc theory. In D. P. Flanagan, J. L. Genshaft, & P. L. Harrison (Eds.), *Contemporary intellectual assessment: Theories, tests, and issues* (pp. 53–91). New York: Guilford.

Inouye, S. K., Albert, M. S., Mohs, R., Sun, K., & Berkman, L.F. (1993). Cognitive performance in a high-functioning community-dwelling elderly population. *Journal of Gerontology, 48*(4), M146–M151.

Jones, J.M. (1991). Psychological models of race: What have they been and what should they be? In J. D. Goodchilds (Ed.), *Psychological perspectives on human diversity in America* (pp. 5–46). Washington, D.C.: American Psychological Association.

Kaufman, A. S. (1990). *Assessing adolescent and adult intelligence.* Boston: Allyn & Bacon.

Kaufman, A. S., McLean, J. E., & Reynolds, C. R. (1988). Sex, race, residence, region, and education differences on the 11 WAIS-R subtests. *Journal of Clinical Psychology, 44*, 231–248.

Kaufman, A. S., McLean, J. E., & Reynolds, C. R (1991). Analysis of WAIS-R factor patterns by sex and race. *Journal of Clinical Psychology, 47*, 548–557.

Klove, H. (1974). Validation studies in adult clinical neuropsychology. In R. M. Reitan & L. A. Davison (Eds.), *Clinical neuropsychology: Current status and applications* (pp. 211–235). Washington, D.C.: V. H. Winston.

Kush, J. C., & Watkins, M. W. (1997). Construct validity of the WISC-III verbal and performance factors for black special education students. *Assessment, 4*, 297–304.

Landrine, H., & Klonoff, E. A. (1995). The African American Acculturation Scale II: Cross-validation and short form. *Journal of Black Psychology, 21*, 124–152.

Landrine, H., & Klonoff, E. A. (1996). *African American acculturation: Deconstructing race and reviving culture.* Thousand Oaks, CA: Sage.

Leon-Carrion, J. (1989). Trail making test scores for normal children: Normative data from Spain. *Perceptual and Motor Skills, 68,* 627–630.

Lichtenberg, P. A., Ross, T., & Christensen, B. (1994). Preliminary normative data on the Boston Naming Test for an older urban population. *The Clinical Neuropsychologist, 8,* 109–111.

Lin, K. M., Poland, R. E., & Nakasaki, G. (1993). Introduction: Psychopharmacology, psychobiology, and ethnicity. In K. M. Lin, R. E. Poland, & G. Nakasaki (Eds.), *Psychopharmacology and psychobiology of ethnicity* (pp. 3–10). Washington, D.C.: American Psychiatric Press.

Lopez, S., & Romero, A. (1988). Assessing the intellectual functioning of Spanish speaking adults: Comparison of the EIWA and the WAIS. *Professional Psychology: Research and Practice, 19,* 263–270.

Maj. M., D'Elia, L., Satz, P., Janssen, R., Zaudig, M., Uchiyama, C., Starace, F., Galderisi, S., & Chervinsky, A. (1993). Evaluation of two new neuropsychological tests designed to minimize cultural bias in assessment of HIV-1 seropositive persons: A WHO study. *Archives of Clinical Neuropsychology, 8,* 123–135.

Manly, J. J. (1996) *The effect of African American acculturation on neuropsychological test performance.* Unpublished doctoral dissertation, University of California, San Diego and San Diego State University.

Manly, J. J., Miller, S. W., Heaton, R. K., Byrd, D., Reilly, J., Velasquez, R. J., Saccuzzo, D. P., & Grant, I. (1998). The effect of African American acculturation on neuropsychological test performance in normal and HIV-positive individuals. *Journal of the International Neuropsychological Society, 4,* 291–302.

McGoldrick, M., Pearce, J. K., & Giordano, J. (1982). *Ethnicity and family therapy.* New York: Guilford.

Melendez, F. (1994). The Spanish version of the WAIS: Some ethical considerations. *The Clinical Neuropsychologist, 8,* 388–393.

Okazaki, S., & Sue, S. (1995). Methodological issues in assessment research with ethnic minorities. *Psychological Assessment, 7,* 367–375.

Omotoso, H. M. (1996). Problems of educational research on tests and measurements in Nigeria. In R. L. Jones (Ed.), *Handbook of tests and measurements for black populations* (Vol. 1; pp. 185–195). Hampton, VA: Cobb & Henry.

Perez-Arce, P., & Puente, A. E. (1996). Neuropsychological assessment of ethnic minorities: The case of assessing Hispanics living in North America. In R. J. Sbordone & C. J. Long (Eds.), *Ecological validity of neuropsychological testing* (pp. 283–300). Delray Beach, FL: GR Press/St. Lucie Press.

Preiss, M. (1994). Klinicke vysetreni pameti u deti. [Clinical examination of memory in children.] *Ceskoslovenska Psychologie, 38,* 545–554. Abstract from Melvyl File: PsychINFO

Preiss, J., & Hynek, K. (1991). Neuropsychologicka baterie Halstead–Reitan: Prvni zkusenosti s ceskym prevodem. [Halstead–Reitan neuropsychological battery. Initial experience with Czech application]. *Ceskoslovenska Psychiatrie, 87,* 249–254.

Reitan, R. M. (1971). Trail Making Test results for normal and brain-damaged children. *Perceptual and Motor Skills, 33,* 575–581.

Reitan, R. M., & Wolfson, D. (1993). *The Halstead–Reitan Neuropsychological Test Battery* (2nd ed.). Tucson, AZ: Neuropsychology Press.

Reynolds, C. R., Chastain, R. L., Kaufman, A. S., & McLean, J. E. (1987). Demographic characteristics and IQ among adults: Analysis of the WAIS-R standardization sample as a function of the stratification variables. *Journal of School Psychology, 25,* 323–342.

Roberts, R. J., & Hamsher, K. D. (1984). Effects of minority status on facial recognition and naming performance. *Journal of Clinical Psychology, 40,* 539–545.

Ross, T. P., Lichtenberg, P. A., & Christensen, B. K. (1995). Normative data on the Boston Naming Test for elderly adults in a demographically diverse medical sample. *The Clinical Neuropsychologist, 9,* 321–325.

Russell, E. W. (1995). The accuracy of automated and clinical detection of brain damage and lateralization in neuropsychology. *Neuropsychology Review, 5,* 1–68.

Spreen, O., & Strauss, E. (1991). *A compendium of neuropsychological tests: Administration, norms, and commentary.* Oxford: Oxford University Press.

Steinmeyer, C. H. (1986). A meta-analysis of Halstead–Reitan test performances of non-brain damaged subjects. *Archives of Clinical Neuropsychology, 1,* 301–307.

Sternberg, R. J. (1997). The triarchic theory of intelligence. In D. P. Flanagan, J. L. Genshaft, & P. L. Harrison (Eds.), *Contemporary intellectual assessment* (pp. 92–104). New York: Guilford.

Unverzagt, F. W., Hall, K. S., Torke, A. M., Rediger, J. D., Mercado, N., Gureje, O., Osuntokun, B. O., & Hendrie, H. C. (1996). Effects of age, education, and gender on CERAD neuropsychological test performance in an African American sample. *The Clinical Neuropsychologist, 10,* 180–190.

van de Vijver, F. (1994). Bias: Where psychology and methodology meet. In A. M. Bouvy, F. van de Vijver, Boski, P., & Schmitz, P. (Eds.), *Journeys into cross-cultural psychology* (pp. 111–126). Berwyn, PA: Swets & Zeitlinger.

van de Vijver, F. (1997). Neuropsychology from a cross cultural perspective. *INSNET, Spring,* 3–4.

Vega. A., & Parson, O. A. (1967). Cross-validation of the Halstead–Reitan tests for brain-damage. *Journal of Consulting Psychology, 31,* 619–625.

Vincent, K. R. (1991). Black/white IQ differences: Does age make the difference? *Journal of Clinical Psychology, 47,* 266–270.

Warner, M. H., Ernst, J., Townes, B. D., Peel, J., & Preston, M. (1987). Relationships between IQ and neuropsychological measures in neuropsychiatric populations: Within-laboratory and cross-cultural replications using WAIS and WAIS-R. *Journal of Clinical and Experimental Neuropsychology, 9,* 545–562.

Wechsler, D. (1968). Escala de inteligencia Wechsler para adultos. New York: The Psychological Corporation.

Welsh, K. A., Fillenbaum, G., Wilkinson, W., Heyman, A., Mohs, R. C., Stern, Y., Harrell, L., Edlans, S. D., & Beekly, D. (1995). Neuropsychological test performance in African-American and white patients with Alzheimer's disease. *Neurology, 45,* 2207–2211.

Xie, Y., & Gong, Y. (1993). The revision and application of the Halstead–Reitan neuropsychological test battery for children in China. *Chinese Mental Health Journal, 7*(2), 49–53. Abstract from: Melvyl File: PsychINFO.

Yee, A. H., Fairchild, H. H., Weizmann, F., & Wyatt, G. (1993). Addressing psychology's problems with race. *American Psychologist, 48,* 1132–1140.

17

Cross-Cultural Applications of the Luria–Nebraska Neuropsychological Test Battery and Lurian Principles of Syndrome Analysis

CHARLES J. GOLDEN AND RHIANNON B. THOMAS

Luria's contributions to neuropsychology were influenced and developed in the context of Soviet psychology which focused specifically on the relationship between the brain and the role of history and culture in human development (Mecacci, 1977/1979). Luria's work has been developed in other countries outside Russia. Continued research has shown that Luria's diagnostic procedure is an effective assessment measure for brain-damaged patients with an accuracy founded on a sound theoretical basis, rather than solely upon the unique clinical skills of Luria himself (Pachalska, Kaczmarek, & Knapik, 1995). Luria's theories from his earliest work emphasized the relationship between behavior and culture, while maintaining the existence of a dynamic brain organization reflective of the integrated efforts of basic brain areas which had specific (although multiple) localized functions.

The Luria–Nebraska Neuropsychological Test Battery (LNNB) (Golden, Hammeke, & Purisch, 1980) standardized Luria's original approach. Based on the basic tenets of Luria's theory along with an attempt to identify objective and scorable aspects of his clinical work, the LNNB attempted to provide a synthesis of quantitative and qualitative approaches to neuropsychology.

Luria's basic theory emphasizes the role of culture and experience in the development of the brain, especially in the secondary and tertiary association areas the development of which are strongly influenced by language, culture, and experience. Despite the theoretical emphasis on the role of environment, Luria also assigned basic functions to each of the areas of the brain.

CHARLES J. GOLDEN AND RHIANNON B. THOMAS • Nova Southeastern University, Fort Lauderdale, Florida 33314.

Handbook of Cross-Cultural Neuropsychology, edited by Fletcher-Janzen, Strickland, and Reynolds. Kluwer Academic/Plenum Publishers, New York, 2000.

These functions are too basic to be reflected in test behavior, but rather these functions are summed together to form functional systems which are actually responsible for the behaviors observed in real life or on a neuropsychological examination.

Thus, while the general functions of brain areas remain the same, their contribution to a given functional system or behavior may vary considerably based on cultural and environmental variables. The more complex the behavior under consideration, the more variable the underlying functional system can be in an individual, group or culture. Conversely, the more basic the behavior the simpler the functional systems and the more likely that the systems are similar across cultural groups.

While simple behaviors may reflect more consistency in process, they may vary in content. Thus, while individuals from different cultural groups may (in the absence of injury) use the same brain systems to discriminate basic and overlearned phonemes, the nature of those phonemes will vary from language to language. As a result, a native speaker of English may have no trouble discriminating an *r* from an *l*, while a native speaker of Japanese may have severe problems making such a discrimination because of the absence of that phonemic differentiation in Japanese. Thus, the failure of the native Japanese speaker to discriminate between these phonemes is not an indication of brain injury but rather a cultural/language-based issue which results in subtle differences within the receptive speech areas of the brain.

When more complex behaviors are involved, differences may be far more extensive. Problem-solving styles differ from culture to culture ranging from the emphasis placed on certain inputs and information to the ways in which logic is recognized and followed. The more these styles differ, the more variable will be the results of tests which demand the use of such processes. Individuals from different cultures may approach problems with radically different functional systems, as will the brain-injured individual forced to reorganize cognitive processes because of the impact of an injury. In one case, those differences are the result of cultural choice and influence on the development of a functional system, while in the other it is forced on the individual by a brain injury.

Luria often addressed a multicultural clientele and had a substantial background in sociology, so he was very aware of the influence of these issues. He was also aware of the impact of such issues on the assessment of brain injury. As individual tests were made more difficult and complex, each test was harder to analyze in terms of the specific brain areas involved and their role in the overall functional system. It became harder to recognize the source of a brain injury, or even whether the behavior reflected choice rather than injury. The identification of cultural influences was very similar, as it became harder in complex behaviors to identify which variations were cultural and which were due to actual brain dysfunction.

As a result, Luria championed a hierarchical approach to assessment that involved demonstration of the intactness of basic functions followed by examination of the ability to combine these functions. Functions were investigated from a variety of perspectives to insure that a deficit was consistently present no matter how one evaluated it. If a deficit was not consistent, then the area under review was likely somewhat intact and other avenues needed to be explored to explain any deficits. If a deficit could be consistently elicited, then its presence was much more likely. By emphasizing basic procedures, the complexity of these processes could be minimized so that a detailed analysis could be completed.

Similarly, if a difference in a given behavior is due to cultural influences, alternate methods of testing the same function would result in evidence that the underlying brain area was likely partially intact and that the behavior did not reflect the outcome of a brain injury. Thus, by isolating each basic function of the brain through a syndrome analysis, each area could be assessed to be functional, arguing against the presence of a brain injury.

Luria's examination was organized into individual, basic pieces that could be used in combination to test a specific brain process. As a result, basic motor skills might be assessed by the client's ability to imitate, follow a command, learn from a demonstration, or from spontaneous movement secondary to another process. Only when a consistent deficit arose could a question be raised about a particular brain injury. The interpretation of such data required a complete understanding of brain–behavior relationships. Luria focused on basic skills that are common to all peoples and cultures as these are the basic skills mediated by the brain, which is not the case with more culturally driven and diverse complex skills.

Luria recognized that while the skills were in common, the content needed to be varied for the items to be appropriate to other cultures. A picture of a telephone could not be used for visual identification in a culture that had never seen a telephone. The same answer could not be expected for logic problems or language construction patterns that were not present or generated different problemsolving approaches. Luria customized each of his examinations to address these issues.

Cross-Cultural Adjustments to the LNNB

The approach to the cross-cultural adjustment of the LNNB is similar to the approach Luria used. Each item of the test must be reviewed for appropriate cultural content with regards to the intention of the item. The items are relatively simple as in Luria's approach, and therefore the identification of such content and possible differences in underlying processes is easier to see and eliminate. Such alterations must not only insure that behavior requested is culturally meaningful but also meets the goals of the original item.

For example, one item requires the spelling of the word *knife*. Knife is included because it contains both beginning and final silent letters. In some languages there is no such thing as a silent letter and so we must eliminate the item altogether. In languages where silent letters occur, we must insure that the frequency and the difficulty of the word and the silent letter are similar to *knife* in English.

Although we cannot cover all possible modifications for all possible cultural groups, we will briefly review the major issues that have arisen to date in the translation of the LNNB.

Motor Scale

The Motor Scale is relatively culture-free in most of the LNNB translations. The basic motor items can remain the same across groups. There is some difficulty in translating such items as "Pretend you are making scrambled eggs" as this is not present in all groups. Substitution requires the use of a common multistep procedure requiring bilateral coordination. The remaining items are very basic (such as simple drawings) that do not seem to present any problems.

Rhythm Scale

These are again simple items that require matching and reproducing very basic rhythms that are easily recognized by all cultures. The client is asked to sing the first line of a common song which must be selected from the culture.

Tactile Scale

This is another simple scale with most of the items looking at basic touch and sensation. Two items assess recognition of numbers written on the back of the wrist. Most cultures recognize Arabic numbers although these must be changed if this is not the case. Two items also require the tactile recognition of letters, which must be adjusted as necessary to languages that use other alphabets (and must be eliminated in languages where an alphabet is not used). The astereognosis items use objects that are common in our culture (e.g., paper clip, nickel, eraser, rubber band) but alternate objects of similar difficulty in tactile identification may need to be used.

Visual Scale

The Visual Scale contains pictures and drawings of objects which are common to many western hemisphere countries but are not present in all cultures. These must be carefully evaluated and replaced as necessary by objects that can be recognized as easily. The more abstract items (such as lock visualization or rotation) appear to be generalizable to many cultural groups.

Receptive Language Scale

Any language-based scale will clearly need translation and substitution in order to be used in different language/culture groups. The first set of items examines the repetition of basic phonemic sounds. These must be modified to include frequent sounds in a given language although the original phonemes were chosen because of their general use across many language groups. Some of the items require matching of phonemes with individual letters which will be inappropriate when the written language is not phonemically based. The next section examines simple commands, using motor responses or picture identification. As the concepts become more abstract, there may be a need to alter the ideas to fit a culture and the pictures used may need to be altered if not immediately recognized by normal individuals in that group.

Of greater concern are the more complex command items that must be translated carefully to preserve the intent of the item. Some involve comparisons, spatial relationships, logical relationships, and double negatives that will usually not translate word for word. Again, maintenance of the original intent of the item as described in the manual and in Luria's work is more important than the exact wording of the question.

Expressive Language

The initial part of this subtest involves repetition of sounds, words, and phrases of increasing complexity to test for fluency. Translation of this material should not be focused on reproducing these words but rather words of similar complexity when pronounced. For example, some use words that have similar beginning sounds but different endings (key–kick), when translated directly, would result in a phrase but not one that tests the same process. In such cases, other words with similar linguistic properties must be chosen. In all cases the relative frequency of the word in the language should be maintained as best as possible. Throughout the scale there is an emphasis on the fluency in the language the client speaks most easily.

Writing

As with the expressive language scale, a direct translation is inappropriate. Substitutions must be made with words of similar frequency and similar difficulty in motor writing. Because of the vast variation in written languages, an exact match will rarely be made but must be approximated. Some of the concepts in some of the items (initial silent letter, for example) may not exist and should be deleted or replaced by an additional item measuring another written language skill. In some languages, the use of tonal changes that alter the written word might be added. Items that involve common phrases must be translated to suitable common phrases of equal difficulty.

Reading

The same issues arise with this scale as seen with other language scales. As before, direct translation of the words is inappropriate but the intent of the item must be maintained. For languages where there is no phoneme–letter correlation, several of the items would be inappropriate and would need to be approximated with simple common words as best as possible.

Arithmetic

This scale translates across most cultures fairly well as long as Arabic numbers are used. In most cases, it can be adopted without change except to translate the instructions into the appropriate language.

Memory

This scale also translates reasonably well. The nonverbal items seem to have little problem when translated. The verbal items need to be translated into similarly simple and frequent words as the words used here. Otherwise, there seem to be few difficulties with this scale.

Intelligence

Translation from both a language perspective and a cultural perspective presents a major challenge to the cross-cultural use of tests. Items must be culturally sensitive, use equally difficult language, and reflect the logical thinking style of each culture. Thus, while the general intent of the items (e.g., picture interpretation, vocabulary, sequencing, proverb interpretation, generalization, discrimination, categorization, and arithmetic reasoning) will remain the same, the content must often be changed to similar items of similar difficulty. The pictures used are appropriate in most western cultures, but may not be appropriate outside this group. Proverbs must be substituted by similar common sayings but they can rarely be translated. Categorization items must be substituted by common categories, although many used (finger/hand, twig/tree, etc.) are common to most cultures and thus can be used fairly easily.

Intermediate Memory

This is the delayed memory component of the test and simply must reflect the changes made in the items themselves when they were first presented. It requires no additional translation efforts.

Scoring

If the test is properly translated to other cultures/languages, scoring follows fairly closely to the American version. A majority of items are simply right or wrong, and appropriate changes in scoring criteria to reflect changes in items will accommodate these items. For items with more complex responses in terms of time and speed, there is a need to validate the current criteria against the performance of formal individuals. However, given the simplicity of many of these items (speed of opening and closing a fist, time to draw a circle) the norms are remarkably stable across cultures with only minor variations. Items in which the scoring is more abstract, involving judgments of appropriate/concrete/inappropriate, require the development of criteria for these judgments that follow the intent of the items. In all of these cases, the simplicity of the items and the basic skills they reflect generally result in only minor changes as long as item difficulty remains equal.

Similarly, scoring for the scales remains the same although norms may differ depending on the difficulty of the translated items compared to the original items. The biggest influence on changes in norms results from using normative samples with different age and educational levels. In addition, the LNNB standardization sample used normal individuals who were hospitalized for nonneurological reasons, arguing that such a group made a better comparison for people with brain injuries as well as a more accurate measure of the accuracy of the test. If a "normal" sample is taken from the population at large, T scores may be as many as 4–7 points lower. This changes cutoff scores from 10 points to 15 points above the average score. When establishing critical levels for identifying brain injury, it is also necessary to include age and education adjustments appropriate to the given population.

Interpretation

Interpretation of the LNNB occurs on several levels that are affected in different ways by translations of the test. The most basic is level of performance. This is based on normative test data and it is essential that normative data be gathered on all the quantitative scoring for each translation. Given the simplicity of the items, there is remarkable consistency in norms across cultures when scores are adjusted for age and education using a critical point comparison as is done in the first version of the test. In some translations, some items may not be included because they have no meaningful translation (e.g., writing letters for sounds in a nonphonetic written language.) This will clearly affect normative data.

The second level is the interpretation of quantitative score patterns. At present, this is the least investigated area of interpretive changes due to the highly specific nature of the samples necessary to validate such patterns. Anecdotal data suggest that the patterns have similar interpretations in cultures similar to our own. It would be expected, however, that in non-Western cultures we would see more deviation in underlying functional systems which would change the functional significance of the scales in some manner. Again, though, the basic nature of the scales would make this less obvious than in some more complex tests.

The third level of interpretation involves item analysis, from both qualitative and quantitative perspectives. Both of these approaches attempt to isolate specific deficits by comparing items which differ in minor ways from one another to determine which variations cause a breakdown of the client's performance. This allows the clinician to isolate specific deficits. However, the neuropsychological significance of those deficits may vary by culture. For example, in our own culture reading and word recognition is a very basic overlearned left-hemisphere skill resistant to the effects of brain injury, while in cultures that use symbols for words rather than a phonemic written language, word recognition is less overlearned and more the product of both hemispheres. In more complex intellectual skills, the underlying functional system may differ considerably in terms of localizing significance so that interpretation must be based on an awareness of how individuals in that culture approach and analyze specific tasks. Early work of ours found significant differences in the approach to specific tasks in Japanese Americans depending on how long they had been in the U.S.: First-generation subjects showed widely different underlying functional systems, while third-generation subjects were identical to the patterns seen in the general American population (Golden, 1973).

Luria emphasized the importance of environment to the development of functional systems and the importance of the roles played by individual brain areas in a given task. As has been noted, his emphasis for assessment was using simple tasks to isolate problems so as to minimize the number of alternate functional systems that might be used to perform a given task. But no matter how simple a task, variations in functional systems as a result of experience (as well as brain injury) are present and must be carefully considered in any neuropsychological analysis.

Research Results

Research on alternate forms is scarce by American standards. Luria's work itself was multicultural and multilanguage, suggesting the appropriateness of the techniques across cultures. The interest in Luria's theories and in developing quantitative versions of the test have contributed to the translation of the Luria–Nebraska Neuropsychological Test Battery into several languages including Spanish, Polish, German, Chinese, Japanese, Greek, Korean, French, Czech, Hungarian, and Portuguese. These represent actual translations of LNNB with some variations to accommodate cultural differences although not all are formally researched or published in scientific journals.

Yun, Xian, and Mathews (1987) presented an extensive Chinese translation of the LNNB. The battery follows the initial test closely with significant variations in 68 items to accommodate cultural variables. The test was able to achieve discriminations of up to 97% in separating brain-injured from normals. The test was able to separate individuals with lateralized damage up to 90% of the time. Split half correlations in the scale ranged from .82 to .97. Overall, the results were remarkably similar to those found with the American version of the test. The Greek version of the test was similarly a detailed retranslation and analysis of the test (Stamati, 1985). Similar results were obtained as with the original LNNB and the Chinese version of the test.

The German version, a translation of the Luria–Nebraska Neuropsychological Battery— Children's Revision is known as the Berlin Luria–Neuropsychological Procedures (BLNP). Neumaeker and Bzufka (1989) used the BLNP to show the benefits of application of neuropsychological concepts to mentally handicapped children.

Application of the Luria–Nebraska Neuropsychological Battery (Form I) has been made to populations experiencing degenerative disease, head injury, cerebrovascular accidents, and epilepsy in India. The LNNB proved to be an accurate assessment for brain damage (Marwaha & Barnes, 1991). Venkatesh, Verma, Santosh, and Siddiqui (1993) utilized the Luria–Nebraska Battery to evaluate intellectual problem solving, memory, perceptuomotor functions, and language.

Researchers in Serbia, Yugoslavia, have used the Luria–Nebraska Battery for study of

Alzheimer's disease to distinguish between the cortical symptoms of early onset and the diffuse cognitive impairment of later onset (Pavlovic & Ocic, 1994). The Spanish version of the LNNB has also been utilized in the study of Alzheimer's disease. Munoz-Cespedes, Iruarrizaga-Diez, Miguel-Tobal, and Cano-Vindel (1995) compared Alzheimer's disease patients with normal controls to measure motor ability, perception of rhythm, tactile sensations, visual and visuospatial perception, language comprehension and expression, reading and writing abilities, arithmetic abilities, memory, and intellectual processes.

Galindo, Paez, Sanchez-de-Carmona, & Wolff (1993) assessed patients at the Mexican Institute of Psychiatry diagnosed with obsessive–compulsive disorders (OCD) using the LNNB to explore the relationship between OCD symptom severity and cognitive impairment.

Baribeau, Laurent, and Decary (1993) in Montreal analyzed tardive dyskinesia (TD) and neuroleptic dosage in relation to cognitive and motor tests of the LNNB and to attentional evoked potentials (Eps). Reading-retarded Icelandic children were given the LNNB (Arnkelsson, 1993). The expressive scale was found to discriminate most highly between the reading-retarded children and the normal controls. Kang (1992) in a preliminary study of the Korean version of the Luria–Nebraska Neuropsychological Battery—Children's Revision examined how effectively brain-damaged children were differentiated from normal ones. Pruneti, Cocci, Marchionni, and Rota (1995) studied the reliability of the LNNB in the functional analysis of Italian school-age children, adolescents, and adults with head injury and subsequent coma.

Glozman and Tupper (1995) presented qualitative and quantitative discussion of evaluation of a closed head injury utilizing the Lurian principle of syndrome analysis to illustrate the findings. A large correspondence was demonstrated between the clinical data and the results obtained via both North American and Russian neuropsychological assessment methods. Luria's qualitative emphasis on syndrome analysis, however, (1) revealed mechanisms underlying the observed defects, (2) provided for analysis and explanation of apparent contradictions in some of the testing results, and (3) whether applied to Lurian assessment methods or more psychometric measures, the principle of syndrome analysis aided in the identification of primary goals of the rehabilitation and in the determination of the optimal strategies to employ. Glozman and Tupper maintain that cross-cultural sharing of neuropsychological methods and approaches strengthens the field on a worldwide basis as well as enhancing the individual's treatment.

A parallel approach to the LNNB is the Polish version of the Luria's neuropsychological investigation known as the Cracow Neurolinguistic Battery of Aphasia Examination (CNBAE). It is comprised of five basic parts assessing general orientation, memory, linguistic functions, visuospatial functions, and abstract thinking. The 27 subtests assess various neurolinguistic functions and component processes. The battery has shown to be useful for assessment of the efficacy of aphasia rehabilitation (Pachalska 1990, 1993). The computerized version of the CNBAE has been shown to discriminate between the four types of aphasia including paradigmatic, syntagmatic, mixed and, global (Pachalska, Kaczmarek, & Knapik, 1995).

Conclusions

While there are many issues in the cross-cultural applications of any neuropsychological or psychological test, the multicultural roots of Luria's theories and syndrome analysis along with the simplicity of the test overall make it a relatively easy instrument to translate across cultures and languages. Success of the battery in versions as diverse as Chinese, Greek and Spanish illustrate the flexibility of the approach and the adapatability of the scoring and interpretive system. As long as such adaptations pay attention to cultural and language issues and do not simply attempt word-for-word translation of items and interpretive statements, the LNNB can be used in a variety of cross-cultural settings.

References

Arnkelsson, G. B. (1993). Reading-retarded Icelandic children: The discriminate validity of psychological tests. *Scandinavian Journal of Educational Research, 37*, 163–174.

Baribeau, J., Laurent, J., & Decary, A. (1993). Tardive dyskinesia and associated cognitive disorders: A convergent neuropsychological and neurophysiological approach. *Brain and Cognition, 23*, 40–55.

Galindo, G., Paez, F., Sanchez-de-Carmona, M., & Wolff, M. (1993). Neuropsychological evaluation of patients with obsessive–compulsive disorder: Evidence of changes in the central nervous system. *Salud Mental, 16*(4), 8–13.

Glozman, J. M., & Tupper, D. E. (1995). Converging impressions in Russian and American neuro-psychology: Discussion of a clinical case. *Applied Neuropsychology, 2*, 15–23.

Golden, C. J. (1973). *Cross-cultural differences in cognitive structure.* Master's thesis, University of Hawaii, Honolulu.

Golden, C. J., Hammeke, T. A., & Purisch, A. D. (1980). *The Luria–Nebraska Neuropsychological Battery.* Los Angeles: Western Psychological Services.

Kang, Y. (1992). A preliminary study for a Korean version of the Luria–Nebraska Neuropsychological Battery—Children's Revision. *Korean Journal of Child Studies, 13*, 203–216.

Marwaha, S. B., & Barnes, B. L. (1991). Application of the Luria–Nebraska Neuropsychological Battery (Form I) to the Indian Population. *Indian Journal of Clinical Psychology, 18*, 19–23.

Mecacci, L. (1979). *Brain and history: The relationship between neuropsychology and psychology in Soviet research* (Henry A. Buchtel, Trans.). New York: Brunner/Mazel. (Original work published, 1977)

Munoz-Cespedes, J. M., Iruarrizaga-Diez, I., Miguel-Tobal, J. J., & Cano-Vindel, A. (1995). Neuropsychological deficits related to Alzheimer's disease. *Psicothema, 7*, 473–487.

Neumaeker, K. J., & Bzufka, M. W. (1989). An evaluation of neuropsychological investigation methods for the mentally handicapped. *European Journal of Child and Adolescent Psychiatry: Acta Paedopsychiatrica, 52*, 307–316.

Pachalska, M. (1990). [Rehabilitation of patients with global aphasia treated by trained and untrained therapists.] *Research Annals, Academy of Physical Education, 24*, 261–272. (in Polish)

Pachalska, M. (1993). The concept of holistic rehabilitation of persons with aphasia. In A. Holland and M. Forbes (Eds.), *Aphasia treatment: World perspectives* (pp. 145–149). San Diego, CA: Singular.

Pachalska, M., Kaczmarek, B. L. J., & Knapik, H. (1995). Cracow Neurolinguistic Battery of Aphasia Examination. Special Issue: Special issue for A. R. Luria. *Aphasiology, 9*, 193–206.

Pavlovic, D. & Ocic, G. (1994). Clinical manifestations of Alzheimer's disease. *Psihijatrija Danas, 26*(2–3), 173–178.

Pruneti, C. A., Cocci, D., Marchionni, M., & Rota, S. (1995). Application of the Luria–Nebraska Neuropsychological Battery in functional analysis of subjects with head injury and subsequent coma. *Giornale di Neuropsichiatria dell'Eta Evolutiva, 15*, 159–165.

Stamati, D. (1985). *The neuropsychological evaluation with the Luria–Nebraska.* Athens: Thessaloniki.

Venkatesh, S., Verma, S. Santosh, K., & Siddiqui, R. S. (1993). Neuropsychological assessment in organic brain pathology: An overview. *Psychological Studies, 38*, 125–134.

Yun, Y., Xian, Y. X., Mathews, J. R. (1987). The Luria–Nebraska Neuropsychological Battery revised for China. *International Journal of Neuropsychology, 9*, 97–101.

V

Special Topics

18

Neuropsychological Differential Diagnosis of Spanish-Speaking Preschool Children

ROBERT L. RHODES, HORTENCIA KAYSER,
AND ROBYN S. HESS

The neuropsychological assessment of preschool children is an exceptionally difficult task because of the rapid cognitive, behavioral, and structural changes characteristic at this age level. The rapid changes which take place during the preschool years are greater than at any other time in an individual's development. In fact, Aylward (1997) uses an original term, early developmental neuropsychology, to describe the practice of working with this age group and to bring attention to the unique aspects of conducting a neuropsychological assessment within the context of a continually expanding repertoire of behaviors. For these reasons, it is critical that practitioners do not attempt to use a "scaling down" approach; that is, applying what is known about adult neuropsychological assessment to preschool-aged children (Aylward, 1997; Hooper, 1991). The neuropsychological assessment of preschool children must proceed only with a clear understanding and knowledge of the unique aspects of working with this population. This is particularly true when conducting a neuropsychological assessment of a Spanish-speaking preschool child.

The Hispanic preschool- and school-age population is the fastest growing children's group in the United States and by the year 2010 is expected to be the largest minority children's group in the nation (U.S. Bureau of the Census, 1994). The service needs of this burgeoning population are unique, especially in regard to the language of assessment and intervention. While not all Hispanic children speak Spanish, many do. In fact, the United States has the fifth-largest Spanish-speaking population in the world, behind only Mexico, Spain, Colombia, Argentina, and Peru (Kayser, 1993; Langdon, 1992). When one considers that immigration from Mexico outnumbers all other host countries by a three-to-one margin (U.S. Immigration and Naturalization Service, 1997a), and that overall immigration from Mexico represents the largest population migration from a single country in the history of the United States (U.S.

ROBERT L. RHODES AND **HORTENCIA KAYSER** • New Mexico State University, Las Cruces, New Mexico 88003-8801.   **ROBYN S. HESS** • University of Colorado at Denver, Denver, Colorado 80211.

Handbook of Cross-Cultural Neuropsychology, edited by Fletcher-Janzen, Strickland, and Reynolds. Kluwer Academic/Plenum Publishers, New York, 2000.

Immigration and Naturalization Service, 1997b), the need to establish clear procedures for the neuropsychological differential diagnosis of Spanish-speaking preschool children takes on particular importance.

The purpose of this chapter is to provide individuals involved in the neuropsychological assessment of Spanish-speaking preschool children with an overview of general and specific assessment considerations when working with this population, a model through which to conduct the assessment process, and an introduction to language development issues which are critical to differential diagnosis. In that, by definition, the neuropsychological assessment of Spanish-speaking preschool children emphasizes the language through which the assessment is conducted, information regarding translating and adapting instruments, the use of interpreters, and suggested procedures for the differential diagnosis of language impairments and normal language differences will be provided.

Considerations in the Neuropsychological Assessment of Preschool Children

While the foundation for implementing a neuropsychological approach to preschool evaluation is quite new, many researchers and clinicians support its utility in providing detailed diagnostic profiles, prognosis, and effective intervention (Aylward, 1988; Hartlage & Telzrow, 1986; Hooper, 1988; Wilson, 1986). Indeed, there is a growing emphasis on the application of neuropsychological assessment to the preschool population. This increased interest is related both to expanding knowledge about the importance of early neurological development as well as the greater numbers of infants surviving insult to the central nervous system including preterm birth, prenatal drug exposure, seizures, intraventricular hemorrhage, hydrocephalus, and prenatal asphyxia. Additionally, while the incidence of major disabilities (e.g., severe mental retardation, cerebral palsy) has leveled off, the occurrence of less-severe disabilities (e.g., learning, attention, and behavior problems) continues to increase (Aylward, 1997).

The neuropsychological assessment of preschool children allows the practitioner to: (1) determine the current neurodevelopmental status of the young child, (2) identify children who might benefit from intervention, (3) evaluate changes in neurodevelopmental status, and (4) predict later levels of functioning (Aylward, 1997). Abnormal neuropsychological findings in preschool children can be related to a number of variables including maturational delay, neural dysfunction, motor deficits, and/or the influence of variables external to the individual (e.g., behavioral state, temperament, environmental influences, or test limitations) (Hynd & Willis, 1988).

Neuropsychological Assessment Models

Most traditional neuropsychological assessment instruments are limited in their ability to provide differential diagnostic information regarding the cause of abnormal neuropsychological findings in early childhood populations because the age norms do not extend downward into the preschool years (i.e., 3–5 years). A common, alternative approach for evaluating neuropsychological functioning in preschool children is an integrative flexible model of assessment in which domains of behavior (e.g., perceptual/sensory, motor functions, intelligence/ cognitive abilities, attention/learning/processing activity, communication/language skills) are evaluated using qualitative and quantitative methods (D'Amato, Rothlisberg, & Rhodes, 1997;

Hooper, 1991). Although this strategy was originally designed with the school-aged child in mind, it is easily adapted to a preschool population.

Aylward (1997) proposes an additional framework for evaluating the neuropsychological functioning of infants and preschool children containing five basic constructs: (1) basic neurological function/intactness, (2) receptive functions, (3) expressive functions, (4) processing, and (5) mental activity. Each construct may be given more or less emphasis depending on the age of the child. For example, neurological function/intactness and mental activity are given more weight in a newborn because of a limited repertoire of behaviors amenable to evaluation and because of their importance to later functioning. In a five-year-old, a broader range of abilities can be measured and the emphasis on neurological functioning would be reduced. Regardless of the specific model adopted by the clinician, a broad range of skills must be evaluated in preschool neuropsychological examinations to obtain the most accurate picture of the child's functioning.

Evaluation of Risk

One of the most important concepts to consider when evaluating preschool children is the level of risk present. The type of risk, length of exposure, and the child's age will all have a decided impact on the child's present level of functioning and the longterm outcome for the child (Aylward, 1997). Tjossem (1976) outlined potential risk factors in terms of three categories: established (medical disorders of known etiology), biological (e.g., low birthweight, asphyxia), and environmental. Although medical and biological factors continue to be seen as the major causative factors for delayed developmental outcomes, a greater recognition of the impact of environmental risks is developing (Aylward, 1990, 1996; Bradley, Whiteside, Mundfrom, & Blevins-Kwabe, 1995).

Established, biological, and environmental risk factors are particularly pronounced for preschool children who live in poverty. Frequently children from low socioeconomic backgrounds are exposed to multiple risk factors due to inadequate prenatal care, low birthweight, environmental toxins, poor nutrition, drugs, and limited access to medical care (Aylward, 1997; Barona & Garcia, 1990). This combination of risk factors (e.g., biological and environmental) is sometimes referred to as double jeopardy (Parker, Greer, & Zuckerman, 1988). The concept of double jeopardy is an important consideration when evaluating culturally and linguistically diverse preschool children because of the large number of culturally and linguistically diverse children that live in poverty (U.S. Department of Commerce, 1994, cited in U.S. Department of Education, 1996).

An example of the double jeopardy which may be encountered by culturally and linguistically diverse preschool children is seen in the migrant and seasonal work setting. Approximately 3 million workers in the U.S. are migrant and seasonal workers, the majority of whom are from culturally and linguistically diverse backgrounds (Mines, Gabbard, & Boccalandro, 1991). Although the number of farm laborers suffering neurotoxic injury annually is not specifically known, it is estimated that the prevalence of pesticide poisoning in the U.S. is 300,000 cases annually, only 1%–2% of which are reported (Office of Technology Assessment [OTA], 1990). Prenatal exposure (via the placenta) is but one method through which children of migrant and seasonal workers contact high levels of neurotoxins; postnatal exposure (through breast milk) can occur as well (Aylward, 1997; Huisman et al., 1995). Higher levels of these toxins are associated with reduced levels of neonatal functioning. Furthermore, an estimated 17% of the U.S. preschool population is exposed to neurotoxic pesticides above the declared "safe" levels established by the Federal government (National Resource Defense

Council [NDRC], 1989; OTA, 1990). In that children absorb more pesticides per pound of body weight, they are considered to be more at risk than adults (OTA, 1990; Singer, 1997).

An Ecological Approach to Risk Evaluation

An ecological approach to the assessment process can provide a framework for considering environmental factors (both risks and buffers) and can help the clinician to better understand the potential impact of these variables on the neuropsychological development of young children (Bronfenbrenner, 1979; Kopp & McIntosh, 1997). The concepts of microsystem, mesosystem, exosystem, and macrosystem are often used to analyze such environmental factors. For example, at the closest level to the child, the microsystem, one needs to consider the parent–child interaction and the family's attitude toward illness. Some families may see a child's disability as a result of their own behavior and others may not see a deficit as a disability but rather as a basic characteristic of their child. Clinicians must try to understand the background and culture of the family and to identify how their personal values and biases may interfere with assessment and treatment (Krefting, 1991; Rhodes & Páez, 1999). Within the mesosystem, the interactions between daily contexts, family interactions, interactions between parents, and day care/preschool environments all must be taken into account.

Environmental risks to a child's development may also occur in settings more distant from the child, yet exert a strong negative impact on the child's overall wellbeing. In considering exosystem risks, it is important to evaluate issues of housing and income, family practices related to medical care and education, and the family's access to medical care. Finally, macrosystem risks might include poverty, stresses related to being a member of a culturally and linguistically diverse group and speaking a language other than English, and even federal and state legislation designed to regulate health care to noncitizens. It is important to note that while the effect of individual or isolated negative environmental factors may be relatively minor, the incremental impact on later cognitive functioning is often quite significant. The accumulation of risk factors presents as a major contributor to negative neurodevelopmental outcomes (Sameroff, Seifer, Barocas, Zax, & Greenspan, 1987). In effect, it is the biological risks that will determine whether a deficit will occur, but it is the environmental factors that will moderate the severity of the deficit (Aylward, 1997).

Neuropsychological Assessment of Spanish-Speaking Preschool Children

The difficult and complex task of assessing preschool children is made even more complex when the child and family are from a limited-English-speaking background (Barona & Santos de Barona, 1987). The appropriate assessment of Spanish-speaking preschool children requires an understanding of the child's native language, life experiences, cultural expectations, and environmental circumstances. This is in no way to insinuate that all Spanish-speaking preschool children are subject to the effects of poverty and limited life experiences, but rather to acknowledge the high percentage of Hispanic children who live in poverty (25% to 40%; U.S. Bureau of the Census, 1997; U.S. Department of Commerce, 1994 cited in U.S. Department of Education, 1996) when structuring the neuropsychological assessment process.

An outline for conducting appropriate neuropsychological assessments of Spanish-speaking preschool children is presented using a modified version of Aylward's (1988) conceptual framework. Issues of differential diagnosis are examined within each conceptual area. The original framework (basic neurological function/intactness, receptive functions, expressive functions, processing, and mental activity) does not include adaptive behaviors (e.g., self-help skills, socialization) because Aylward (1997) noted that neuropsychological assessment typically places less emphasis on these types of behaviors. It is the authors' experience that when evaluating Spanish-speaking preschool children it is critical to include adaptive and social information, as it will help the clinician to understand how the child is functioning within his or her environment, to develop culturally sensitive interventions, and to work more effectively with culturally and linguistically diverse families. Without a thorough examination of this domain, important components of the child's overall functioning might often be overlooked. The assessment of adaptive behavior is therefore included as a modification to Aylward's conceptual framework.

Prior to examining the proposed assessment model, it is important to note that in the area of neuropsychological assessment there are not adequate norm-referenced measures available for use with Spanish-speaking children (Puente, Sol Mora, & Munoz-Cespedes, 1997). Although specific tests are mentioned throughout this chapter, it is the authors' recommendation that they be utilized to measure particular aspects of functioning and as an avenue through which to examine a child's responses, rather than as an absolute determination of ability. With this caveat in mind, the following is an outline of a neuropsychological assessment model for use with Spanish-speaking preschool children and age-specific information regarding language development to aid in the differential diagnosis of language impairments and normal language differences.

Basic Neurological Functions/Intactness

Assessment of this aspect of functioning involves a review of the child's basic neurological functioning including early reflexes, muscle tone, asymmetries, head control, and absence of abnormal indicators (e.g., excessive drooling, motor flow) (Aylward, 1997). This component of a child's functioning is examined most closely during infancy and therefore will not be covered in-depth within this chapter. Although it is unlikely that these areas of functioning will vary greatly based on the child's cultural or linguistic background, it should be noted that exposure to environmental toxins and other environmental risks (e.g., low socioeconomic status [SES]) might create delays and deviance in developmental levels. Thus, if the clinical interview process or other evaluation efforts so indicate, it is critical that an in-depth medical and developmental history be completed to evaluate potential negative influences in the child's environment.

Receptive Functions

Receptive functions describe how information enters into the central processing system through sensation and perception. For example, how well does the child understand and discriminate sounds and language or accurately perceive what is presented visually. Sensory-perception skills are vital to an individual's understanding and response to the environment because they form the basis of each individual's interaction with the world (D'Amato et al., 1997). Assessment in this area can take place by using extensive interviews (in the parent or caregiver's language of choice) in conjunction with observations and data from traditional tests (e.g., Bayley Scales of Infant Development-II [Bayley, 1993], WPPSI-R, [Wechsler, 1989]), supplemented by instruments designed to measure discrete areas of function (e.g., Motor-Free Visual Perception Test [Colarusso & Hammill, 1996], PPVT-III, [Dunn & Dunn, 1997]). The clinician should keep in mind that certain developmental areas, such as receptive verbal skills, are more greatly impacted by environmental factors than other areas (e.g., expressive motor) (Aylward, 1997; Kayser, 1995), and thus use extreme caution when interpreting the results of language-based assessments. The accurate assessment of language skills has special importance not only because it represents a critical area of development but also because it is necessary to know a child's linguistic competence in both their native language and English in order to facilitate the interpretation of test results (Barona, 1991; Puente, Sol Mora, & Munoz-Cespedes, 1997).

Expressive Functions

Expressive functions refer to behaviors produced by the child and include both fine/gross motor functioning as well as the ability to produce sounds and language. Medical/biological factors tend to be most strongly related to neurological and perceptual–performance functions (Aylward, Verhulst, & Bell, 1994). Basic neurological functions and gross and fine-motor expressive skills are typically relatively unaffected by negative environmental influences. Despite this generalization, the clinician must rule out for exposure and opportunity issues. For example, some children might not be able to manipulate seemingly common objects like pencils or scissors as they have not had experiences with these items. As with receptive functions, the clinician can use comprehensive measures such as the Bayley II (Bayley, 1993) or McCarthy (McCarthy, 1972) to measure fine and gross-motor functioning and expressive verbal skills and/or specific tests such as the Bruininks–Oseretsky Test of Motor Proficiency (Bruininks, 1978) or the Developmental Test of Visual Motor Integration (Beery, 1989).

Language and Receptive and Expressive Functions

There are a number of variables which affect the development of language and the preschool child's mastery of receptive and expressive functions and each of these variables will differ depending upon the child's environment and exposure to English. Clinicians assessing Spanish-speaking preschool children must understand these issues concerning bilingualism and assessment of individuals who use two languages or who are learning English as a second language. The following section will provide a detailed discussion of the language development of Spanish speaking preschool children.

Communicative Competency

Communicative competency for Spanish-speaking monolingual and bilingual preschool children is determined by the norms that have been accepted by the community of speakers of the language(s). Kessler (1984) states that children, in becoming communicatively competent, must learn the grammatical, sociolinguistic, discourse, and strategic competencies necessary to successfully communicate in their group. Grammatical, or linguistic, competence refers to the knowledge of the phonologic, syntactic, and lexical features of the language. Sociolinguistic competence refers to the knowledge of the cultural rules of language-use and appropriateness for the context. Discourse competence is concerned with the skills necessary to connect utterances to form conversations, narratives, and other speech events. Strategic competencies refer to the strategies used by the bilingual preschool child to compensate for breakdowns in communication that may result from imperfect knowledge of the rules, fatigue, memory lapses, distraction, and/or anxiety.

Communicative competence is the interaction of these four components: grammatical, sociolinguistic, discourse, and strategic competencies. For Spanish-speaking children the interaction of the two languages and exposure to the two cultures will shape their bilingualism. This communicative competence framework will be used to describe the development of Spanish-speaking preschool children.

Linguistic Competency (Phonologic Development)

Spanish has a simpler phonologic system than English (Stockwell and Bowen, 1965), therefore Spanish-speaking children appear to develop their sound-system earlier than English-speaking children. The following is a summary of the phonemic and phonologic development of Spanish-speaking children.

The majority of the Spanish phonemes are mastered by age four. Acevedo (1989), Jimenez (1987), Linares (1981), and Terrero (1979) agree that /j/, /l/, /r/, /rr/, /s/, /t/ appear to be more difficult for Spanish-speaking children to produce. Goldstein (1995) states that by 3 years of age Spanish-speaking children will typically use the dialect features of the community and have the vowel and the majority of the consonant system in place.

The use of phonologic processes (rules for combining consonants in a language) by Spanish-speaking children is still a new area of research, although some initial studies have been reported. For Spanish-speaking children, it appears that developmental phonologic processes occur at or before the age of four. Goldstein (1995) summarizes phonological development by stating that Spanish-speaking preschoolers may occasionally exhibit cluster reduction (reducing *blanco* to *banco*), unstressed syllable deletion (*escuela* to *cuela*), stridency deletion (*esto* to *eto*), and tap/trill /r/ deviations (*carro* to *cado*).

Linguistic Competency (Morphosyntactic Development)

A significant difficulty in assessing Spanish-speaking preschool children within the United States stems from the additional variable that they are exposed to English as well. Spanish-speaking preschool children may not be monolingual Spanish speakers but may understand English as well and be incipient bilinguals without the knowledge of their parents. Children are often exposed to English-speaking siblings, an English-speaking community, and English-language programs on television. This English influence has a great impact on the development of Spanish and in turn on the use of Spanish during the neuropsychological assessment process.

Spanish-speaking children typically use single words before age two, two-word utterances by age two, and simple three-word constructions by age three. Spanish-speaking preschoolers should be intelligible to strangers by the age of 3 years. Additionally, Spanish-speaking preschool children are most often asking questions and using compound sentences with conjunctions by age 4½. Garcia and Gonzalez (1984) state that by age 4½, the Spanish-speaking preschool child should be using approximately 38 different syntactic structures. Children have great variation in normalcy, therefore, the individual's style in language learning should be kept in mind (Owens, 1988).

Some areas of concern for Spanish-speaking children are noun and article gender-agreement, dialectal variations, and the linguistic complexity of the utterances. The use of the article in Spanish is different from English. The speaker must use the correct gender-article for the noun that is to be expressed. If plurality is used, both article and noun must be marked. An example would be the phrase "the red car." In Spanish, the child must learn that *carro* (car) is a masculine word and must have a masculine article (*el carro rojo*). If the phrase becomes plural, as in "the red cars," the child must mark the article, noun, and adjective as plural: *los carros rojos*. Spanish-speaking children may have difficulty with gender and number agreement as late as age six (Garcia & Gonzalez, 1984; Garcia, Maez, & Gonzalez, 1984). The acquisition of article and gender agreement may be affected by the complexity in use, the influence of English, and the possibility that some children may be losing proficiency in Spanish.

Complexity of language form (syntax and morphology) is an area that is looked at in monolingual English-speaking children to determine if a language disorder exists. But for Spanish-speaking children who are exposed to English in uncertain amounts, complexity *may not* be an indicator of a language disorder. For example, Leopold (1939) observed in his daughter Hildegarde an avoidance of difficult words and constructions in the weaker language. For Hildegarde, the weaker language shifted from German to English and back to German, depending upon the child's dominant language environment. Avoidance of difficult words and constructions is a communicative strategy that bilingual children and adults use for efficiency and ongoing communication. Additionally, Anderson (1995) reports that children may be using the dialectal variation of the parent who may be second- to fourth-generation Hispanic, born in the United States. That is, the parent may use a nonstandard variety of Spanish that is acceptable within the community context.

In summary, the child that is learning Spanish acquires simple structures first and uses a variety of these structures by age 4½. The child's utterances increase from one word to compound sentences using conjunctions within the same approximate time that English-speaking children develop these constructions. The use of articles and noun gender, dialectal variations, and morphosyntactic complexity are areas that should be monitored but will vary for each child depending upon the amount of exposure the child has to English. One must keep in mind that the development of Spanish in an English-speaking community will have an effect on these language areas.

Linguistic Competency (Semantic Development)

Development of an awareness of the meaning of words and the use of specific vocabulary is closely tied to the child's socialization within the family unit. Parents instruct their children on what they believe is important to know. Slobin (1983) describes the social context of three Mexican American families who used Spanish as the language of the home. He described that the words learned were related to topics that adults felt children should know. Slobin (1983) identified four major topics as: 1) labels for objects and names of individuals, 2) the identity of the donor of an object, 3) the location or activity of relatives, and 4) the birth of a new sibling. He states that it was important to teach who is important to the children and whom they should know within the family. This semantic knowledge was reinforced by the frequency with which this type of information was asked for outside the home by other people. Therefore, first words for Spanish-speaking children may be names of people who are important to the family.

Quinn (1995) reports that 22-month-old Spanish speaking infants responded differently than English-speaking children on the Sequenced Inventory of Communication Development (SICD) (Hedrick, Prather, & Tobin, 1990). The highest category of single words used by the children were in family members' names. This was followed by categories for animal names, household objects, verbs, foods, and social words.

Specific information concerning concept development and vocabulary development in Spanish-speaking children is not fully known. We do know that knowledge of colors, numbers, and letters is not part of what many Hispanic parents believe is important information for their preschool-age children to know. Respect and politeness is emphasized and with these ideals follow the socialization of rituals and specific formulas for social interaction. Specific vocabulary that is considered important by mainstream society may not be part of the child's semantic knowledge. This may be a particular limitation for many Spanish-speaking preschool children when faced with items from norm-referenced, standardized tests. Culturally different semantic knowledge may also prove to be a limitation when direct translations of tests are used in the assessment process. In this case, although the words are in the child's native language, the meaning may still be unknown.

Strategic Competency

Children utilize a variety of strategies to help them learn a language. Peters (1977) discusses the analytic versus gestalt strategies of the young language learner, Nelson (1973) refers to the referential versus the expressive strategies used by children, and Snyder-McLean and McLean (1978) discuss the metalinguistic strategies of children for language learning. Imitation has been used as a strategy in the acquisition of words, morphology, and syntactic–semantic structures (Bloom, Hood, & Lightbrown, 1974). These same strategies appear in children who are learning two languages (Corder, 1967). Corder suggests that bilingual children have two strategies: learning and communicative. Communicative strategies are used to communicate effectively, while learning strategies are mental processes to help construct the rules of the language. Similar to Corder's communicative and learning strategies are Wong-Fillmore's (1979) social and cognitive strategies. Social strategies include joining groups and acting as if you understand, using choice words to give the impression of expressive abilities in the language, and counting on friends for help when a topic is not understood. Cognitive strategies include the assumption that speech is related to the context, guessing, analysis of repeated phrases, and focusing on the big picture rather than the finer parts of the language. Older children use a number of other strategies, such as imitation, deferred practice, asking informants, reading, observation, using a dictionary, silent practice, asking for repetition, and many others. All of these are strategies, whether they are social, learning, or cognitive, that the second language learner uses to become communicatively competent.

Processing

The ability to process information includes two key components: memory/learning and thinking/reasoning. Many of these skills can be measured using various items on cognitive developmental instruments (e.g., Bayley II [Bayley, 1993] Battelle [Newborg et al., 1984]) or through more traditional tests of intelligence, such as the Differential Abilities Scale (DAS) (Elliot, 1990). As previously mentioned, these results are not considered an absolute index of cognitive functioning, but instead should be viewed as an estimate of the child's current level of functioning based on the level and types of skills that the child has demonstrated relative to other children (Barona, 1991).

Differential diagnosis is especially critical in this domain of functioning as environmental factors most strongly influence verbal and general cognitive outcomes (Aylward et al., 1994). The importance of various risk factors changes depending upon the developmental level of the child, with mother–child interaction exerting more influence at the earliest ages and environmental factors becoming more important as a child enters toddlerhood (18 to 24 months) (Aylward, 1997). In particular, correlations between cognitive scores and environment increase with age, while the relationship between cognitive scores and biological variables decreases as the child gets older. Motor and neurological functioning may stay relatively stable (Aylward, Gustafson, Verhulst, & Colliver, 1987), while cognitive functioning (which is affected by environmental factors) can decline dramatically. Thus, when environmental risks are present, it is especially important that effective and appropriate interventions designed to strengthen cognitive and verbal development be implemented in addition to more specific strategies aimed at the specific area(s) of delay.

Mental Activity

Conclusions about a child's general level of attention and mental activity will largely rely on observation and qualitative judgments regarding age-appropriate behavior (Aylward, 1996). Because of the subjective nature of this component of the evaluation, it is especially important to consider cultural and linguistic variables that might impact clinical findings. For example, a Spanish-speaking child's style of interaction with an adult might differ from those of majority culture children in terms of eye contact or speaking to an adult unless spoken to (Barona, 1991). These differences might be interpreted as a lack of attention, distractibility, or lack of focus on pertinent environmental stimuli.

Adaptive/Social

An examination of adaptive behavior and social skills are key components of a neuropsychological examination for linguistically diverse preschoolers. This information can be combined with other types of data to help the clinician determine whether delays in performance are related to specific impairments or cultural and language differences. In all cases, the clinician must keep in mind that adaptive behavior is dependent on the expectations of the child's culture. Although a clinician monitors risk factors throughout the assessment, it is critical not to make automatic assumptions that the lower scores of children from low-SES homes, for example, are related purely to environmental factors. It is always imperative to rule out other possibilities because of the strong biological and environmental interface. Measures which are frequently used to assess the adaptive/social functioning of preschool children and which are available in Spanish include the Vineland Adaptive Behavior Scales (Sparrow, Balla, & Cicchetti, 1984) and the Behavior Assessment System for Children (Reynolds & Kamphaus, 1984/1992).

Recommendations for Differential Diagnosis

The following are suggested procedures to aide in the differential diagnosis of a language impairment and normal language development among Spanish-speaking preschool children during the neuropsychological assessment process:

1. Identify parent or student concerns. Hispanic parents recognize communication impairments in their children.
2. The characteristics of acquired aphasia, dysarthria, apraxia, and traumatic brain injury will be present in both languages.
3. Collect information through questionnaires and interviews from all preschool teachers and parents as well as observations by the speech-language pathologist. These data should all support the diagnosis of a language impairment.

4. Observe sequencing, memory, and attention span. Language-impaired children have difficulty in these areas in both languages. Assessment of sequencing, memory, and attention span should consider the familiarity of the test items on the part of the child. If a Spanish-speaking preschool child does not know numbers, do not use digits to test these abilities.
5. Document the possibility of language loss. Children may lose their ability to speak their first language as they are exposed to English. If school language dominance records document this phenomenon, the child's communicative abilities in both languages may appear impaired.
6. Observe the variety of forms (syntax and phonology), use, and content (semantics) in different contexts. Hispanic children with language impairments typically have restricted abilities in both languages, regardless of the context.
7. Observe code switching and language mixing as the child speaks with other bilingual speakers. A bilingual child will typically not switch or mix languages with a monolingual English speaker.

Standardized Instrument Translation, Adaptation, and Interpretation

A single standardized measure for many culturally and linguistically diverse populations in the United States is not possible. The demographics for the different cultural populations, census within a region, generational shifts in cultural ideologies, language, levels of bilingualism, education, and other variables all contribute to invalidating the process of standardizing a measure for individuals from any specific group. Therefore, measures may need to be modified through translation, adaptation, and/or an interpreter. The following are brief discussions and suggestions for each of these areas.

Translating and Adapting Instruments

Test instruments written in English are frequently translated for use by clinicians and their agencies. The purpose of this activity is to measure the individual's neuropsychological functioning by using the standardized instrument's theoretical and language framework. Merely translating the test does not, however, equate to an appropriate assessment instrument (Erickson & Iglesias, 1986; Kayser, 1989). A translated test used for specifying an impairment does not take into consideration differences in languages in areas such as honorifics, gender markers, semantics, structural rules, registers, dialectal variations, and cultural norms for who speaks what to whom and when. If these language areas are not addressed in the translation, it is possible to have a child respond incorrectly to an inappropriately translated item because of any of the above language differences. Thus the measure becomes an unreliable means of measurement (Kayser, 1995).

A second concern is cultural variation. Translations of instruments often neglect complex variables such as cultural norms, beliefs, life expectations and experiences, roles, and acceptable and unacceptable inter- and intragroup relationships. A direct translation of a measure will need to be adapted so that a true measure of a child's performance can be obtained.

Adapting a test instrument requires that the tasks and content of the original instrument are changed to include culturally appropriate items (Gavillan-Torres, 1984; Kayser, 1989) and are, therefore, less biased for the child from a culturally and linguistically different background. The content is reviewed and revised to reflect the needs of the population served. For example, the vocabulary may be altered to reflect dialectal variations. These changes may be made through group discussions with focus groups from the community who could act as the informants of acceptable and unacceptable questions concerning the development of the measure. As with any norm-referenced, standardized measure, however, the direct translation of an instrument or alteration to include culturally appropriate items changes the nature of the measure and as such the reliability and validity of the results.

Using Interpreters

Frequently, the terms *interpreter* and *translator* are used by professionals interchangeably, but they have different meanings and functions. An interpreter is one who conveys information from one language to the other in the oral modality. A translator is one who conveys information in the written modality (Langdon, 1992). This discussion is limited to the term interpreter because neuropsychologists are more likely to depend on interpreters in clinical practice.

Interpreters are an important link between the clinician and the child. Their skills in interpreting information conveyed by the clinician are crucial for accurate assessment of child outcomes. To maintain high quality of service, there should be clearly established educational, clinical, and linguistic competencies for interpreters in all clinical settings. Langdon (1992) suggests that interpreters should have a minimum of a high school diploma with communication skills that are adequate for the tasks assigned by the professional. They should have oral and written abilities in English and the minority language. Langdon (1992) states that the role of the interpreter requires an ability to stay emotionally uninvolved with the discussions and an ability to maintain confidentiality and neutrality. When an untrained individual serves in this role, there may be omitted, misinterpreted, or misunderstood information relayed to the family (Kayser, 1993). An example of the type of difficulty an untrained interpreter might face is found in the process of code switching.

Code Switching

Code switching is the alternating use of two languages at the word, phrase, and sentence level with a complete break between languages in phonology (Valdes-Fallis, 1978). This phenomenon is developed and encouraged in children who live in bilingual communities. McClure (1981) states that child code switching begins early in children and is different from adult code switching. She notes that Spanish-speaking children produce different kinds of code switching depending upon age. Young children tend to mix codes by inserting single items from one language into the other. Usually English nouns, followed by adjectives, have the highest frequency of mixing into Spanish utterances; for example, "*Quiero comer un hot dog*" ("I want to eat a hot dog") or "*Me gusta la red pelota*" ("I like the red ball"). At three years of age code switching is used to resolve ambiguities, clarify statements, and attract attention; for example, "*Mira aqui*, look here." At 6 years, mode shifting, such as moving from narration to commentary, is seen through code switching; and at 8 years, code switching is used for emphasis, commands, and elaboration, for example, when during an English dialogue the child emphasizes a negation: "*Te dije que no*" ("I told you no"). By the time bilingual children are 9 years of age, code switching may occur at the phrase and sentence levels (McClure, 1981), for example, "*Give me the pencil que tiene un arco*" ("that has a rainbow").

An important point for clinicians is that Genishi (1976) found that children generally choose the language that the interlocutor spoke better. If the addressee was English dominant or monolingual, the children would use English only. On the other hand, if the addressee was Spanish dominant or monolingual, the children chose to use Spanish only. Children may not use their home language with individuals who do not have fluent proficiency in their home language. This has special relevance for both marginally fluent interpreters and clinicians.

Zentella (1981) states that children learn the rule "follow the leader," which is expected of capable bilinguals beyond the age of five. Children can accurately determine the language preference of peers and will use English, Spanish, or both. Zentella states children use more intrasentential (within sentence) code switching during the interviews with adults but more extrasentential (between sentences) code switching among themselves. She found that children were skilled by the age of eight at code switching if the addressee switched codes, using their repertoire in two languages for communication. Children readily interact in Spanish with Hispanic clinicians and English with Anglo clinicians. Children appear to identify all non-Hispanics as English-speakers. Zentella adds that it was considered abnormal to speak Spanish to a non-Hispanic. She also noted that switching to mark ethnicity and group membership appeared later. Therefore, young children may not speak Spanish to a non-Hispanic who is not fluent in the Spanish language.

Some children of school age learn English because of necessity and their situation and therefore switch codes. Valdes-Fallis (1978) suggest that monolingual Spanish-speaking children who are in a monolingual English classroom normally remain silent in the classroom unless forced to speak. The child may begin to speak in English but switch languages as an emergency attempt to continue communication. English is understood to be the norm for the classroom, therefore, code switching may not be heard by the monolingual teacher. Bilingual children do not alternate between two languages with people who speak only one of the languages. Valdes-Fallis state that it is reasonable to assume that children who begin to switch codes follow the adult rules for when it is appropriate to switch codes.

Code switching among preschool children is an area of research that has not yet provided a complete picture of how children learn to alternate between two languages and the occurrence of code switching among children with language impairments. This will continue to be an important area of research as clinicians attempt to make differential diagnosis between language impairments and normal language differences among Spanish-speaking preschool children.

Conclusion

There are a number of issues and factors that may affect the neuropsychological differential diagnosis of Spanish-speaking preschool children. These include language environments, cultural beliefs, environmental risks, culturally and linguistically appropriate measures, translation and adaptation of instruments, and the use of interpreters. Hispanic groups may view impairment, disability, and handicapping conditions differently from other cultural groups. The use of standardized instruments validated on mainstream populations are often limited in their application. However, without adequate replacement, their adaptation and translation will most likely persist as the usual practice. Interpreters can assist in the majority of child–clinician interactions, but both the interpreter and the clinician must have clinical and educational competencies that will best serve the client.

The results of neuropsychological assessments with Spanish-speaking preschool children should provide the clinician with a good understanding of the child's current level of functioning. The assessment results, however, must be carefully evaluated in order to identify aspects of the child's performance which might be related to factors other than the child's ability. It is especially critical that the practitioner bring together all available data in determining the degree that cultural, linguistic, and environmental variables affect the assessment data (Puente et al., 1997). Both biological and environmental risks will affect the findings of neuropsychological evaluations, and these findings will, in turn, determine the focus of interventions. It is critical that clinicians develop strategies to differentiate between delay, deviance, and difference among members of the Spanish-speaking preschool population.

References

Acevedo, M. (1989, November). *Typical Spanish misarticulations of Mexican-American preschoolers*. Presented at the annual meeting of the American Speech-Language-Hearing Association, St. Louis.

Anderson, R. T. (1995). Spanish morphological and syntactic development. In H. Kayser (Ed.), *Bilingual speech-language pathology: An Hispanic focus* (pp. 41–74). San Diego, CA: Singular Publishing Group.

Aylward, G. P. (1988). Infant and early childhood assessment. In M. G. Tramontana & S. R. Hooper (Eds.) *Assessment issues in child neuropsychology* (pp. 225–248). New York: Plenum.

Aylward, G. P. (1990). Environmental influences on developmental outcome of children at risk. *Infants and Young Children, 2,* 1–9.

Aylward, G. P. (1996). Environmental risk, intervention and developmental outcome. *Ambulatory Child Health, 2,* 161–170.

Aylward, G. P. (1997). *Infant and early childhood neuropsychology*. New York: Plenum.

Aylward, G. P., Gustafson, N., Verhulst, S. J., & Colliver, J. A. (1987). Consistency in the diagnosis of cognitive, motor, and neurologic function over the first three years. *Journal of Pediatric Psychology, 12,* 77–98.

Aylward, G. P., Verhulst, S. J., & Bell, S. (1994). Enhanced prediction of later "normal" outcome using infant neuropsychological assessment. *Developmental Neuropsychology, 10,* 377–394.

Barona, A. (1991). Assessment of multicultural preschool children. In B. A. Bracken (Ed.), *The psychoeducational assessment of preschool children* (2nd ed., pp. 379–391). Boston: Allyn & Bacon.

Barona, A., & Garcia, E. E. (1990). *Children at risk: Poverty, minority status, and other issues in educational equity*. Washington, DC: NASP.

Barona, A., & Santos de Barona, M. (1987). A model for the assessment of limited English proficient students referred for special education services. In S. H. Fradd & W. J. Tikunoff (Eds.), *Bilingual education and bilingual special education: A guide for administrators* (pp. 183–210). Boston: College-Hill.

Bayley, N. (1993). *Bayley Scale of Infant Development-II*. San Antonio, TX: Psychological Corporation.

Beery, K. E. (1989). *Developmental Test of Visual-Motor Integration*. Odessa, FL: Psychological Assessment Resources.

Bloom, L., Hood, L., & Lightbrown, P. (1974). Imitation in language development: If, when and why. *Cognitive Psychology, 6,* 380–420.

Bradley, R. H., Whiteside, L., Mundfrom, D. J., & Blevins-Kwabe, B. (1995). Home environment and adaptive social behavior among premature, low birth weight children: Alternative models of environmental action. *Journal of Pediatric Psychology, 20,* 347–362.

Bronfenbrenner, U. (1979). *The ecology of human development: Experiments by nature and design*. Cambridge, MA: Harvard University Press.

Bruininks, R. H. (1978). *Bruininks-Oseretsky Test of Motor Proficiency*. Circle Pines, MN: American Guidance Service.

Colarusso, R. P., & Hammill D. D. (1996). *Motor-Free Visual Perception Test—Revised*. Novato, CA: Academic Therapy.

Corder, S. P. (1974). The significance of learner's errors. In J. C. Richards (Ed.), *Error analysis: Perspectives on second language acquisition* (pp. 155–177). London: Longman.

D'Amato, R. C., Rothlisberg, B. A., & Rhodes, R. L. (1997). Utilizing a neuropsychological paradigm for understanding common educational and psychological tests. In C. R. Reynolds & E. Fletcher-Janzen (Eds.), *Handbook of clinical child neuropsychology* (2nd ed., pp. 271–295). New York: Plenum.

Dunn, L. M., & Dunn, L. M. (1997). *Peabody Picture Vocabulary Test-III*. Circle Pines, MN: American Guidance Service.

Elliot, C. D. (1990). *Differential Abilities Scale*. San Antonio, TX: Psychological Corporation.

Erickson, J. G., & Iglesias, A. (1986). Assessment of communication disorders in non-English proficient children. In O. Taylor (Ed.), *Nature of communication disorders in culturally and linguistically diverse populations* (pp. 181–218). San Diego: College-Hill.

Garcia, E., & Gonzalez, G. (1984). The interrelationship of Spanish and Spanish/English language acquisition in the Hispanic child. In J. L. Martinez & R. H. Mendoza (Eds.), *Chicano psychology* (2nd ed., pp. 427–451). New York: Academic.

Garcia, E. E., Maez, L. F., & Gonzalez G. (1984). *A national study of Spanish/English bilingualism in young Hispanic children of United States*. Los Angeles: California State University, National Dissemination and Assessment Center.

Gavillan-Torres, E. (1984). Issues of assessment of limited-English-proficient students and of truly disabled in the United States. In N. Miller (Ed.), *Bilingualism and language disability: Assessment and remediation* (pp. 131–153). San Diego, CA: College-Hill.

Genishi, C. (1976). *Rules for code-switching in young Spanish-English speakers: An exploratory study of language socialization*. Thesis: University of California, Berkeley.

Goldstein, B. A. (1995). Spanish phonological development. In H. Kayser (Ed.), *Bilingual speech language pathology: An Hispanic focus,* (pp. 17–40). San Diego, CA: Singular.

Hartlage, L. C., & Telzrow, C. F. (1986). *Neuropsychological assessment and intervention with children and adolescents*. Sarasota, FL: Professional Resource Exchange.

Heath, S. B. (1986). Social cultural contexts of language development. In C. F. Leyba (Ed.), *Beyond language: Social and cultural factors in schooling language minority students* (pp. 143–186). Los Angeles: Evaluation Dissemination and Assessment Center, California State University, California State Department of Education, Bilingual Education Office.

Hedrick, D., Prather, E., & Tobin, A. (1990). *Sequenced inventory of communication development*. Los Angeles: Western Psychological Services.

Hooper, S. R. (1988). The prediction of learning disabilities in the preschool child. A neuropsychological perspective. In M. G. Tramontana & S. R. Hooper (Eds.), *Assessment issues in child neuropsychology* (pp. 313–335). New York: Plenum.

Hooper, S. R. (1991). Neuropsychological assessment of the preschool child: Issues and procedures. In B. A. Bracken (Ed.), *The psychoeducational assessment of preschool children* (2nd ed., pp. 465–485). Boston: Allyn & Bacon.

Huisman, M., Koopman-Esseboom, C., Fidler, V., Hadders-Algra, M., Van der Paauw, C. G., Tuinstra, L. G., Weisglas-Kuperus, N., Sauer, P. J., & Touwen, B. C. L. (1995). Perinatal exposure to polychlorinated biphenyls and dioxins and its effect on neonatal neurological development. *Early Human Development, 41*, 111–127.

Hynd, G. W., & Willis, W. G. (1988). *Pediatric neuropsychology*. Boston: Allyn & Bacon.

Jimenez, B. C. (1987). Acquisition of Spanish consonants in children. *Language, Speech, and Hearing Service in the Schools, 18*, 357–363.

Kayser, H. (1989). Speech and language assessment of Spanish-English speaking children. *Language, Speech, and Hearing Services in Schools, 20*, 226–244.

Kayser, H. (1993). Hispanic cultures. In D. Battle (Ed.), *Communication disorders in multicultural populations* (pp. 114–157). Boston, MA: Andover Medical Publishers.

Kayser, H. (1995). Assessment of speech and language impairments in bilingual children. In H. Kayser (Ed.), *Bilingual speech-language pathology: An Hispanic focus* (pp. 243–264). San Diego: Singular.

Kessler, C. (1984) Language acquisition in bilingual children. In N. Miller (Ed.), *Bilingual and language disability*. San Diego: College-Hill.

Kopp, C. B., & McIntosh, J. M. (1997). High-risk environments and young children. In J. D. Noshpitz (Series Ed.), S. Greenspan, S. Wieder, & J. Osofsky (Volume Eds.), *Handbook of child and adolescent psychiatry, Vol. 1: Infants and preschoolers: Development and syndromes* (pp. 160–176). New York: Wiley.

Krefting, L. (1991). The culture concept in the everyday practice of occupational and physical therapy. In S. K. Campbell & I. J. Wilhelm (Eds.), *Meaning of culture in pediatric rehabilitation and health care*. New York: Haworth.

Langdon, H. W. (1992). *Interpreter/translator process in the educational setting: A resource manual*. Sacramento, CA: Resources in Special Education.

Leopold, W. F. (1939). *Speech development of bilingual child: A linguist's record* (4 Vols.). Evanston, IL: Northwestern University Press.

Linares, T. A. (1981). Articulation skills in Spanish-speaking children. In R. V. Padilla (Ed.), *Ethnoperspectives in bilingual education series. Vol. III: Ethnoperspectives in bilingual education research: Bilingual education technology* (pp. 363–367). Ypsilanti, MI: Eastern Michigan University Press.

McCarthy, D. (1972). *McCarthy Scale of Children's Abilities*. New York: Psychological Corporation.

McClure, E. (1981). Formal and functional aspects of the code-switched discourse of bilingual children. In R. Duran (Ed.), *Latino language and communicative behavior* (pp. 69–95). Norwood, NJ: Ablex.

Mines, R., Gabbard, S., & Boccalandro, B. (1991). *Findings from the National Agricultural Workers Survey 1990: A demographic and employment profile of perishable crop farm workers*. Washington, DC: Office of Program Economics, U.S. Department of Labor.

National Resources Defense Council (1989). *Intolerable risk: Pesticides in our children's food*. Washington, DC: Author.

Nelson, K., (1973). Structure and strategy in learning to talk. *Monographs of the society for research in child development, 38*(1–2). Chicago: University of Chicago Press.

Newborg, J., Stock, J. R., Wnek, L., Guidubaldi, J., & Svinicki, J. (1984). *Battelle Developmental Inventory*. Allen, TX: DLM Teaching Resources.

Office of Technology Assessment (1990). *Neurotoxicity. Identifying and controlling poisons of the nervous system (OTA-BA-436)*. Washington, DC: Office of Technology Assessment, U.S. Congress.

Owens, R. (1988). *Language development: An introduction* (2nd ed.). Columbus, OH: Merrill.

Parker, S., Greer, S., & Zuckerman, B. (1988). Double jeopardy: The impact of poverty on early child development. *Pediatric Clinics of North America, 35*, 1227–1240.

Peters, A. (1977). Language-learning strategies: Does the whole equal the sum of the parts? *Language, 53*, 560–573.

Puente, A. E., Sol Mora, M., Munoz-Cespedes, J. M. (1997). Neuropsychological assessment of Spanish-speaking children and youth. In C. R. Reynolds & E. Fletcher-Janzen (Eds.), *Handbook of clinical child neuropsychology* (2nd ed., pp. 371–383). New York: Plenum.

Quinn, R., (1995). "Early intervention? Que decir eso?" … What does that mean? In H. Kayser (Ed.), *Bilingual speech language pathology: An Hispanic focus* (pp. 75–96). San Diego, CA: Singular.

Rhodes, R. L., & Páez, D. (1999). Cultural attitudes towards special education. In C. R. Reynolds and E. Fletcher-Janzen (Eds.), *Encyclopedia of Special Education* (2nd ed., pp. 496–500). New York: Wiley.

Reynolds, C. R., & Kamphaus, R. W. (1992). *Behavior Assessment System for Children*. Circle Pines, MN: American Guidance Service. (Original published in 1984)

Sameroff, A. J., Seifer, R., Barocas, R., Zax, M., & Greenspan, S. (1987). Intelligence quotient scores of 4-year-old children: Social environmental risk factors. *Pediatrics, 79*, 343–349.

Singer, R. (1997). Neuropsychological assessment of toxic exposures. In A. MacNeill Horton Jr., D. Wedding, & J. Webster (Eds.), *The neuropsychology handbook* (2nd ed.). Vol. 2: *Treatment issues and special populations* (pp. 357–373). New York: Springer.

Slobin, D. (1983). *The acculturation and development of language in Mexican-American children [final grant report NIE-G-81-0103]*. Washington, DC: National Institute of Education.

Snyder-McLean, L., & McLean, J. (1978). Verbal information-gathering strategies: The child's use of language to acquire language. *Journal of Speech and Hearing Disorders, 43*, 306–325.

Sparrow, S. S., Balla, D. A., & Cicchetti, D. V. (1984). *Vineland Adaptive Behavior Scales*. Circle Pines, MN: American Guidance Service.

Stockwell, R. P., & Bowen J. D. (1965). *The sound of English and Spanish*. Chicago, IL: University of Chicago Press.

Taylor, O. L. (1987). Clinical practice as a social occasion. In L. Cole & V. Deal (Eds.), *Linguistic diversity in multicultural populations*. Rockville, MD: ASHA.

Teller, C. A. (1988). Physical health status and health care utilization in the Texas Borderlands. In S. R. Ross (Ed), *Views across the border* (pp. 147–155).

Terrero, I. (1979, November). *Spanish phonological acquisition*. Paper presented at the annual meeting of the American Speech-Language and Hearing Association, Atlanta.

Tjossem, T. (1976). *Intervention strategies for high risk infants and young children*. Baltimore: University Park Press.

U.S. Bureau of the Census. (1994). *Population projections of the United States by age, sex, race, and Hispanic origin: 1995–2050*. Washington, DC: U.S. Department of Commerce, Economics and Statistics Administration.

U.S. Bureau of the Census. (1997). *Selected characteristics of the population by citizenship for selected states*. Washington, DC: U.S. Department of Commerce, Economics and Statistics Administration.

U.S. Department of Education. (1996). *The pocket condition of education 1996, NCES 96-305. National Center for Education Statistics*. Washington, DC: Thomas J. Smith.

U.S. Immigration and Naturalization Service. (1997a). *Characteristics of legal immigrants*. Washington, DC: U.S. Department of Justice.

U.S. Immigration and Naturalization Service. (1997b). *Immigration fact sheet*. Washington, DC: U.S. Department of Justice.

Valdes-Fallis, G. (1978). *Code switching and the classroom teacher. Language in education: Theory and practice* (Vol. 4). Arlington, VA: Center for Applied Linguistics.

Wechsler, D. (1989). *Wechsler Preschool and Primary Scale of Intelligence—Revised.* San Antonio, TX: The Psychological Corporation.

Wilson, B. C. (1986). An approach to the neuropsychological assessment of the preschool child with developmental deficits. In S. B. Filskov & T. J. Boll (Eds.), *Handbook of clinical neuropsychology* (Vol. 2, pp. 121–171). New York: Wiley.

Wong-Fillmore, L. (1979). Individual differences in second language acquisition. In C. Fillmore, D. Kempler, & W. Wang (Eds.), *Individual differences in language ability and language behavior* (pp. 202–228). New York: Academic.

Zentella, A. (1981). Ta bien, you could answer me en cualquier idioma: Puerto Rican codeswitching in bilingual classrooms. In R. Duran (Ed.), *Latino language and communicative behavior* (pp. 109–131). Norwood, NJ: Ablex.

19

Neuropsychological Assessment of the Criminal Defendant

The Significance of Cultural Factors

ROBERT J. SBORDONE, TONY L. STRICKLAND,
AND ARNOLD D. PURISCH

Introduction

Neuropsychologists are often asked to evaluate complex cases involving the neurobehavioral consequences of brain injury with numerous etiological and modulating considerations beyond the injury indicated in the referral. Though many of these patients have sustained a serious compromise in their intellectual, behavioral, and cognitive functioning, the magnitude of their impairment and its relationship to their disability is often difficult to ascertain. Examining patients in a forensic context is even more challenging given the myriad of variables that potentially affect the assessment process. Moreover, specific modulating factors such as low motivation, low education, nonorganic or functional disturbances, concurrent medical disorders (e.g., hypertension, pulmonary, cardiovascular disease), socioeconomic status, cultural and/or ethnic influences, and a history of chemical dependency can further complicate this complex differential diagnostic process (Lezak, 1995; Sbordone, 1991; Strickland et al., 1993).

Neuropsychological assessment has typically considered premorbid factors such as prior medical history, educational attainment, occupational history, familial and interpersonal functioning, in formulating an impression regarding residual neurocognitive impairment secondary to brain injury (Lezak, 1995). Although patients are generally queried about their substance-abuse history, the incorporation of knowledge regarding the sustained effects that drugs of abuse may have on neuropsychological functioning has not been applied to the neuropsychological evaluative process in any systematic manner. Moreover, neuropsychology has generally lagged behind in its appreciation of the extent that altered neurochemical

ROBERT J. SBORDONE AND ARNOLD D. PURISCH • Irvine, California 92718.   TONY L. STRICKLAND • Charles R. Drew University of Medicine and Science, Los Angeles, California 90059; and UCLA School of Medicine, Los Angeles, California 90095.
Handbook of Cross-Cultural Neuropsychology, edited by Fletcher-Janzen, Strickland, and Reynolds. Kluwer Academic/Plenum Publishers, New York, 2000.

substrates influence our dependent measures of interest (Hartman, 1995). Since a high correlational between substance abuse and criminal behavior exists, therefore, it is crucial for neuropsychologists examining patients in the forensic context to be knowledgeable about how drugs effect the brain and cognitive function.

Neuropsychological Assessment of Criminal Defendants

While neuropsychological assessment has been frequently utilized to detect subtle organic brain pathology and cognitive deficits, many neuropsychologists have implicitly assumed that a criminal defendant's performance on these tests can simply be compared to normative standards to determine whether they are mentally retarded, cognitively impaired, or "brain damaged." Strict reliance on standardized test norms is clearly inappropriate when the defendant's cultural, ethnic, educational, and/or linguistic background differs significantly from the subjects upon which the tests were normed. Furthermore, such invidious comparisons are likely to result in inaccurate diagnoses (e.g., mentally retarded, brain damaged, etc.) and/or treatment recommendations (e.g., continued incarceration, denial of probation, etc.). While there has been a growing recognition of the importance of obtaining a detailed history in forensic cases which includes developmental, educational, medical, psychiatric, and psychosocial factors, relatively little attention has been paid to cultural, ethnic, linguistic, educational, socioeconomic, and acculturation factors. This practice is often more problematic when the criminal defendant is not perceived as being part of mainstream society.

The neuropsychological tests which are typically administered to the criminal defendant are frequently the same tests that are utilized in clinical or private practice settings (e.g., Halstead–Reitan Battery), even though the background of the defendant, the purpose of testing, and the conditions present during assessment are typically dramatically different from patients who are seen in clinical settings. For example, patients suspected of having brain dysfunction in clinical settings are usually tested in quiet environments that are relatively free of extraneous or distracting stimuli, so as to optimize their test performance. This type of environment has been a standard in the field in order to reduce the extraneous negative influences that occur during the evaluation process (Cronbach, 1984). A key issue, however, is whether we can legitimately apply the normative test data obtained in clinical settings to the setting under which many criminal defendants are tested. For example, the criminal defendant may be seated behind an imposing metal grate or a thick plexiglass window in a rather cold, inhospitable, and often noisy environment (e.g., guards yelling at prisoners, prisoners laughing in the background, announcements being made over the PA system, etc.). Furthermore, the conditions inherent in this situation make it difficult to establish any rapport with the defendant, particularly since physical contact is not allowed. For example, the tests which are administered to the defendant are occasionally passed through a thin slot while the defendant and the examiner are usually sitting on very uncomfortable metal stools, facing each other with an imposing physical barrier between them in a locked room, with prison guards located nearby. This environment frequently causes the inexperienced examiner to feel uncomfortable (if not paranoid), and is likely to make the defendant feel uncomfortable, mistrustful, less cooperative, and unwilling to perform to the best of his or her ability. Not only is this testing environment dramatically different from the standard clinical environment, but there are no normative data available for individuals who are tested under such conditions.

While the choice of which specific neuropsychological tests to be administered to criminal defendants should reflect their cultural, ethnic, socioeconomic, educational, and linguistic background, it is essential that the neuropsychologist determine whether a defendant's test performance has adequate ecological validity (e.g., Is the test data consistent with the defendant's cognitive and behavioral functioning in their environment prior to the instant offense?). Thus, the defendant's test performances should be compared to their expected functioning in their particular ecological niche. In order to accomplish this, the neuropsychologist should be sufficiently "culturally competent" to compare the defendant's test data with the observations of the defendant's family and/or significant others to determine its "goodness of fit."

Neuropsychologists should not rely solely on the defendants' test scores to determine their mental status or whether they are competent to stand trial. It is essential for the neuropsychologist to seek out convergent and consistent sources of information to increase his or her understanding of the defendant's mental capacity and/or competence in their particular ecological niche. *There is no one specific neuropsychological test measure which can accurately be utilized to determine a criminal defendant's mental capacity or competency to stand trial if their cultural, ethnic, linguistic, educational, and socioeconomic background is dramatically different from the published test norms and the examiner's background or experience.* Impaired performances on such measures may not be necessarily indicative of impaired functional skills or even remotely predictive of the defendant's competence to stand trial. Neuropsychological testing, however, may have more predictive value if the measures used during testing more closely match or simulate the defendant's functioning in everyday or real-world settings. However, there are at present few such assessment measures available that will provide the examiner with this opportunity (Sbordone & Guilmette, 1999).

Executive Functioning in Assessment of Violent Behavior

The executive functions of the brain can be defined as the complex process by which an individual goes about performing a novel problem-solving task from its inception to its completion. This process includes: (1) the awareness that a particular problem exists, (2) an evaluation of the particular problem, (3) an analysis of the conditions of the problem, (4) the formulation of specific goals, (5) the development of a set of plans which determine which specific actions are needed to solve this problem, (6) evaluation of the potential effect of using such plans, (7) the selection and initiation of a particular plan to solve the problem, (8) evaluation of any progress made toward solving the problem, (9) modification of the plan if it has not been effective, (10) eliminating ineffective plans and replacing them with more effective plans, (11) comparing the results achieved by the new plan with the conditions of the problem, (12) terminating the plan when the conditions of the problem have been met, and (13) storing the plan, or retrieving it later when the same or similar problem appears (Sbordone, 2000).

Damage to the orbital frontal cortex has been reported to produce a neurobehavioral syndrome characterized by a lack of social tact, use of crude or coarse language, an inability to regulate one's behavior or emotions (disinhibition), emotional lability, insensitivity to the needs and welfare of others, and antisocial and criminal acts (Blumer & Benson, 1975; Cummings, 1985; Stuss & Benson, 1986). Similar behaviors, however, can also be produced by lesions in nonfrontal cortical and subcortical structures since the orbital frontal cortex receives input from the dorsolateral prefrontal regions, temporal pole, and the amygdala. For example, the amygdala receives input from the medial dorsal and central anterior nuclei of the thalamus. Since the orbital frontal cortex also regulates the activity of the dorsal prefrontal cortex, temporal pole, and amygdala, it forms what has been described as an orbitofrontal–subcortical circuit (Cummings, 1995).

A variety of psychiatric and subcortical disorders can impair the executive functions as a result of either lesions in the frontal–subcortical structures or alterations in their metabolic activity. For example, alcohol (Moscovich, 1982), attention deficit disorder (Barkley, Grodzinsky, & DuPaul, 1992), head trauma (Mattson & Levin, 1990), inhalation of organic solvents (Arlien-Soborg, Bruhn, Gyldensted, & Melgaard, 1979; Hawkins, 1990; Tsushima & Towne, 1977), stimulant abuse (Strickland et al., 1993), mania (Cummings & Mendez, 1984), psychosis (Cummings, Gosenfeld, Houlihan, & McCaffrey, 1983), and schizophrenia (Morris, Rushe, Woodruff, & Murray, 1995) have been reported to produce significant alterations in the executive functions of the brain.

Neuropsychologists have frequently relied on one or more of the following psychological tests to assess the executive functions of the brain: Wisconsin Card Sorting Test, Halstead Category Test, Verbal Concept Attainment Test, Oral Word Association Test, Thurstone Word Fluency Test, Design Fluency, Ruff Figural Fluency Test, Austin Maze, Porteus Maze Test, Tinker Toy Test, Stroop Test, Trail Making Test, Rey Complex Figure Test, and various motor tests such as Finger Tapping, Purdue Pegboard, and Grooved Pegboard tests. While these tests may possess some sensitivity to the frontal lobes or the executive functions of the brain, a patient's performance on these tests may not provide us with accurate information about whether their executive functions are intact since they may only assess one or two of the many steps that are involved in the complex process served by the executive functions of the brain (Cripe, 1996).

A number of investigators have stressed that behavioral changes associated with frontal–subcortical circuits tend to be exceedingly complex, variable, difficult to determine in technical terms, or almost impossible to quantify by our current neuropsychological measures (e.g., Mesulam, 1986). Damasio (1985) has stressed that the standardized neuropsychological tests which are commonly used by neuropsychologists are inadequate to assess the executive functions of the brain. For example, he described a 42-year-old patient whose computed tomography scan showed clear evidence of bilateral damage to the frontal lobes and revealed that the orbitofrontal surface and the frontal polar cortex of both hemispheres were almost entirely missing as a consequence of extensive surgical ablation in order to remove a brain tumor. Although the patient's neuropsychological test scores were almost completely normal, this patient exhibited a lack of awareness of his numerous cognitive and behavioral deficits which included diminished sexual and exploratory behavior, an inability to focus his attention, marked confabulation, a loss of originality and creativity, inappropriate social and emotional behavior, and the inability to organize his thoughts and behavior and engage in planning for the future.

The neuropsychologist is frequently called upon in forensic settings to establish a functional relationship between a criminal defendant's neuropsychological deficits and instant offense behavior such as in a mental capacity assessment. Any link between the defendant's violent criminal behavior and the defendant's neuropsychological deficits is likely to have considerable relevance to the accused's mental capacity at the time of the alleged offense, particularly if the test data demonstrates that the defendant is incapable of suppressing or modulating his emotions or behavior. Thus, any of the above psychiatric or subcortical disorders described above may be used to explain the patient's impaired executive functions which contributed to the instant offense behavior.

One of the inherent difficulties with this approach is that poor performance on tests of "executive functioning" may be due to a variety of cultural, ethnic, socioeconomic, educational, situational, and acculturation factors. Thus, neuropsychologists who ignore these factors are likely to overpathologize the defendant's executive functions and are likely to incorrectly attribute the defendant's poor neuropsychological test performance as evidence of impaired executive functions or frontal lobe pathology, even when the defendant's executive functions are relatively intact. Furthermore, defendants who are inaccurately identified as "brain-damaged" or as having "frontal lobe pathology" may be perceived as poor risks for probation/rehabilitation.

Assessment of Distortion, Deception, and Malingering

There are a number of considerations in applying the *Diagnostic and Statistical Manual of Mental Disorders*, 4th edition (DSM-IV) (American Psychiatric Association, 1994) criteria for malingering to individuals in which socioeconomic, ethnic, and cultural factors distinguish them from the dominant cultural and ethnic group. Use of the word "minority" in this context is simply meant to indicate the overrepresentation of cultural and ethnic minority groups within low socioeconomic circumstances rather than referring to minority status in general.

Certainly, the DSM-IV definition of malingering would appear appropriate across groups, independent of ethnic minority status, but the application of the four "suspicion indices" have potential for misclassification and abuse. Focus, then, will be upon the suspicion indices rather than the definition of malingering.

As conceived, the definition of malingering has three components. The first component specifies that an individual who is malingering must be either feigning or grossly exaggerating symptoms or disability. The second component requires that such symptom exaggeration or feigning be done on a voluntary and intentional basis. The third component is a designation of a clearly specified external incentive which is presumed to motivate and reinforce the malingering. According to the DSM-IV schema, malingering should be considered when various factors, or suspicion indices, are present. These four indices include referral within a medical–legal context, the presence of an antisocial personality disorder, subjective complaints markedly discrepant from objective findings, and poor compliance with treatment and evaluation.

Unfortunately, these four criteria are ineffective in identifying malingering. Rogers (1990a) examined their sensitivity and specificity in a forensic population. Sensitivity, the proportion of malingerers correctly identified by these criteria, was moderate. Two-thirds of malingerers met two or more of the four criteria. However, specificity, the proportion of nonmalingerers correctly identified, was discouragingly poor. About 80% of the nonmalingerers met two or more of the suspicion indices. Thus, use of these four indices carries with it an unacceptably high rate of false identifications of nonmalingerers as being malingerers.

Rogers (1990b) discusses limitations of the DSM criteria of malingering, which is based upon a criminological model. Such a model assumes the "badness" of character and behavior of the malingerer. However, Rogers proposes that many malingerers may be motivated to such behavior as a way to cope with a negative situation rather than any inherent "badness." This alternative adaptational model assumes that malingering is more likely to occur under circumstances that are adversarial, in which the individual believes that there is more to lose from disclosure than to gain from malingering, and/or he or she does not perceive a more effective means to achieve the goal. Clearly, such an explanatory model may be more applicable to individuals who find themselves under negative circumstances such as poverty, or perceived or real discrimination, as is more common for minority groups, as this designation is being used.

The criminological model also runs the risk of raising undue suspicion of malingering in ethnic minority groups who may fit the various criteria for reasons other than "badness." Each of the four indices will be discussed within this context.

The first index refers to presentation within a medical–legal context. Such a specification is based upon the presence of obvious external incentives within such a context such as the potential for monetary award in civil litigation, compensation in disability situations, housing or other basic needs when an individual has few tangible means, or avoidance of conviction in the criminal arena, among others. Thus, contextual factors, not just those present in a medical–legal situation, are relevant, particularly those that carry with them an external secondary gain.

Ethnic minorities are overrepresented in situations related to the criminal justice system. Also, on the average, they have a lower educational level and socioeconomic status, and thus would have comparatively fewer vocational alternatives. Moreover, they would be more highly represented in jobs that require physical labor and other hazardous situations in which the potential for physical injury is greater than in more sedentary clerical and office-based jobs, often resulting in pursuit of disability compensation.

The designation of presentation within a medical–legal context or one in which there is potential for secondary gain, while a reasonable suspicion index, is one which, nonetheless, has low sensitivity to malingering. While individuals within such contexts may have more incentive to malinger than individuals not presenting under such circumstances, the vast majority of individuals do not malinger. In criminal proceedings, for example, the evidence for malingering was found to be only 3%–8% (Cornell & Hawk 1988; Rogers 1986, 1988). The sensitivity of the medical–legal context index to the presence of malingering, therefore, is low.

The second suspicion index is the presence of an antisocial personality disorder. The reasoning in designating this as a suspicion index relates to the fact that malingering may be construed as an antisocial behavior. Such a behavior would be consistent with a general personality style in individuals with an antisocial personality disorder and, as such, the individual would have fewer misgivings about malingering. However, there is a problem with the DSM-IV criteria for diagnosing the presence of antisocial personality disorder which undermines its effectiveness as a correlate of malingering. The DSM-IV criteria relate primarily to antisocial behavior. However, definitions of antisocial behavior may, at times, be culturally relative and need to be judged within the socioeconomic context.

For example, some ethnic minority members growing up in poverty are likely to be exposed to a number of criminal activities within their environment. However, such criminal behaviors may be motivated by the need to adapt to very difficult life circumstances. There may be few options, or at least the perception of limitations, for advancement within society at large, such that behaviors may be motivated by a need to cope with a difficult situation. As such, antisocial behavior, a basis for diagnosis of antisocial personality disorder, may not correlate with manipulation and deception implicit in the reasoning behind designation of antisocial personality disorder as a suspicion index.

The DSM-IV fails to specify underlying characterological traits associated with core psychopathy in its definition and specification of criteria for antisocial personality disorder. Hare (1991) has found that the psychopathic personality consists of two factors, only one of which relates to various antisocial behaviors as per the DSM-IV. The other factor relates to core personality characteristics including underdeveloped conscience, conning and manipulative behavior, callousness, and pathological lying. It is these characteristics, rather than a history of antisocial behavior, which should logically raise suspicion of malingering, particularly when considering cultural context. For example, theft would be considered antisocial behavior, but what if such an individual was stealing food to provide for his starving family? Similarly, a homeless person feigning illness to be admitted to a hospital or other institution may also be engaging in malingering to cope with a desperate situation. Thus, antisocial behaviors can be motivated as circumstances dictate, but not identify the individual as a psychopath in which malingering might be more readily suspected.

The third suspicion index designated by the DSM-IV is the presence of subjective complaints markedly discrepant from objective findings. This criterion, by itself, cannot distinguish between a number of psychiatric disorders in which symptoms are legitimate but not necessarily medically or physiologically based, versus malingering, in which the subjective complaints are purposefully exaggerated or even feigned. Epidemiological studies demonstrate a higher rate of psychopathology (Narrow, Regier, Rae, Mandershceid, & Locke, 1993) in minorities compared to the majority population. Thus, the likelihood of suffering a psychiatric disorder in which there are few objective physical or "objective" findings but considerable subjective complaints is greater in minority groups. The risk of misdiagnosis of malingering based on the belief that there is a purposeful exaggeration or feigning of symptoms needs to be considered greater under such circumstances.

The fourth index considers poor compliance with evaluation and treatment as suspicion of malingering. Utilization of health services is less for minority groups (Lin & Poland, 1994). Such underutilization may have several explanations independent of malingering. Lower socioeconomic areas are underserved by medical and psychiatric services, they generally receive inferior quality of services (Cole & Pilisuk, 1976), and there may be a reluctance of various minority groups to utilize mainstream medical and psychiatric services due to financial reasons and suspicion (Sue, McKinney, Allen, & Hale, 1974).

Reviewing the above considerations, many ethnic minorities would qualify for one or more of these suspicion indices. However, the reason for meeting these factors may be unrelated to malingering itself and, therefore, there is a greater chance of minority individuals being misdiagnosed as malingerers as a result of blindly using these criteria.

Obviously, there are other approaches to identifying malingering in addition to the DSM-IV definitions and criteria. Attempts to identify malingering of neuropsychological impairment and disability also utilize test performance. Some interpretive principles and strategies would appear to be largely unaffected by cultural, ethnic, or socioeconomic status. When such strategies rely upon a comparison of performance to chance, such as symptom validity testing (Pankratz, 1979) and other forced-choice procedures. In symptom validity testing, an individual is typically presented with a relatively easy task in which they are required to identify one of two response alternatives as the correct answer. For example, a number of tests utilize a format in which the individual is presented with a five-digit number followed by a delay period in which they are then presented with two five-digit numbers, one of which is a foil and the other which is a match to the five-digit number that they had been shown earlier; for example, the Victoria Symptom Validity Test (Slick, Hopp, Strauss, & Thompson, 1997). Simple guessing or a random response style should result in approximately 50% accuracy. A performance significantly below chance provides strong evidence of malingering in that, in order to do so, it is quite likely that the test-taker knew the correct response but purposefully decided to respond incorrectly. Such tests would appear to be free of cultural or socioeconomic influences as a cause related to malingering. However, the majority of individuals malingering score at least at chance or above. Thus, the sensitivity of a below-chance performance is low, although the specificity is rather high.

The neuropsychological performance of malingerers often is not consistent with a known pathological process. For example, following a mild traumatic brain injury, it is highly unusual to have significant aphasia or severe sensory–motor difficulties. Similarly, many forms of brain injury which result in sensory–motor difficulties are lateralized to one side of the body. To the extent that the pattern of test results conforms with expectation of the etiology in question, the effort and motivation a person puts forth on testing is certainly less suspect, and should aid in determining the credibility of performance in ethnic-minority populations.

Studies of malingering using the Halstead–Reitan and Luria–Nebraska Neuropsychological Batteries have revealed that individuals feigning brain damage tended to produce sensory–motor disturbance that was not lateralized and also did not show an expected negative performance slope (Golden & Grier, 1998; Heaton, Smith, Lehman, & Vogts, 1978). A negative slope indicates that, as tests become more difficult or challenging, performance tends to deteriorate. Analysis of the Halstead–Reitan performance in individuals feigning brain damage revealed that they frequently performed more poorly on easy tasks than would be predicted based upon their better performance on complicated tasks (Reitan & Wolfson, 1998). Such a performance is also found on the Luria–Nebraska. In fact, McKinzey, Podd, Krehbiel, Mensch, and Tromblea (1997) identified two sets of items discriminating malingerers from brain damaged individuals in which malingerers performed disproportionately more poorly on easy items compared to complicated items, while the nonmalingering brain-injured individuals showed the expected negative performance slope. The absence of a negative performance slope should raise suspicions of malingering in anyone, regardless of ethnic status.

Another commonly used criterion employed to identify malingering is the presence of excessive impairment or pathology shown on cognitive tests, particularly when judged relative to external criteria. For example, an individual who has suffered from a mild head injury should demonstrate relatively benign findings on neuropsychological tests. When such an individual produces a moderately to severely-impaired profile, suspicion is naturally raised as to the validity of performance, with purposeful exaggeration or feigning being one consideration to explain the results. However, there are many potential explanations for this disparity other than a purposeful attempt to manipulate the data. One such issue has already been discussed previously and relates to the dangers of interpreting test performances in individuals who differ from the normative group on factors such as language, culture, and other related variables. In addition, the association between minority status and lower socioeconomic status, as defined for this discussion, is associated with a higher prevalence of various medical illnesses, physical injuries, brain injuries, psychiatric disorders, academic deficiencies, substance abuse, and other such factors (Strickland, Jenkins, Myers, & Adams, 1998). Each factor, in its own right, can exert a negative influence upon neuropsychological performance. Performance on the neuropsychological tests may represent an amalgam of factors in addition to the injury in question and result in greater impairment in test scores than would be expected on the basis of the injury in question by itself (Sbordone & Purisch, 1996).

Thus, reliance upon neuropsychological testing to identify malingering in ethnic minorities is fraught with hazards and runs the clear risk of excessive false-positive diagnoses. Greater reliance needs to be placed upon the full clinical neuropsychological examination including interview, review of records, obtaining information from collateral sources, and behavioral observations. It is only after an analysis of the consistencies and inconsistencies developed from this richer and larger data pool, that the test results can be placed in a larger context. Inconsistencies need to be examined for motivation and are usually reflected in a self-serving pattern. For example, an individual who reports a loss of consciousness after a head injury may differ in the length of time in which this persisted when evaluated by different examiners. However, if initial reports indicate that he or she claims an hour loss of consciousness, followed by later reports in which he or she reduces this estimate, such an inconsistency likely is not motivated by secondary gain. On the other hand, if an individual, over time, extends the length in which he or she was unconscious excessively such an inconsistency may serve the goal of representing his or her injury as more serious than it really was. Such principles would appear to apply regardless of minority status.

A diagnosis of malingering requires considerable converging points of information and data and should only be offered with considerable caution. Such a label can be quite damaging and may negatively affect the reaction of individuals toward the identified malingerer in the future. Such individuals, in fact, may be significant providers of services or other benefits, and such a misdiagnosis may result in unjust treatment and stigmatization. With individuals who are ethnic minorities, the risk of false identification of malingering is heightened, making it mandatory to consider and rule out the multiple competing explanations of factors that could account for inconsistent or suspicious results before applying such a pejorative label.

References

American Psychiatric Association. (1994). *Diagnostic and statistical manual of mental disorders* (4th ed.). Washington, DC: Author.

Arlien-Soborg, P., Bruhn, P., Gyldensted, C., & Melgaard, B. (1979). Chronic Painter's syndrome. *Acta Neurologica Scandinavica, 60,* 149–156.

Barkley, R., Grodzinsky, G., & DuPaul, G.J. (1992). Frontal lobe functions and attention-deficit disorder with and without hyperactivity: A review and research report. *Journal of Abnormal Clinical Psychology, 20,* 163–188.

Blumer, D., & Benson, D. F. (1975). Personality changes with frontal and temporal lobe lesions. In D. F. Benson & D. Blumer (Eds.), *Psychiatric aspects of neurologic disease* (pp. 151–170). New York: Grune & Stratton.

Cole, J., & Pilisuk, M. (1976). Differences in the provision of mental health services by race. *American Journal of Orthopsychiatry, 46,* 510–525.

Cornell, D. G., & Hawk, G. L. (1988, August). *Malingerers diagnosed in pretrial evaluations: Clinical presentations.* Paper presented at the Annual Meeting of the American Psychological Association, Atlanta.

Cripe, L. I. (1996). The ecological validity of executive function testing. In R. J. Sbordone & C. J. Long (Eds.), *Ecological validity of neuropsychological testing* (pp. 171–202). Delray Beach: GR/St. Lucie.

Cronbach, L. J. (1984). *Essentials of psychological testing* (4th ed.). New York: Harper & Row.

Cummings, J. L. (1985). *Clinical neuropsychiatry.* New York: Grune & Stratton.

Cummings, J. L. (1995). Anatomic and behavioral aspects of frontal-subcortical circuits. *Annals of the New York Academy of Sciences, 769,* 1–13.

Cummings, J. L., Gosenfeld, L. F., Houlihan, J. P., & McCaffrey, T. (1983). Neuropsychiatric disturbances associated with idiopathic calcification of the basal ganglia. *Biological Psychiatry, 18,* 591–601.

Cummings, J. L., & Mendez, M. F. (1984). Secondary mania with focal cerebrovascular lesions. *American Journal of Psychiatry, 141,* 1084–1087.

Damasio, A. R. (1985). The Frontal Lobes. In K. M. Heilman & E. Valenstein (Eds.), *Clinical neuropsychology* (2nd ed., pp. 339–375). New York: Oxford University Press.

Golden, C. J., & Grier, C. A. (1998). Detecting malingering on the Luria–Nebraska neuropsychological battery. In C. R. Reynolds (Ed.), *Detection of malingering during head injury litigation* (pp. 133–162). New York: Plenum.

Hare, R. D. (1991). *The Hare Psychopathy Checklist—Revised manual.* North Tonawanda, NY: Multi-Health Systems.

Hartman, D. E. (1995). *Neuropsychological toxicology.* New York: Plenum.

Hawkins, K. A. (1990). Occupational neurotoxicology: Some neuropsychological issues and challenges. *Journal of Clinical and Experimental Neuropsychology, 12,* 664–680.

Heaton, R. K., Smith, H. H., Jr., Lehman, R. A., & Vogts, A. T. (1978). Prospects for faking believable deficits on neuropsychological testing. *Journal of Consulting and Clinical Psychology, 46,* 892–900.

Lezak, M. D. (1995). *Neuropsychological assessment* (3rd ed.). New York: Oxford University Press.

Lin, K. M., & Poland, R. (1994). Ethnic differences in the response to psychotropic drugs. In S. Friedman (Ed.), *Anxiety disorders in African Americans* (pp. 203–204). New York: Springer.

Mattson, A. J., & Levin, H. S. (1990). Frontal lobe dysfunction following closed head injury. *Journal of Nervous and Mental Diseases, 178,* 282–291.

McKinzey, R. K., Podd, M. H., Krehbiel, M. A., Mensch, A. J., & Trombka, C. C. (1997). Detection of malingering on the LNNB: An initial and cross validation. *Archives of Clinical and Neuropsychology, 12,* 505–512.

Mesulam, M. M. (1986). Frontal cortex and behavior: Editorial. *Annals of Neurology, 19,* 320–325.

Morris, R. G., Rushe, T., Woodruff, P. W. R., & Murray, R. M. (1995). Problem solving in schizophrenia: A specific deficit in planning ability. *Schizophrenia Research, 14,* 235–246.

Moscovich, M. (1982). Multiple dissociations of function in amnesia. In L. Cermack (Ed.), *Human memory and amnesia* (pp. 337–370). Hillside, NJ: Erlbaum.

Narrow, W. E., Reiger, D. A., Rae, D. S., Manderscheid, R. W., & Locke, B. Z. (1993). Use of services by persons with mental and addictive disorders. *Archives of General Psychiatry, 50*, 95–107.

Pankratz, L. (1979). Symptom validity testing and symptom retraining: Procedures for the assessment and treatment of functioning sensory deficits. *Journal of Consulting and Clinical Psychology, 47*, 409–410.

Reitan, R. J., & Wolfson, D. (1998). Detection of malingering and invalid test results using the Halstead–Reitan Battery. In C. R. Reynolds (Ed.), *Detection of malingering during head injury litigation* (pp. 163–208). New York: Plenum.

Rogers, R. (1986). Malingering and deception. In R. Rogers (Ed.), *Conducting insanity evaluations* (pp. 61–76). New York: Van Nostrand Reinhold.

Rogers, R. (1988). *Clinical assessment of malingering and deception.* New York: Guilford.

Rogers, R. (1990a). Development of a new classificatory model of malingering. *Bulletin of the American Academy of Psychiatry and Law, 18*, 323–333.

Rogers, R. (1990b). Models of feigned mental illness. *Professional Psychology: Research and Practice, 21*, 182–188.

Sbordone, R. J. (2000). The executive functions of the brain. In G. Groth-Marnat (Ed.), *Neuropsychological assessment in clinical practice: A practical guide to test interpretation and integration* (pp. 437–456). New York: Wiley.

Sbordone, R. J., & Guilmette, T. J. (1999). Ecological validity: Prediction of everyday and vocational functioning from neuropsychological test data. In J. Sweet (Ed.), *Forensic neuropsychology: Fundamentals and practice* (pp. 227–254). Royersford, PA: Swets & Zeitlinger.

Sbordone, R. J., & Purisch, A. D. (1996). Hazards of blind analysis of neuropsychological test data in assessing cognitive disability: The role of confounding factors. *Neurorehabilitation, 7*, 15–26.

Slick, D., Hopp, G., Strauss, E., & Thompson, G. B. (1997). *Victoria Symptom Validity Test, Version 1.0: Professional manual.* Odessa, FL: Psychological Assessment Resources.

Strickland, T. L., Mena, I., Villanueva-Meyer, J., Miller, B. L., Cummings, J., Mehringer, C. M., Satz, P., & Myers, H. (1993). Cerebral perfusion and neuropsychological consequences of chronic cocaine use. *Journal of Neuropsychiatry and Clinical Neuroscience, 5*, 419–427.

Strickland, T. L., & Stein, R. (1995). Cocaine-induced cerebrovascular impairment: Challenges to neuropsychological assessment. *Neuropsychology Review, 5*(1), 69–79.

Strickland, T. L., Jenkins, J. O., Myers, H. F., & Adams, H. E. (1998). Diagnostic judgments as a function of client and therapist race. *Journal of Psychopathology and Behavioral Assessment, 10*, 141–151.

Stuss, D. T., & Benson, D. F. (1986). *The frontal lobes.* New York: Raven.

Sue, S., McKinney, H., Allen, D., & Hall, J. (1974). Delivery of community mental health services to black and white clients. *Journal of Consulting and Clinical Psychology, 42*, 241–344.

Tsushima, W. T., & Towne, W. S. (1977). Effects of paint sniffing on neuropsychological test performance. *Journal of Abnormal Psychology, 86*, 402–407.

20

Trends in American Immigration

Influences on Neuropsychological Assessment and Inferences with Ethnic-Minority Populations

ANTOLIN M. LLORENTE, I. MARIBEL TAUSSIG,

PAUL SATZ, AND LISSETTE M. PEREZ

Recent large-scale American migrations continue to shape the face of this nation, revitalizing and reweaving the foreign fabric that characterized American society during the early part of the twentieth century (Portes & Rumbaut, 1990). The effects of these immigrations have sweeping consequences for American psychology (Rogler, 1994).

With regard to the impact of these migrations upon neuropsychology, demographic variables, including age, education, and ethnicity, significantly influence the outcome of neuropsychological (NP) assessments (Adams, Boake, & Crain, 1982; Badcock & Ross, 1982; Botwinick, 1967; Heaton, Grant & Matthews, 1986; Rosselli, Ardila, & Rosas, 1990). Therefore, a phenomenon capable of modulating demographic characteristics of ethnic-minority groups comprising normative samples would be of significant interest to cross-cultural neuropsychology. A logical candidate would be capable of affecting the procurement and application of neuropsychological norms, as well as the overall NP assessment process.

American immigration patterns indirectly influence demographic characteristics during the acquisition of normative standards for certain minority groups within the United States (Llorente, 1997; Llorente, Ponton, Taussig, & Satz, 1998). These influences are the indirect impact of migrational patterns upon demographic characteristics and on the subsequent availability of adequate and suitable reference and comparison groups. Aside from factors associated with the acquisition and application of normative data, migrations are inextricably associated with levels of acculturation and assimilation (Montgomery & Orozlo, 1984; Portes & Bach, 1985), differences in levels of educational attainment capable of impacting test-taking strategies (Rey, Feldman, Rivas-Vazquez, Levin, & Benton, 1998; Rosselli et al., 1990), perceptions of the immigrant as an individual and of the immigration process proper (Malz-

ANTOLIN M. LLORENTE • Baylor College of Medicine, Houston, Texas 77030.   I. MARIBEL TAUSSIG • University of Southern California, Los Angeles, California 90089.   PAUL SATZ • UCLA School of Medicine, Los Angeles, California 90095; and Charles R. Drew University of Medicine and Science, Los Angeles, California 90059.   LISSETTE M. PEREZ • Texas A&M University, College Station, Texas 77843-4225.

Handbook of Cross-Cultural Neuropsychology, edited by Fletcher-Janzen, Strickland, and Reynolds. Kluwer Academic / Plenum Publishers, New York, 2000.

berg & Lee, 1956; Ødegaard, 1932; Sanua, 1970), and the clinical inferences made about these groups.

A Brief Glance at Patterns of American Immigration

A brief examination of American immigration trends for Hispanics and their relation to neuropsychology has been presented elsewhere (Llorente, 1997; Llorente et al., 1998). However, it is proper to review, in a broad fashion, the biased nature of migrations as they relate to various ethnic-minority groups in an attempt to understand with greater insight their subsequent impact on the acquisition and application of neuropsychological standards. Close scrutiny of migrational patterns reveals that American immigration (legal migration to the U.S. from abroad) is not the result of chance processes (Hamilton & Chinchilla, 1990; U.S. Immigration and Naturalization Service, 1991; Portes & Rumbaut, 1990; Portes & Borocsz, 1989). The nonrandom nature of migratory patterns is the result of selective factors associated with both the sending and host countries (Portes & Rumbaut, 1990). With regard to factors associated with the host country, Garcia (1981) has argued convincingly that the United States government has had specific and select immigration aims in the past that were arbitrary by their very nature.

Revisions in American immigration laws during the past three decades also served as impetus behind recent changes in migrational patterns. According to the Immigration and Naturalization Service (U.S. Immigration and Naturalization Service, 1991), the predominant shift has been in eliminating "country specific quotas," replacing them with quotas partially based on "humanitarian concerns," shifting American migrational patterns from "European to Asian and Latin American immigration." This change in immigration policy altered the profile that typified U.S. migrations for "over 200 years." This shift in migrational trends is illustrated in Figure 1.

The substantial variability observed in the number of immigrants allowed to enter the U.S during the past nine decades is another marker capable of elucidating the nonrandom and shifting nature of American migrational patterns. Figure 2 clearly shows the toll that various socioeconomic and historical events (e.g., the Great Depression, World War II) had on the total number of immigrants allowed to enter the U.S. between the early 1930s and the mid-to-late 1940s. This figure additionally depicts the increasing number of legal immigrants that have been allowed to enter the U.S. in the last 3 or 4 decades and the sudden shifts in total migration that have taken place over time.

Closely associated with education, Figure 3 shows the reported occupational allegiance of legal immigrants entering the U.S. from 1976 to 1990. These data indicate that the various occupational categories (and most likely the educational attainment) encompassed by legal immigrants during those two decades were not proportionally represented. Although great variability in immigrants' occupational and educational attainment is observed in the literature, disproportionate occupational representations are more pronounced for certain ethnic groups relative to others (see Llorente et al., 1998).

Absolute and Relative Migrations

Table 1 depicts the number of *legal* immigrants entering the United States from Argentina, mainland China, Cuba, Haiti, and Mexico by decade between 1931 and 1990. Table 1 shows that the total number of immigrants from Mexico exceeded 3 million during the past 60

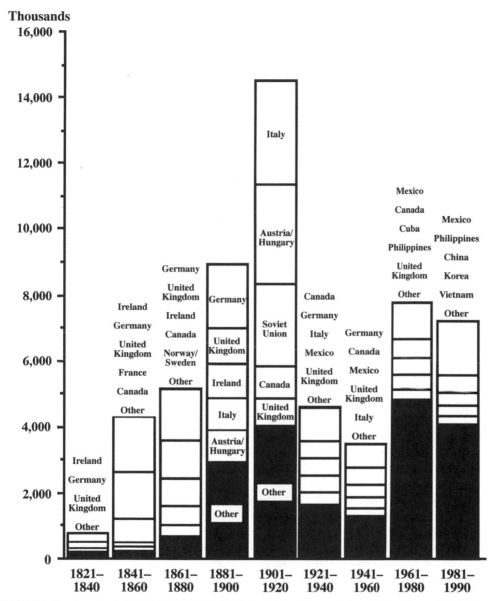

FIGURE 1. Immigrants admitted to the U.S., 1821–1990, from the top five countries of last residence (adapted from INS, 1991).

years, while the total number of immigrants from Argentina during the same period was only about 131,000. During the same period, the total numbers of immigrants from Haiti, China, and Cuba were approximately 234,000, 537,000, and 732,000, respectively. A great deal of variability was observed in timing of migration climax and the magnitude of maximum immigration. Whereas immigration from Mexico peaked at approximately 1.5 million between 1981 and 1990, Chinese and Haitian migrations peaked during the same period but in signifi-

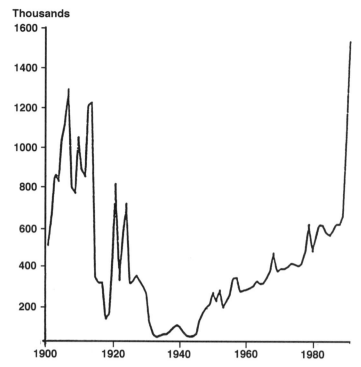

FIGURE 2. Total legal American immigration, 1901–1990 (adapted from INS, 1991).

cantly smaller numbers, approximately 347,000 and 138,000 immigrants, respectively. Migration from Cuba peaked at approximately 264,000 during 1971–1980 while migration from Argentina to the United States reached approximately 50,000 legal immigrants between 1961 and 1970. With regard to absolute migration, the number of Argentinean immigrants is approximately 24 times less than the number of Mexican immigrants and approximately six times less than the number of Cubans immigrating to the United States over the same period. The total number of immigrants from China and Cuba are six and four times less, respectively, than the total number of immigrants from Mexico during the same six decades. In the same vein, migration from Haiti is approximately 13 times less than the migration to the U.S. from Mexico between 1931 and 1990.

Although analyses could have been conducted to determine whether the expected number of immigrants from each nation under investigation differed statistically for the five countries across the six decades, such analyses are beyond the scope of this chapter. However, it should be noted that analyses conducted in the past with Hispanics have easily reached statistical significance (Llorente et al., 1998) indicating that the expected distribution of absolute number of immigrants changed significantly over time and for each country. It is also clear from the data presented above that the relationship for these nations is statistically significant in all likelihood. These data also underscore the biased nature of American immigration patterns.

As critical as an examination of the absolute number of emigrants was to an attempt to understand American migratory patterns, a study of the proportion of emigrants for three decades (1961–1970, 1971–1980, and 1981–1990) relative to the total population of each country at the end of those decades was just as important. This analysis was thus conducted for

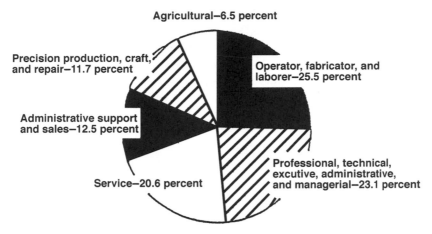

FIGURE 3. Percentage based on proportion of total number of legal immigrants reporting occupation upon U.S. entry, 1976–1990) (adapted from INS, 1991).

each country. In 1970, Argentina had a population of about 24,300,000 and a migration to the U.S. (1961–1970) of 50,000 or .2% of its population. China had a population of about 800,000,000 in 1970 and an American migration of 34,000 between 1961 and 1970 or .004% of its population. Haiti had a total population of 4,000,000 inhabitants in 1970 and an American emigration (1961–1970) of 34,000 or .01% of its population. In contrast, in 1970 Cuba and Mexico had populations of 8,500,000 and 48,000,000 and American emigrations of 208,000 and 454,000, respectively, between 1961 and 1970 of 3% and 1% of their populations.

In 1980, Argentina had a population of 27,300,000 and an American emigration of about 30,000 or .1% of its population. China had an estimated 1 billion inhabitants and a migration of 124,300 or .0001% of its population. Cuba's population was 9,980,000, with a U.S. migration of 264,863, 2.6% of its population, while Haiti, with a population of 5,100,000, had emigration to the U.S. of 56,300, 1.1% of its population. Mexico's emigration was 1% of its population (total U.S. emigration, 1971–1980 = 640,294/total estimated population, 1980 = 71,900,000).

TABLE 1. Total Number of Immigrants (Absolute Migration) across Six Decades (1931–1990) for Argentina, Mainland China, Cuba, Haiti, and Mexico

Decade	Country and number of legal immigrants				
	Argentina	China	Cuba	Haiti	Mexico
1931–1940	1,349	4,928	9,575	191	22,319
1941–1950	3,338	16,709	26,313	911	60,589
1951–1960	19,486	9,657	78,948	4,442	299,811
1961–1970	49,721	34,764	208,536	34,499	453,937
1971–1980	29,897	124,326	264,863	56,335	640,294
1981–1990	27,327	346,747	144,578	138,379	1,655,843

Source: Adapted from U.S. Immigration and Naturalization Service (1991).

For 1981–1990, the percentages of the 1990 populations of Argentina, China, Cuba, Haiti, and Mexico that had emigrated to the U.S. were .1%, .003%, 1.3%, 2.1%, and 1.8%, respectively.

In summary, in terms of proportions of emigrants relative to each country's total population, migrations to the United States from Argentina and China remained relatively constant and small in magnitude over the last three decades. Cuban emigration reached its peak during the decade between 1971 and 1980 with decreasing American emigration in the last decade, while Haiti's migration declined in the middle decade with similar numbers in the first and last decades under investigation. In contrast, although Mexico's relative emigration to the U.S. has steadily decreased during the same period, the decrease has been less pronounced.

Immigration and Occupational Allegiance

Table 2 presents the "occupational group allegiance" for legal immigrants in 1990 for the same nations. It is clear from these data that the occupational (and most likely educational) levels of these five migrational groups were substantially different. Whereas Haitian and Mexican immigrants reporting occupations were primarily classified under precision/craft, operator/fabricator, farming/forestry, and service categories, with few immigrants from the professional/technical, executive/managerial, sales, and administrative support sectors, Argentinean, Chinese, and Cuban immigrants reporting occupational status showed greater diversity. Specifically, Argentinean, Chinese, and Cuban immigrants represented the entire occupational spectrum including those from the professional/technical (with less representation from Cuba), executive/managerial, sales, administrative support, precision/craft and all other occupational ranks. Immigrants from Argentina had the most even representation across all occupational categories of the five countries.

Previous studies with Hispanics (Llorente et al., 1998) have revealed statistical significance in reported occupational allegiance when a randomly selected year (1990) was chosen for analysis. In that investigation, Argentinean and Cuban immigrants reported occupational allegiance from across the entire occupational spectrum within the range of expectation with underrepresentation in the farming/forestry category while immigrants from Mexico were underrepresented for most occupational categories in the same year, except for farming/

TABLE 2. Percentage of Total Legal Immigration and Reported Occupational Allegiance at Time of U.S. Entry for 1990[a]

| Occupation | Country and percent of total immigration | | | | |
	Argentina	China	Cuba	Haiti	Mexico
Professional/technical	9.2	9.9	4.0	2.8	.88
Executive/managerial	7.9	6.0	1.7	1.0	1.4
Sales	3.6	1.8	2.6	1.0	1.7
Administrative/support	6.5	4.0	4.0	2.6	2.7
Precision/craft	8.1	2.7	7.7	6.0	9.2
Operator/fabricator	6.7	9.8	16.2	10.2	24.0
Farming/forestry	0.5	10.8	0.4	6.8	12.0
Service	10.2	8.7	10.6	16.0	17.4

Source: Adapted from U.S. Immigration and Naturalization Service (1991).
[a]Excludes immigrants not reporting occupation (e.g., children).

forestry category, where they were overrepresented at twice the rate of expectation (Portes & Rumbaut, 1990).

These findings suggest that occupational migratory configurations (and possibly education) for these nations are indeed different. These data also suggest that either these nations had been differentially targeted for decades by the U.S. government to satisfy occupational manpower needs in the U.S. (host country) or the sending nation had undergone major changes requiring large scale migrations. These selective recruitment and exodus impetuses are partly responsible for each country's demographic differences as it relates to occupational status (see Portes & Rumbaut [1990] for specific U.S. government recruitment aims of Mexican nationals relative to occupational allegiance). Regardless of the etiology for the differences in reported occupational allegiance, it is clear from the data that discrepancies do exist in occupational and possibly educational migratory patterns. The discrepancy between these data and that depicted in Figure 3 (all immigrants entering U.S.) also deserves attention.

Immigration and Residential Preference

Table 3 shows the number of legal immigrants admitted to this country from mainland China, Cuba, Haiti, and Mexico for 1990 and their intended area of initial residence for five major metropolitan regions. As was the case for Hispanics (Llorente et al., 1998), these data indicated that immigrants tend to have a predilection for certain geographical areas within the United States, but not for others. Whereas 11% and 34% of Chinese and Mexican immigrants, respectively, reported Los Angeles, California as their preference for initial residence in 1990, only 2.5% and .3% of immigrants from Cuba and Haiti, respectively, reported Los Angeles as their intended initial residence. In sharp contrast, 72% and 18% of Cuban and Haitian immigrants reported Miami, Florida as their intended residence as opposed to only 8.5% and .2% of immigrants from China and Mexico (U.S. Immigration and Naturalization Service, 1991). With respect to New York, immigrants from China and Haiti represented the largest immigration from these countries with 28% and 38%, respectively, in 1990 while only 3.4% and 1% of immigrants from Cuba and Mexico, respectively, planned to move to New York. Chicago, Illinois and Houston, Texas had relatively low percentages of immigrants, although Mexico, due to its large absolute migration had a large numbers of its immigrants reporting these cities as their intended area of initial residence.

Discrepant patterns of selective immigration were not only observed for the major metropolitan cities listed in Table 3. They were also present for immigrants from other

TABLE 3. Percentage and Total Number of Legal Immigrants Reporting Intended Metropolitan Region of Initial Residence for Four Countries for 1990—Five Selected Regions

Metropolitan region	Country, percent, and (total number) of immigrants			
	China	Cuba	Haiti	Mexico
Chicago, Illinois	2.6 (838)	0.8 (84)	0.98 (199)	6.2 (41,846)
Houston, Texas	1.5 (473)	0.3 (31)	0.1 (24)	5.2 (34,973)
Los Angeles, California	11 (3,525)	2.5 (274)	0.27 (55)	34 (231,267)
Miami, Florida	8.5 (157)	72 (7,685)	17.9 (3,635)	0.2 (1,273)
New York, New York	28.4 (9,030)	3.4 (358)	37.7 (8,066)	0.9 (6,436)

Source: Adapted from U.S. Immigration and Naturalization Service (1991).

countries as well. As was the case for Hispanics (Llorente et al., 1998), all minority groups examined (Table 3) as part of the present investigation exhibited significant geographical predilection. These results suggest that certain groups of immigrants have historically selected specific metropolitan areas of residence different from those chosen by other groups of immigrants (Portes & Rumbaut, 1990).

The migrational data presented thus far show that the total number of immigrants (absolute migration) to the U.S. varies substantially for each country and fluctuates over time for each nation as a result of variables affecting both the host and sending countries. Therefore, migrational patterns must be considered dynamic nonrandom processes that change over time as a result of selective factors. The variability of these patterns of immigration may be the result of various social, political, and economic trends affecting all countries sharing migrations (i.e., the host and the sending country). The range of occupational status of foreign immigrants also varies extensively among nations regardless of the total size of their migration. This variation may be, among other factors, the result of selective recruitment policies or similar nonrandom variables adopted by the host country to satisfy certain of its unmet occupational classification requirements (Garcia, 1981; Portes & Rumbaut, 1990). For this reason, occupational allegiance from immigrants entering the U.S. cannot be assumed to be random as a certain degree of selectivity for specific vocational groups was observed for some nations. Instead, nonrandom shifts in the occupational choice of immigrants from foreign countries should be expected longitudinally, including the occupational choice of immigrants from the same country. Finally, considerable affinity for certain geographical/residential areas was observed for most immigrant groups across the time span under investigation. In sum, and as previously argued (Llorente, 1997; Llorente et al., 1998), a review of the migrational literature reveals that American immigration is *not* the result of chance processes (U.S. Immigration and Naturalization Service, 1975, 1981, 1991; Portes & Rumbaut, 1990), but rather the result of shifting and changing migrational patterns.

American Migratory Trends: Impact on the Acquisition and Application of Neuropsychological Norms for Ethnic-Minority Groups

The norm acquisition process for ethnic minorities is not free from potential biases. A host of possible confounds could distort these standards, invalidating future inferences made on the basis of these norms. Three of the potential sources of bias are subsequently reviewed while addressing the demographic characteristics of the ethnic-minority groups previously presented.

Potential Confounds Associated with Demographic Characteristics

The effects of demographic variables, including education, on neuropsychological performance are well established in the literature (Adams, Boake & Crain, 1982; Ardila, 1993; Ardila, Rosselli, & Rosas, 1989; Heaton et al., 1986; Laosa, 1984). A comparison of neuropsychological performance between a patient and a normative cohort differing in educational attainment would be inappropriate under most circumstances. This issue is best exemplified with ethnic-minority populations through research recently conducted by Ponton and associates (1996). In their sample, individuals of similar age attained higher levels of performance on measures assessing neuropsychological functions as a result of greater educational attainment across all groups. Similarly, Rey and colleagues (1998), while conducting research to develop psychological instruments for Hispanics, have shown that differences in neuropsychological performance existed between Cuban and Mexican normative samples in Dade County, Florida. Although at first glance the differences between these two seemingly similar Hispanic groups could have been attributed to differences in brain functions consequent to ethnic differences (Jensen, 1980), a closer look at the demographic characteristics of the samples revealed *selection biases* associated with lower levels of education in the Mexican cohort available to researchers in Dade County, Florida (see Table 3) relative to the Cuban cohort. The demographic differences of these two groups were most probably the result of distinct immigration patterns. Nevertheless, when subjects were matched on age, gender, and education, the discrepancies observed in neuropsychological performance between the two groups of participants disappeared.

These findings suggest that potential confounds associated with certain demographic characteristics, modulated by migrations in the case of certain ethnic-minority groups, must be carefully monitored to avoid the introduction of putative sources of systematic error from entering the norm-acquisition process. Careful consideration of these factors is also required to avoid attributing differences in neuropsychological performance within minority groups or mainstream versus ethnic groups to nonexistent abnormal brain–behavior relationships rather than differences in demographic characteristics. These potential sources of error not only apply to age and education but to other demographic factors as well.

Potential Confounds Associated with Site Selection Biases

Standardization populations differ according to region (Anastasi, 1988; Ponton et al., 1996). These differences are probably accentuated for certain ethnic-minority groups as a result of their tendency to concentrate in certain regions of the United States after immigrating to this country. This issue is best depicted by the intended area of initial residence data presented in Table 3. These findings are significant for neuropsychology because they suggest that differential geographic migrational patterns and predilection for certain residential areas may have a substantial impact on the collection and subsequent application of neuropsychological norms for ethnic groups (Rey et al., 1998).

Neuropsychological data has traditionally been collected in academic and medical centers in or near metropolitan areas around the U.S. where the majority of neuropsychologists live and conduct research with urban ethnic-minority populations. While keeping in mind that the observed pattern of geographical settlement of immigrants from China has been historically typical of that observed during the year depicted in Table 3 (1990), the figures in this table suggest that neuropsychological data collected in Houston, Texas, by its very nature, will most likely underrepresent people from China or of Chinese descent living in the U.S. due to their small numbers there. Consequently, unless procedures are established during the collection of norms in Houston to preclude biases from entering into the acquisition process, such procurement could very well result in invalid inferences were the norms to be applied later to people from China or of Chinese origin in New York City. People from China or of Chinese descent living in New York comprise one of the largest populations of immigrants from that country.

A similar scenario could occur with immigrants from Mexico. Neuropsychological data collected in Miami will most likely underrepresent individuals from Mexico or Mexican nationals due to their small population there. Consequently, unless procedures are established during the collection of norms in Miami to preclude biases from entering into the acquisition process, such procurement could very well result in invalid inferences were the norms to be applied at a later date to individuals from Mexico or of Mexican origin in Los Angeles where the number of Mexican immigrants is extraordinarily large. The obverse is also plausible. Normative data ascertained in Los Angeles where the prevalent Hispanic population is of Mexican background would probably not be representative of Cubans, hardly available to researchers there.

Site selection bias also has significant implications when making inferences about ethnic-minority populations living in the U.S. on the basis of foreign norms. As depicted by the migrational data, most populations in the U.S. from foreign countries do not represent a demographic cross-sectional sample of their nation. Therefore, when foreign norms do not represent minority individuals in the U.S. (or even individuals from that country living in the U.S.), the accuracy of the inferences made on the basis of those norms may be compromised due to their lack of inferential validity.

In summary, it should be recognized that ethnic-minority groups tend to exhibit geographical affinity for certain areas within the U.S. and that this geographical predilection may affect the acquisition and application of neuropsychological norms. Geographical predilection may also affect the acquisition process as a result of the effects that specific migratory patterns may have upon the assimilation of American culture by specific ethnic-minority groups (e.g., limiting their exposure to American customs and language).

Potential Confounds Associated with Interactions between Demographic Variables

Education and geographical region most probably interact with other demographic characteristics (modulated by migrations) to create specific patterns of neuropsychological performance captured through the normative process capable of encroaching upon subsequent inferences. For example, although Haitian populations may be available to researchers in New York City, different levels of acculturation may, as a result of poor sampling or other factors, lead to an inadequate representation of this ethnic group regardless of the number of participants comprising the normative cohort. The same could be said of Cuban populations living in Miami in spite of the fact that this metropolitan region is home to so many Cubans.

Other potential confounds, such as level of acculturation (Marin & Marin, 1991), interacting with demographic characteristics known to affect neuropsychological performance (Heaton et al., 1986), and modulated by the immigration process, may play a moderating role in the acquisition and inferential process.

Immigration, Acculturation, and Assimilation

The process of immigration is inextricably intertwined with acculturation (Portes & Rumbaut, 1990) and with the acquisition and application of neuropsychological norms for ethnic-minority groups. Llorente et al. (1998) have argued that, depending on the level of acculturation and assimilation, norms acquired in the United States for certain minority groups may not be representative of individuals from their country of origin if the standardization group differs from recent immigrants in levels of acculturation. All other variables held constant, norms ascertained from individuals living in the U.S. whose countries of origin are cross-sectionally represented in the U.S. with varying levels of acculturation would probably make for a more valid inferential tool. In contrast, normative data for minority groups of foreign nationals (individuals born in the U.S. of foreign ancestry) should be representative of such populations.

Level of acculturation and assimilation is also closely associated with language, particularly for ethnic-minority groups whose language of origin is not English living in the U.S. It is clear that immigrants with greater assimilation and acculturation would in all likelihood have greater language proficiency. Greater language proficiency, in turn, would allow for a more valid NP comparison with existing norms from mainstream populations. It is also critical to note that bilingualism can affect NP test performance (Paradis, 1978).

The question of level of acculturation and language proficiency, however, should not be left to armchair speculation. Instead, a data-based assessment approach should be used to establish level of language proficiency and acculturation for each patient; scales for both of these purposes are available. The language proficiency of Hispanics can be assessed using the scales developed by Woodcock (1981). Several investigators have also developed instruments capable of providing an index of acculturation for specific minority groups (adults and children; see Franco, 1983; Marin, Sabogal, Marin, & Otero-Sabogal, 1984; Suinn, Richard-Figueroa, Lew, & Vigil, 1987). These instruments take into consideration variables known to significantly affect acculturation and assimilation such as age, context of immigration, generational differences in migration, ethnic identification, and length of U.S. residence.

In sum, neuropsychologists serving ethnic-minority populations should be cognizant of the effects of acculturation on the NP evaluation process. They should be aware of the methods available to them to determine the level of acculturation and language proficiency of a specific patient prior to the commencement of such an examination.

Perceptions of the Immigrant and Neuropsychological Assessment

Data documenting examiner and patient characteristics capable of biasing an evaluation abounds in the psychological literature. In particular, examiners' expectancy effects (e.g., halo effects) may infringe upon the validity and outcome of a psychological assessment (Donahue & Sattler, 1971; Grossman, 1978; Sattler & Winget, 1970). The patient's history can also have significant impact on how an examiner conducts, scores, and interprets the results of a psychological evaluation (Auffrey & Robertson, 1972). These issues take on greater significance with immigrants because they may possess more pronounced characteristics (observable or otherwise) (e.g., anxiety associated with no prior contact with psychological professionals; Egeland, 1967) capable of enhancing the expectancy effects of the examiner.

Many stereotypes about immigrants have permeated American society, affecting lay as well as professional circles. These stereotypes can have a deleterious impact on an NP evaluation despite their unsubstantiated nature and the fact that they have insufficient weight to withstand the rigor of scientific scrutiny. Within American society, the perceptions of the immigrant have been less than favorable, even within the mental health professions (Ødegaard, 1932; Sanua, 1970). During earlier large-scale migrations to the U.S., a correlation was initially proposed between immigrants and innate marginality or psychopathology, and between the process of immigration and mental illness. Although misguided, these perceptions were the result of early epidemiological studies indicating the presence of higher incidence of mental illness among immigrants on the basis of hospital admissions (Jarvis, 1866; Rothman, 1971; Sanua, 1970), greater suicide rates among immigrants in the U.S., U.S. versus European differential suicide rates in groups of individuals of the same nationality (Faris & Dunham, 1939), and differential patterns and rates of mental disorders in metropolitan areas with large immigrant populations relative to suburban areas with small numbers of immigrants (Faris & Dunham, 1939). On the basis of these findings, researchers concluded that immigration was associated with mental disorders (Ødegaard, 1932). Unfortunately, these investigations suffered from poor methodology marked by biased samples and similar confounds, and sound research later demonstrated that the effects of objective variables such as age, poverty, and area of residence (Hollingshead & Redlich, 1958; Kessler & Cleary, 1980; Kohn, 1973; Srole, Langner, & Mitchell, 1962) accounted for most of the differences observed. Despite the significant shortcomings of the earlier investigations, these findings found their way into mainstream culture and became part of the perception of the immigrant, held not just by lay people but by mental health providers alike, regarding the mental abilities of the immigrant. These stereotypes can bias the outcome of a neuropsychological examination.

Unfortunately, there is no reason to believe, despite our present level of knowledge with regard to which factors affect immigrants and large-scale migrations (e.g., context of immigration, socioeconomic status of the immigrant, reasons for immigration; see Portes & Rumbaut, 1990), that new generations of clinicians will behave differently toward these populations than did past generations of clinicians, unless the former become cognizant of the biases against these populations and the factors capable of compromising their assessments. Although immigration can be one of the greatest stressors that any individual will experience in life, immigration per se, is not necessarily responsible for mental illness or the etiology behind abnormal brain–behavior relationships.

Conclusion

Although the effects of certain demographic variables have been known to significantly affect neuropsychological performance (Laosa, 1984; Heaton et al., 1986), the etiology behind differences in demographic characteristics has not been well researched, especially among ethnic-minority groups. The present chapter examines a plausible candidate capable of modulating demographic variables, namely, American immigration trends.

With regard to immigration proper, examination of this process revealed nonrandom, shifting, selective, and dynamic mechanisms affecting patterns of American immigration. Regardless of the causes for the nonrandom nature of immigration (e.g., economic, immigration laws of the host country), absolute and relative migration to this country were observed to vary dramatically. Fluctuations over time for migrations within the same country of origin were also evidenced. Similarly, the occupational affiliation of immigrants from foreign nations to the U.S. varied extensively. More important, occupational status and possibly educational attainment differed significantly for immigrants from various nations, independent of absolute migration. Finally, selective patterns of geographical settlement within the U.S. were observed for most immigrant groups.

These results have significant implications for neuropsychology. They suggest that migration trends are capable of modulating demographic characteristics, partly compromising the acquisition and application of norms for ethnic groups. This compromise could bias normative data and their application (e.g., assessment or rehabilitation results). Such biases could invalidate studies comparing intellectual functioning or other NP domains in research participants or patients between sites. Similarly, such selective factors could render invalid norms or research comparing ethnic groups at the same or different geographical sites.

The present findings also suggest that differences in demographic characteristics are capable of mimicking abnormal brain–behavior relationships (Rey et al., 1998). Therefore, care should be exercised not to attribute NP differences to nonexistent brain–behavior relationships when those differences can be accounted for by more objective variables such as demographic characteristics modulated by trends in American immigration in the case of specific ethnic-minority groups.

These results also argue in favor of comparing an individual's performance to multiple normative data sets (when available), especially to those with similar demographic characteristics to that of the individual undergoing evaluation, treatment, or both. The present results additionally support an assessment posture favoring the use of longitudinal examinations. This type of assessment allows the individual being evaluated to establish his or her own baseline, thus reducing reliance on the nomothetic approach.

The present findings also have implications for private and government bodies responsible for the development of policies funding neuropsychological research and norm development. For example, the geographical predilections of certain ethnic-minority groups for select metropolitan areas suggest that funded attempts to acquire norms for these groups should be conducted at several centers throughout the United States. Multicenter acquisition would allow for proportional stratification according to U.S. Bureau of the Census data with full representation of specific ethnic groups and subgroups. In the same vein, these data suggest that the racial definitions used by government bodies, including the U.S. Bureau of the Census, do not accurately reflect the complexity of ethnic differences found in the U.S., confounding ethnicity with racial characteristics. This finding suggests that new categorical definitions should be created by Bureau of the Census and by the Immigration and Naturalization Service to account for these differences.

The current results buttress the need for the development of standards and guidelines for the appropriate acquisition of normative data for minority groups. Future normative studies with ethnic minority groups should be required to describe in more detail their research cohorts while alerting potential users of their possible shortcomings and possible misapplication(s). In addition to information historically critical to normative data sets in neuropsychology (age, education [parental education in the case of children], gender, lateralization, medical criteria, sample size, etc.), norms for ethnic-minority populations should at least report the level of acculturation of the sample, location of data collection, language fluency, and broad stratification information of the sample.

Finally, these results place limitations on the assumptions neuropsychologists may be able to make when using normative data sets for ethnic-minority groups. Under most circumstances, it would be inappropriate for neuropsychologists to assume that norms ascertained in one geographical region of the U.S., or in a foreign country, would be applicable to individuals (and interchangeable with norms) from other geographical areas in the U.S. solely because the normative cohort was predominantly similar (e.g., African American) to the patient (e.g., Haitian) undergoing assessment.

ACKNOWLEDGMENTS.   Portions of this work were presented at the 105th Annual Convention of the American Psychological Association in August 1997. This research was supported in part by a grant from the UCLA CIRID-Fogarty AIDS International Foundation #TW00003-07 to Antolin M. Llorente.

The authors would like to express their sincere thanks to Professors Vicki Green, Department of Psychology, University of Northern Arizona, Nora Hamilton, Department of Political Science, University of Southern California, and Marcel O. Ponton, Department of Psychiatry and Biobehavioral Sciences, University of California, Los Angeles for their assistance and suggestions on a preliminary draft of this manuscript. The authors also thank the staffs at the University of California, Los Angeles (UCLA), University Research Library (URL, Government Documents Division) and the City of Houston Public Library (Downtown Branch, Government Documents and Humanities Sections) for their assistance in locating immigration information.

References

Adams, R. L., Boake, C., & Crain, C. (1982). Bias in neuropsychological test classification related to education, age and ethnicity. *Journal of Consulting and Clinical Psychology, 50,* 143–145.

Anastasi, A. (1988). *Psychological Testing* (6th ed.). New York: Macmillan.

Ardila, A. (1993). Future directions in the research and practice of cross-cultural neuropsychology. *Journal of Clinical and Experimental Neuropsychology, 15*(1), 19. (Abstract)

Ardila, A., Rosselli, M., & Rosas, P. (1989). Neuropsychological assessment of illiterates: Visuo-spatial and memory abilities. *Brain and Cognition, 11,* 147–166.

Auffrey, J., & Robertson, M. (1972). Case history information and examiner experience as determinants of scoring validity on the Wechsler intelligence tests. *Proceedings of the 80th Annual Convention of the American Psychological Association, 7,* 553–554.

Badcock, K. A., & Ross, M. W. (1982). Neuropsychological testing with Australian aborigines. *Australian Psychologist, 17,* 297–299.

Botwinick, J. (1967). *Cognitive processes in maturity and old age.* New York: Springer.

Donahue, D., & Sattler, J. M. (1971). Personality variables affecting WAIS scores. *Journal of Consulting and Clinical Psychology, 36,* 441.

Egeland, B. (1967). Influence of examiner and examinee anxiety on WISC performance. *Psychological Reports, 21,* 409–414.

Farris, R. E. L., & Dunham, H. W. (1939). *Mental disorders in urban areas.* Chicago: University of Chicago Press.

Franco, J. N. (1983). An acculturation scale for Mexican-American children. *Journal of General Psychology, 108,* 175–181.

Garcia, M. (1981). *Desert immigrants: The Mexicans of El Paso, 1880–1920.* New Haven, CT: Yale University Press.

Grossman, F. D. (1978). The effect of an examinee's reported academic achievement and/or physical condition on examiner's scoring and of the WISC-R Verbal IQ. *Dissertation Abstracts International, 38,* 4091A. (University Microfilms No. 77-28,462).

Hamilton, N., & Chinchilla, N. S. (1990). Central American migration: A framework for analysis. *Latin American Research Review, 25,* 75–110.

Heaton, R. K., Grant, I., & Matthews, C. G. (1986). Differences in neuropsychological test performance associated with age, education, and sex. In I. Grant & K. M. Adams (Eds.), *Neuropsychological assessment of neuropsychiatric disorders* (pp. 100–120). New York: Oxford University Press.

Hollingshead, A. B., & Redlich, F. C. (1958). *Social class and mental illness: A community study.* New York: Wiley.

Jarvis, E. (1866). Influence of distance from and nearness to an insane hospital on its use by the people. *American Journal of Insanity, 22,* 361–406.

Jensen, A. (1980). *Bias in mental testing.* New York: Free Press.

Kessler, R. C., & Cleary, P. D. (1980). Social class and psychological distress. *American Sociological Review, 45,* 463–478.

Kohn, M. L. (1973). Social class and schizophrenia: A critical review and reformulation. *Schizophrenia Bulletin, 7,* 60–79.

Laosa, L. M. (1984). Ethnic, socioeconomic and home language influences upon early performance on measures of abilities. *Journal of Educational Psychology, 76,* 1178–1198.

Llorente, A. M. (August, 1997). *Neuropsychologic assessment of Hispanic populations: The influence of immigration on assessment.* Paper presented at the 105th Annual Convention of the American Psychological Association, Chicago, IL.

Llorente, A. M., Ponton, M. O., Taussig, I. M., & Satz, P. (1998). Patterns of American immigration and their influence on the acquisition of neuropsychological norms for Hispanics. *Archives of Clinical Neuropsychology, 14,* 603–614.

Malzberg, B., & Lee, E. S. (1956). *Migration and mental disease: A study of first admissions to hospitals for mental disease, New York, 1939–1941.* New York: Social Science Research Council.

Marin, G., & Marin, B. V. (1991). *Research with Hispanic populations.* Newbury Park, CA: Sage.

Marin, G., Sabogal, F., Marin, B., & Otero-Sabogal, R. (1984). Development of a short acculturation scale for Hispanics. *Hispanic Journal of Behavioral Sciences, 9,* 183–205.

Montgomery, G. T., & Orozlo, S. (1984). Validation of a measure of acculturation for Mexican Americans. *Hispanic Journal of Behavioral Sciences, 6,* 53–63.

Ødegaard, Ø. (1932). Emigration and insanity: A study of mental disease among the Norwegian-born population of Minnesota. *Acta Psychiatrica et Neurologica Scandinavica, 4* (Suppl.), 1–206.

Paradis, M. (Ed.). (1978). *Aspects of bilingualism.* Columbia, SC: Hornbeam.

Ponton, M. O., Satz, P., Herrera, L., Ortiz, F., Urrutia, C. P., Young, R., D'Elia, L. F., & Namerow, N. (1996). Normative data stratified by age and education for the Neuropsychological Screening Battery for Hispanics (NeSBHIS): Initial report. *Journal of the International Neuropsychological Society, 2,* 96–104.

Portes, A., & Bach, R. L. (1985). *Latin Journey: Cuban and Mexican Immigrants in the United States.* Berkeley: University of California Press.

Portes, A., & Borocsz, J. (1989). Contemporary immigration: Theoretical perspectives on determinants and modes of incorporation. *International Migration Review, 23,* 606–630.

Portes, A., & Rumbaut, R. G. (1990). *Immigrant America: A portrait.* Los Angeles: University of California Press.

Rey, G. J., Feldman, E., Rivas-Vazquez, R., Levin, B. E., & Benton, A. (1998). Neuropsychological test development for Hispanics. *Archives of Clinical Neuropsychology, 14,* 593–601.

Rogler, L. H. (1994). International migrations: A framework for directing research. *American Psychologist, 49,* 701–708.

Rosselli, M., Ardila, A., & Rosas, P. (1990). Neuropsychological assessment of illiterates: II. Language and praxic abilities. *Brain and Cognition, 12,* 281–296.

Rothman, D. J. (1971). *The discovery of the asylum.* Boston: Little, Brown.

Sanua, V. D. (1970). Immigration, migration, and mental illness. In E. B. Brody (Ed.), *Behavior in new environments: Adaptation of migrant populations* (pp. 291–322). Beverly Hills, CA: Sage.

Sattler, J. M., & Winget, B. M. (1970). Intelligence testing procedures as affected by expectancy and IQ. *Journal of Clinical Psychology, 26,* 446–448.

Srole, L., Langner, T. S., & Mitchell, S. T. (1962). *Mental health in the metropolis: The Midtown Manhattan Study.* New York: New York University Press.

Suinn, R. M., Richard-Figueroa, K., Lew, S., & Vigil, P. (1987). The Suinn–Lew Asian Self-Identity Acculturation Scale: An initial report. *Educational and Psychological Measurement, 6,* 103–112.

U.S. Immigration and Naturalization Service. (1975). *1974 statistical yearbook of the Immigration and Naturalization Service.* Washington, D.C.: U.S. Government Printing Office.

U.S. Immigration and Naturalization Service. (1981). *1980 statistical yearbook of the Immigration and Naturalization Service.* Washington, D.C.: U.S. Government Printing Office.

U.S. Immigration and Naturalization Service. (1991). *1990 statistical yearbook of the Immigration and Naturalization Service.* Washington, D.C.: U.S. Government Printing Office.

Woodcock, R. W. (1981). *Bateria Woodcock de Proficiencia en el Idioma.* Allen, TX: DLM Teaching Resources.

21

Neurobehavioral Disorders and Pharmacologic Intervention

The Significance of Ethnobiological Variation in Drug Responsivity

TONY L. STRICKLAND AND GREGORY GRAY

Introduction

The Epidemiological Catchment Area Study has determined that the lifetime prevalence of any mental disorder in the United States is 33% (Marzuk, 1993). More than half of the patients with mental disorders are treated by primary care physicians and fewer than 20% receive treatment in specialized mental health settings (Simon, 1992). This is particularly true for anxiety and depression, which are among the most common of the mental disorders (Simon, 1992). Family physicians treat approximately 90% of anxiety disorders (Narrow, Regier, Rae, Manderscheid, & Locke, 1993). Surveys of outpatients in primary care settings demonstrate 6%–8% are suffering from a major depressive disorder (Walley, Beebe, & Clark, 1994) that is frequently associated with high levels of medical utilization (Depression Guideline Panel of the Agency for Healthcare Policy and Research, 1994). This pattern of health care delivery is also true of African American patients (Lin & Poland, 1994). While these disorders are clearly treatable, they can be difficult to manage and may require attention to many patient variables, including interethnic pharmacogenetic, pharmacokinetic, and pharmacodynamic differences. When primary care physicians refer their patients to mental health specialists, as many as half do not complete the referral (Schulberg, 1991; Schulberg, Coulchan, Black, et al., 1993). Also, pharmacotherapy with elderly populations is a significant concern as this patient population typically presents with multiple compounds on board and is at high risk for renal and hepatic pathologies that have profound implications for safety.

Patients who present for neuropsychological evaluation generally are treated with multiple medications. Traumatic brain-injured patients may receive anxiolytics, antidepressants,

TONY L. STRICKLAND AND GREGORY GRAY • Charles R. Drew University of Medicine and Science, Los Angeles, California 90059; and UCLA School of Medicine, Los Angeles, California 90095.

Handbook of Cross-Cultural Neuropsychology, edited by Fletcher-Janzen, Strickland, and Reynolds. Kluwer Academic/Plenum Publishers, New York, 2000.

and antiepileptics, as well as other compounds to treat a range of neurobehavioral sequelae of their injuries (Stein & Strickland, 1998).

Ethnicity and Drug Responsivity

There has been an emerging interest in the study of relationships between mental disorders, cultural influences, and subsequent pharmacological treatment interventions. Although considerably more study of ethnic differences to pharmacologic treatment have been accomplished with nonpsychoactive medications (Flaherty & Meagher, 1980), recent research developments in psychopharmacology reveal significant ethnobiologic differences in response to a number of different psychotropic compounds (Lin, Poland, & Chien, 1990; Strickland et al., 1991; Strickland, Lin, Fu, Anderson, & Zheng, 1995; Wood & Zhou, 1991). Pharmacokinetic properties of psychotropics and nonpsychotropics share similar metabolic pathways (Kalow, Goedde, & Agarwal, 1986; Kalow, 1982). As a result, it is not surprising that ethnic differences also have been reported to occur with psychoactive compounds. Historically, most comparative studies that have demonstrated pharmacokinetic and pharmacogenetic differences contrasted Asian and Caucasian populations. Yet, the importance of understanding the contrast with African Americans is clear considering that this group is prescribed a greater volume of sedating compounds (Lin, Poland, & Lesser, 1986) and are at greater risk for being misdiagnosed despite no greater prevalence of psychiatric disorders when standardized diagnostic systems are used (Adebimpe, 1980, 1981).

The focus of this chapter will be on ethnic related factors that should be considered in the pharmacotherapy of anxiety and mood disorders in African American patients, and suggest some general guidelines for the use of psychotropic compounds with African Americans. Although most interethnic differences will be genetically determined, it should be noted that additional influences such as nutritional status, diet, smoking behavior, alcohol, and illicit or prescribed drug use, may singularly or collectively modify a medication's effect.

Genetic Basis for Pharmacokinetic Differences

Most psychotropic drugs are metabolized by one of the hepatic cytochrome P-450 isoenzymes. Genetic polymorphism in the functional expression of these isoenzymes underlies the well documented interpatient variability in drug metabolism (Meyer, Zanger, Grant, & Blim 1990; Pollock, 1994). Two of the most often encountered P-450 isoenzymes are the IID6 (debrisoquine hydroxylase) and IIC19 (mephenytoin hydroxylase) and are also polymorphic in nature (Kalow, 1992). The IID6 isoenzyme is responsible for the metabolism of many tricyclic antidepressants (TCAs), selective serotonergic reuptake inhibitors (SSRIs), and most antipsychotics. While only 2.9% to 10% of European Americans are IID6-mediated "poor metabolizers," a study by Kalow (1993) suggests that as many as 33% of African Americans have a "gene alteration" in this isoenzyme which results in a slower metabolic rate. Thus, the metabolism of the TCAs, SSRIs and antipsychotics may be significantly reduced in approximately one-third of African American patients. The IIC19 isoenzyme is involved in the metabolism of diazepam, and the demethylation of the tertiary TCAs (Goldstein, Faletto, Romkes-Sparks, et al., 1994). While only 3% of European Americans are IIC19 poor metabolizers, approximately 18%–22% of African Americans are IIC19 poor metabolizers, suggesting a slower rate of metabolism of some benzodiazepines and tertiary TCAs in African Americans. There is, however, no evidence of genetic polymorphism in the 3A4 isoenzyme, which metabolizes alprazolam, triazolam, midazolam, and some TCAs.

Tricyclic Antidepressants

Asians

Much of the study of interethnic differences in the pharmacokinetics and pharmacodynamics of psychotropic medications has involved tricyclic antidepressants and differences between Asians and Caucasians (Pi, Wang, & Gray, 1993). There are anecdotal reports indicating that Asians require lower doses of tricyclic antidepressants (Murph, 1969), although other studies of prescribing patterns have failed to confirm this (Pi, Jain, & Simpson, 1986). It has also been suggested that Asians show a therapeutic response at lower blood levels of tricyclic antidepressants (Yamashita & Asano, 1979).

The tricyclic antidepressant clomipramine is metabolized by CYP 2D6 and CYP 2C19. Given the high percentage of Asians who are CYP 2D6 "slow metabolizers" (33–60%) and CYP 2C19 "poor metabolizers" (20%), it would be expected that a greater percentage of Asians than Caucasians would metabolize clomipramine slowly (Pi & Gray, 1998). Pharmacokinetic studies of clomipramine have confirmed that Asian Indian or Pakistani subjects had significantly higher mean plasma levels of clomipramine and appeared to be more sensitive to adverse drug effects than English subjects (Allen, Rack, & Vaddadi, 1977).

Desipramine is also metabolized by CYP 2D6. It, too, would therefore be expected to be metabolized slowly by a greater percentage of Asians than Caucasians. Rudorfer and colleagues (Rudorfer, Lane, Chang, et al., 1984) studied the pharmacokinetics of a single oral dose of despiramine in Chinese and Caucasian volunteers and found that all of the Chinese subjects were slow or intermediate metabolizers, while all of the Caucasian subjects were intermediate or fast metabolizers. The authors suggested that Asians who were slow metabolizers were at risk of toxicity from standard doses of tricyclic antidepressants. Similar results were reported by Pi and associates (Pi, Tran-Johnson, Walker, et al., 1989). These results are perhaps not surprising, given what we now know of CYP 2D6 activity: relatively few Asians are CYP 2D6 poor metabolizers, but a high percentage of the Asian "extensive metabolizers" have a form of the enzyme that is less active than the form found in Caucasians (Pi & Gray, 1998). The slower clearance of desipramine was most likely due to the "slow metabolizer" form of the enzyme, rather than the "poor metabolizer" form.

African Americans

Studies involving psychopharmacologic responses to TCAs in African American populations have only recently received systematic investigation. However, the few studies which have been performed reveal significant differences in the pharmacokinetics between African Americans and European Americans.

Raskin, Thomas, and Crook (1975) studied the differential effects of chlorpromazine and imipramine in 159 African American and 555 European American inpatients. They used a number of standard psychometric scales to assess the symptomatology and the response to different medications administered. The study suggested that African Americans manifest more rapid improvement and African American men were therapeutically more responsive to imipramine. Methodological difficulties notwithstanding, it is important to note that the more rapid improvement among African American patients treated with TCAs is not an isolated finding. Earlier, large-scaled, multicentered studies (Henry, Overall, & Markette, 1971; Overall, Hollister, & Kimball, 1980) also demonstrated "by chance" similar differences in the response rates in African American patients.

In the often cited study of Ziegler and Biggs (1977), there were no ethnic differences in the rate of demethylation of amitriptyline to nortriptyline or the steady state plasma levels of amitriptyline. However, African American patients had significantly higher (50%) nortrip-tyline plasma levels compared to European Americans. This difference (higher levels of secondary amine TCAs) is proposed as a plausible reason for the more rapid response to TCAs in the African American patients.

In a retrospective chart review, Livingston, Zucker, Isenberg, and Wetzel (1983) studied 125 psychiatric inpatients (102 European American and 23 African American) treated with TCA. While African Americans comprised 18% of the sample, of the 10 patients that devel-oped delirium, half were African American. The researchers concluded that delirium was significantly more common in African American patients, older patients, and those with higher TCA plasma levels. However, it is not clear from the authors' summary of the data how race is significantly related to delirium independent of age and plasma TCA levels.

In another retrospective chart review (Rudorfer & Robins, 1982), 19 patients who had overdosed on amitriptyline were studied. Subjects included were 13 European Americans (5 males and 8 females) and 6 African American females. Results revealed significant ethnic differences in the level/dose ratio between African American and European American females and higher plasma concentrations in African Americans.

In a study of indigenous African outpatients from Tanzania, the patients responded to clomipramine in much lower doses than those recommended in western textbooks (Kilonzo, Kaaya, Rweikiza, Kassam, & Moshi, 1994). Yet, at the low-to-moderate dose of 125 mg, drowsiness and tremulousness were notable.

Although these clinical reports suffer from significant methodological concerns, taken together they do consistently suggest that African Americans treated with TCAs will have higher plasma levels per dose, more side effects with equivalent plasma levels, and earlier onset of action than European Americans. The issue of side effects is particularly noteworthy because they are the major reasons for patient noncompliance. Side effects and noncompliance may be minimized, without compromise of efficacy, by using lower than generally recom-mended doses of TCAs. Based on the above reviewed literature and the authors' clinical experience, the following modified TCA prescribing guidelines are proposed for African American patients. Begin African American patients with 25 to 50 mg of TCA at bedtime (with the notable exceptions of protriptyline which should be started at 10–15 mg). Increase dose by 25 mg/day every 2 to 3 days until the patient is taking 100–150 mg/day, or side effects preclude further increases, or the patient exhibits significant clinical response to lower doses. If side effects develop and/or the patient does not exhibit a therapeutic response at 150 mg/day, order TCA plasma levels to ensure that the patient does not have unexpected plasma levels before increasing the dose. Although monitoring of the electrocardiogram is recommended for all patients on TCAs, this may be particularly important for African American populations who may have a tendency to have higher plasma levels and may be more sensitive to the adverse cardiotoxic effects.

Hispanics

Several studies have also found Hispanics to respond to lower doses of antidepressant medications. For example, Marcos and Cancro (1982) found that Hispanic (predominantly Puerto Rican) women responded to doses of tricyclic antidepressants that were only half those prescribed to Caucasian women. However, significantly more of the Latinos complained of side effects. Similarly Escobar and Tuason (1980) found that Colombian patients receiving imipramine complained of more anticholinergic side effects than did Caucasians or African Americans in the United States.

This increased sensitivity to tricyclic antidepressants is most likely pharmacodynamic. There do not appear to be differences in CYP 2D6 activity (Pi & Gray, 1998). Unfortunately, there has been only one study of tricyclic antidepressant pharmacokinetics in Latinos, and that study by Gaviria, Gil, and Javaid (1986) found no difference in nortriptyline pharmacokinetics between Latinos and non-Latino Caucasians.

Serotonergic Antidepressants

A computer search of the recent literature yields no data on ethnic differences in the pharmacokinetic, pharmacodynamic, or pharmacotherapeutic effects of SSRIs in African American patients. Recent FDA approvals for new SSRIs and their tremendous popularity as alternatives to TCAs suggest an acute need for studies of ethnic variations in their biological activity. An important clue as to the potential importance of such research is found in the review by Preskorn (1994) on metabolism of SSRIs which described substantial inhibitory impact on the P-450 enzyme system. Fluoxetine and paroxetine, at effective minimum doses, were found to have a profound inhibitory impact on the hepatic isoenzyme CYP2D6, with fluoxetine also inhibiting CVP3A4 (Crewe, Lennard, Tucker, Woods, & Haddock, 1994; Preskorn, 1993). Both of these enzymes in the P-450 class are important in the hepatic metabolism of a variety of drugs (e.g., TCAs, some neuroleptics, beta-blockers, alprazolam, carbamazepine). Fluoxetine and paroxetine at the common dose of 20 mg/day cause a decrease in clearance of the TCA desipramine by approximately 80%. This pharmacological impact of fluoxetine on desipramine is expressed in greater cognitive impairment and psychomotor functioning (Lasher, Fleishaker, Steenwyck, & Antal, 1991). Interestingly, another SSRI, sertraline, showed minimal (< 30%) impact on the metabolism of desipramine. The effect of fluoxetine on CYP3A4 is relevant for this enzyme's role in the metabolism of drugs such as alprazolam and carbamazepine (Greenblatt, Preskorn, Cotreau, Horst, & Harmatz, 1992; Lasher et al., 1991).

Given that the SSRIs are metabolized and/or inhibit the P-450 isoenzymes, and the genetic polymorphism of these enzymes in African Americans, we can predict that there may be at least some pharmacokinetic differences in a significant minority of African American patients. It is the clinical observations of the authors that many African American female patients will report significant side effects when prescribed the generally recommended dose of paroxetine (20 mg) and fluoxetine (20 mg) and will better tolerate the medication, as well as have an adequate therapeutic response, when prescribed at half of the recommended adult doses. It is unclear if this suggests purely pharmacokinetic effects or hints to a more sensitive pharmacodynamic effect as well. We propose the following dosing guidelines for African American patients taking SSRIs. Begin with one-half the recommended starting dose. Increase to full dose after three to four days unless significant side effects develop. If side effects develop, continue at the lower dosage for two to three weeks and then increase if the patient has not responded.

Antianxiety Compounds

A review of the existing research suggests slowed clearance and greater adverse cognitive side effects from benzodiazepines in African Americans may exist. Additionally, it appears that African Americans show more anxiety reduction with anxiolytics than European Americans (Henry, Overall, & Markette, 1971). Interestingly, several epidemiological studies suggest that African Americans receive benzodiazepines less often than Caucasians whether the data is from a national database (Olfson & Pincus, 1994), a southern community (Swartz et al., 1991), or a university hospital database of medical and surgical patients (Zisselman, Rovner, Kelly, & Woods, 1994).

In a recent study of the pharmacokinetics of adinazolam (Flashaker & Phillips, personal communication), a triazolo-benzodiazepine currently being investigated as an antidepressant and anxiolytic, 8 African American and 8 European American normal volunteers were included in the study. The results showed that African Americans had increased clearance of adinazolam. Concurrently, however, the C_{max} and area under the curve of N-demethyladinazolam, the metabolite of adinazolam, were significantly higher in African Americans. Along with these pharmacokinetic findings, African Americas also manifested significantly larger drug effects on psychomotor performance. N-demethyladinazolam has been shown to exclusively mediate the benzodiazepine-like side effects, including effects on psychomotor performance, after adinazolam. This may be responsible for the larger drug effects on African Americans despite their higher metabolic capacity for adinazolam.

Other Neuropsychiatric Medications

While antiepileptics (e.g., dilantin and carbamazepine) have long been used for neurological conditions, they have become increasingly popular in psychopharmacotherapy. This use of antiepileptics would suggest that ethnic differences should be attended to by primary care physicians. Hundt, Aucamp, Muller, and Potgieter (1983) studied carbamazepine and its major metabolites by monitoring plasma levels in patients over a period of eight years. The sample included 451 African American and 2,225 European American patients who were monitored for carbamazepine, and the metabolites carbamazepine-10,11-epoxide and 10,11-dihydroxycarbamazepine. Mean carbamazepine and carbamazepine metabolite levels found in the African American group were found to be significantly lower than the European American group. This observation indicates a difference in the monooxygenase enzyme activity, but not for epoxide hydroxylase activity, which is probably the same for both groups. These findings are important in that the therapeutic use of carbamazepine is increasing, being used either alone or in combination with other antimania agents. Also, carbamazepine is particularly indicated for patients with severe mania, a history of rapid cycling, mixed states with symptoms of depression or anxiety, or schizoaffective symptoms, all of which correlate with poor response to lithium therapy (Chou, 1991).

Phenytoin has long been demonstrated to exhibit differential ethnic biologic activity. Arnold and Gerber (1969) reported a 43% longer plasma half-life in African Americans (26.5 hours) than in Caucasians (18.5 hours). Interestingly, this effect was not found in South African blacks (Buchanan, Bill, Moodley, & Eyberg, 1977) suggesting that the effect in African Americans could be a result of genetic differences. Alternatively, differences in diet, possibly from the role of regional differences in fat intake, may contribute to the ethnic differences (Kulow, Goedde, & Agarwal, 1986).

Summary and Conclusions

Increased interest and scientific advances in psychopharmacology have facilitated some interesting and provocative ethnobiologic comparisons of pharmacogenetic, pharmacokinetic, and pharmacodynamic differences. Though there exists some methodologic and other research design concerns that make more definitive impressions premature, there is nevertheless an emerging body of data which identify significant differential patterns of genetic, kinetic, and dynamic responsivity to various psychotropics among Asian, African American, and Hispanic populations.

Tricyclic antidepressants activity in African Americans appears to be mediated by significant pharmacogenetic and pharmacokinetic influences, and results in higher plasma TCA levels and a faster therapeutic response, though with more toxic side effects compared to European Americans. Problems with appropriate diagnosis of mood disturbance in this population continues to be a major issue relative to accurate assessment of the efficacy of TCAs in African Americans. The SSRI class of antidepressants have shown tremendous popularity, in part because of the perception that they are safer than TCAs with fewer side effects. While there is no literature directly addressing ethnic differences in pharmacological effects of SSRIs, their interaction with drugs that do show ethnic differences raises concerns regardless of any potential direct effects of ethnicity on SSRIs.

Benzodiazepines have not been well-studied in African Americans, but there is some data to suggest slowed clearance and greater adverse cognitive effects. As for anticonvulsants, carbamazepine levels in African Americans tend to be lower while phenytoin levels are commonly higher.

In general, the psychopharmacology literature on African Americans reveals important differential trends along a number of important pharmacogenetic, pharmacokinetic, and pharmacodynamic parameters. Much work remains to be done to clearly delineate these important ethnobiologic differences. Future psychopharmacology studies should control for patient nutritional status, diet, alcohol and other drug use. Also, due to problems with accurate diagnosis of mood disturbance in African Americans, efforts to improve assessment in this area should be undertaken. Finally, we noted few studies of benzodiazepine use in this population despite their widespread use. Research relevant to kinetic and dynamic responses to anxiolytics in African Americans is much needed.

References

Adebimpe, V. R. (1980). Psychopharmacological norms in blacks and whites. *American Journal of Psychiatry, 137,* 870–871.

Adebimpe, V. R. (1981). Overview: White norms and psychiatric diagnosis of black patients. *American Journal of Psychiatry, 138,* 279–285.

Allen, J. J., Rack, P. H., & Vaddadi, K. S. (1977). Differences in the effets of climipramine on English and Asian volunteers: Preliminary report on a pilot study. *Postgraduate Medical Journal, 53*(Suppl. 4), 79–86.

Arnold, K., & Gerber, N. (1969). The rate of decline of diphenylhydantoin in human plasma. *Clinical Pharmacological Therapeutics, 11,* 121–134.

Buchanan, N., Bill, P., Moodley, G., & Eyberg, C. (1977). The metabolism of phenobarbitone, phenytoin and antipyrine in black patients. *South African Medical Journal, 52,* 394–395.

Chou, J. C. Y. (1991). Recent advances in treatment of acute mania. *Journal of Clinical Pharmacology, 11,* 3–21.

Crewe, H. K., Lennard, M. S., Tucker, G. T., Woods, F. R., & Haddock, R. E. (1994). The effect of selective serotonin re-uptake inhibitors on cytochrome P4502D6 (CYP2D6) activity in human liver microsomes. *British Journal of Clinical Pharmacology, 34,* 262–265.

The Depression Guideline Panel of the Agency for Healthcare Policy and Research. (1994). Synopsis of the clinical practice guidelines for diagnosis and treatment of depression in primary care. *Archives of Family Medicine, 3,* 85–92.

Escobar, J. I., & Tuason, V. B. (1980). Antidepressant agents: A cross-cultural study. *Psychopharmacology Bulletin, 16,* 49–52.

Flaherty, J. A., & Meagher, R. (1980). Measuring racial bias in inpatient treatment. *American Journal of Psychiatry*, *127*, 679–682.

Gaviria, M., Gil, A. A., & Javaid, J. I. (1986). Nortriptyline kinetics in Hispanic and Anglo subjects. *Journal of Clinical Psychopharmacology*, *6*, 227–231.

Goldstein, J. A., Faletto, M. B., Romkes-Sparks, M., et al. (1994). Evidence that CYP2C19 is the major (S)-mephenytoin 4′-hydroxylase in humans. *Biochemistry*, *33*, 1743–1752.

Greenblatt, D. J., Preskorn, S. H., Cotreau, M. M., Horst, W. D., & Harmatz, J. S. (1992). Fluoxetine impairs clearance of alprazolam but not of clonazepam. *Clinical Pharmacological Therapeutics*, *52*, 479–486.

Henry, B. W., Overall, J. E., & Markette, J. (1971). Comparison of major drug therapies for alleviation of anxiety and depression. *Diseases of the Nervous System*, *32*, 655–667.

Hundt, H. K., Aucamp, A. K., Muller, F. O., & Potgieter, M. A. (1983). Carbamazepine and its major metabolites in plasma: A summary of eight years of therapeutic drug monitoring. *Therapeutic Drug Monitor*, *5*, 427–435.

Kalow, W. (1982). Ethnic differences in drug metabolism. *Clinical Pharmacokinetics*, *7*, 373–400.

Kalow, W., Goedde, H. W., & Agarwal, D. P. (Eds.). (1986). *Ethnic differences in reactions to drugs and xenobiotics*. Proceedings of a meeting held in Titisee, Federal Republic of Germany, October 1985. New York: Liss.

Kalow, W. (1992). *Pharmacogenetics of drug metabolism*. New York: Pergamon.

Kalow, W. (1993). Pharmacogenetics: Its biologic roots and the medical challenge. *Clinical Pharmacological Therapeutics*, *54*, 235–241.

Kilonzo, G. P., Kaaya, S. F., Rweikiza, J. K., Kassam, M., & Moshi, G. (1994). Determination of appropriate clomipramine dosage among depressed African outpatients in Dar es Salaam, Tanzania. *Central African Journal of Medicine*, *40*(7), 178–182.

Lasher, T. A., Fleishaker, J. C., Steenwyck, R. C., & Antal, E. J. (1991). Pharmacokinetic pharmacodynamic evaluation of the combined administration of alprazolam and fluoxetine. *Psychopharmacology*, *104*, 323–327.

Lin, K. M., Poland, R. E., & Lesser, I. M. (1986). Ethnicity and psychopharmacology. *Culture, Medicine, and Psychiatry*, *10*, 151–165.

Lin, K. M., Poland, R. E., & Chien, C. P. (1990). Ethnicity and psychopharmacology: Recent findings and future research directions. In E. Sorel (Ed.), *Family, culture and psychobiology*. New York: Legas.

Lin, K. M., & Poland, R. (1994). Ethnic differences in the response to psychotropic drugs. In S. Friedman (Ed.), *Anxiety disorders in African Americans*. New York: Springer.

Livingston, R. L., Zucker, D. K., Isenberg, K., & Wetzel, R. D. (1983). Tricyclic antidepressants and delirium. *Journal of Clinical Psychiatry*, *44*, 173–176.

Marcos, L. R., & Cancro, R. (1982). Pharmacotherapy of Hispanic depressed patients: Clinical observations. *American Journal of Psychotherapy*, *36*, 505–513.

Marzuk, M. R. (1993). Progress in psychiatry. *New England Journal of Medicine*, *329*, 552–560.

Meyer, U. A., Zanger, U. M., Grant, D., & Blim, M. (1990). Genetic polymorphism of drug metabolism. *Advances in Drug Research*, *19*, 197–241.

Murph, H. B. M. (1969). Ethinic variations in drug responses. *Transcultural Psychiatric Research Review*, *6*, 6–23.

Narrow, W. E., Regier, D. A., Rae, D. S., Manderscheid, R. W., & Locke, B. Z. (1993). Use of services by persons with mental and additive disorders. *Archives of General Psychiatry*, *50*, 95–107.

Olfson, M., & Pincus, H. A. (1994). Use of benzodiazepines in the community. *Archives of Internal Medicine*, *154*, 1235–1240.

Overall, J. E., Hollister, L. E., & Kimball, I., Jr. (1980). A pilot study of racial differences in erythrocyte lithium transport. *American Journal of Psychiatry*, *137*, 120–121.

Pi, E. H., Jain, A., & Simpson, G. M. (1986) Review and survey of different prescribing practices in Asia. In C. Shagass, R. C. Josiassen, W. H. Bridger, et al. (Eds.), *Biological psychiatry*. New York: Elsevier.

Pi, E. H., Tran-Johnson, T. K., Walker, N. R., et al. (1989). Pharmacokinetics of desipramine in Caucasian and Asian volunteers. *Psychopharmacology Bulletin 2*, 483–487.

Pi, E. H., Wang, A. L., & Gray, C. E. (1993). Asian/non-Asian transcultural tricylcic antidepressant psychopharmacology: A reivew. *Progress in Neuropsychopharmacology and Biological Psychiatry*, *17*, 691–702.

Pi, E. H., & Gray, G. E. (1998). A cross-cultural perspective on psychopharmacology. *Essential Psychopharmacology*, *2*, 233–262.

Pollock, B. G. (1994). Recent developments in drug metabolism of relevance to psychiatrists. *Harvard Review of Psychiatry*, *2*, 204–213.

Preskorn, S. H. (1993). The pharmacokinetics of antidepressants: Why and how they are relevant to treatment. *Journal of Clinical Psychiatry*, *54*(Suppl.), 5–18.

Preskorn, S. (1994). Targeted pharmacotherapy in depression management: Comparative pharmacokinetics of fluoxetine, paroxetine and sertraline. *International Clinical Psychopharmacology*, *9*(Suppl. 3), 13–19.

Raskin, A., Thomas, H., & Crook, M. A. (1975). Antidepressants in black and white inpatients. *Archives of General Psychiatry*, *32*, 643–649.

Rudorfer, M. V., & Robins, E. (1982). Amitriptyline overdose: Clinical effects on tricyclic antidepressant plasma levels. *Journal of Clinical Psychiatry, 43,* 457–460.

Rudorfer, M. V., Lane, E. A., Chang, W. H., et al. (1984). Desipramine pharmacokinetics in Chinese and Caucasian volunteers. *British Journal of Clinical Pharmacology, 17,* 433–440.

Schulberg, H. C. (1991). Mental disorders in the primary care settings: Research priorities for the 1990s. *General Hospital Psychiatry, 13,* 156–164.

Schulberg, H. C., Coulehan, J. L., Block, M. R., et al. (1993). Clinical trials of primary care treatment for major depression: Issues in design, recruitment and treatment. *International Journal of Psychiatric Medicine, 23,* 29–42.

Simon, G. E. (1992). Psychiatric disorder and functional symptoms as predictors of health care use. *Psychiatric Medicine, 10,* 49–50.

Stein & Strickland, T. L. (1998). A review of the neuropsychological effects of commonly used prescription medicactions. *Archives of Clinical Neuropsychology, 13,* 254–284.

Strickland, T. L., Ranganath, V., Lin, K.-M., Poland, R. E., Mendoza, R., & Smith, M. W. (1991). Psychopharmacologic considerations in the treatment of black American populations. *Psychopharmacology Bulletin, 27,* 441–448.

Strickland, T. L., Lin, K.-M., Fu, P., Anderson, D., & Zheng, Y. (1995). Comparison of lithium ratio between African American and Caucasian bipolar patients. *Society of Biological Psychiatry, 37,* 325–330.

Swartz, M., Landerman, R., George, L. K., Melville, M. L., Blazer, D., & Smith, K. (1991). Benzodiazepine antianxiety agents: Prevalence and correlates of use in a southern community. *American Journal of Public Health, 81,* 592–596.

Walley, E. J., Beebe, D. K., & Clark, J. L. (1994). Management of common anxiety disorders. *American Family Physician, 50,* 1745–1753.

Wood, A. J., & Zhou, H. H. (1991). Ethnic differences in drug disposition and responsiveness. *Clinical Pharmacokinetics, 20,* 1–24.

Yamashita, I., & Asano, Y. (1979). Tricyclic antidepressants: Therapeutic plasma level. *Psychopharmacology Bulletin, 15,* 40–44.

Ziegler, V. E., Clayton, P. J., & Biggs, J. T. A comparison study of amitriptyline and nortriptyline with plasma levels. *Archives of General Psychiatry, 34,* 607–612.

Zisselman, M. H., Rovner, B. W., Kelly, K. G., & Woods, C. (1994). Benzodiazepine utilization in a university hospital. *American Journal of Medical Quality, 9*(3), 138–141.

Index